PROCEEDINGS OF THE VI INTERNATIONAL CONFERENCE ON SARCOIDOSIS

Proceedings of the VI International Conference on Sarcoidosis, 6th, Tokyo, 1972.

Edited by
KAZURO IWAI
YUTAKA HOSODA

UNIVERSITY PARK PRESS

UNIVERSITY PARK PRESS
Baltimore · London · Tokyo

Library of Congress Cataloging in Publication Data
International Conference on Sarcoidosis, 6th, Tokyo, 1972.
Proceedings.

Conference held Sept. 11–15, 1972.
    1. Sarcoidosis—Congresses. I.   Iwai, Kazurō, ed.
II. Hosoda, Yutaka, ed. [DNLM : 1. Sarcoidosis—
Congresses. W3IN191D 1972p/[WR500 I61 1972p]]
RC182. S14I5 1972   616.9   74–3228
ISBN 0-8391-0689-0

© UNIVERSITY OF TOKYO PRESS, 1974
UTP 3047-67973-5149

Originally published by
UNIVERSITY OF TOKYO PRESS

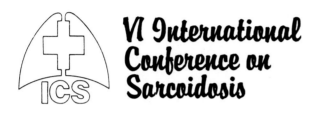

VI International Conference on Sarcoidosis

Chairman
KANEHIKO KITAMURA

Organized by
THE JAPAN SARCOIDOSIS COMMITTEE

Under the Sponsorship of
THE INTERNATIONAL COMMITTEE
ON SARCOIDOSIS

SECRETARIAT

JAPAN SARCOIDOSIS COMMITTEE
c/o J.N.R. CENTRAL HEALTH INSTITUTE
YOYOGI 2–1, SHIBUYA, TOKYO 151

SCHEDULE OF CONFERENCE
September 11–15, 1972
Tokyo Metropolitan Festival Hall

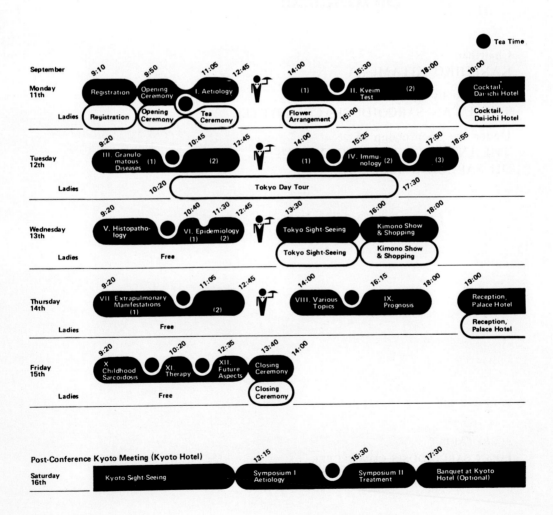

OFFICERS OF THE CONFERENCE

JAPAN SARCOIDOSIS COMMITTEE

Honorary Chairmen:	DONOMAE, I.
	NOBECHI, K.
Chairman:	KITAMURA, K.
Vice-Chairmen:	CHIBA, Y.
	SHIGEMATSU, I.
	TSUJI, S.
Treasurers:	FUJITA, S.
	OHIRA, I.
Secretaries General:	HOMMA, H.
	HOSODA, Y.

ADVISORY COMMITTEE

FUKUSHIRO R.
GOMI, J.
HIBINO, S.
HIGUCHI, K.
IWASAKI, T.
KAWAMURA, T.
KIRISAWA, N.
KITAMOTO, O.
KOJIMA, R.
MIKAMO, Y.
NAITO, M.
NAKAO, K.
OKINAKA, S.
OSAMURA, S.
SATO, H.
SHIKANO, S.
SODA, T.
SUNAHARA, S.
TAKAHASHI, Y.
TATENO, S.
UEDA, H.
YANAGISAWA, K.

ORGANIZING COMMITTEE

HAGIWARA, T.
HAMASHIMA, Y.
IKUI, H.
KATSUKI, H.
KAWABE, H.
KAWAMORI, Y.

KAWAI, T.
KIMURA, T.
KINOSHITA, Y.
KITAMURA, T.
KUKITA, A.
MAEKAWA, N.
MATSUSHIMA, M.
MISHIMA, S.
MIURA, Y.
MASAKI, M.
MIZUNO, N.
MORIKAWA, K.
MUROHASHI, T.
NAKAGAWA, Y.
NISHIMOTO, Y.
OBUCHI, S.
OHTAKE, H.
OIKE, Y.
OSHIMA, S.
OSHIMA, Y.
SASAMOTO, H.
SAWASAKI, H.
SUGIYAMA, K.
TACHIIRI, H.
TAKAHASHI, T.
TAKAMATSU, T.
TANIOKU, K.
TATEISHI, T.
TERAMATSU, T.
UESAKA, I.
UMEZAWA, T.
YAMASHITA, H.

YAMAMURA, Y.
YASUHIRA, K.
ZENDA, I.

EXECUTIVE COMMITTEE

Secretaries
NIITU, Y.
MURAO, M.

Scientific Programme
MIKAMI, R.
AKISADA, M.
DOHI, I.
FUKUSHIMA, Y.
HIRAGA, Y.
SHIGEMATSU, N.
TACHIBANA, T.
KOBAYASHI, F.
YAMAMOTO, M.

Proceedings and Recording
IWAI, K.
AOKI, K.
ASAKAWA, M.
FUJII, K.
HIRAKO, T.
HIRASAWA, I.
HOSODA, H.
ISHIDA, O.
IZUMI, T.
UYAMA, M.
KUMAKURA, K.
MATSUDA, M.

vii

Mikata, A.
Morii, H.
Soejima, R.
Suzuki, S.
Yoneda, R.
Yoshida, K.
Watanabe, M.
Kato, M.

Language
Goodman, A.
Saito, L. H.

Hall Management
Kosuda, T.
Aruga, H.
Emdo, A.
Fukuda, Y.
Furuie, T.
Furuta, M.
Hashimoto, T.
Hijikata, F.
Ishidate, T.
Ito, Y.
Kondo, K.

Maeda, Y.
Masaoka, K.
Matsumoto, M.
Minami, O.
Nukada, H.
Ogawara, M.
Okui, S.
Osada, H.
Shikanai, K.
Shimo, T.
Takahashi, H.
Takahashi, M.
Takahashi, H.
Takeuchi, S.
Tanaka, S.
Tanishima, M.
Yamada, M.
Yamamoto, T.
Yanagawa, T.

Exhibition
Kataoka, T.
Matsui, Y.
Mochizuki, H.

Okano, H.
Tamura, M.
Tanimoto, S.

Social Programme
Hongo, O.
Fukuhara, S.
Takahara, T.

Liaison
Odaka, M.
Kobara, Y.
Tsukamoto, T.

Ladies Programme
Mrs. Shigematsu, I.
Mrs. Fujita, S.
Mrs. Hiraga, Y.
Mrs. Hongo, O.
Mrs. Hosoda, Y.
Mrs. Kosuda, T.
Mrs. Mikami, R.
Mrs. Ohira, I.

Art Director
Hagihara, Y.

INTERNATIONAL COMMITTEE ON SARCOIDOSIS
EXECUTIVE COMMITTEE

Executive Secretary
Siltzbach, L. E.   New York

Chapman, J. S.   Dallas
Cummings, M. M.   Bethesda
Hosoda, Y.   Tokyo
Hurley, T. H.   Melbourne
Israel, H. L.   Philadelphia

James, G.   London
Jones-Williams, W.   Cardiff
Levinsky, L.   Prague
Löfgren, S.   Stockholm
Turiaf, J.   Paris
Uehlinger E., A.   Zurich

CONTENTS

I AETIOLOGY

II KVEIM REACTION

1

2

IV IMMUNOLOGY

1

2

V HISTOPATHOLOGY

VI EPIDEMIOLOGY

1

2

VII EXTRAPULMONARY INVOLVEMENT

1

2

VIII VARIOUS TOPICS

IX PROGNOSIS

XII FUTURE ASPECTS

RELATED EVENTS

The Post-Conference Kyoto Meeting

Other Meetings

LIST OF PARTICIPANTS

A

AKANO, AKIYUKI
JNR Shizuoka Hospital, Morishitamachi, Shizuoka, Japan

AKITA, JUNKO
Kitano Hospital, 3 Nishiogi-machi, Kita-ku, Osaka, Japan

ANSZAI, TUNEO
Nagai Hospital, 5–511 Aokicho Kawaguchi-shi, Saitama, Japan

AOKI, KOKI
Hokkadoi University, N. 16 W. 4, Sapporo, Hokkaido, Japan

AOYAGI, KAZUHIRO
JNR Moji Health Service, 1–1 Takada 2 chome Moji-ku, Kitakyushu-shi, Fukuoka, Japan

AOYAGI, TERUO
Keio University, 35 Shinanomachi, Shinjuku-ku, Tokyo, Japan

ARAI, TOSHIO
84 Minami-tsuji, Iwatsuki-shi, Saitama, Japan

ARATAKE, KAZUHIKO
Osaka Prefectural Hospital, 4 chome, Bandai Higashi, Sumiyoshi-ku, Osaka, Japan

ARUGA, HIKARU
Kawatetsu Hospital, Minami-cho, Chiba-shi, Japan

ASAKAWA, MITSUO
Sapporo Medical College, S. 1 W. 16, Sapporo, Hokkaido, Japan

B

BABA, HARUKATA
National Nakano Chest Hospital, 3–14–20 Egota, Nakano-ku, Tokyo, Japan

BEHREND, HORST
Medizinishe Hochschule Hannover, Abteilun

BERGQVIST, SVEN
Central Dispensary, Stockholm, Sweden

BLASI, ANTONIO
Clinic of Tuberculosis and Respiratory, University of Naples, Napoli, Italy

BOVORNKITTI, SOMACHI
Siriraj Hospital, Mahidol University, Bangkok 7, Thailand

BRACKERTZ, D.
Rhuematologische Universitätsklinik, Felix Platter-Spital, Burgfelderstraße 101, CH-4000 Basel, Switzerland

BYRNE, EARL B.
Jefferson Medical College of Thomas Jefferson University, Philadelphia, Pa. 19107, U.S.A.

C

CARLENS, ERIC
Karolinska Hospital, 10401 Stockholm, Sweden

ÇELİKOGLU, İ. SEYHAN
University of Istanbul, Turkey

CHIBA, YASUYUKI
JNR Central Hospital, 2–1 Yoyogi, Shibuya-ku, Tokyo, Japan

D

DALEN, ANDERS
Central-despensãr, Törnrosvägen 10 B, S-181 61 Lindingö, Sweden

DJURIĆ BRANISLAV
Institute TBC, 21107 Novi Sad, Yugoslavia

DOI, ICHIRO
JNR Central Hospital, 2–1 Yoyogi, Shibuya-ku, Tokyo, Japan

DONOMAE, IMASATO
Sumitomo Hospital, 15–5 Nakanoshima, Kita-ku, Osaka, Japan

DOUGLAS, A. C.
City Hospital, Greenbank Drive, Edinburgh EH10 5SB, Scotland

E

EJIMA, HIROKO
University of Tokyo, 7-3-1 Hongo, Bunkyo-ku, Tokyo, Japan

EWERT, GÜNTHER
Waldsanatorium Höchenschwand, 7821
Höchenschwand, Panoramastr. 17, Federal
Republic of Germany

F

FIEZ-VANDAL, PANE-VES
2 Rue Amiral Courber, St. Mondé 94,
France

FIGUEROA-LEBRON, RAMON E.
Veterans Administration Hospital, GPO
Box 4867 San Juan, Puerto Rico 00936,
U.S.A.

FUERTES, SYLVIA A.
207 Pesante Street, Santurce, Puerto Rico
00912, U.S.A.

FUJIE, HIROTADA
3-31-11 Hongo, Bunkyo-ku, Tokyo, Japan

FUJII, CHIAKI
100 Higashi Fukatsu-shi, Fukuyama, Japan

FUJII, KOH
Nagoya University School of Medicine,
65 Tsuruma-cho, Showa-ku, Nagoya,
Japan

FUJIMORI, IPPEI
Kawasaki Municipal Hospital, 70 Shinkawa-dori, Kawasaki-shi, Kanagawa, Japan

FUKUSHIMA, YASUYOSHI
Ohizumigakuen 193, Nerima-ku, Tokyo,
Japan

FUJITA, SHINNOSUKE
Tokyo Teishin Hospital, 2-14-23 Fujimi,
Chiyoda-ku, Tokyo, Japan

FUKUDA, YASUHEI
JNR Central Health Institute, 2-1 Yoyogi,
Shibuya-ku, Tokyo, Japan

FUKUHARA, SUSUMU
Tokyo Medical College, 7-71 Nishishinju-
ku, Shinjuku-ku, Tokyo, Japan

FUKUSHIRO, RYOICHI
Kanazawa University, 13-1 Takaramachi,
Kanazawa, Japan

FURUKAWA, Takeharu

Ministry of Health and Welfare, 2-1
Kasumigaseki, Chiyoda-ku, Tokyo, Japan

FURUTA, MAMORU
Shritsu Akita Sogo Hospital, 12 Hodono
Haranomachi, Akita, Japan

FURUIYE, TAKASHI
Tokyo Teishin Hospital, 2-16-1 Fujimi,
Chiyoda-ku, Tokyo, Japan

FUSE, YUSUKE
Sapporo Hospital of Japanese National
Railway, N. 3, E. 1, Chuo-ku, Sapporo,
Hokkaido, Japan

G

GOMAA, TAHA
Faculty of Medicine, Cairo University, 33
Sarwat Street, Cairo, Egypt

GOMI, JIRO
Keio University School of Medicine, 35
Shinanomachi, Shinjuku-ku, Tokyo, Japan

GONDA, NOBUYUKI
Kawasaki City Hospital, 1480 Tomioka-
cho, Kanazawa-ku, Yokohama, Japan

H

HAGIHARA, TADAFUMI
Nihon University School of Medicine, 30
Oyaguchikami-machi, Itabashi-ku, Tokyo,
Japan

HAMADA, NOBORU
Osaka City University, Abeno, Osaka,
Japan

HANNGREN, ÅKE
Karolinska sjukhuset, S-104 01 Stockholm
Sweden

HARA, KAZUO
Chest Diseases Research Institute, Kyoto
University, Kawara-machi, Shogoin, Sa-
kyo-ku, Kyoto, Japan

HARA, KOHEI
Nagasaki University School of Medicine,
7-1 Sakamoto-machi, Nagasaki, Japan

HARADA, KUNIO
JNR Tosu Hospital, 3 chome Akiba-cho,
Tosu-shi, Saga, Japan

HASHIMOTO, TSUTOMU
JNR Central Health Institute, 2-1 Yoyogi,
Shibuya-ku, Tokyo, Japan

HATTA, KOJI
I.P.C. Clinic, Hirakawa-cho 2–7–5, Chiyoda-ku, Tokyo, Japan

HAYASHI, HIROSHI
Ministry of Health and Welfare, 2–1 Kasumigaseki, Chiyoda-ku, Tokyo, Japan

HIBINO, SUSUMU
National Nagoya Hospital, 2–44 Meigetsu-cho, Showa-ku, Nagoya, Japan

HIGUCHI, KENTARO
Fukuoka University, Hamamatsucho, 979 Maeda-shi, Fukuoka, Japan

HIJIKATA, FUMIO
Akita Kenritsu Chuo Hospital, Chiaki Kubota-cho, Akita, Japan

HIRAGA, YOMEI
JNR Sapporo Hospital, N. 3, E. 1, Chuo-ku, Sapporo, Hokkaido, Japan

HIRAKO, TADASHI
National Leprosarium Tama Zenshoen, Minamiakitsu, Higashimurayama-shi, Tokyo, Japan

HIRASAWA, ISAKICHI
Fujimi Hospital, Miyakami, Shimizu-shi, Shizuoka, Japan

HIRONE, TAKAE
Kanazawa University, Kanazawa, Japan

HOMMA, HIOMI
Juntendo University School of Medicine, 2 1 1, Hongo, Bunkyo-ku, Tokyo, Japan

HONDA, KATSUGI
Kawasaki City Hospital, 70 Shinkawa-dori, Kawasaki-shi, Kanagawa, Japan

HONGO, OSAMU
Komagome Hospital, 3–18–22 Honkomagome, Bunkyo-ku, Tokyo, Japan

HORIKAWA, MASAHIRO
Tohoku University, 4–12 Hirosemachi, Sendai, Japan

HORSMANHEIMO, MAIJA
University of Helsinki, Haartmaninkatu 3, Helsinki 29, Finland

HOSHINO, TOMOH
JNR Central Hospital, 2–1 Yoyogi, Shibuya-ku, Tokyo, Japan

HOSODA, MEGUMI
Nihon University School of Medicine, Oyaguchi, Itabashi-ku, Tokyo, Japan

HOSODA, YUTAKA
JNR Central Health Institute, 2–1 Yoyogi, Shibuya-ku, Tokyo, Japan

HURLEY, T. H.
University of Melbourne, Royal Melbourne Hospital, Post Office 3050, Victoria, Austrailia

I

IMAI, KIYOSHI
Shionogi Research Laboratory, Shionogi Seiyaku, 2–47 Sagisu Fukushimaku, Osaka, Japan

ISHIDA, OSAMU
Osaka University School of Medicine, Dojima-Hamadori, Fukushima-ku, Osaka, Japan

ISHIDATE, TAKUZO
Department of Pathology Akita University School of Medicine, Senshu Kubota-cho 6–10, Akita-shi, 010, Japan

ISRAEL, HAROLD L.
Thomas Jefferson University, Philadelphia, Pa. 19107, U.S.A.

ITO, MASAHARU
Ministry of Health and Welfare, 2–1 Kasumigaseki, Chiyoda-ku, Tokyo, Japan

ITO, YOSHIO
Niigata University School of Medicine Asahimachi-dori, Niigata, Japan

IWAI, KAZURO
Japan Anti-Tuberculosis Association Research Institute, 2–4–24 Matsuyama, Kiyose-shi, Tokyo, Japan

IWASAKI, TATSURO
Japan Anti-Tuberculosis Association Research Institute Matsuyama Kiyose-shi, Tokyo, Japan

IZUMI, TAKATERU
Chest Diseases Research Institute, Kyoto University, Kawara-machi, Shogoin, Sakyoku, Kyoto, Japan

J

JAMES, D. GERAINT
Royal Northern Hospital, London NN 7, Great Britain

JOHNS, CAROL JOHNSON
Johns Hopkins University and Hospital, 601 N. Broadway, Baltimore Md. 21205 U.S.A.

JOHNES WILLIAMS, WILLIAM
Welsh National School of Medicine Department of Pathology, Cardiff, Great Britain

K

KALDEN, JOACHIM ROBERT
Medizinische Hochschule Hannover, D 3000 Hannover, Roderbruchstrasse 101, Federal Republic of Germany

KAMMERLING, K.
2307 Hungary Rd., Richmond, Va. U.S.A.

KANATOMI, MASUO
JNR Moji Railway Division, R-23-22 Kamimaiso 1 chome, Moji-ku, Kitakyushu-shi, Fukuoka, Japan

KATAOKA, TETSURO
National Institute of Health, 2–10–35 Kamiosaki, Shinagawa-ku, Tokyo, Japan

KATAYAMA, SHINICHI
JNR Central Hospital, 2–1 Yoyogi, Shibu-ya-ku, Tokyo, Japan

KATO, SHIRO
Research Institute for Microbial Deseases, Osaka University, Yamadakami, Suita, Osaka, Japan

KATSU, MASATAKA
Kawasaki City Hospital, 70 Shinkawa-dori, Kawasaki, Japan

KAWABE, HIDEO
St. Luke's International Hospital, 10–1 Akashi-cho, Chuo-ku, Tokyo, Japan

KAWAMURA, TARO
Saitama Medical College, Morohongo, Moroyama-cho, Iruma-gun, Saitama, Japan

KAWAZOE, DAISHIRO
Nagoya University, School of Medicine, 65 Tsuruma-cho, Showa-ku, Nagoya, Japan

KEDIG, EDWIN L.
Virginia Commonwealth University, 3603 Grove Avenue, Richmond, Va. 23221 U.S.A.

KINOSHITA, YASUTAMI
Niigata University School of Medicine, Asahi-cho, Niigata-shi, Japan

KIRA, SHIRO
Tokyo University School of Medicine, 7–3–1 Hongo, Bunkyo-ku, Tokyo, Japan

KITAHARA, TAKI
1487–1 Akaho Komagane-shi, Nagano, Japan

KITAMOTO, OSAMU
Kyorin University School of Medicine, 6–20–2 Shinkawa, Mitaka-shi, Tokyo, Japan

KITAMURA, KANEHIKO
Tokyo Medical College, 1–412 Higashi-okubo, Shinjuku-ku, Tokyo, Japan

KIYONAGA, GOICHI
Center for Adult Disease, 1 chome, Naka-machi, Higashinari-ku, Osaka City, Osaka, Japan

KOBARA, YUKINOBU
Chest Diseases Research Institute, Kyoto University, Kawara-machi, Shogoin, Sakyo-ku, Kyoto, Japan

KOBAYASHI, FUMIKO
Toranomon Hospital, 2 chome, Aoi-cho, Minato-ku, Tokyo, Japan

KOIZUMI, HIROSHI
Kawasaki City Hospital, 6–5 Miyamotocho, Kawasaki-ku, Kawasaki-shi, Kanagawa, Japan

KOJIMA, RIICHI
Tokyo Medical College, 6–7–1 Nishisin-juku, Shinjuku-ku, Tokyo, Japan

KONDO, KIWAMU
JNR Central Health Institute, 2–1 Yoyogi, Shibuya-ku, Tokyo, Japan

KONO, TOSHINAO
Tokyo North Railway Operation Division, Japan National Railways, 1–6–5 Maruno-uchi, Chiyoda-ku, Tokyo

KOSUDA, TATSUO
Kanto-chuo Hospital, 5–25–1 Kami-yoga, Setagaya-ku, Tokyo, Japan

KOTEDA, TSUNETOSHI
Nagasaki University School of Medicine, 7–1 Sakamoto-cho, Nagasaki, Japan

KUKITA, ATSUSHI
Sapporo Medical College, S. 1, W. 16, Sapporo, Hokkaido, Japan

KURATA, AKIHIKO
Kitano Hospital, 3 Nishiogi-machi, Kita-ku, Osaka, Japan

KURIHARA, TADAO
JNR Central Health Institute, 2–1 Yoyogi, Shibuya-ku, Tokyo, Japan

L

LEE, JAE R.
Central NFLD Hospital, Union St., Grand Fails, NFLD, Canada

LEE, JAY Q.
Lee Chest Clinic, 50 Myung-Dong 2 Ka, Seoul, Korea

LITTLE, T. O.
6955 Montauk Drive, Richmond, Va. 23225 U.S.A.

LUNDAR, JOHAN
H. Heyerdahlsgt. 1, Oslo 1, Norway

M

MAEDA, MIKI
Matsushita Denki Health Service Shonan Blockcenter, Tsujido Motomachi 6-4-1, Fujisawa, Kanagawa, Japan

MAEDA, YUTAKA
JNR Central Health Institute, 2-1 Yoyogi, Shibuya-ku, Tokyo, Japan

MAEKAWA, NOBUO
Chest Diseases Research Institute, Kyoto University, Kawara-machi, Shogoin, Sakyo-ku, Kyoto, Japan

MAJIMA, JIHEI
Kitano Hospital, 3 Nishiogi-machi, Kita-ku, Osaka, Japan

MASAKI, MIKIO
St. Luke's International Hospital, 10-1 Akashicho, Chuo-ku, Tokyo, Japan

MASAOKA, KAZU
Tokyo Metropolitan Health Bureau, 3-5-1 Marunouchi, Chiyoda-ku, Tokyo, Japan

MATSUBA, KENICHI
JNR Moji Hospital, 1-1 Takada 2 chome Moji-ku, Kitakyushu-shi, Fukuoka, Japan

MATSUDA, MINORU
Center for Adult Disease, 1 chome Naka-machi, Higashinari-ku, Osaka, Japan

MATSUI, AKIRA
St. Luke's International Hospital, 10-1 Akashicho, Chuo-ku, Tokyo, Japan

MATSUI, YASUO
Japan Red Cross Central Hospital, 4-1-22 Hiroo, Shibuya-ku, Tokyo, Japan

MATSUMOTO, MASAHARU
JNR Central Hospital, 2-1 Yoyogi, Shibu-ya-ku, Tokyo, Japan

MATSUMOTO, MASANOBU
Tochigi National Sanatorium, 2-160 Shimookamoto, Kawachi machi, Kawachi-gun, Tochigi, Japan

MATSUOKA, TAKASHI
Nihon University School of Medicine, Oyaguchikami-machi, 30-2, Itabashi-ku, Tokyo, Japan

MATSUSHIMA, HIDENO
Toho University, Ohashi Hospital, 2-17-6 Ohashi, Meguro-ku, Tokyo, Japan

MATSUSHIMA, MASAMI
Gunma University School of Medicine, 4-20-8 Iwagamicho, Maebashi, Gunma, Japan

MEDINA, GLORIFICATION
8425 E. Twelve Mile, Warren, Michigan 48093 U.S.A.

MIKAMI, JIRO
The First Tokyo National Hospital, 1 Toyamacho Shinjuku-ku, Tokyo, Japan

MIKAMI, RIICHIRO
Tokyo University School of Medicine, 7-3 1 Hongo, Bunkyo-ku, Tokyo, Japan

MIKAMO, YOSHIO
Kanto-chuo Hospital, 5-21-5 Kami-yoga, Setagaya-ku, Tokyo, Japan

MILLER, ALBERT
The Mount Sinai Hospital, Fifth Avenue and 100th Street, New York, N.Y. 10029, U.S.A.

MINAMI, OSAMU
Nissei Hospital, 4-11 Minami-dori, Uch-bori, Noshi-ku, Osaka, Japan

MITCHELL, DONALD N.
MRC Tuberculosis and Chest Diseases Unit Brompton Hospital, Fulham Road, London SW 36 HP, Great Britain

MIURA, OSAMU
Nihon University Hospital, 1-8-13 Suruga-dai, Kanda, Chiyoda-ku, Tokyo, Japan

MIURA, SHOJI
JNR Moji Health Service, 1-1 Takada 2 chome, Moji-ku, Kitakyushu-shi, Fukuoka, Japan

MIURA, YUSHO
Hokkaido University, N. 14, W. 5, Sapporo, Hokkaido, Japan

MIYAMURA, MINORU
Tsubakimoto Chain Co. Ltd., Tsurumicho, Joto-ku, Osaka, Japan

MIZUNO, NOBUYUKI
Nagoya City University School of Medichine, Mizuhocho, Mizuho-ku, Nagoya, Japan

MOCHIZUKI, HIROYUKI
Nisso Nihongi Hospital, Nakago-mura, Naka-kubiki-gun, Niigata,Japan

MOORE, HARRY
21 Storthes Street, Mt. Lawley, West Australia 6050, Australia

MORII, HIROTOSHI
Toranomon Hospital, 2 Aoi-cho, Akasaka, Minato-ku, Tokyo, Japan

MORIOKA, SHIGEHARU
Kochi Hospital, 15–2 Takaracho, Kochi-shi, Japan

MURAO, MAKOTO
Hokkaido University School of Medicine, N. 16, W. 6, Sapporo, Hokkaido, Japan

MURATA, YOSHIO
Osaka Prefectural Hospital, 4 chome, Bandai Higashi, Sumiyoshi-ku, Osaka, Japan

MUROHASHI, TOYOHO
National Institute of Health Japan, 10–35 Kamiosaki 2 chome, Shinagawa-ku, Tokyo, Japan

MUROMOTO, HITOSHI
Kitano Hospital, 3 Nishiogimachi, Kita-ku, Osaka, Japan

N

NAGANO, HIROSHI
St. Luke's International Hospital, 10–1 Akashi-cho, Chuo-ku, Tokyo, Japan

NAGASHIMA, AKIRA
JNR Central Health Institute, 2–1 Yoyogi, Shibuya-ku, Tokyo, Japan

NAITO, MASUKAZU
10–15 Kitadacho, Kamitakano, Sakyo-ku, Kyoto, Japan

NAKAGAWA, YOSHIMASA
Tokyo Metropolitan Government, 3–5–1 Marunouchi, Chiyoda-ku, Tokyo, Japan

NAOE, SHIRO
St. Malianna School of Medicine, 2095 Sugao Takatsu-ku, Kawasaki, Kanagawa, Japan

NAKAMURA, EICHI
Tokyo Metropolitan Government, 3–5–1 Marunouchi, Chiyoda-ku, Tokyo, Japan

NAKAO, KIKU
Jiji Medical College, 3311–1, Yakushiji, Minamikawa-chi, Tochigi, Japan

NAKASHIMA, TOSHIRO
Nishi Beppu Hospital, 4548 Turumi, Beppu, Japan

NAKAYAMA, SHUZO
Kumamoto Health Center, 1–13–16 Kubonji-cho, Kumamoto, Japan

NIEMISTÖ, MARKUS
Mjölbolsta Hospital, 10350 Mjölbolsta, Finland

NIESCHULZ, OTTO
Hermal-Chemie Kurt Herrmann, 2057 Reinbek, Danziger Street 5, Federal Republic of Germany

NIITU, YASUTAKA
Tohoku University, 5–12 Hirosemachi, Sendai, Japan

NISHIMOTO, YUKIO
Hiroshima University School of Medicine, 1–2–3 Kasumi, Hiroshima, Japan

NOBECHI, KEIZO
Nishiogi-minami 2–148, Suginami-ku, Tokyo, Japan

NOGUCHI, YOSHIKUNI
Yushima 3–18–12, Bunkyo-ku, Tokyo, Japan

NOMURA, YASUO
Tokai Central Hospital, 1–26 Nakasakura-cho, Kagamihara-shi, Gifu, Japan

NORIMATSU, YOSHIMASA
Minami Kyushu Hospital National Sanatorium, 1–882 Kida Kagikicho, Kagoshima, Japan

NUKADA, HIKARU
The Nukada Institute for Medical and Biological Research, 5–18, Inage-machi, Chiba, Japan

NUKADA, HISAKO
Toho University School of Medicine Omori Hospital, 4–7–14 Sanno, Ota-ku, Tokyo, Japan

O

OBUCHI, SHIGEYOSHI
Tokyo Medical Dental College, 3–1 Yushima, Bunkyo-ku, Tokyo, Japan

ODAKA, MINORU
  JNR Central Health Institute, 2–1 Yoyogi,
  Shibuya-ku, Tokyo, Japan

OGASAWARA, YOSHIO
  Toyohashi Hospital, 2–73 Kawara-cho-
  dori, Toyohashi, Japan

OGIHARA, MASAO
  Tokyo Jikeikai University School of Medicine, 106 Izumi Komae-shi, Tokyo, Japan

OGIMA, ISAMU
  Niigata University School of Medicine,
  Asahimachi-dori, Niigata, Japan

OHIRA, ICHIRO
  Tokyo Jikeikai University School of Medicine, 106 Izumi Komae-shi, Tokyo, Japan

OHNISHI, TOSHIO
  St. Luke's International Hospital, 10–1
  Akashi-cho, Chuo-ku, Tokyo, Japan

OHTAKE, HACHIRO
  JNR Central Health Instititate, 2–1 Yoyogi,
  Shibuya-ku, Tokyo Japan

OIKE, YASABURO
  Hirosaki University School of Medicine,
  Zaifu-cho, Hirosaki, Japan

OKADA, SHIZUO
  Japan Antituberculosis Association Osaka
  Branch, 2 chome Yokobori, Higashi-ku,
  Osaka, Japan

OKAMOTO, TERUO
  Osaka City University, Abeno, Osaka,
  Japan

OKANO, HIROSHI
  Toranomon Hospital, 2 Aoi-cho, Akasaka,
  Minato-ku, Tokyo, Japan

OKAYASU, MASAHITO
  Nihon University, 30 Ohyaguchikami-
  machi, Itabashi-ku, Tokyo, Japan

OKUI, SHINJI
  National Kasumigaura Hospital, 760
  Shimotakatsu, Tsuchiura, Ibaraki, Japan

OLIVIERI, DARIO
  Clinic of Tuberculosis and Respiratory
  Diseases University of Naples, Napoli,
  Italy

OSADA, HIROSHI
  JNR Central Hospital, 2–1 Yoyogi, Shibuya-ku, Tokyo, Japan

OSAMURA, SHIGEYUKI
  Tokyo Medical College, 6–71 Nishishin-
  juku, Shinjuku-ku, Tokyo, Japan

OSHIMA, KAZUYOSHI
  Tokyo Metropolitan Government, 3–5–1
  Marunouchi, Chiyoda-ku, Tokyo, Japan

OSTERMAN, KARIN
  Department of Pulmonary Diseases University Hospital, Uppsala, Sweden

OSTERMAN, PER OLOF
  Department of Neurology University Hospital, Uppsala, Sweden

P

PAIK, YONG H,
  John J. Kane Hospital, Pittsburgh, Pa.
  15243, U.S.A.

PAIK, HEE HAE
  John J. Kane Hospital, Pittsburgh, Pa.
  15243, U.S.A.

PATTERSON, JOHN R.
  Jefferson Hospital, No. 16 Concord
  Avenue, Havertown, Penn. 19083, U.S.A.

PENG, ALRED
  St. Luke's Hospital, 421 W. 113 St.,
  U.S.A.

Q

QUINTILANI, RICHARD
  Hartford Hospital, Conn., U.S.A.

R

RUPEC, MLADEN
  Dermatologische Klinik und Poliklinik der
  Philipps-Universität, 355 Marburg a.d.
  Lahn, Deutschhausstr 9, Federal Republic
  of Germany

S

SAKUMA, KOHSHI
  JNR Central Health Institute 2–1 Yoyogi,
  Shibuya-ku, Tokyo Japan

SASAMOTO, HIROSHI
  Keio University School of Medicine, 35
  Shinanomachi, Shinjuku-ku, Tokyo, Japan

SATO, ATSUHIKO
  Chest Diseases Research Institute, Kyoto
  University, Kawara-machi, Shogoin, Sa-
  kyoku, Kyoto, Japan

SATO, HIKOJIRO
Kitasato University, 5–9–1 Shirokane, Minato-ku, Tokyo, Japan

SAWASAKI, HIROTSUGU
Izu Teishin Hospital, Hirai, Kannami machi, Takata, Shizuoka, Japan

SBAR, SIDNEY
Veteran's Hospital Administration, Brooklin, New York, U.S.A.

SEIFERT, ISABELLA
8004 Lohhof, Oberbayern, Buchenstr. 12, Federal Republic of Germany

SELROOS, OLOF
Helsinki University Central Hospital, 00170 Helsinki 17, Finland

SHIGEMATSU, ITSUZO
National Institute of Public Health, 1 Shirokanedai-machi, Minato-ku, Tokyo, Japan

SHIGEMATSU, NOBUAKI
Research Institute for Diseases of the Chest Kyushu University School of Medicine, 1276 Katakasu, Higashi-ku, Fukuoka, Japan

SHIGEMATSU, NORIO
Kitano Hospital, 3 Nishiogi-machi, Kita-ku, Osaka, Japan

SHIKANAI, KENKICHI
Seirei Hospital, 34353 Mikatabara, Hamamatsu, Shizuoka, Japan

SHIMA, KIYOSHI
Kumamoto University School of Medicine, 1–1–1 Honjo, Kumamoto, Japan

SHIMIZU, SUGURU
Institute of Brain Research School of Medicine, University of Tokyo School of Medicine, Motofuji 1, Bunkyo-ku, Tokyo, Japan

SHIMO, TADAKO
Kanda Health Center, 3–10 Kanda Nishiki-cho, Chiyoda-ku, Tokyo, Japan

SHIMOKATA, KAORU
Nagoya University School of Medicine, 65 Tsuruma-cho, Showa-ku, Nagoya, Japan

SHINKAI, AKIHIKO
National Nakano Chest Hospital, 3–14–20 Egota, Nakano-ku, Tokyo, Japan

SHINOHARA, SHUNJI
Tokyo Hospital, 1–4–3 Mita Minato-ku, Tokyo, Japan

SOEJIMA, RINZO
Kumamoto University School of Medicine, 1–1–1 Honjo, Kumamoto, Japan

SONODA, SETSUYA
Tokyo Medical College, 6–7–1 Nishishin-juku, Shinjuku-ku, Tokyo, Japan

SPIELMAN, STUART
United States Army, USA Meddac, APO S.F., Calif. 96346, U.S.A.

STÅHLE, INGVAR
Komardssjukhuset, 610 23 Kolmården, Sweden

STAVENOW, SVEN
St Göran Hospital, S-112 81 Stockholm, Sweden

STORK, WALTER J.
Jefferson Davis Hospital, 180 Allen Parkway, Houston, Texas 77019, U.S.A.

SULAVIK, STEPHEN B.
St. Francis Hospital, 114 Woodland Street, Hartford, Conn. 06105 U.S.A.

SUNAHARA, SHIGEICHI
Tokyo National Chest Hospital, 3–1–1 Takeoka, Kiyose-shi, Tokyo, Japan

T

TACHIBANA, TERUO
OSAKA Prefectural Hospital, 4 chome Bandai, Higashi Sumiyoshi-ku, Osaka, Japan

TACHIRI, HIROMU
Osaka University School of Medicine, 553 Dojimahama-dori, Fukushima-ku, Osaka, Japan

TADA, HIROSHI
St. Luke's International Hospital, 10–1 Akashi-cho, Chuo-ku, Tokyo, Japan

TAKAHARA, TADASHI
JNR Central Health Institute, 2–1 Yoyogi, Shibuya-ku, Tokyo, Japan

TAKAHASHI, HAKKO
JNR Central Health Institute, 2–1 Yoyogi, Shibuya-ku, Tokyo, Japan

TAKAHASHI, MASAYOSHI
JNR Central Hospital, 2–1 Yoyogi, Shibu-ya-ku, Tokyo, Japan

TAKAHASI, TZIHIRO
Health Control Institute in Kawasaki Ajinomoto Co. Inc., Kawasaki Factory, Suzukicho, Kawasaki-ku, Kawasaki, Japan

TAKAMATSU, HIDEO
Chest Diseases Research Institute, Kyoto
University, Kawara-machi, Shogoin,
Sakyo-ku, Kyoto, Japan

TAKASHIMA, HISASHI
JNR Central Health Institute, 2–1 Yoyogi,
Shibuya-ku, Tokyo, Japan

TAKEUCHI, FUMIKO
JNR Moji Health Service, 1–1 Takada 2-
chome, Moji-ku, Kitakyushu-shi, Fukuoka,
Japan

TAKEUCHI, SATORU
JNR Osaka Health Institute, Ofuka-cho,
Kita-ku, Osaka, Japan

TAMAKI, TAKESHI
Ministry of Health and Welfare, 2–1
Kasumigaseki, Chiyoda-ku, Tokyo, Japan

TAMESHIGE, TETSUO
JNR Moji Health Institute, 1–1 Takada 2-
chome, Moji-ku, Kitakyushu-shi, Fukuoka,
Japan

TAMURA, MASASHI
Toranomon Hospital, 2 Aoicho, Akasaka,
Minato-ku, Tokyo, Japan

TANAKA, AKIRA
Tokyo Metropolitan Government, 3–5–1
Marunouchi, Chiyoda-ku, Tokyo, Japan

TANAKA, MOTOICHI
Tokyo Teishin Hospital, 2–16–1 Fujimi,
Chiyoda-ku, Tokyo, Japan

TANAKA, NOBORU
Chiba Cancer Center, 666–2 Nitona-machi,
Chiba, Japan

TANAKA, SHIRO
Insurance Naruwa Hospital, Ohi-machi
3–1, Kanazawa, Japan

TANAKA, TAKAO
JNR Sendai Hospital, 7–27 Kitame-machi,
Sendai, Japan

TANIMOTO, HIROKAZU
Toranomon Hospital, 2 Aoicho, Akasaka,
Minato-ku, Tokyo, Japan

TANISHIMA, MORIJU
Sumitomo Electric Industries, 1 Miya-
higashi, Koya, Itami, Hyogo, Japan

TATEISHI, NORITAKA
First Dep. of Internal Medicine Kuma-
moto University Medical School, 1–1–1
Hojo, Kumamoto, Japan

TATEISHI, TAKERU
Gumma University School of Medicine
Showa-machi, Maebashi, Gumma, Japan

TATENO, SEIGO
Sapporo Medical College, S. 1, W. 16,
Sapporo, Hokkkaido, Japan

TAUB, ROBERT N.
The Mount Sinai School of Medicine,
Fifth Avenue and 100th Street, New York
10029, U.S.A.

TEIRSTEIN, ALVIN S.
The Mount Sinai Hospital, Fifth Avenue
and 100th Street, New York 10029, U.S.A.

TERAMATSU, TAKASHI
Chest Diseases Research Institute, Kyoto
University, Kawara-machi, Shogoin,
Sakyo-ku, Kyoto, Japan

THYGESEN, KRISTIAN
Bispebjerg Hospital, Copenhagen, Denmark

TOKUNAGA, TOHRU
National Institute, Kamiosaki, Shinagawa-
ku, Tokyo, Japan

TSUJI, SHUSUKE
Chest Diseases Research Institute, Kyoto
University, Kawara-machi, Shogoin,
Sakyo-ku, Kyoto, Japan

TSUKAMOTO, TSUTOMU
Metropolitan Police Department, 2–1–1
Kasumigaseki, Chiyoda-ku, Tokyo, Japan

TURIAF, J.
Université Paris VII, Hôpital Bichat, 170
Bd Ney, Paris 18e, France

U

UEDA, HIDEO
JNR Central Hospital, 2–1 Yoyogi,
Shibuya-ku, Tokyo, Japan

UESAKA, ICHIRO
Chest Diseases Research Institute, Kyoto
University, Kawara-machi, Shogoin,
Sakyo-ku, Kyoto, Japan

UMEDA, HIROMICHI
Tokyo Medical & Dental University 1–5–
45 Yushima, Bunkyo-ku, Tokyo, Japan

UMEZAWA, TSUTOMU
Metropolitan Police Department, 2–1
Kasumigaseki, Chiyoda-ku, Tokyo, Japan

URABE, HARUKUNI
Kyushu University Schol of Medicine,
1276 Katakasu, Fukuoka, Japan

URICH, HENRY
The London Hospital, London E1, 1BB,
Great Britain

UYAMA, MASANOBU
Department of Opthalmology Kyoto
University School of Medicine, Kawara-
machi, Shogoin, Sakyo-ku, Kyoto, Japan

V

VILLAR, THOMÉ GEORGE
Lisbon University, Faculty of Medicine
Lisbon, Portugal

VISKUM, KAJ
Bispebjerg Hospital Dept. P., Copenhagen
2400 NV., Denmark

W

WAKABAYASHI, ICHIJI
Veterrans Administration Hospital 1601
Perdido St., New Orreans, La. 70114,
U.S.A.

WAKABAYASHI, MASAKO
Touro Infirmary, N.O., La. U.S.A. 1400
Foucher 87 New Orleans, La. 70115,
U.S.A.

WASHIZAKI, MAKOTO
Toranomon Hospital, 2 Aoicho, Akasaka,
Minato-ku, Tokyo, Japan

WATANABE, YASUSHI
JNR Central Hospital, 2–1 Yoyogi, Shibuya-ku, Tokyo, Japan

WIDSTRÖM, OLLE
Karolinska sjukhuset Medical Clinic, S-
10401 Stockholm 60, Sweden

WILLIAMS, EIRIAN
Pembroke County War Memorial Hospital,
Haverfordwest, Pembrokshire, Great
Britain

WIMAN, LARS-GÖSTA
University Hospital Department of Lung
Diseases, S-901 85 Umeå, Sweden

WURM, KARL
Universität Freiburg, 7821 Höchenschwand
Schwarzwald, Federal Republic of Ger-
many

WU, MIN-CHIEN
National Taiwan University Hospital,
Taipei, Taiwan, Republic of China

Y

YACHI, MICHIKO
JNR Central Hospital, 2–1 Yoyogi,
Shibuya-ku, Tokyo, Japan

YAMADA, MICHITAKA
Kanto Teishin Hospital, 5–55 Gotanda,
Shinagawa-ku, Tokyo, Japan

YAMAGUCHI, AKIRA
Tokyo Jikeikai University School of Medicine, 106 Izumi, Komae-shi, Tokyo, Japan

YAMAMOTO, MASAHIKO
Nagoya City University School of Medicine, Mizuho-ku, Nagoya, Japan

YAMASHITA, HIDEAKI
Fujimi Hospital, Shimizu-shi, Shizuoka,
Japan

YANAGAWA, HIROSHI
National Institute of Public Health, 1
Shirokanedaimachi, Minato-ku, Tokyo,
Japan

YANAGISAWA, KEN
National Institute of Health, 2–10–35
Kamiosaki, Shinagawa-ku, Tokyo, Japan

YANAKA, MAKOTO
JNR Central Hospital, 2–1 Yoyogi, Shibuya-ku, Tokyo, Japan

YASUHIRA, KIMIO
Chest Diseases Research Institute, Kyoto
University, 606 Kawara-machi, Shogoin,
Sakyo-ku, Kyoto, Japan

YI, SANG-YOL
Honam Hospital, Kwangsan-kun, Cholla-
namdo, Korea

YOKOZAWA, NOBORU
Tokai Bank Institute of Public Health,
Ohtemachi, Chiyoda-ku, Tokyo, Japan

YONEDA, RYOZO
Tokyo National Chest Hospital, 3–1–1
Takeoka, Kiyose-shi, Tokyo, Japan

YOSHIMOTO, SEIICHI
Kyushu University Hospital, 1276 Katakasu, Fukuoka, Japan

YOUNG, ROSCOE C., Jr.
Howard University Freedmen's Hospital,
Washington D.C., 20001, U.S.A.

Yoshizawa, Yasuyuki
  Tokyo Teishin Hospital, Fujimi 2–14,
  Chiyodaku, Tokyo, Japan

Z

Zenda, Ichiro
  JNR Hiroshima Hospital, 3–1–36 Futaba-
  nosato, Hiroshima-shi, Japan

OPENING CEREMONY

Kanehiko Kitamura

*Chairman of the Sixth International Conference on Sarcoidosis
Tokyo Medical College, Tokyo, Japan*

Respectable Guests,
Dear Colleagues,
Ladies and Gentlemen:

In 1869, more than 100 years ago, the skin lesions of sarcoidosis were first observed merely as a skin disease by Hutchinson in England and around the same time also by Carl William Boeck in Norway. And over 50 years have elapsed since Schaumann in Sweden 1914 first conceived of the systemic character of sarcoidosis from simultaneous involvement of several organs.

In recent years general concern about this extremely protean disease of unknown cause has increased remarkably, leading to the successive international conferences on sarcoidosis since 1958 and the establishment of the International Committee on Sarcoidosis as a standing body of the conferences in 1966. Needless to say, these international organizations have greatly and really effectively supported, promoted and coordinated international sarcoidosis research.

In Japan, sarcoidosis research can be traced back to Takeya's report on two cases of so-called Boeck's sarcoid published 1921. However, studies on sarcoidosis as a systemic disease commenced much later, in about 1960 with the participation of Dr. Nobechi, one of our honorary chairmen, in the Washington Conference of that year. Soon after, those interested in this disease set up the Japan Sarcoidosis Committee. The three following studies should be mentioned as products of our collaboration in this committee: 1. Epidemiological studies of 1,752 cases of sarcoidosis observed in Japan until 1969. 2. Evaluation of Kveim test with special reference to antigens of our own making. 3. Double blind test and follow-up of corticoid treatment of sarcoidosis.

It seems that the attention of the world's sarcoidologists to the works of Japanese colleagues has risen gradually in the last ten years. And this encouraged us to hold, under the auspices of the International Committee, the Sixth International Conference in Tokyo and to extend invitation universally to all researchers of sarcoidosis in the world. Fortunately it was accepted by many, both at home and abroad, and now we have gathered here over 300 participants from 22 countries.

We fervently wish that the Conference be carried out successfully with your cooperation and that your presentations, discussions and exhibitions would disclose complete aspects of sarcoidosis, namely the clinical, immunological, epidemiological and other findings, and their present interpretations, besides some new acquisitions in its treatment. We have no doubt that in succession to the achievements of the previous conferences, this will also induce further progress of sarcoidology. Especially, we have great expectations that some more light will be thrown on the solution of pathogenesis and aetiology of sarcoidosis, the longstanding and most fundamental questions. Three years ago in Prague, Chairman Levinsky stated in his opening address that the Conference would open the door to the last, fourth stage of sarcoidosis research, according to Dr. James, research on aetiology.   We now hope, the investigation of pathogenesis and aetiology will further be another step.

Quite recently in Japan, eight diseases were designated officially as "hardly curable diseases".   Together with other seven diseases, such as Behçets disease, systemic lupus erythematosus, etc., sarcoidosis was put in this category and the Ministry of Health and Welfare organized eight project teams, one for each disease, to study its epidemiology, diagnostic criteria, treatment, etc.   I am confident that what will be gained here will help this plan.

In closing my address, I would like to express our sincere thanks for the kind assistance given us by the Japan Medical Association.   I would also like to thank the International Committee on Sarcoidosis for the most helpful advices and suggestions.   Furthermore, I should like to return my deep appreciation to the staff of the Japan Sarcoidosis Committee who have devoted themselves to the arrangement of this Conferences for the past three years.

Dear colleagues, on this occasion, I am sure, you will renew old friendship and cultivate new acquaintances.   You may also be afforded a good opportunity for enjoying views and highlights of old and modern Japan with its traditional cultures and natural scenic beauties.   Lastly, I hope you will enjoy your stay in the ancient capital of Kyoto where our colleagues there are looking forward to seeing you at the Post-Conference Sarcoidosis Meeting.

In conclusion, I regret to say that Professor Levinsky, Chairman of the last Conference in Prague in 1969 is not here and accordingly we are not able to hear his address to us.

TARO TAKEMI

President, Japan Medical Association

It is a great honour for me to offer my greetings on behalf of the Japan Medical Association on the occasion of the Sixth International Conference on Sarcoidosis. Sarcoidosis was discovered 100 years ago, but because it is a disease which has numerous facets and follows a peculiar pattern of development, no definitive therapy has been discovered yet. I believe that this conference can make a new contribution to the welfare of mankind by conducting an international study of this serious disease.

In Japan we have witnessed the emergence of new diseases that defy medical treatment, such as Smon. The government is now launching a new research programme to cope with such diseases. This an International Conference on Sarcoidosis raises our expectations for solutions to new medical problems.

I wish to take this opportunity to express my fervent hope that this conference will produce many results. It would also give me great pleasure if the foreign participants in this conference would gain a new understanding of Japanese medical science. I wish all of you a very pleasant stay here during and after the conference.

LADISLAV LEVINSKY

Chairman of the Fifth International Conference on Sarcoidosis at Prague
Charles University, Prague, Czhechoslovakia

Your Excellencies,
Mister Chairman,
Members of the Sixth International Conference on Sarcoidosis,
Ladies and Gentlemen,
Dear Friends :

It is a great honour for me that the Japanese Committee on Sarcoidosis asked me, as the organiser and chairman of the Fifth International Conference which was held in Prague in 1969, to greet the participants of the Sixth International Conference on Sarcoidosis in Tokyo.

Before the Prague Conference I asked—for the first time—my distinguished friend Professor Turiaf, chairman of the Fourth Conference in Paris, to address our opening ceremony in Prague.

It was due to the efforts of Professor Turiaf, Professor Löfgren and Dr James that we were able to welcome in the old Aula Magna of Charles University in Prague researchers from all parts of the world interested in sarcoidosis.

At the Conference in Paris we felt uncertain whether the International Committee on Sarcoidosis would accept the proposal to hold the next conference in such a small country as Czechoslovakia. Professor Turiaf declared : " Il n'y a pas de petits pays " (there are no small countries), and it was his convincing enthusiasm and warm sympathy with our proposal that decided the situation in our favor.

Dr Hosoda, to whom I am joined in close friendship since we met in Prague, believes that it should become a tradition that the chairman of the last conference should address the assembly at the opening session of a present conference. All those who have a high esteem for Japan as a typical country of wise traditions would certainly welcome the establishement of this new tradition in our international co-operation, which would be helpful in maintaining our mutual friendly relations in future.

May I suggest on this occasion that the future organizers and chairmen should impress on future conferences their way of thinking, i.e., the thinking pertinent to that part of the world where the conference is being held. I believe that the Conference in Tokyo has the best prerequisites to fulfill this demand.

Surprisingly, numerous Japanese colleagues attended the Conference on Sarcoidosis in Prague. Japan was third in number of participants from 32 nations, including Czechoslovakia, and in number of reports Japan was fifth. Considering the great distance between our countries, these figures illustrate the deep interest of our Japanese colleagues in the problems posed by sarcoidosis. Therefore we supported the proposal of the International Committee to organize the next conference in Tokyo, even though we were well aware of the fact that we would probably not be able to attend a conference so far from our country. Of course, we were deligted too that so many Japanese colleagues and their charming wifes travelled from the biggest metropolis of the world to a much smaller town in the heart of Europe, and that they liked Prague.

The mutual relations between Czechoslovakia and Japan have been going on for many years. Their culmination was represented by the visit of the Czechoslovak President General Ludvik Svoboda to Japan in 1970. Mr. Kenzo Kono the President of the Upper Chamber of the Japanese Parliament visited Czechoslovakia two weeks ago.

I would like to mention that Japan has attracted more and more of our musicians in recent times because of the highly refined esthetic sense of the Japanese people. An exhibition of Japanese paintings at Prague with many Hiroshige's, Hokusai's and other pictures documented this sense to our artists some forty years ago. The famous Hokusai picture " The Wave " remains forever fixed in my mind.

Finally the representants of Japan are being admired by the whole world now at the Olympic Games in Munich.

An old tale says that Japan was created by a miracle when the god of the seas with his halberd disturbed the waters of the Ocean and some corals which dropped back from the edge of the halberd into the sea gave origin to several islands. These islands subsequently became the cradle of a nation which has been within the last twenty-five years admired by the whole world for its miraculous industrial development. However in contrast to the accidental action of the mythical god, this modern miracle was achieved by intensive intentional efforts.

One hundred and two million of modest, well-disciplined Japanese transformed by their immense efforts and courage a relatively small area consisting of several islands into one of the most important industrial, scientific and cultural centres on our planet.

All these facts most certainly should exert an influence on the present International Conference which opens today. It was prepared with the same calm concentration and thoughfulness which are characteristics of the Japanese nation. They aimed not only at a successful competition with other highly developed industrial countries, but equally at a better understanding between nations. This is an extremely favorable medium for scientific work. Therefore all who attend this opening ceremony of the Sixth International Conference on Sarcoidosis are certainly impatiently awaiting to hear the reports on the recent results of the research work in the field of sarcoidosis from various countries and, in particular, the numerous reports from this country of ingenious invention, diligence and marvellous hospitality.

D. Geraint James

*Representing the International Committee on Sarcoidosis
Royal Northern Hospital, London, Great Britain*

This Olympic movement originated in 1958 in London. Until that time we had read each other's articles, but we did not know each other. And when we got together, we got together in a spirit of cordiality and camaraderie. And it is a most unique international council because fourteen years later, we are all close friends. Because of that spirit of cordiality and camaraderie, it was not difficult to continue the movement once it had started. London was followed by Washington (Marty Cummings), Stockholm (Sven Löfgren), Paris (Jude Turiaf) Prague (Ladislav Levinsky).

Is there any point in an International Conference on Sarcoidosis? Could we not just carry on with national meetings? The answer is this. Firstly, the internationalism of medicine is so strong that it breaks down barriers, and it is important to have an international body to guide conferences. Secondly, the International Committee has a moral responsibility to choose congresses in places where there is serious scholarship on sarcoidosis. So, at our last congress, it was not difficult to choose Japan for the next congress. There was practically no discussion on where we should hold it because you have demonstrated over the years, for many years, serious scholarship and high academic standards in your investigation of sacoidosis.

In order to make a success of a conference, at least two factors are necessary; namely good facilities and a dynamic driving force to see it through. You have the most wonderful facilities; and you have a splendid driving force in Yutaka Hosoda. There is no doubt about that. And so, there can be very little doubt about the success of this congress. We appreciate your efforts. You have put a lot of hard work into it's organisation.

From the first congress onwards we have always maintained the principle of being hard-hitting during these scientific meetings. We can get up and say that somebody is talking rubbish or nonsense and that is good for the congress, but in the evenings we are still very good friends and enjoy a drink. This is important. You don't want a congress in which everybody gets up and agrees with everybody else. That is a sterile conference. And I hope there will be a lot of active discussion in the daytime followed by geniality in the evening.

The last point I make on behalf of the International Committee on Sarcoidosis, is to mourn the absence of a few members. And it is an absence not through choice, but because of compelling other reasons. If Ladislav Levinsky could have walked here, he would have been here. If Marty Cummings could have got away, he would have been here. Seven would have been here from Stockholm but for other compelling factors. But I leave until last probably the greatest omission here today, and I name Louis Siltzbach. Louis Siltabach has been the backbone of the movement, and it must have taken severe ill-health to prevent him from coming. On behalf of all of you, we will send him our greetings, and our earnest wish that he will soon be fully fit and thinking about sarcoidosis again.

I   AETIOLOGY

Nocardia-like Organisms Isolated from Lesions of Sacroidosis

Ichiro Uesaka, Takateru Izumi and Shusuke Tsuji

Chest Diseases Research Institute, Kyoto University, Kyoto, Japan

In order to determine whether any organism could be found in sarcoidosis lesions or not, 65 specimens were taken from 36 cases of the disease admitted to the Sarcoidosis Clinic of our Institute.

Specimens were emulsified in saline and examined microscopically and culturally. No organisms were found in smears stained with Ziehl-Neelsen or Gram.

Each specimen was cultured in 15 to 20 different kinds of medium and incubated at 37°C, 30°C, and room temperature for up to 3 months.

Among 17 organisms isolated from 65 specimens, 4 cultures which were isolated from 3 cases and which resembled each other in their morphological and physiological charactersistics have successfully been maintained up to now. Two of them were isolated from the scalene and mediastinal lymph nodes of a patient and were identical in their characteristics so far as could be ascertained from the tests. Minor differences were observed between other isolates.

Characteristics common to the 4 isolates were as follows: growth was generally poor in all media tested, Sabouraud's glucose agar was better for growth than brain-heart infusion glucose agar and the optimum pH range for growth was 6 to 7. It took more than 1 week for primary isolation, but after serial transfer, growth became faster. Growth was better at 37°C than at 30°C. Trimethylene diamine was not used as the sole source of nitrogen and carbon. Aryl-sulfatase was negative. Tyrosine was decomposed, but xanthine and hypoxanthine were not. Acid was produced from mannose, but not from mannitol or inositol. Milk was liquified after 2 weeks. Colonies on the agar were thin, transparent, moist, and colorless. Slight turbidity and a small amount of sediment appeared in the liquid medium. Microscopically, they had branched hyphae, ca. 1 micron in width, in the early stage of growth, but soon fragmented into rods and coccoids. They were non-acid fast and gram-positive.

These results indicate that they belong to *Nocardia* or are closely related to *Nocardia*. Whether they have any relation to the etiology of sarcoidosis or not remains to be studied.

Isolation of a Mycoplasma from Sarcoid Tissue

MATTI HANNUKSELA

The Department of Dermatology, University Central Hospital,
Helsinki, Finland

AND

ELLI JANSSON

Minerva Foundation, Institute for Medical Research, Helsinki, Finland

INTRODUCTION

At the Fifth International Conference on Sarcoidosis, Homma and his coworkers[1] presented their preliminary studies on attempts to isolate mycoplasma in sarcoidosis. From throat swabs they found unidentified mycoplasma significantly more often than in controls On the other hand, they did not succeed in isolating organisms from sarcoid tissues.

We have also made trials to isolate mycoplasmas from sarcoid tissues. The results of these successful attempts as well as the results of the determination of mycoplasma antibody titers by the indirect hemagglutination technique are presented here.

MATERIAL AND METHODS

Biopsy specimens of sarcoid skin lesions were obtained from 7 patients and specimens of sarcoid lymph nodes from 2 further patients. Three skin biopsies and 18 muscle biopsies taken from controls were studied in the same way as the sarcoid tissues.

The biopsy specimens, after addition of some broth, were crushed in a mortar. Then a loopful of the suspension was inoculated into 3 ml of Marmion's[2] enriched diphasic broth medium. The cultures were incubated at 37°C and subcultures were made on solid media* after 10 and 20 days, inoculating 0.1 ml of the broth culture on solid medium in Petri dishes 5 cm in diameter. The agar plates were incubated in an anaerobic milieu at 37°C for 10 days. Subcultures from the broth tubes were made by transferring 0.3 ml of the culture into new broth tubes. The agar plates were examined under a high-power microscope.

* The medium was the solid and diphasic PPLO medium described by Marmion (2) with the following modifications: 1. Brain-heart infusion broth was used instead of PPLO broth; for solid medium, 1.1% agar was added. 2. The broth medium was further enriched with egg yolk pasteurized at 60°C for 50 minutes and added in amounts of 0.1 ml to 10 ml of broth medium.

Biochemical, growth inhibition, and indirect hemagglutination tests were made to identify the isolated strains (see ref. 3).

RESULTS

Attempts to isolate mycoplasmas

An organism resembling mycoplasma was isolated from 4 out of 7 skin biopsy speci-

Table 1. Isolation of mycoplasmas from sarcoid tissues.

Patient No.	Sex	Age yrs.	Duration of the disease	Sarcoid manifestations						Isolation of mycoplasma			IHA titer against strain 215-M	Skin tests	
				BHA±lung	lymph node	skin	liver	spleen	bone	organ	result	strain		Kveim	Tuberculin TU of PPD
1	M	20	2 mon.	+	+	−	−	−	−	LN	+	215-M	<8	+	100+
2	F	53	6 yrs.	−	+	+	−	−	−	LN skin	+ −	336-M	1024	+	10+
3	F	56	3 yrs.	+	+	+	−	−	−	skin	−		32	+	100−
4	F	45	11 mon.	+	−	+	−	−	−	skin	+	191-M	ND	+	1+
5	F	59	3 yrs.	+	−	+	−	−	+	skin	+	192-M	<8	−	0.1+
6	F	51	2 yrs.	+	−	+	−	−	−	skin	−		<8	+	10+
7	F	51	2 mon.	+	−	+	−	−	−	skin	+	227-M	32	ND	10+
8	M	39	5 mon.	+	−	+	−	−	−	skin	+	239-M	ND	+	1+

BHA=bilateral hilaradentis.
LN=lymph node.
ND=not done.

mens and from both lymph nodes examined (Table 1).

The isolated strains did not convert to bacteria when penicillin and thallium acetate were omitted from the culture medium. They required sterol for growth. The isolates did not ferment glucose or split urea, but they were arginine-positive.

The isolates did not form colonies visible to the naked eye. Antisera against 5 strains were prepared in rabbits. The immune sera inhibited the growth of M. orale type 1 with an inhibition zone of 3 mm, which was equal to that obtained with homologous

Table 2. Mycoplasma (strain 215-M) antibody titers.

	No. of cases	Antibody No.	Titer ≥16 percent	Highest titer
Sarcoidosis				
Subacute +EN	71	5	7	2048
Subacute −EN	116	20	17	2048
Chronic	43	7	16	2048
Probable	14	2		2048
Total	244	34	14	2048
Comparison Series				
Nonsarcoid EN	49	4	8	128
Tbc	34	1		32
Collagenoses	6	1		32
Granulomatosis disciformis (Miescher)	6	2		256
Malignomas	4	1		2048
Tularemia	1	1		128
Other diseases	60	3	5	64
Total	160	13	8	2048
Controls	355	2	0.6	16

EN=erythema nodosum.

immune serum. M. hominis, M. salivarium, M. fermentans, M. pulmonis, M. arthritidis, and M. gallinarum were not inhibited.

Mycoplasmas could not be isolated from any of the control specimens.

Mycoplasma antibodies

Using the indirect hemagglutination technique (IHA), 230 patients with definite sarcoidosis, 14 patients with probable sarcoidosis, 160 patients with other diseases (comparison series), and 355 blood donors were tested for antibodies against an isolated mycoplasma (strain 215-M). The results are shown in Table 2.

A titre of 2048 was found in 5 cases. One of them had acute sarcoidosis with erythema nodosum (EN), another had a very acute form of the disease but without EN, one had chronic smoldering sarcoidosis with pulmonary manifestations, one had probable pulmonary sarcoidosis, and one had acute lymphatic leukemia with fatal outcome.

As a group, the patients with sarcoidosis showed higher IHA titers against the isolated strain 215-M than the others. The number of patients with elevated antibody titer among those with sarcoidosis and EN was smaller (8%) than among those with other forms of sarcoidosis (17%).

DISCUSSION

Mycoplasma was isolated from 2 sarcoid lymph nodes and 4 skin biopsy specimens. Growth inhibition tests showed them to be related to M. orale type 1. This mycoplasma has been found in the throat in 25% of healthy persons.[4] The possibility that the isolated strains were laboratory pickups was small because there was no growth either from the skin specimens or from the muscle biopsies of the nonsarcoid patients. Moreover, M. orale type 1 reference strain was not handled in the laboratory during this study. M. gallinarum and M. gallisepticum, mycoplasmas occurring occasionally in hens' eggs, were not found as contaminants during this investigation.

The patients with sarcoidosis and those with nonsarcoid EN were Kveim-tested. It is not impossible that the Kveim material may have influenced the mycoplasma antibody titer. Further studies to solve this problem have been started already.

The role of mycoplasma in the pathogenesis of sarcoidosis is obscure. Further studies on its occurrence and pathogenicity are needed. It is possible that mycoplasmas found in sarcoid tissues are able to survive there due altered immunity in this disease. The organism may increase in number in sarcoidosis and other chronic diseases with impaired cellular and/or humoral immunity, such as collagen diseases and malignomas. The results of the determination of mycoplasma antibodies favour this suggestion.

SUMMARY

A mycoplasma closely related to M. orale type 1 was isolated from sarcoid skin lesions in 4 out of 7 cases and from both sarcoid lymph nodes examined. Elevated antibody titers (IHA) against the isolated strain (215-M) were found more often in sarcoidosis (14%) than in a comparison series (8%) and in blood donors (0.6%). It is possible that mycoplasmas are able to increase in number in sarcoidosis and other diseases with impaired immunity.

REFERENCES

1. Homma, H., Okano, H., and Mochizuki, H. 1971. An attempt to isolate mycoplasmas from patients with sarcoidosis. *Proc. Fifth Int. Conf. on Sarcoidosis.* Prague: Univ. Karlova, p. 101.

2. Marmion, B. P. 1967. The mycoplasmas: new information on their properties and their pathogenicity for man. In Recent Advances in Medical Microbiology (ed. A. P. Waterson). London: Churchill, pp. 170–253.

3. Jansson, E., Makisara, P., Vainio, K., Snellman, O., and Tuuri, S. 1971. Further studies on mycoplasma in rheumatoid arthritis. *Acta Rheum. Scand.* **17**: 227–235.

4. Taylor-Robinson, D., Canchola, J., Fox, H., and Chanok, R. M. 1964. A newly identified oral mycoplasma (M. orale) and its relationship to other human mycoplasmas. *Amer. J. Hyg.* **80**: 135–148.

Is Sarcoidosis due to an Infectious Interaction Between Virus and Mycobacterium?

Å. Hanngren, G. Biberfeldt, E. Carlens, E. Hedfors, B. S. Nilsson,
E. Ripe, and B. Wahren

Karolinska Hospital, Stockholm, Sweden

Following Scadding's advice[1] not to include any reference to aetiology in the definition of sarcoidosis we have reconsidered the relationship of sarcoidosis to mycobacterial infections. The main reasons for doing so have been the increasing amount of information concerning immunology in general and also the immunology of tuberculosis and of sarcoidosis. The immune system consists of 2 cell types: 1) Bone marrow or Bursa equivalent-derived lymphocytes, so-called B cells, which are responsible for humoral antibody production. 2) Thymus-derived lymphocytes, so-called T cells, which are responsible for delayed-type immune reactions (Fig. 1). The relatively new concept of the pathogenesis of tuberculosis brought about by a great number of investigators during the sixties indicates that the tuberculous lesion is the result of an interaction between antigen and sensitized lymphocytes of T cell type. The present views about the events involved may, in a simplified way, be described as follows (Fig. 2).

Thymus-derived lymphocytes, so-called T cells, with receptors specific for tuberculin initiate the reaction when stimulated by the antigen. The T cells multiply, secret biologically active substances, and some of them are transformed to so-called killer cells with cytolytic activity which cause the necrosis. Macrophages become involved in the reaction, possibly due to some of the secreted substances, and are transformed to epitheloid cells.[2] The reaction constitutes the tuberculous lesion as well as the tuberculin reaction. In sarcoidosis we find a sort of defective epitheloid cell granuloma without necrosis and a depressed tuberculin reaction, suggesting a defective T cell function. This has also been found in several in vitro studies using a specific T cell stimulator[3-6].

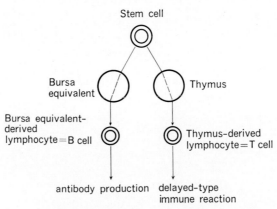

B/T=20/80 (normal value in peripheral blood)

Fig. 1.

Pathogenesis of tuberculosis?

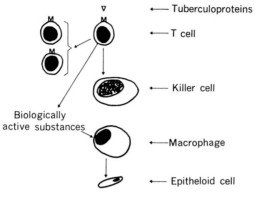

FIG. 2.

In earlier considerations on the relationship of sarcoidosis to tuberculosis (for a review see ref.[7] several facts have been considered to argue against such a relationship. Among these facts are the histological picture of epitheloid cell granuloma without necrosis, devoid of tubercle bacilli in most cases, and a negative turberculin reaction, sometimes combined with a clinical hyperergic symptom such as erythema nodosum. However, there have been other (clinical, laboratory and epidemiological) observations suggesting that the 2 diseases are associated. If we include BCG in the relationship of sarcoidosis to mycobacterium there are some findings in favour of a relationship, namely the finding of Mitchell and collaborators[8] that nonreactors to tuberculin became Kveim reactors following serial BCG vaccination, and that of Gormsen[9] who found disseminated epitheloid cell granulomas in many organs at autopsy up to 3 years following a BCG vaccination. However, bacilli were only found in regional lymph nodes which may contraindicate BCG as the cause of the widespread lesions in sarcoidosis. Also arguing against BCG as a cause are many epidemiological investigations where no increase of sarcoidotic cases was found among vaccinated people.

When some years ago it was found that sarcoidosis patients had elevated titers of antibodies to EB virus[10, 11], considered to cause infectious mononucleosis, and other viruses belonging to the herpes group, it did not arouse much discussion concerning its possible rōle as an etiological agent.

We can understand this if we put together the pros and cons for a virus etiology. Against virus as a cause is the fact that elevated titers are also found in other diseases of different kinds as well as in many healthy persons. The EB viral antigen in sarcoidotic lymph glands has been found in other diseases too. We know that virus infections and virus vaccines depress tuberculin reactivity and that EB virus probably does the same thing, but there are several conditions not connected with sarcoidosis where we find depressed tuberculin reactivity. In infectious mononucleosis, where EB virus is believed to be the causal factor, we find lymphoglandular enlargement, including BHL in some cases, but findings of epitheloid cell granulomas have not been reported. Thus, there is no convincing evidence that viruses may be the causal factor for sarcoidosis. Nevertheless a virus infection may offer a satisfactory explanation of what is found in sarcoidosis.

In infectious mononucleosis there is a depression of tuberculin reactivity[12]. In 17

EB virus infection (or other virus)

↓

IM or subclinical type of IM
(Defective T cell function=depressed PPD reactivity
Undisturbed B cell function=increased immunoglo-
   bulins)

↓ ←— Antigen, e.g. BCG or tbb

Atypical lymphocyte reaction
(Defective T cell response
Stimulation of unaffected B cells by, e.g. BCG as B
   cell stimulator)

FIG. 3.   Hypothesis.

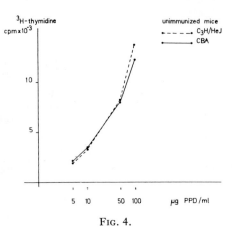

FIG. 4.

consecutive cases of verified infectious mononucleosis, no skin reactions were noted to 2 TU PPD. All patients had been BCG vaccinated earlier in life and the tuberculin reactions, known in 14 cases, had been positive from 1 month to 2 years before the onset of mononucleosis. After recovery, tuberculin tests could again be performed in 10 patients. In 8 patients the test became positive from 2 to 19 months after the disease, in 2 it remained negative. Earlier in vitro studies had shown that lymphocytes from these patients cannot be stimulated by phytohaemagglutinin, which is a T cell stimulator. Taken together, the findings suggest a transient functional T cell defect. The B cell function, on the other hand, seems to the undisturbed as judged from increased immunoglobulin levels and the production of heterophile antibodies. A patient with this type of selective T cell defect may not react normally to an antigen that otherwise gives rise to a T cell response, for example tuberculoproteins from a BCG vaccination or tuberculous infection. Perhaps a hypothesis can be formulated as follows (Fig. 3):

A virus infection, for example an EB infection, depresses the T cell function but leaves the B cells undisturbed, resulting in depressed tuberculin reactivity and increased antibody production. A BCG vaccination or a tuberculous infection may induce an atypical immune response due to the defective T cell function. Instead of a normal T cell response, a B cell-stimulating property of the tuberculoproteins will dominate. It has recently been found that tuberculin is a B cell stimulator.[13–14] In nonimmunized mice (Fig. 4) of 2 different strains, spleen cells responded strongly to PPD stimulation. The same stimulatory effect was also found in newborn guinea pigs, rabbits and rats and in mice having only B cells. (The B cell-stimulating effect was found to be stronger than LPS).

Thus, our hypothesis is built on 1 assumption and 2 facts. The assumption is that tuberculoproteins (not bacilli) are spread throughout the body after BCG vaccination or tuberculous infection. The facts are 1) that tuberculin is a strong B cell stimulator and 2) that sarcoidosis patients show signs of infection with viruses that can depress T cell function. The hypothesis may explain the following clinical findings in sarcoidosis:

1) The generalized disease may be explained by the spread of tuberculoproteins (not bacilli) throughout the whole body, best seen in the reticuloendothelial system of the filtering organs; lungs, spleen and liver.

2) The formation of epitheloid cell granuloma without necrosis can be explained

by stimulated macrophage activity but without any transformation of T lymphocytes to killer cells. They are depressed by viral infection.

3) The B cell-stimulating effect of tuberculoprotein causes an increase of the immunoglobulins found in stage I.

4) The hyperergic reaction, erythema nodosum, which is in contrast to the hypoergic negative tuberculin reaction can perhaps be explained by an antigen-antibody-complement reaction caused by a B cell-stimulating effect.

5) The depressed PPD reactivity is explained by the defective T cell function.

We have formulated the hypothesis that virus may act as a T cell depressor and tuberculoprotein as a B cell stimulator. However, we feel that the essential pathogenetic event in this disezse is a disturbance of the balance of the 2 components of the immune system, T and B lymphocytes. Whatever agents which, in cooperation, fulfil the conditions of depressing T cells and stimulating B cells have to be considered in a discussion of the etiology.

REFERENCES

1. Scadding, J. G. 1970. The definition of sarcoidosis. *Postgrad. Med. J.* **46**: 465–467.
2. Sutton, J. S., and Weiss, L. 1966. Transformation of monocytes in tissue culture into macrophages, epitheloid cells and multinucleated cells. An electron microscopic study. *J. Cell. Biol.* **28**: 303–332.
3. Hirschhorn, K., Schreibman, R. R., Bach, F. H., and Silitzbach, A. E. 1964. In vitro studies on lymphocytes from patients with sarcoidosis and lymphoproliferative diseases. *Lancet ii*: 842–843.
4. Sharma, O. P. 1969. Correlation of in vivo delayed-type hypersensitivity with in vitro lymphocyte transformation in sarcoidosis. Proc. of the Thor. Soc. *Thorax* **24**: 510.
5. Buckley, C. E., Nagaya, H., and Sieker, H. O. 1966. Altered immunologic activity in sarcoidosis. *Annals of Internal Med.* **64**: 508–520.
6. Topilsky, M., Williams, M., Siltzbach, L. E., and Glade, P. R. 1972. Lymphocyte response in sarcoidosis. *Lancet* **i**: 117–120.
7. Scadding, J. G. 1967. Sarcoidosis. London: Eyre & Spottiswoode.
8. Mitchell, D. N., Siltzbech, L. E., Sutherland, I., and A'Arcy Hart, P. 1967. Some further observations on the Kveim test in relation to BCG vaccination and tuberculin sensitivity. *La Sarcoidose Rapp. IVe Conf. Intern.* Paris: Masson & Cie. 154–161.
9. Gormsen, H. 1956. On the occurence of epitheloid cell granulomas in the organs of of BCG-vaccinated human beings. *Acta Path. et Microbiol. Scand.* suppl. **111**: 117.
10. Hirshaut, Y., Glade, P., Viera, L. O., Ainbender, E., Dvorak, D., and Siltzbach, L. E. 1970. Sarcoidosis, another disease associated with serologic evidence for Herpes-like virus infection. *New Engl. J. Med.* **283**: 502–506.
11. Wahren, B., Carlens, E., Espmark, Å., Lundbeck, H., Löfgren, S., Madar, E., Henle, G., and Henle, W. 1971. Antibodies to various herpesviruses in sera from patients with sarcoidosis. *J. Nat. Cancer Inst.* **47**: 747–756.
12. Lantorp, K., Wahren, B., and Hanngren, Å. 1972. Depression of the tuberculin reaction in infectious mononucleosis. *Brit. Med. J.* **4**: 668.
13. Sultzer, B., and Nilsson, B. S. 1972. PPD-tuberculin, a B cell mitogen. *Nature.* **240**: 198–200.
14. Nilsson, B. S., Sultzer, B. M., and Bullock, W. W. 1973. PPD-tuberculin induces immunoglobulin production in normal mouse spleen cells. *J. Exp. Med.* **137**: 127–139.

The Production of Granulomas in Mice by Sarcoid Tissue Suspensions

D. N. MITCHELL

MRC Tuberculosis and Chest Diseases Unit, Brompton Hospital,
London, Great Britain

AND

R. J. W. REES

National Institute for Medical Research, London, Great Britain

INTRODUCTION

Although the presentation and clinical evolution of the more common forms of sarcoidosis are now well-recognised, the etiology and pathogenesis remain unknown and no specific causal agent has been found. We have previously reported[1] our earlier attempts to transmit sarcoidosis directly to animals by inoculating homogenates of human sarcoid lymph nodes into the footpads of normal and immunologically deficient mice prepared by adolescent thymectomy followed by whole-body irradiation, (T/900r). We are currently undertaking a reappraisal of the use of immunologically deficient (T/600r, but without syngeneic mouse bone-marrow cell replacement) mice;[2] meanwhile, we have substantially extended our studies using normal in preference to immunologically deficient (T/900r) mice, since these showed no significant advantages in our earlier studies.

MATERIALS AND METHODS

Sarcoid tissues

Fresh lymph nodes were obtained by mediastinoscopy[3] from patients with sarcoidosis; fresh splenic tissue was obtained at splenectomy for hypersplenism. Each tissue showed characteristic microscopic changes.

Control tissues

Fresh lymph nodes were obtained from the groin at operations for ligation of varicose veins or during the course of vascular surgery in otherwise healthy subjects. Microscopically, each showed an essentially normal structure although simple inflammatory changes were present in some instances. Splenic tissue was obtained from a Kveim-negative patient with recurrent illness in whom splenectomy was undertaken for gross splenomegally, but who showed no other evidence suggestive of sarcoidosis. Microscopically, the spleen showed focal and diffuse granulomatous infiltration.

Homogenates

These were prepared in an identical manner from each fresh unfrozen tissue in 1% bovine albumin in saline solution, yielding approximately a 13.5% suspension. Prior to intravenous injection, homogenates were filtered through nylon to remove coarse particles and diluted 1:3 or 1:4 as required to avoid toxicity. For passage, homogenates

12

were prepared in an identical manner from mouse footpad tissues showing epithelioid cell granulomas 18 months following the inejction of human sarcoid homogenate, and as controls, from the footpad tissues of mice receiving homogenates from normal lymph nodes after the same interval following footpad inoculation. The homogenate for a second passage was similarly prepared from the footpads of mice showing epithelioid cell granulomas 6 months following the inoculation of these footpads with a first passage of 'sarcoid' mouse footpad homogenate. All homogenates were injected into guinea pigs and cultured on Lowenstein-Jensen medium. No mycobacteria were detected.

Inoculation

Each sarcoid or nonsarcoid homogenate was injected into the hind footpads, (0.03 ml) intraperitoneally, (0.5 ml) or intravenously, (0.07 ml) into normal female and in some instances additionally into immunologically deficient (T/900r) female CBA strain mice of 12 weeks of age.

Biopsy specimens and tissues

In order to assess the nature and development of the cellular response in the footpad we have continued to sample a proportion of footpads from each experiment after varying intervals of time. An initial assessment of cellular changes (e.g. 0–6 months) and of Kveim reactivity was made histologically by full thickness biopsy of a footpad and by biopsy of a Kveim test given in the ear using a skin biopsy (Hayes-Martin) punch. The late changes (e.g. 7–24 months or more) were assessed by biopsy of the contralateral footpad and of a further Kveim test site in the contralateral ear. In some instances the footpads from which the early changes were assessed were re-examined after a prolonged interval. Mice were killed when they became sick or after prolonged intervals of time; the footpads and viscera were examined histologically.

Kveim tests

Lots 0025, 004 and 005 of Hurley (Type 1) test suspension were used. Tests were given in the ear after similar intervals of time following inoculation with sarcoid or nonsarcoid homogenates. Tests sites were assessed macroscopically and microscopically 6 weeks after injection.

Microscopic assessments

These were assessed 'blind' according to conventionally accepted criteria.[9] Thus, in mice with 'positive' histology the appearances closely resembled those seen in sections from spontaneous sarcoid lesions in man.

RESULTS

Table 1 shows cumulative results for footpad histology and Kveim tests in the ear among normal and immunologically deficient mice inoculated with fresh sarcoid or nonsarcoid homogenates. Sarcoid granulomas have thus far been seen in 44 footpads from 114 mice. Kveim tests were made in 111 of these mice; 21 showed a microscopically positive response and these were all associated with a positive or equivocal footpad histology. Conversely, only 1 positive and 6 equivocal footpads were encountered in 164 footpad tissues examined from 69 mice after varying intervals of time following inoculation with nonsarcoid homogenates. All 69 had microscopically negative Kveim tests.

TABLE 1. Histological assessments of footpads and of Kveim tests in the ears of normal and immunologically deficient mice inoculated with sarcoid or nonsarcoid homogenates.

Mean interval following inoculation (months)	Site	Sarcoid			Nonsarcoid		
		Pos.	Equiv.	Neg.	Pos.	Equiv.	Neg.
12	Footpad	44	36	75	1	6	157
12	Ear	21	28	62	0	0	69

TABLE 2. Histological assessments of footpads and of Kveim tests in the ears of normal mice inoculated with fresh sarcoid or nonsarcoid homogenate or their derivatives into footpads.

Nature of fresh homogenate	No. mice	Histology*					
		Footpad			Ear Kveim		
		Pos.	Equiv.	Neg.	Pos.	Equiv.	Neg.
Sarcoid							
Whole	12	10	3	9	10	4	3
Autoclaved whole	12	0	0	20	0	0	20
Supernatant (400 g/5 min)	12	0	5	11	0	4	12
Supernatant filtered (0.2 μm)	12	0	1	14	0	0	15
Nonsarcoid							
Whole	12	0	0	12	0	0	12
Autoclaved whole	12	0	0	16	0	0	16
Supernatant (400 g/5 min)	12	0	0	15	0	0	15
Supernatant filtered (0.2 μm)	12	0	0	16	0	0	16

* After a mean interval of 15 months.

TABLE 3. Histological assessments of footpads and of Kveim tests in the ears of normal mice inoculated with fresh sarcoid or nonsaroid homogenate or their derivatives, intravenously.

Nature of fresh homogenate	No. mice	Histology†					
		Footpad			Ear Kveim		
		Pos.	Equiv.	Neg.	Pos.	Equiv.	Neg.
Sarcoid							
Whole*	53	2	17	43	5	9	48
Autoclaved*	12	0	0	18	0	0	18
Supernatant (400 g/5 min) ↓ Filtered (0.2 μm)	6	0	3	9	0	1	11
Nonsarcoid							
Whole*	23	0	0	36	0	0	21
Autoclaved*	6	0	0	6	0	0	6
Supernatant (400 g/5 min) ↓ Filtered (0.2 μm)	4	0	0	4	0	0	4

† After a mean interval of 15 months.
* Crudely filtered and diluted.

TABLE 4. Histological assessments of footpads and of Kveim tests in the ears of normal mice inoculated with fresh sarcoid or nonsarcoid homogenate, intraperitoneally.

Nature of fresh homogenate	No. mice	Histology*					
		Footpad			Ear Kveim		
		Pos.	Equiv.	Neg.	Pos.	Equiv.	Neg.
Sarcoid							
Whole	27	1	5	31	5	7	26
Autoclaved	5	0	0	9	0	0	9
Nonsarcoid							
Whole	11	0	0	11	0	0	10
Autoclaved	6	0	0	6	0	0	6

* After a mean interval of 15 months.

TABLE 5. Histological assessments of footpads and of Kveim tests in the ears of normal mice inoculated with fresh or irradiated sarcoid lymph node homogenate into footpads, or intravenously.

Months following inoculation	Site of inoculation	No. mice	Tissue examined	Nature of homogenate					
				Fresh			Irradiated (2.5 mega.r)		
				Pos.	Equiv.	Neg.	Pos.	Equiv.	Neg.
12	Footpad	6	Footpad	2	3	1	0	0	6
			Ear	0	4	2	0	0	6
12	I. V.	6	Footpad	0	2	4	0	0	6
			Ear	1	1	4	0	0	6

TABLE 6. Histological assessments of footpads and of Kveim tests in the ears of normal and immunologically deficient mice inoculated with a first passage of mouse 'sarcoid' or 'nonsarcoid' mouse footpad tissue homogenates into footpads or intravenously.

Mean interval following inoculation (months)	Site	'Sarcoid'			'Nonsarcoid'		
		Pos.	Equiv.	Neg.	Pos.	Equiv.	Neg.
15	Footpad	3	11	9	0	0	36
15	Ear	3	4	13	0	0	36

In separate experiments, mice have been inoculated with whole fresh or fresh auto-claved sarcoid or nonsarcoid homogenates or their derivatives into the hind footpads, intravenously or intraperitoneally. Tables 2, 3 and 4 show the interim results of these experiments, according to the route of inoculation and the nature of the homogenate injected. Table 5 shows interim results of experiments in which fresh whole or irradiated (2.5 mega. r) sarcoid homogenate was inoculated into footpads or intravenously. In all these experiments sarcoid granulomas were again associated with Kveim reactivity among mice receiving fresh sarcoid homogenates, irrespective of the route of inoculation. Conversely, granulomas were not present in the footpads of mice receiving nonsarcoid homogenates or their derivatives, or among mice receiving autoclaved or irradiated homogenates by any of these routes and Kveim tests in the ears of all these mice were negative.

TABLE 7. Histological assessments of footpads and of Kveim tests in the ears
of normal mice inoculated with a second passage of 'sarcoid'
mouse footpad tissue homogenate into footpads

Nature of fresh homogenate	No. mice	Histology*					
		Footpad			Ear Kveim		
		Pos.	Equiv.	Neg.	Pos.	Equiv.	Neg.
Whole	6	1	7	3	1	1	9
Supernatant (400 g/5 min)	6	1	3	9	1	5	7
Supernatant filtered (0.2 μm)	6	0	3	2	0	4	9
Autoclaved	6	0	0	6	0	0	6

* After a mean interval of 13 months.

The findings among mice receiving supernatant or filtered supernatant homogenates by each of these routes were equivocal or negative.

Table 6 shows interim results following the inoculation of a first passage of mouse 'sarcoid' or 'nonsarcoid' footpad homogenate into footpads or intravenously. Of 18 mice receiving 'sarcoid' homogenate 3 showed positive and 11 equivocal footpad histology after a mean interval of 15 months following inoculation. Kveim tests in the ear were positive in 3 and equivocal in 4 of these mice. Conversely, no granulomas were found in the footpads of the 18 mice receiving 'nonsarcoid' mouse footpad homogenate and Kveim tests in the ears of these mice were negative.

Table 7 shows interim results following a second passage of 'sarcoid' mouse footpad homogenate after a mean interval of 13 months following inoculation into footpads. Positive footpad histology was encountered among mice receiving whole fresh or fresh supernatant homogenate and was again associated with positive Kveim tests in the ear. Equivocal changes were seen in the footpads and in Kveim tests made in the ear among mice receiving filtered (0.2 μm) supernatant homogenate; conversely, the footpads of mice receiving autoclaved homogenate were negative and were all associated with negative Kveim tests in the ear.

SUMMARY AND CONCLUSIONS

This report summarises our findings following further controlled experiments in which mice were inoculated with fresh human sarcoid or nonsarcoid homogenates or with a first or second passage of mouse 'sarcoid' or 'nonsarcoid' homogenate or their derivatives into footpads, intraperitoneally or intravenously. Evidence is presented to confirm our earlier finding of a transmissible agent for mice from human sarcoid tissue. Moreover, we were able to show that the transmissible agent concerned is viable since it can be passed successfully and is inactivated when the human sarcoid or mouse footpad 'sarcoid' homogenate is autoclaved or irradiated. In addition to positive footpad histology (Fig. 1) and positive Kveim tests in the ear (Fig. 2) systemic lesions have been encountered in regional and hilar lymph nodes and in other organs, (e.g. liver, lung, spleen or tail) of mice receiving fresh human sarcoid or a first or second passage of mouse 'sarcoid' footpad homogenate (Figs 3, 4 and 5). We are at present unable to say whether or not the transmissible agent concerned can be passed through a membrane

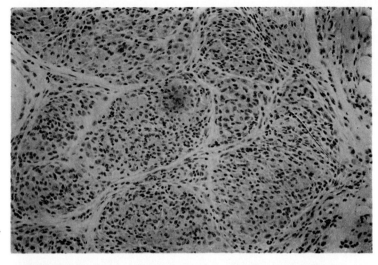

Fig. 1.

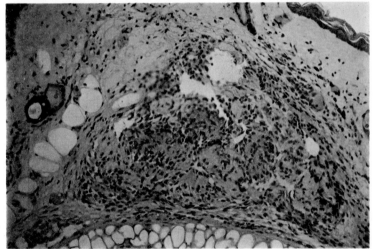

Fig. 2.

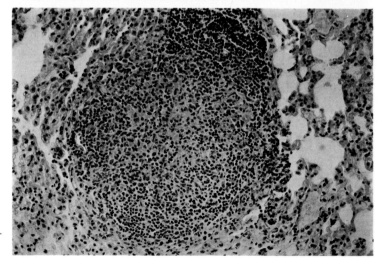

Fig. 3.

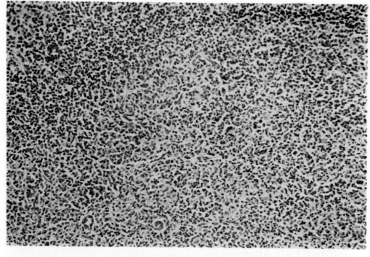

FIG. 4.

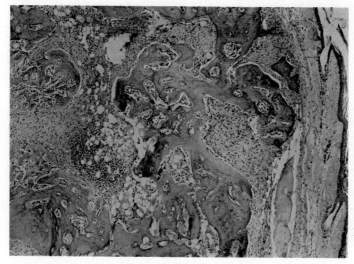

FIG. 5.

filter, (0.2 μm Sartorius) but we have as yet no firm evidence that it will do so. Further extensive and controlled studies using modern sophisticated culture techniques are required in an endeavour to isolate a specific infective agent from human sarcoid tissue.

ACKNOWLEDGEMENTS

We thank Dr J. R. Mikhail, Mr J. F. Newcombe, and Miss Mary Shephard for the lymphnodes. Dr T. H. Hurley Kindly Supplied the Kveim test material.

REFERENCES

1. Mitchell, D. N., and Rees, R. J. W. 1969. A transmissible agent from sarcoid tissue. *Lancet* **2**: 81.
2. Mitchell, D. N., and Rees, R. J. W. 1972. *Sixth Int. Conf. on Sarcoidosis* (Kyoto).
3. Carlens, E. 1959. Mediastinoscopy: a method for inspection and tissue biopsy in the superior mediastinum. *Diseases Chest* **36**: 343.

Induction of Granulomas in Mice by Injection of Human Sarcoid and Ileitis Homogenates

ROBERT N. TAUB AND LOUIS E. SILTZBACH

Mount Sinai School of Medicine, City University of New York, New York, U.S.A.

The etiology of sarcoidosis is unknown. Although at one time M. tuberculosis, atypical mycobacteria, viruses, and airborne allergens have been cited as causative, proof that sarcoid-like diseases can be transmitted by these or other agents has been lacking. Recently Mitchell and Rees[1,2] reported that lymphoid tissues from patients with active sarcoidosis or regional ileitis will induce granulomas after injection into mouse footpads. Accordingly, we attempted to determine if affected tissues of patients with either sarcoidosis or regional ileitis contain substances that are capable of inducing granulomas in mice. Granulomatous lymph nodes were obtained from patients with either of these disorders, and involved bowel from patients with exacerbated ileitis at the time of surgery. Normal lymph nodes were removed from control patients undergoing thoracic surgery. The excised tissues were homogenized for 3 to 15 minutes at 4°C and made into a 13.5% V/V saline suspension. 0.05 cc of the suspension was injected into each hind footpad of 6 to 8 CBA mice. Injections were made with a 26-gauge needle introduced along the dorsum and side of the foot. Two types of material were used: fresh material which was injected within 3 hours after removal from the patient and material frozen for several days or longer at −25°C before homogenization. Three-mm punch biopsies of the injected footpads were studied 1, 5, and 8 months after inoculation.

RESULTS

No abnormalities were seen in the footpads of 16 mice injected with lymph-node homogenates of 2 normal patients. (Table 1) Furthermore, no abnormalities were detected in the footpads of close to 100 mice injected with frozen sarcoid or normal homogenates.

TABLE 1.

Patient	DX	No. mice with granulomas	Days p. injection
VH	normal	0/8	230
MK	normal	0/8	150
GE	sarcoid	2/7	225
RS	sarcoid	2/7	35
CH	ileitis	2/6	225
AG	ileitis (node)	2/6	35
AG	ileitis (ileum)	1/4	35

This work was supported by the National Foundation for Ileitis and Colitis, Inc. and a research grant from the National Heart and Lung Institute, Public Health Service (HE–13853–14). R.N.T. is a Scholar of the Leukemia Society of America, Inc.

20

In contrast, after periods of 1 to 8 months, 4 of 14 sarcoid-injected and 5 of 16 ileitis-injected mice showed slowly evolving epithelioid granulomas not characteristic of foreign-body reactions. In several mice, the granulomas showed bony invasion.

The lymph nodes draining the injection site were hyperplastic in both sarcoid- and ileitis-injected groups as compared to the control groups. In addition there was hyperplasia of the nodes distant from the injection site. As determined by syngeneic transfer assay[3] neither experimental group showed any evidence of depletion of thymus-derived recirculating lymphocytes. There appeared to be no dissemination of granulomas to the spleen, liver or lung in the mice.

Six to 8 months after injection, all mice were tested with Kveim suspensions injected intradermally into the ear. Neither unreactive mice nor those showing granulomas in the footpad with sarcoid or ileitus tissue showed positive Kveim ear tests.

Our data partially confirm and extend those of Mitchell and Rees. They allow the speculation that the affected lymph nodes of sarcoidosis and regional ileitis may harbor transmissible agents that play a role in granuloma formation.

REFERENCES

1. Mitchell, D. N., and Rees, R. J. W. 1969. *Lancet* **ii**: 81.
2. Mitchell, D. N., and Rees, R. J. W. 1970. *Lancet* **ii**: 168.
3. Taub, R. N., Lance, E. M. 1972. *Transplantation* **11**: 36.

Familial Occurrence of Sarcoidosis

Lars-Gösta Wiman

Department of Lung Diseases, University Hospital, Umeå, Sweden

Planned family studies concerning sarcoidosis are not commonly reported in the literature, but some observations on separate families and sarcoidosis found in twins suggest that genetic factors play a definite part in the etiology.

In an extensive study made in the German Federal Republic in 1965, Jörgensen, on the examination of 2,471 patients with sarcoidosis, found the disease among near relatives of 3.7% of the series. He considered sarcoidosis to be a special form of tuberculosis and believed in a hereditary predisposition determined by a sort of "multifactorial system of inheritance".

During a 20-year period, 1951–1971, in the Västerbotten County of Northern Sweden 299 patients suffering from sarcoidosis were detected (Fig. 1). These patients showed an interesting pattern. An unusual sex ratio was found, 125 women and 174 men. At the time of diagnosis the mean age for women surprisingly exceeded 50 years of age—for men it was below 50. Histopathological diagnosis was achieved in two-thirds of all patients.

In this actual geographic district (Fig. 6), not far from the arctic circle, the familial occurrence of sarcoidosis was fairly high, and some families were concentrated in isolated areas. The patients presented clinical symptoms or were detected among contacts of tuberculous patients.

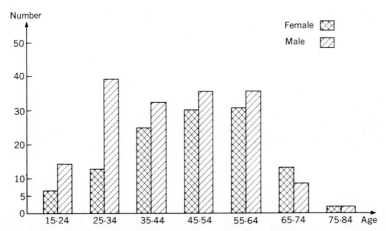

Fig. 1. Sarcoidosis, 1951–71, University Hospital, Umeå, Sweden: Distribution according to sex and age in 299 patients.

Family I (Fig. 2)

In this family with 10 children, 1 brother and 2 sisters suffered from sarcoidosis. One had a positive tuberculin test, and the remaining 2 a negative test. In all of them, chest X-rays showed hilar enlargement and parenchymatous lesions. The brother also de-

22

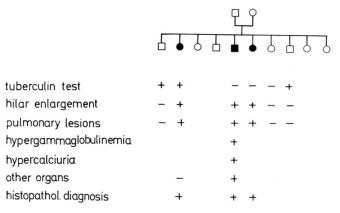

	tuberculin test	+ +	− − − +
	hilar enlargement	− +	+ + − −
	pulmonary lesions	− +	+ + − −
	hypergammaglobulinemia		+
	hypercalciuria		+
	other organs	−	+
	histopathol. diagnosis	+	+ +

FIG. 2.   Familial occurrence of sarcoidosis. Family I.

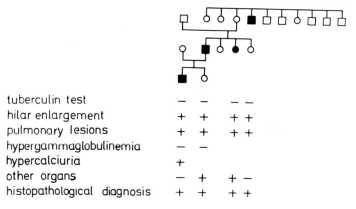

	tuberculin test	− −	− −
	hilar enlargement	+ +	+ +
	pulmonary lesions	+ +	+ +
	hypergammaglobulinemia	− −	
	hypercalciuria	+	
	other organs	− +	+ −
	histopathological diagnosis	+ +	+ +

FIG. 3.   Familial occurrence of sarcoidosis. Family II.

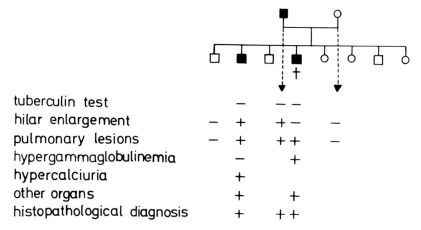

	tuberculin test	−	− −	
	hilar enlargement	− +	+ −	−
	pulmonary lesions	− +	+ +	−
	hypergammaglobulinemia	−	+	
	hypercalciuria	+		
	other organs	+	+	
	histopathological diagnosis	+	+ +	

FIG. 4.   Familial occurrence of sarcoidosis. Family III.

veloped skin lesions, hypercalciuria and hypergammaglobulinemia. Histopathological confirmation was found in all 3 patients. Two sisters died very young, and 1 brother was treated once for pleurisy, without tubercle bacilli, but with a tuberculin test that turned from negative to positive. One brother and 1 sister were not examined.

Family II (Fig. 3)

In this family, 2 out of 4 children suffered from sarcoidosis, as did 5 cousins, a brother to the mother and a boy in the next generation. The tuberculin test was negative throughout, and everybody displayed hilar adenopathy and pulmonary lesions, some of them hypergammaglobulinemia and hypercalciuria as well. Extrapulmonary manifestations were found in the skin, eyes and parotid gland. A histopathological diagnosis was obtained in åll these patients.

Family III (Fig. 4)

The father and his 2 sons had a histopathologically confirmed disease. Both sons had an advanced form of sarcoidosis. One of them presented sarcoid lesions on biopsy from the kidney, liver and muscle, and extensive pulmonary changes were apparent. In the other son, the disease ran a very bad course, terminating in a serious respiratory insufficiency with cor pulmonale and death at the age of 40. Six children remained in normal condition, and were not examined.

Although a cousin was found to have only slight pulmonary lesions and hilar enlargement, clinically he had a constant cough, asthenia, long periods of headache, renal colic and urinary calculi. His urinary excretion of calcium exceeded 600 mg in 24 hours on a normal diet. However, mediastinoscopy did not show lymphomas, and the diagnosis could not be histopathologically confirmed as sarcoidosis.

Family IV (Fig. 5)

In this family, the mother, 6 children and 6 cousins were suffering from sarcoidosis, confirmed by biopsy in all but 2. Hilar lymphomas, along with pulmonary lesions, were found on chest X-ray. Some patients developed a high urinary excretion of calcium, and a high serum level of gammaglobulin. Other organs were not affected, except in respect of 1 cousin, who presented a history of bilateral parotid enlargement in adult age. Though all the children were BCG-vaccinated at birth, the tuberculin test proved

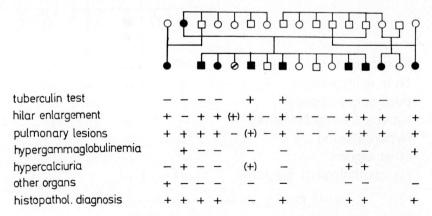

tuberculin test	−	−	−	−	+		+				−	−	−	−
hilar enlargement	+	−	+	+	(+)	+	−	+	−	−	−	+	+	+	+
pulmonary lesions	+	+	+	+	−	(+)	−	+	−	−	−	+	+	+	+
hypergammaglobulinemia	+	−	−		−		−				−	−		+
hypercalciuria	−	+	−	−	(+)		−				+	+	
other organs	+	−	−	−		−		−				−	−		−
histopathol. diagnosis	+	+	+	+		−		+				+	+		+

FIG. 5. Familial occurrence of sarcoidosis. Family IV.

negative, with the exception of 2 sons. A sister exhibiting suspected hilar lymphomas on mass radiography has not yet been fully investigated. The remaining 4 children, and the father, had normal chest X-rays and were found to be free of symptoms.

All these families—with the exception of the first—displayed a very close relationship. (Fig. 6). Two grandfathers and 1 grandmother were siblings, and thus originated from the same family. Moreover, 2 grandmothers were sisters. However, it was not possible to examine the grandparents, and all information concerning their health and disease is uncertain.

Also, the investigation is incomplete in the parental generation, since some are dead, and others are out of reach. There are many large families, and 3 brothers from 1 family married 3 sisters from another. Two patients with sarcoidosis were found at this level, both confirmed histopathologically.

Most of the people in the third generation are now between the ages of 30 and 50, and many of them have been carefully examined. Only in 2 cases is a histopathological diagnosis missing, but clinical and laboratory findings of sarcoidosis were conclusive. All stages of the disease were represented, from symptom-free hilar lymphomas to confluent parenchymatous lesions, with extensive destructions of both lungs, many other organs being simultaneously affected. Spontaneous regression was sometimes observed, but most of the patients required treatment with corticosteroids, usually with good results. In some patients, however, it was impossible to stop a progressive pulmonary fibrosis.

With the exception of some families on the left and right wings of the family tree, all people originated from a couple of nearby villages. For many years the outer communications of this area have been very poor, and the isolated geographic location has—no doubt—contributed to better inner communications.

The population of this area consists of 3 main ethnic groups: Lapps, Finns and people originating from the South of Sweden. This results in a marked genetic hetero-

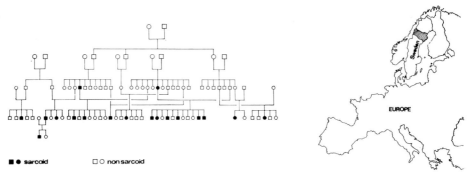

■ ● sarcoid   □ ○ non sarcoid

Sweden

Area: 411,405 square km

Population: 8,013,696 inhabitants

Capital: Stockholm

Sarcoidosis rates (Prevalence): 64 Cases per 100,000 mass chest radiographies (in Northern Sweden 100–150/100,000)

Tuberculosis rate (Prevalence): 310 Cases per 100,000 inhabitants (in Northern Sweden 487/100,000)

FIG. 6. Familial occurrence of sarcoidosis.

geneity showing considerable variations in gene frequencies, as is found in blood groups, serum proteins and in red blood cell enzymes.

Where variations in gene frequencies cannot be explained by ethnic heterogeneity only, they might also be ascribed to *genetic drift* or genetic random variation. When a small area is colonized by a small group of people, a rare genetic trait may be present, e.g. as a somatic malformation or a mental defect. If there is a normal reproduction concerning the carrier of this rare genetic trait, and the original population remains isolated and grows continually, the rare trait or defect may later be present in a high frequency. This is also called the *founder effect*.

The high rate of some other diseases in this part of Sweden has been explained in this way. Therefore, genetic drift may be of importance also in the familial occurrence of sarcoidosis, at least in combination with ethnic heterogeneity and geographic isolation.

REFERENCES

1. Jörgensen, G. 1965. Untersuchungen zur Genetik der Sarkoidose. Heidelberg: Hüthig Verlag.
2. Beckman, L. 1959. A contribution to the physical anthropology and population genetics of Sweden. *Hereditas* **45**: 1–189.
3. Beckman, L., Cedergren, B., Collinder, E., and Rasmusson, M. 1972. Population studies in Northern Sweden III. Variations of ABO and Rh blood group gene frequencies in time and space. *Hereditas* **72**: (in press).

Familial Occurrence of Sarcoidosis

HIDEO KAWABE, HIROSHI TADA AND HIROSHI NAGANO

St. Luke's International Hospital, Tokyo, Japan

At present the cause of sarcoidosis is still unknown, and the question of familial occurrence arises. Does it occur because the family has been exposed to the same pathogenic substance[1] (whether it is infective or noninfective) or is it in relation to the problem of familial disposition[2]?

In 1961 we experienced a case of a mother with sarcoidosis which was clinically cured. But in 1966 she developed pyelonephritis and died. Five years later, in 1971, sarcoidosis was diagnosed in the patient's eldest daughter who is at present under treatment. We would like to make a report relating to previous work on the cause of sarcoidosis.

Case 1. 35-year-old mother (housewife)

In 1957, the patient was operated upon for uterine cancer and hysterectomy and ovarectomy were carried out. After the operation, the patient had an injection of "Ovahormon Depo" in both arms alternately, at 2-monthly intervals over a period of 4 years. In August 1961, painless swellings were found on the lateral sides of both upper arms where the injections had been made. Upon her admittance in November 1961, the patient's development and nutrition were average. There was no swelling of the superficial lymph nodes and no signs of uveitis. Chest X-rays revealed a mild enlargement of the hilum lymph nodes, but no abnormalities in the lung. Mild hyperemia of the bronchial mucous membrane was observed by bronchoscopy. On biopsy, an induration of the upper arm was found in subcutaneous tissue and was histologically compatible with sarcoidosis. Tuberculin skin test was negative and the Kveim reaction was positive. Treatment was not given but the induration healed gradually when injections were stopped. The patient was under close observation, but in May 1963, about a little over a year later, she developed fever, a swelling of the parotid gland on the right side and again an induration of both upper arms. Also eruptions appeared on the skin of both patellar regions of the knee joints and a small nodule 1 mm in diameter developed in the lower right palpebral conjunctiva. A biopsy of these specimens histologically revealed sarcoidosis. Predonisolon treatment was given and the patient improved.

In January, 1966, the patient developed pyelonephritis and died in February, 1966 in another hospital, where no autopsy was performed. The point of interest in this case is that sarcoid changes seem to have developed strongly at the "Ovahormon" injection site.

Case 2. 17-year-old student, daughter of the above patient

On May 1, 1971, the girl suddenly developed right facial palsy and was cured in 2 weeks without treatment. Swelling of both parotid glands appeared on May 26, especially in the right side and she complained of lack of taste. Again facial palsy developed on both sides. On biopsy of the right parotid gland, sarcoidosis was histologically confirmed. A swelling of the supraclavicular lymph node and the right inguinal lymph node appeared. White spots appeared in both iries with a turbid vitreous body. The papilla of the eye fundus were hyperemic and turbid. Chest X-rays revealed a mild bilateral hilar lymph gland swelling and fine nodular and fibrotic lesions in the lower part of both lung fields. A right paratracheal lymph-node swelling was also noticed. By bronchoscopy, hyperemia of the bronchial mucous membrane was seen and also fine granular changes were found in the left upper bronchi. A biopsy specimen was taken from this region but was not histologically confirmed as sarcoidosis. There was no anemia and the white blood count was normal. The spinal fluid was normal. Tuberculin skin test was negative, and the Kveim reaction positive. Blood chemistry was within normal limits.

After the result of the Kveim reaction, Predonisolon treatment was started and is still being continued. Symptoms have almost disappeared except for the eye findings, and the patient seems to be much improved.

In this familial occurrence, the daughter developed sarcoidosis 9 years and 9 months after the onset of sarcoidosis in the mother, and 5 years and 3 months after the mother's death. The mother and daughter lived together for 12 years until the mother's death.

DISCUSSION

According to some of the lung biopsy findings, sarcoid granuloma were found in asymptomatic patients who by X-ray had bilateral hilar lymphadenopathy with no lung parenchymal mottling[3]. This fact suggests the possibility that the inhalation of pathogenic substances may be a cause of sarcoidosis.

By observing familial occurrences we may find clues by which we may determine whether sarcoidosis occurs as a familial disposition or through environmental factors. More than 60 cases of familial occurrences of sarcoidosis have been reported abroad, and 10 cases in Japan. It seems there are more familial occurrences in this disease than in other diseases. Sarcoidosis could be cured naturally without treatment, so there may be many cases not diagnosed. Many cases of sarcoidosis are found in mass chest X-ray examinations. If a case of sarcoidosis is found, the family should be X-rayed. By this means more familial occurrence cases may be diagnosed. In other countries, there have been reports of 6 familial occurrences involving a parent and child, 9 sets of twins, 9 sisters, 8 brothers and 7 brother-sister pairs. In Japan there have been 2 parent-and-child, 4 involving sisters, 1 instance of brothers and 4 brother-and-sister pairs. The period of time during which the occurrences were reported in the respective families was: 1 instance simultaneous; 3 instances within 1 year; 2 within 2 years; 1 case within 5 years and 2 within 9 years. In 1 case of a brother and a sister having lived separately over the last 7 years, the period of occurrence was 6 years.[4] In Japan, the period of occurrence among members of a femily seems to be longer, while in other countries familial occurrence seems to be more common in twins, which leads us to consider the existence of hereditary disposition.

The inhalation of pathogenic substance and hereditary disposition, may both conceivably constitute a cause of sarcoidosis.

REFERENCES

1. Iwai, K. 1964. *Am. Rev. Resp. Dis.* **90**: 612.
2. Iwai, K. 1972. *Saishin Igaku* **27**: 1265.

3. Mikami, R. 1969. *Saishin Igaku* **19**: 104.
4. Gomi, J. 1968. *Nihon Iji Shinpoh* No. 2301: 14.

Familial Sarcoidosis in Japan

Yoshio Ito, Isamu Ogima and Yasutami Kinoshita

*The Second Department of Internal Medicine, Niigata University
School of Medicine, Niigata, Japan*

Although about 100 years have elapsed since sarcoidosis was discovered, its etiology is still unknown. Among the many ways by which we may pursue its origin, data for the study of familial occurrence are easily available and important. Investigators have reported 3 types of familial sarcoidosis: in parent and offspring, in siblings, and in married couples. In the present study, the authors have analysed 16 instances of familial sarcoidosis reported in Japan.

RESULTS

Sex and Age

As shown in Table 1, 12 cases were male and 21 cases, female. Nine cases ranged in age from 10 to 19 and 15 cases, from 20 to 29.

TABLE 1. Sex and age

Sex	No. of cases	Age	No. of cases
Male	12	0~9	1
Female	21	10~19	9
		20~29	15
Sex (33 cases)		30~39	2
		40~49	2

Age { 14 families, 29 cases

Tuberculin Test

Positive	7 cases
Equivocal	2 cases
Negative	16 cases
Unknown	4 cases

Negative cases outnumbered the others.

Number of siblings

The number of family members varied from 2 to 10. In 4 cases there were 6 siblings.

Combination of siblings

2 sisters	5 pairs
2 brothers	2 pairs
A brother and a sister	7 pairs

A combination of 2 brothers was relatively rare. The examples of sarcoidosis in parent and offspring have been reported. One example is a combination of a mother, her son and her daughter; another, now, reported by Dr Kawabe, is of a mother and her daughter.

Symptoms

In 16 groups patients reported some complaints. In 13 groups patients reported no complaints at all. In 2 groups a half of the patients reported some complaints.

Diagnostic criteria

The diagnostic criteria according to the International Sarcoidosis Committee are as follows:

Group I	4 cases
Group II	3 cases
Group III	13 cases
Group IV	13 cases

The number of patients in Groups III and IV was greater than the others, but recently the number of patients in Groups I and II has been increasing.

The interval between discovery of the disease in 2 members of a familial group is given in Table 2.

TABLE 2.   Interval of discovery (17 pairs).

Interval (yr)	No. of cases
Simultaneous	3
< 1 yr	0
1 ~ 2 yr	4
2 ~ 3	3
3 ~ 4	1
4 ~ 5	2
5 >	4

In 3 groups, simultaneous development of the disease was observed. In 1 of these 3 groups both patients were found to be suffering from uveitis.

DISCUSSION

Tables 3 and 4 show all cases of familial sarcoidosis reported up to the present time. There were 16 examples of these cases, 13 of which were sarcoidosis in siblings. Two examples were those of parent and offspring. One example was that of a husband and wife. In these instances, data distributions for sex, age, tuberculin test, and symptoms revealed nothing remarkable.

The fact that 3 hospitals had reported 2 or more familial sarcoidosis cases suggested that these hospitals had been actively engaged in the diagnosis of this disease, and that widespread incidence is higher than previously believed.

Cases with an earlier onset were inclined to be more severe than those with a later onset. At the present time, sarcoidosis in the same family is not uncommon, but there were only 8 examples of the parent-and-offspring type previously reported in the liter-

TABLE 3. Familial sarcoidosis cases.

	Sex	Age	Relation	Tuberculin reaction	Biopsy	BHL	Ocular Sympt.	Subj complaint	Interval of discovery	Reason for exam.	Kveim reaction	Year of report
Yamada	♂○	41		−	+	+	+	+	8yr	eye pain blurred vision, fever	−	1962
	♂	24		−	−		+	+			−	
Sugiyama	♀○	12		−	+	○ +○	−	−	4yr	mass exam		1968
	♀	14		−	+		−	−				
	♀○	13		+	+	+	+	−	9yr	mass exam.		1968
	♂	13		+	−		−					
Hirasawa	♂○	22		−	−	+	+	+	1yr 8m	eye involv. mass exam.		1968
	♀	20		+	+		−	−				
Arai	♂	19		?	?	+	?	?	simultaneous	?		1968
	♀	10										
	♀	14		?	?	+	?	?	2yr 6m	?		1968
	♀	8										
Gomi	♂○	24	† Apo.	±	±	+○	−	−	1yr 5m	mass exam. back ache Iritis	not done	1968
	♀	23		−	−	+●	+	+			+	
Yamamoto	♀○	33	† Ca.	−	−	+	−	+	1yr 3m	abdominal pain dyspnea mass exam.	+	1970
	♀	20		−	−		−	−			−	
Ito	♂	29		−	−	○ +○	+	+	simultaneous	eye involv.	+	1971
	♀	26		−	+		+	+			−	

○ early onset ● Pulm. infiltration +
○ " −

TABLE 4. Familial sarcoidosis cases.

	Sex	Age	Relation	Tuberculin reaction	Biopsy	BHL	Ocular Sympt.	Subj complaint	Interval of discovery	Reason for exam.	Kveim reaction	Year of report
Niitsu	♀	27		−	−	○ +○	−	−	3yr 8m	mass exam.	−	1970
	♀○	15		+	+		−	−			not done	
Tachibana	♀○	31		−	+	+● ●	+	+	2yr 3m	general malaise mass exam.	not done	1970
	♀	25		+	+		−	−			−	
Tsuchiya Matsushima	♂	23		−	+	+● ●	+	+	1yr 10m	mass exam.	+	1972
	♂○	13		±	+		+				−	
Hiraga	♂○	20		+	+	+● +○	+	+	4yr	eye involv.	−	1972
	♀	20		+	+		+	+			+	
Kinoshita	Mother	45	†♂	−	+		−	+	2yr Simul- taneous	palpitation mass exam. eye involv.	not done	1966
	♂	23		−	−	+○	−	−				
	♀	21				○	+	+				
Kawabe	Mother○	35		−	+	+●	+	+	9yr 9m	arm swelling facial palsy	+	1972
	♀	17		−	+	+●	+	+			+	
Ito	Wife○	49	†♂	+	+	○ +○	−	−	8yr	mass exam.	not done	1972
	Husband○	53		±	−		+	+			−	

○ early onset ↓ ● Pulm. infiltration + ●
○ " −

ature. It is interesting to note that a combination of father and offspring has never been reported. The present authors have noted a case of sarcoidosis in a husband and wife without consanguinity (Table 5). This case is very instructive in the study of the etiology of sarcoidosis. Upon diagnosis of the disease, only 3 pairs showed simultaneous development, while others were diagnosed independently. In 1 of these 3 pairs, the initial symptoms of the partners were also similar. Even though the onset or discovery of the disease is not always simultaneous, sarcoidosis does have a tendency to develop at about the same age. In Japan the number of cases of sarcoidosis reported is about

TABLE 5. Comparison of cases (married couple).

	Husband	Wife
Age on discovery	53 (1961, Oct.)	49 (1969, Sept.)
Reason for exam.	mrss exam.	mass exam.
Interval of discovery	8 yr	
Subj. compl.	eye involv.	(−)
Tuberculin reaction {before	(−) → (+)	(卌) N
{after	6×7 mm	20×20 mm
Chest X-ray	BHL	BHL
Kveim reaction	not done	(−)
Biopsy	(−)	(+)
Clinical course	BHL disappear	BHL persistent
Therapy	steroid.	steroid.

TABLE 6. Expected number of familial sarcoidosis cases in Japan. According to binomial distribution:

Family number	Number of households	Expected value
5	2×10^7	0.5
10	10^7	1.125
15	6.7×10^6	1.759

Japanese population: 10^8, Number of patients: 5000, Prevalence rate: 5×10^{-5}.

2,700, but there are probably 10 to 20 times this number undiagnosed. If this is so, the incidence of familial sarcoidosis appears to be significantly greater than the incidence of sarcoidosis in the general population (Table 6). Therefore, when sarcoidosis is discovered, it is important to investigate carefully both the family and the background of the patient. Although familial occurrence of sarcoidosis has been discussed from the constitutional point of view,[1] it should also be considered from the viewpoint of infection regarding personal contact, because of the presence of the disease in a married couple (Table 5) and in the population in a limited area.[2]

It may be by mere chance that sarcoidosis occurs in a family, but statistically its occurrence definately much higher than expected (Fig. 6).

REFERENCES

1. Merchant, R. K., and John, P. 1960. Familial sarcoidosis. *Arch. Intern. Med.* **106**: 116–122.
2. *Ito, Y., Ogima, I., and Kinoshita, Y. 1973. Diseased population with sarcoidosis in a limited area. *Jap. J. Thorac. Dis.* **11**: 103.

* Written in Japanese.

DISCUSSION

Chairmen: M. HORSMANHEIMO AND N. SHIGEMATSU

DR ISRAEL: I believe the demonstration by Hanngren and his associates of the anergy caused by infectious mononucleosis is very important and is consistent with the possibility that a slow virus is an etiologic factor in sarcoidosis. I should like to raise objections to their hypothesis that mycobacteria are involved. Hannuksuela, both in his monograph and in the slide presented today, showed that a majority of patients in Finland who have sarcoidosis have positive tuberculin reactions. Thus it is not essential to have anergy to get sarcoidosis.

Secondly, if mycobacteria were an important factor in the development of sarcoidosis, there should not be much sarcoidosis in the United States, where natural infection with tuberculosis and BCG vaccination are both infrequent; yet we see no sign of a decline in the incidence of sarcoidosis.

DR HANNGREN: I said that mycobacteria are one example that may give a B cell stimulation, and I stressed that sarcoidosis was an immunological reaction which is characterised by T cell depression and B cell stimulation. Whatever agents that can depress T cell function, on the one hand, and stimulate B cell function, on the other, will create the sarcoidosis reaction. The mycobacterium is one of those to be found in Sweden. BCG. vaccination is a common event in Sweden, and because this may stimulate B cells, maybe this is the reason why we in Sweden have such a high prevalence of sarcoidosis.

Concerning the condition in the United States, I may be wrong in this, but isn't tuberculosis in the New York area at least connected with sarcoidosis epidemiologically among negroes but not among whites? And doesn't sarcoidosis have a higher incidence among negroes in the New York area, too?

DR JONES WILLIAMS: I would like to ask Professor Hanngren a few more questions. I think his work suggests that we must look for other factors which depress the T cells, as we have already heard mentioned tuberculosis may do. If his hypothesis is correct, then perhaps we ought to look for and find virus infections much more commonly in sarcoid than has previously been reported.

One thing I would like to question is another topic, his statement that macrophages become epithelioid cells. I'm not at all sure that this is proven, and some of the work my group is doing suggests it may not be so. About his comments on glandular fever, infectious mononucleosis, I think this is most interesting, and histologically I have looked at a series of about 50 cases. They are very difficult to obtain but quite often you find small collections of 3 or 4 epithelioid cells. However, I have not seen really good sarcoid granulomas. If there is a relationship, perhaps one might expect to find this more often. In how many glandular fever cases have you done Kveim tests? Have you found many positive Kveim tests in glandular fever?

Another point possibly in criticism of your theory is that in Drs Mitchell and Rees' work, and also now reported by Dr Taub and Dr Siltzbach, no difference in incidence in immunologically deficient mice was found, and those are mice that have had T cell depression. Perhaps you would say, maybe it needs T cell depression plus B cell stimulation.

DR. HANNGREN: Yes, I think that B cell stimulation for example by the tuberculin is an important thing, as you pointed out. Dr Mitchell, in his experiments on immunodeficient mice as far as I can remember, did not succed in transferring sarcoidosis lesions with the Kveim material. I hope Dr Mitchell can answer this. The main point is, however,

34

that tuberculo-protein may act as a B-cell stimulator during the T-cell depressing period.

DR MITCHELL: The immunologically deficient mice used in our earlier work were prepared by adolescent thymectomy followed by whole-body irradiation (900 r), but these mice received partial syngeneic stem-cell replacement from normal CBA mice of single-line stock. We didn't get a better yield of either local or multisystem lesions among them and since their life span is considerably shorter, it is all rather more difficult. That is why we have preferred to use normal mice in our more recent work.

We are currently reappraising the use of immunologically deficient mice prepared by adolescent thymectomy followed by whole-body irradiation (600 r) but without subsequent syngeneic stem-cell replacement. We have some early results which I shall comment on later. That's one point. Another point is that we have been very surprised how late Kveim reactivity amongst both normal and immunologically deficient (T/900 r) mice, can develop in animals showing evidence of epithelioid cell granulomas in the foot pad following the inoculation of sarcoid tissue homogenates. From the point of view of the Kveim test in man, an important practical point that has emerged this morning is the fact that neither we nor Dr Siltzbach have observed the development of granulomas in the mouse foot pad following the inoculation of homogenates prepared from deep-frozen as distinct from fresh sarcoid tissue.

DR OSHIMA: We tried to produce sarcoidosis experimentally with nocardia-like organisms isolated from sarcoidosis patients by Dr Uesaka. We used Hartley strain female guinea pigs. We injected 1 mg of living cells with Freund's complete adjuvant into the foot pad. At the same time 1 mg of cells was injected intravenously into the same animal. Three weeks later a remarkable granulomatous change was seen in both lungs of

about 40% of the experimental animals. There were macrophages and epithelioid cells but there was no caseous reaction. On the other hand in 2 control groups, 1 with an intravenous injection only, and the other with a foot pad injection only, we did not see such remarkable granulomatous changes in the lungs.

DR. NOGUCHI: I would like to ask Dr Hanngren about 2 things. Firstly, Dr Hanngren, you evaluated the T cell system only by using lymphocyte transformation. Are you employing any other test such as the macrophage migration inhibition test (MIF)? Secondly, what is your opinion about the role of neutrophils in the pathogenesis of sarcoidosis?

We have had 2 cases with attenuated response to the nitroblue tetrazolium (NBT) reduction test for neutrophils which may imply participation of a nonspecific immunologic defect.

DR JAMES: I think I can help here. The nitroblue tetrazolium test is normal in sarcoidosis. We have used it. The test indicates a defect within the neutrophil as a response to a bacterial infection. When there is a bacterial infection, the first thing that happens is a tremendous eruption within the neutrophil of oxygen, and that gives you the test. If there is a defect, you don't produce the oxygen, then you get a positive one. The only time you get a positive nitroblue tetrazolium test is in chronic granulomatous disease of childhood. In fact it is pretty well diagnostic of that disease. You (Dr Noguchi) say you had it in 2 cases of sarcoidosis. I wonder if these patients were children, were they? Yes, because this is a most fascinating condition in which you get children, predominantly boys aged 5 or so, presenting with eczema, sinuses, miliary mottling of the lungs, and wherever you biopsy, the skin, or the lung, or the liver, you will find sarcoid granuloma. Many years ago I used to see these patients and do Kveim tests, and they were always negative.

II KVEIM REACTION

The in Vitro Kveim Reaction in Sarcoidosis and Other Diseases
—An evaluation of the specificity of the test—

J. R. KALDEN, F. W. BECKER, P. KRULL AND H. DEICHER

Medizinische Hochschule Hannover, Hannover, Federal Republic of Germany

The Kveim skin test, regarded as highly specific for sarcoidosis, has lately been shown—although not unequivocally[1, 2]—also to be positive in Crohn's disease[3], glandular tuberculosis[4] and different lymphadenopathies[9]. Likewise an in vitro Kveim reaction utilizing the leucocyte migration technique[5] has also been shown not to give exclusively positive results in sarcoidosis. Using a Kveim spleen preparation migration inhibition could be observed in Crohn's disease[3], in glandular tuberculosis, in Hodgkin's and collagen diseases[6].

The present paper deals with an evaluation of the in vitro Kveim reaction using the leucocyte migration technique and a type I Kveim spleen preparation as antigen. An identical spleen preparation from a healthy person who died in a road accident served as control tissue. Both preparations were phenol-free.

The migration technique was as follows[5]. In brief: peripheral blood leucocytes were isolated and packed into capillary tubes with a diameter of 1.2–1.3 mm. The tubes were placed into culture chambers containing Eagle's minimum essential medium and the different test antigens. Physiological saline, 70 μg of Kveim antigen or 70 μg of a normal spleen preparation were added to the medium. After 24-hr incubation the migration of the cells into the medium was measured by planimetry, and the % migration was calculated using the formula:

$$\frac{\text{Area of migration in presence of antigen}}{\text{Area of migration in absence of antigen}} \times 100$$

Leucocyte migration tests were performed in 36 sarcoidosis and in 22 Hodgkin patients of different clinical stages; in 17 patients with solid tumors (including bronchial and uterine carcinoma, melanoma and two cases of kidney tumors), in 10 patients with Crohn's disease and 10 patients suffering from ulcerative colitis, in 12 patients with rheumatoid arthritis, 10 with SLE, and in 10 patients with nontumorous lymphatic diseases including infectious mononucleosis, unspecific lymphadenitis and 2 patients with an acute erythema nodosum of unknown etiology.

RESULTS

Based on the percentage migration obtained with normal spleen in normal controls a migration inhibition of more than 21% seemed to be unlikely (p<0.01). Therefore 19 of the 36 sarcoidosis patients had a significant migration inhibition as compared with 1 normal control, 1 patient with infectious mononucleosis, 1 of Crohn's disease and 1 of the ulcerative colitis group, 3 patients suffering from rheumatoid arthritis, 1 patient

TABLE 1. The incidence of positive migration inhibition in sarcoidosis and different clinical disorders. Note that only in sarcoidosis patients a significant test result was obtained.

Disease	Histology	Incidence of L.M.T.	Significance χ^2
20 Normal controls	—	1/20	—
22 Hodgkin's disease	—	6/22	NS*
17 Solid tumors	—	1/17	NS
21 Gut diseases	—	2/21	NS
25 Collagen disease	—	4/25	NS
10 Non-tumorous Lymphatic diseases	—	1/10	NS
36 Sarcoidosis	26/26	19/36	p<0,01

* NS=not significant

with Horton's disease, 5 Hodgkin patients and 1 patient with melanoma (Table I).

The frequency of migration inhibition with Kveim antigen in sarcoidosis was significantly higher (p<0.01) than that in the controls (clinical and normal)—(Table I).

When the incidence of positive migration inhibition was correlated with the clinical stages no clear correlation was found either in sarcoidosis or in Hodgkin's disease. This may be partly due to the small number of patients tested with clinical stages II and III and IV in the case of Hodgkin's disease.

A fair correlation, however, was observed between in vivo and in vitro Kveim reactions.

SUMMARY

A significant incidence of positive migration inhibition was found in sarcoidosis patients as compared with different normal and clinical controls. This result is in agreement with previous findings[6-8] but is in contrast to a recent report by Topilsky et al.[9].

With the exception of Hodgkin's disease (5 out of 22) and rheumatoid arthritis (3 out of 12) only in single cases of the different clinical control groups positive migration inhibition was observed with Kveim spleen as antigen. These findings, however suggest that the LMT is as specific, but not more sensitive or specific, as the in vivo Kveim test, when the same antigen preparation is used in both test systems.

REFERENCES

1. Williams, W. J. 1965. *Gut* **6**: 503.
2. Siltzbach, L. E., Vicira, L. O. B. D., Topilsky, M., and Janowitz, H. D. 1971. *Lancet* **2**: 634.
3. Mitchell, D. N., Cannon, P., Dyer, N. H., Hinson, K. F. W., and Willoughby, J. M. T. 1969. *Lancet* **2**: 571, 1970. *Lancet* **2**: 496.

4. Israel, H. L., and Goldstein, R. A. 1971. *New Engl. J. Med.* **284**: 345
5. Sberg, M., and Bendixen, G. 1967. *Acta Med. Scand.* **181**: 247.
6. Becker, F. W., Krull, P., Deicher, H., and Kalden, J. R. 1972. *Lancet* **1**: 120.
7. Hardt, F., and Wanstrup, J. 1969. *Acta Path. Microbiol. Scand.* **76**: 493.
8. Williams, W. J. 1971. *Proc. Europ. Symp.* on Sarcoidosis, Genf.
9. Topilsky, M., Siltzbach, L. E., Williams, M., and Glade, P. R. 1972. *Lancet* **1**: 117.

Reactivity of Lymphocytes from Sarcoidosis Patients to Kveim Antigen in vitro

ROBERT A. GOLDSTEIN, BERNARD W. JANICKI AND KAREN E. SCHULTZ

VA George Washington University Medical Center, Washington, D.C., U.S.A.

INTRODUCTION

Although the diagnostic specificity of the Kveim reaction has recently been questioned[1] few doubt that elucidation of the basic mechanism involved would be of immunological and possibly etiological significance in sarcoidosis. Early attempts at defining the active principle in Kveim suspension were impeded by the necessity for an in vivo biological test of activity. More recently however a variety of in vitro immunologic methods have been utilized in an attempt to develop a diagnostic test for sarcoidosis. In an attempt to clarify the immunology of the Kveim reaction, we used a modification of the in vitro David assay for migration inhibition factor (MIF)[2].

MATERIALS AND METHODS

Column-purified peripheral blood lymphocytes from sarcoidosis patients were incubated in tissue culture medium which contained 200 μg/ml of Commonwealth Serum Laboratories Kveim antigen. The cell-free supernatant fluids were collected daily for 4 days after which they were pooled, dialyzed, concentrated by freeze-drying, and assayed for migration inhibition factor (MIF) using oil-induced peritoneal exudate cells from normal guinea pigs. Significant MIF production in this assay is defined as $<80\%$ migration of peritoneal exudate cells in test supernates as compared with controls.

RESULTS

Seven patients with sarcoidosis were tested. In vitro Kveim tests were positive in 5 with hilar lymph node involvement and negative in 2 with pulmonary parenchymal damage only. MIF production was consistently found in the former 5 but not in the latter 2 persons. One subject with repeatedly positive in vitro Kveim tests was used to determine whether centrifugation might separate biological activity of the Kveim suspension. When the particulate fraction alone was suspended in tissue culture media, consistent MIF production was demonstrated. When the supernatant from the Kveim suspension was used, no MIF production was found.

DISCUSSION

A major obstacle to the widespread study of Kveim reactions in sarcoidosis patients has been the chronic shortage of validated test suspensions. The necessity to conduct large clinical studies, to say nothing of the 4–6 week delay and need for expert histopathologic interpretation, has prompted several investigators to utilize in vitro immunological assay systems to test for Kveim reactivity. At the Fifth International Sarcoidosis Conference, Hardt and Wanstrup[3] reported an in vitro Kveim test using a leucocyte migration assay. Subsequently several investigators have reported successful applications of a variety of in vitro immunological methods. Unfortunately, variation in methodology combined with differences in Kveim test suspensions has precluded development of a single satisfactory assay system.

Nevertheless, our results, as well as others[4], suggest that there may indeed be a valid in vitro immunologic correlate of the Kveim reaction and that lymphocyte-mediated production of MIF may be involved. Our findings that the active principle resides in the particulate and not in the soluble portion of Kveim antigen suspension is consistent with results of previous in vivo experiments by others[5].

In conclusion, we have found significant MIF production in 5 patients with sarcoidosis and hilar adenopathy when their purified lymphocytes were exposed to Kveim antigen in vitro. Our preliminary results, as well as others, suggest that such an in vitro assay for Kveim reactivity might serve as a reasonable alternative for in vivo testing and may be useful for comparison and standardization of Kveim antigen preparations.

REFERENCES

1. Israel, H. L., and Goldstein, R. A. 1971. Relationship of Kveim antigen to lymphadenopathy: study of sarcoidosis and other diseases. *New Eng. J. Med.* **284**: 345.
2. Rocklin, R. E., Rosen, F. S., and David, J. R. 1970. Macrophage migration inhibition test. *New Eng. J. Med.* **283**: 493.
3. Hardt, F., and Wanstrup, J. 1971. Leucocyte migration test (LMT) used as an "In-Vitro Kveim Test", *Proc. Fifth Int. Sarcoidosis Conf.* Prague: Univ. Karlova, p. 459.
4. Becker, F. W., Krull, P., Deicher, H., and Kalden, J. R. 1972. Leucocyte migration test in sarcoidosis. *Lancet* **1**: 120.
5. Cohn, Z. A., Fedorko, M. E., Hirsch, J. G. Morse, S. I., and Siltzbach, L. E. 1967. The distribution of Kveim activity in subcellular fractions from Sarcoid lymph nodes. *La Sarcoidose* Rapp. IVe Conf. Int. Paris: Masson et cie. p. 14.

In Vitro Kveim-Induced Macrophage Inhibition Factor, KMIF Test, in Sarcoidosis, Crohn's Disease and Tuberculosis

W. Jones Williams, E. Pioli, D. J. Jones,
B. Calcraft, A. J. Johnson and H. Dighero

*Welsh National School of Medicine, Cardiff, Great Britain and Colindale
Public Health Laboratory, London, Great Britain*

INTRODUCTION

The continuing interest in the cutaneous Siltzbach-Kveim test for the diagnosis of sarcoidosis has stimulated the search for alternative rapid in vitro methods. These are based on the work of Bendixen and Soborg[1], who showed that sensitized lymphocytes as a result of antigen stimulation produce a soluble leucocyte migration inhibition factor (MIF) which correlates with the results of in vivo skin tests of delayed hypersensitivity.

Earlier workers, using the leucocyte migration test (LMT) with Kveim antigen from various sources, have demonstrated reactivity in sarcoidosis, tuberculosis, Crohn's, Hodgkin's and collagen disease and dermatitis herpetiformis[2-8].

We wish to present the results of in vitro Kveim testing using Colindale, type I, K12, batch 14 antigen, in sarcoidosis, tuberculosis and Crohn's disease. We have used guinea pig macrophages as the indicator system and refer to the test as the Kmif test (Kveim-induced macrophage, migration, inhibitor factor). Our results are correlated with the cutaneous Kveim test and the clinicopathological features of the disease.

MATERIAL AND METHODS

Antigens

Both the sarcoid spleen, Kveim antigen and normal control spleen suspensions were prepared by the method of Chase[9]. The sarcoid spleen suspension used was Colindale K12 type I, batch 14, unphenolised, for the in vitro and phenolised batches 15–19 for the skin tests.

Patients

Sarcoidosis: 30 patients with clinical and radiological features of sarcoidosis were investigated. All subjects were Kveim skin-tested, and 25 were positive; the group was composed of 29 Caucasians and 1 Negro, aged 22–65; 17 females and 13 males. The duration of the disease ranged from 3 months to 20 years. In 12 patients the disease was radiologically confined to the hilar lymph nodes. One patient showed clinical evidence of extrathoracic disease and the remainder showed radiological involvement of lung fields with or without hilar lymphadenopathy. Five patients were tested while on steroid therapy, 1 of whom was tested before and after commencement of treatment. Tuberculin skin testing was negative (100 T.U.) in 15 of 23 subjects tested.

Tuberculosis: Eleven patients with bacteriologically proven post primary pulmonary disease were investigated. One patient had developed miliary tuberculosis and one suffered from tuberculous cervical adenitis with pulmonary fibrosis. The series consisted of 2 females and 9 males, aged 20–67. All were tuberculin positive and were on chemotherapy but not steroids. Two were Kveim-positive on skin testing.

Crohn's disease: The test was performed on 27 patients, 14 male and 13 female, aged 13–70, with clinical, radiological and laboratory evidence of active disease[10]. Twenty-two were histologically confirmed—13 showed sarcoid type granulomas and 9 showed nonspecific inflammation. The duration of the disease ranged from 1–21 years. In 10 the disease was confined to the ileum, in 6 confined to the colon and in 11 involved both sites. Of 25 patients skin-tested, 1 was Kveim-positive but Mantoux tests were not performed. Nine patients were receiving steroids at the time of testing.

The control group consisted of 20 apparently healthy adults aged 20–50, with no clinical evidence of disease. Four of the 20 were Mantoux-negative (10 T.U.), the remainder Mantoux-positive. One of the former was skin-tested and gave a negative Kveim test (Colindale K12, batch 19).

Lymphocyte separation and MIF production

Twenty ml of venous blood with 200 i.u. of heparin was mixed with carbonyl iron and methyl cellulose and allowed to stand[11]. The lymphocyte-rich supernatant was washed several times using Eagle's minimal essential medium containing 20% foetal calf serum, the cells counted and finally resuspended in the above medium at a concentration of approximately 1×10^6 cells/ml. The cells were then cultured for 72hr in 1 ml aliquots, half containing either 0.2 ml Kveim antigen (250 μg/ml as measured by protein content) or 0.2 ml of the normal spleen suspensions. After 72 hr the supernatants were removed and duplicates pooled. The supernatants were equilibrated by the addition of 0.2 ml Kveim antigen to the control tubes and 0.2 ml normal spleen to the experimental tubes. All tests were done in duplicate and some in triplicate, depending on the number of lymphocytes available.

Assay for MIF

Macrophages were obtained from nonsensitized guinea pigs by innoculating 20 ml of Eagle's medium (containing heparin) intraperitoneally and withdrawing the fluid after 10 minutes. The cells were washed 3 times in Eagle's medium and transferred to capillary tubes at a concentration of approximately 2 million cells per tube. After centrifugation and cutting within the cell-containing part, these were placed in Mackanesstype chambers, (2 per chamber) and the equilibrated supernatants added. The migration areas were measured after 48 hours by planimetry. The results are expressed as the Mean Migration Index, $M.I.=Ax/Ac$. $Ax=$migration area in chambers containing supernatant from lymphocytes cultures with Kveim antigen. $Ac=$area, as above cultured with normal spleen. The total duration of the test is 5/6 days.

RESULTS

Positive Kmif tests ($M.I.<0.8$) were found in 21 of 30 sarcoid patients (70%), 4 of 11 patients with tuberculosis (36%), and in 5 of 27 patients with Crohn's disease (18%), as compared to 1 of 20 normal subjects, (5%), Fig. 1.

Steroid therapy affected the results. 4 of 5 sarcoid patients and 8 of 9 Crohn's patients

W. JONES WILLIAMS ET AL.

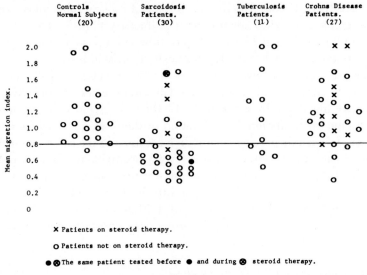

FIG. 1.

TABLES 1a–c. Relationship of Kmif to Kveim tests in patients not on steroids. (Sarcoidosis—26 patients)

		Kveim test	
		+	−
Kmif test	+	18	2
	−	3	3

TABLE 1b. Tuberculosis—11 patients.

		Kveim test	
		+	−
Kmif test	+	1	3
	−	1	6

TABLE 1c. Crohn's disease—16 patients.

		Kveim test	
		+	−
Kmif test	+	0	4
	−	0	12

on steroids were Kmif negative and in 1 sarcoid patient tested before and during therapy the Kmif test changed from positive to negative. None of the tuberculous patients was on steroid treatment. We have therefore analysed the relationship of the Kmif to the Kveim test in patients not on steroids (Tables 1a–c).

In sarcoidosis (Table 1a) the Kmif test was positive in 20/26 (77%) and the Kveim test in 21/26 (80%). Using both tests, 90% were positive. In 21 of the 26 patients the results of the 2 tests were in agreement (80%). Of the 5 patients with discordant results, 2 were Kmif-positive, Kveim-negative and 3 Kmif-negative, Kveim-positive.

In tuberculosis (Table 1b) the Kmif test was positive in 4 of 11 patients (36%) 1 of whom was Kveim-positive. One of the 7 Kmif-negative subjects was Kveim-positive.

In Crohn's disease (Table 1c) the Kmif test was positive in 4 of 16 subjects (25%) and the Kveim test negative in all (The 1 Kveim positive patient was on steroids and so is not included in this table). In 12 of 16 patients the results of the 2 tests were in agreement (75%). In 4 the results were discordant as all were Kmif-positive but Kveim-negative.

We have found (Table 2) that positive Kmif tests in sarcoid patients not on steroids are more frequent in subjects with disease radiologically confined to hilar glands than in those with involvement of other sites. In Crohn's disease (Table 2) there appears to be no relationship between the site affected and the incidence of positive Kmif tests. In tuberculosis, the 4 Kmif-positive subjects all had post-primary active pulmonary tuberculosis.

Our results were affected by the known duration of the illness, prior to Kmif testing (Table 3). In sarcoidosis and in Crohn's disease positive tests were more frequent in patients with a duration of more than 18 months.

TABLE 2. Correlation of Kmif test with distribution of disease;
in patients not on steroids
(26 Sarcoidosis, 18 Crohn's disease)

Disease	Categories	Kmif test	
		+	+
Sarcoidosis	BHL+EN*	10	1
	Others	10	5
Crohn's disease	Ileum	1	5
	Colon	1	3
	Ileum+colon	2	6

* BHL—bilateral hilar adenopathy.
EN —erythema nodosum.

TABLE 3. Correlation of Kmif tests to duration of disease; sarcoidosis and crohn's disease
(not on steroids).

Duration	Kmif test			
	Sarcoidosis		Crohn's disease	
	+	−	+	−
Less than 18 mths	8	4	0	2
More than 18 mths	12	2	4	12

TABLE 4. Correlation of Kmif test with histology
of crohn's disease not on steroids.

Sarcoid-type granuloma	Kmif test	
	+	−
+	0	7
−	3	4
Not examined	1	3

In Crohn's disease positive Kmif tests were not associated with sarcoid-type granulomas (Table 4). In sarcoidosis, tuberculosis and Crohn's disease, age did not affect the results, and in Crohn's disease only, positive results were more frequent in females (4/8) than in males (1/4).

DISCUSSION

Sarcoidosis

In sarcoidosis, our results, 70% positive overall, 77% in patients not on steroids, are in close agreement with those found by Becker et al.[7]—71%, and support the original observations of Hardt and Wanstrup[2] who found that all 7 subjects tested were positive. This is doubly interesting in that Becker et al used their own antigen, Hardt and Wanstrup used Hurley (Australian) antigen, batch 0025, and both used the alternative technique (LMT). Topilsky et al.[8], however, using Siltzbach type 1 spleen J antigen and the LMT technique, obtained negative results in all of 6 patients tested. As the Siltzbach antigen is so well proven, it is unlikely that this divergent result is due to the nature of the antigen, but may be explained by the concentration used, 8 μg/ml, as compared to Becker et al. 70 μg/ml. and our 250 μg/ml. The above findings show that the Kmif test provides comparable results in sarcoidosis with 3 Kveim antigens from different sources.

As in the Kveim test, Siltzbach and Waraich[12], steroid treatment considerably influenced our results. Three of 5 cases on steroids were Kmif-negative and 1 case tested before and during treatment, converted from positive to negative. In contrast, Brostoff and Walker's[4], vide infra, results were unaffected by steroids.

In patients not on steroids, the results of the Kmif (77%) and the Kveim tests (80%) were in close agreement, and in 21 of 26 patients the results were identical (80%). Hardt and Wanstrup[7] showed a 100% correlation in 7 cases and Becker et al.[7] a 90% correlation in 31 patients tested. We thus consider that the Kmif test is a useful alternative to the Kveim tests and when combined with the latter, provided a 90% positive rate and thus considerably increases the diagnostic value of Kveim antigen in sarcoidosis. At the moment we have no clinical or technical explanation for our 5 discordant results which were evenly distributed between the 2 tests and can only be solved by testing larger numbers.

We confirm the findings of Becker et al.[7] and Goldstein et al.[6] who showed a higher positive rate of in vitro Kveim tests in patients with disease confined to hilar lymph glands which agrees with cutaneous Kveim testing. We also confirm the rather surprising finding[7] that the in vitro test is more often positive in patients with a longer rather than a shorter duration of disease and is thus at variance with the cutaneous Kveim test.

Tuberculosis

Our findings of 4 positive tests in 11 patients is greater than Becker et al.[7] findings of 1 positive of 5 tested. In this series, in vivo tests were positive in 2 patients, 1 Kmif-positive and 1 Kmif-negative. Thus with both in vivo 18% and in vitro 36% Kveim tests we obtained positive results, which are much higher than the incidence of 3 of 200 skin tests reported by Siltzbach[13]. With the small numbers examined we are unable to assess the relationship of positive tests to the distribution of disease, though the 4 were in cases of pulmonary and not glandular tuberculosis.

Crohn's disease

In non-steroid treated patients with active disease, the 4 of 16 (25%) Kmif-positive results are in marked contrast to our uniformly negative skin tests.

Our results contrast with those of Brostoff and Walker[4], 47% positive, using the same antigen and batch as ourselves, and Willoughby and Mitchell[3], 66% positive, using Colindale K12, batch 19. Both these reports are based on the leucocyte migration test and are thus not completely comparable with our findings.

As in our sarcoid group, positive reaction tended to be associated with disease of more than 18 months' duration. The absence of correlation between positive reactors and the presence of sarcoid granulomas is noteworthy as Jones Williams et al.[14] showed a positive correlation between granulomas and negative skin tuberculin reactions.

The findings of positive in vivo but negative in vitro Kveim reaction in these 3 diseases mimics the findings with PHA in sarcoidosis[15]. However, as we also found the reverse situation, negative in vivo and positive in vitro reactions, it is difficult to find an adequate explanation. The former may be dependent on the proportion of antigen responsive cells in the circulation and the latter on the concentration of antigen in the 2 tests.

There have been a number of unexplained reports of positive Kveim leucocyte migration tests in a variety of other diseases; dermatitis herpetiformis, 16/17 and coeliac disease 4/10[5], Hodgkin's disease, 6/19 and 'collagen' diseases, 3/3[7]. Positive in vitro Kveim tests have also been previously reported in normal subjects; Becker et al.[7] 2/10. Our 1 positive result in 20 tested, a male aged 24, Mantoux-negative (10 T.U.), Kveim-negative, showed no evidence of disease. The tests will be repeated to exclude the interesting possibility of future development of sarcoidosis.

Finally, despite the various shortcomings, the Kmif test provides a rapid alternative to the Kveim test, avoids biopsies and difficulties in histological interpretations.

SUMMARY

We have analysed the results of in vitro Kveim testing, Kmif tests, in sarcoidosis, tuberculosis and Crohn's disease. The Kmif test is dependant on the detection, using guinea pig macrophages, of a macrophage migration inhibition factor (MIF) produced by the action of Kveim antigen on peripheral lymphocytes.

The Kmif test, in patients not on steroids, was positive in 20/26 (77%) sarcoidosis, 4/11 (36%) tuberculosis, 4/16 (25%) Crohn's disease and 1/20 (5%) of normal subjects.

In sarcoidosis and tuberculosis the results showed a good correlation with skin Kveim tests. This could not be assessed in Crohn's disease as all were Kveim-negative.

In conclusion, we consider that the Kmif test in sarcoidosis is a useful rapid alternative to the Kveim test; though, using Colindale K12 batch 14 Kveim reagent it is not specific for sarcoidosis.

REFERENCES

1. Bendixen, G., and Soborg, M. 1969. *Danish Med. Bull.* **16**: 1.

2. Hardt, F., and Wanstrup, J. 1969. *Acta. Path. Microbiol. Scand.* **76**: 493.
3. Willoughby J. M. T., and Mitchell, D. N. 1971. *Brit. Med. J.* **iii**: 155.
4. Brostoff, J., and Walker, J. G. 1971. *Clin. Exp. Immunol.* **9**: 707.
5. Pagaltsos, A. S., Kumar Parveen J., Willoughby J. M. T., and Dawson, A. M. 1971. *Lancet* **ii**: 1179.
6. Goldstein, R. A., Janick, B. W., and Schultz, K. E. 1971. *Lancet* **ii**: 1204.
7. Becker, F. W., Krull, P., Deicher, H., and Kalden, J. R. 1972. *Lancet* **i**: 120.
8. Topilsky, M., Siltzbach, L. E., Williams, M., and Glade, P. R. 1972. *Lancet* **i**: 117.
9. Chase, M. W., 1961. *Amer. Rev. Resp. Dis.* **84**: 186.
10. Rhodes, J., Bainton, D., Beck, P., and Campbell, H. 1971. *Lancet* **ii**: 1273.
11. Dolby, A. E. 1969. *Immunology* **17**: 709.
12. Siltzbach, L. E., and Waraich, B. A. 1969. *Amer. Rev. Resp. Dis.* **99**: 614.
13. Siltzbach, L. E. 1967. *La Sarcoidose*. Rep. Fouth Int. Conf. Paris (1966) (J. Turiaf and J. Chabot), p. 129.
14. Jones Williams, W. 1965. *Gut* **6**: 503.
15. Bonforte, R. J., Topilsky, M., Siltzbach, L. E., and Glade, P. R. 1972. *Lancet* **i**: 959.

On the Active Principle in the Kveim Antigen

Erik Ripe, Åke Hanngren, Takateru Izumi, Bengt S. Nilsson
and Gunnar Unge

Department of Thoracic Medicine, Karolinska Hospital, Stockholm, Sweden

Even since the Kveim test was introduced it has been an important element for the diagnosis of sarcoidosis in Sweden. At the Karolinska Hospital, Stockholm, we use our own Kveim suspension made from sarcoid hilar lymph nodes obtained through mediastinoscopy. The supply of these lymph nodes together with the increasing knowledge of immunological mechanisms have brought about our interest in the study of the reaction inducing granuloma formation. Therefore, there were two aims of our experiments. Firstly, in consequence of the supposed particle nature of the active principle, we wanted to investigate whether a concentrated particle fraction would constitute a more potent antigen than the conventional one. Secondly, we were interested to see if the soluble part of the antigen, which does not normally give rise to positive reactions, could do so when coupled to synthetic particles.

We used hilar lymph nodes from patients with biopsy-verified pulmonary sarcoidosis for preparation of the extracts. The conventional antigen was made in the usual way by homogenizing the lymph nodes in physiological saline solution. Part of this material was further disintegrated in the X-press described by Edebo[1]. The X-press operated at −25°–30°C and the material was forced through a 2.5 mm hole, which required a pressure of 2–4 tons/cm². This was accomplished with the aid of a hydraulic jack. When examined electron microscopically, it was found that the disintegration had brought about a fracturing of the cell walls, nuclei and most of the vacuoles and the mitochondria. The disintegrated material was then thawed, shaken in a supermixer and centrifuged. The supernatant thus obtained was called the cytoplasma fraction and the sediment the membrane fraction. Part of the cytoplasma fraction was then coupled to Sephadex G-25 ultrafine® (Pharmacia, Sweden) activated with cyanbromide—size about 7 microns[2]. The protein in the cytoplasma fraction was thereby bound to Sephadex in

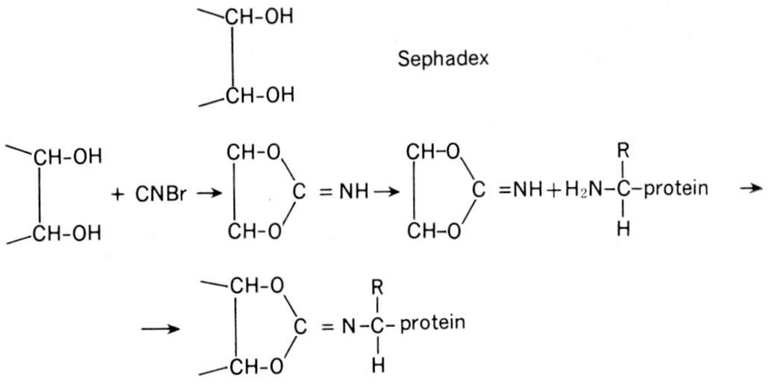

Fig. 1.   The chemical coupling of cyanbromide activated Sephadex G-25 ultrafine to the proteins in the cytoplasma fraction.

the way shown in Fig. 1. Nitrogen determinations of this fraction showed that an amount of amino acids equivalent to virtually all proteins were linked to Sephadex by the procedure used. The main amino acids, based on molecular ratios, were glycine, glutamic acid and proline. The different preparations obtained were sterilized and the dry weight was adjusted to 10 mg/ml.

The test was performed and evaluated in the usual way, utilizing the conventional criteria for a positive test. The only modification made was that the injection sites were examined both after 48 hours and 6 weeks.

In the first series of experiments, in which 22 patients with pulmonary sarcoidosis participated, the epitheloid cell granuloma-developing effect of the membrane fraction was compared with that of the conventional antigen. Table 1 shows that the incidence of positive reactions was much higher after tests with the membrane fraction than with the conventional antigen. In 12 of the 22 cases of sarcoidosis only the membrane fraction produced epitheloid cell granulomas. Tests with the membrane fraction on 29 control cases were all negative.

Another finding of interest was that reactions could be registered after 48 hours in a considerable number of patients (20/38) given the membrane fraction. Since no similar reactions could be seen in the control cases we think that this "early" reaction could be regarded as a prediction of a positive Kveim test. However, the biopsy did not show

TABLE 1. Results of the comparison between the granuloma-producing effect of the membrane fraction and the conventional antigen tested on 22 patients (0.15 ml, 10 mg/ml) with different stages of sarcoidosis. The patients are divided according to the size of the Kveim nodule (>4 mm and <4 mm).

The size of the Kveim nodle after 6 weeks	Number of positive Kveim reactions					
	Stage I		Stage II		Stage III	
	Membrane	Conventional	Membrane	Conventional	Membrane	Conventional
> 4 mm	8	3	6			
< 4 mm	2	4	4	5	2	
Total number tested (negative reactions in parentheses)	10 (0)	7 (3)	10 (0)	5 (5)	2 (0)	0 (2)

TABLE 2. ^{14}C-thymidine incorporation (c.p.m., mean ± S.E.) by peripheral lymphocytes from patients with various stages of pulmonary sarcoidosis. The protein concentration in the Kveim preparations was 0.1 mg/ml except *=0.5 mg/ml and **=1.0 mg/ml.

Patient	Age	Sex	Stage	Added material					
				None	"Conventional antigen"	"Membrane-fraction"	"Cytoplasmafraction"	PHA (10^{-2})	PPD $(10\ \mu g/ml)$
M.N	37	♀	I	15±3	—	19±4*	23±3	1039±75	954±69
T.S	36	♂	II	40±9	46±5	36±6*	35±5	893±72	46±8
I.B	22	♀	II	37±11	31±3**	33±2*	45±7	1808±189	399±13
C.J	31	♂	II	22±4	35±2	32±5*	33±6	1454±188	288±17
V.B	46	♀	III	39±6	27±5**	32±4*	33±5	1313±101	864±30
G.E	47	♂	III	28±3	—	18±1	25±5	551±123	26±3

any typical signs of a delayed reaction, but only a beginning collagenisation and accumulation of poly- and mononuclear cells around the injected extract. Nor did any increasing thymidine uptake using lymphocytes from these patients and the membrane fraction support the hypothesis of a delayed reaction (Table 2).

From the results it can be said that the active principle causing epitheloid cell granuloma was concentrated in the membrane fraction and resisted the disintegrating forces of the X-press. The results thus further supported the view that the active principle is of particle form. There is, however, a certain discrepancy between evidence indicating that the active principle consists of a macromolecule and that showing that it is resistant to many biochemical compounds and, as shown here, also resistant to the forces of the X-press. If the active principle was of high molecular nature, even of particle form, it should be reasonable to expect that the activity of the Kveim suspension should decrease when exposed to enzymes or very high pressure. One explanation of the discrepancy might be that the active principle, in spite of the results of earlier studies, is of low molecular character and therefore less influenced by enzymes, but that it only exerts its effect bound to a macromolecule, for example, part of the cell membrane. Such a mechanism would be in analogy with well-documented findings which have shown that aggregated antigens are much more immunogenic than soluble antigens. Even if the active principle only exerts its granuloma-developing effect when bound to a macromolecule there is nothing indicating that it could not be released from the cell membrane or form structures in the cytoplasma or the nuclei and be found again in the supernatant. The reason why this has not been shown earlier might be that it is reabsorbed too fast from the injection site before exerting a granuloma-developing effect. Bearing this hypothesis in mind, we coupled the cytoplasma fraction to Sephadex G-25® in the way mentioned and injected it intracutaneously. Sephadex G-25® alone was used as control. The investigation showed that the cytoplasma fraction itself did not give any granulomas, but coupled to Sephadex, positive reactions were obtained in 5 of 13 patients with sarcoidosis. While Sephadex G-25® alone caused epitheloid cell granulomas in 2 of 13 patients with sarcoidosis the results are as yet inconclusive but may suggest that the hypothesis about a low molecular active principle, which gives rise to Kveim reactions only when bound to a macromolecular carrier could be correct.

REFERENCES

1. Edebo, L. 1961. Disintegration of microorganism: Uppsala: Thesis.
2. Axén, R., Porath, J., and Ernback, S. 1967. Chemical coupling of peptides and proteins to polysaccharides by means of cyanogen halides. *Nature* **214**: 1302–1304.

Electron Microscopy of Kveim Biopsies in Sarcoidosis

S. D. DOUGLAS AND L. E. SILTZBACH

Mount Sinai School of Medicine, City University of New York, New York, U.S.A.

We have studied positive Kveim biopsies from 11 patients with sarcoidosis by electron microscopy. These biopsies were obtained at intervals from 1–18 weeks after inoculation (8 specimens were studied at 6 weeks). The biopsies were cut to blocks approximately 1 mm³ and fixed in 1.5% glutaraldehyde buffered with sodium cacodylate. The material was then postfixed in 1% osmium tetroxide, embedded in epon, and stained en bloc with 1% aqueous uranyl acetate. These sections were stained with uranyl acetate followed by lead citrate and examined in a Siemens 101 electron microscope. The areas for detailed study by electron microscopy were selected by phase-contrast examination of 1 micron thick epon sections.

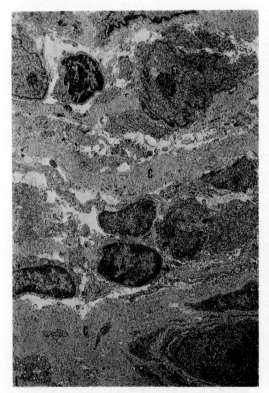

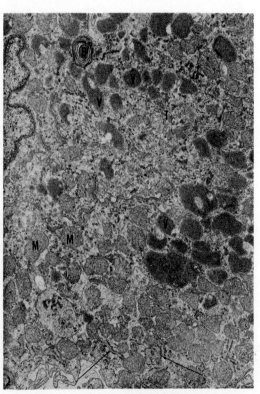

FIG. 1. Low-power electron micrograph of a 6-week Kveim biopsy showing several lymphocytes (L), epithelioid cells (E) and surrounding collagen fibrils (C). Mag. × 7,200.

FIG. 2. Portion of epithelioid showing several homogeneous electron-dense bodies which resemble typical lysosomes (V), a lamellated myelin-like structure (B), mitochondria (M), microtubules (T) and strands of rough-surfaced endoplasmic reticulum (arrows) Mag. × 20,000.

Supported by USPHS NIH Grants, AI–09338, 1 K04–HL 42575 and HL–13853.

Characteristic features which have been described by other investigators[1-3] namely, giant epithelioid cells, occasional lymphocytes and plasma cells were present within the granulomas (Fig. 1). Collagen within these lesions frequently appeared to show loss of its characteristic periodicity. Epithelioid and giant cells contained numerous well-developed cytoplasmic organelles, including many mitochondria, lysosomes and well developed Golgi zones. Some of the epithelioid cells showed well-developed and dilated rough-surfaced endoplasmic reticulum. The nuclei had many infoldings of the nuclear envelope and nucleoli were frequently observed. Golgi zones were extensively developed and contained numerous vacuoles vesicles and saccules. Many of the epithelioid cells showed extensively developed projections of the plasma membrane (microvilli).

The most striking feature of the epithelioid cells in the Kveim biopsies was the presence of abundant pleomorphic cytoplasmic bodies of several types. These included: 1. homogeneous electron-dense bodies from 0.2 to 0.8 microns in diameter, which resembled typical lysosomes. 2. lamellated myelin-like structures which were frequently 1 or more microns in diameter. 3. Structures which resembled autophagic vacuoles containing cytoplasmic organelles and 4. A more numerous type of structure which appears to be unique to this type of epithelioid cell. These vacuoles were about 0.3 to 1.0 microns in diameter and contained material which is intermediate in electron density. Some of these structures are illustrated in Figs. 2–4.

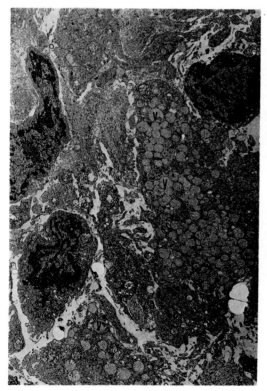

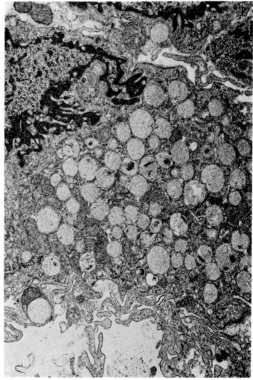

FIG. 3. Epithelioid cell and adjoining lymphocytes present in a Kveim biopsy taken after 6 weeks. Numerous cytoplasmic vacuoles (V) of intermediate electron density are present in several cells. Mag. ×12,0000.

FIG. 4. Electron micrograph of an epithelioid cell showing cytoplasmic bodies of intermediate electron density which are about 0.3 to 1.0 microns in diameter. Mag. ×20,000.

The observations indicate extensively developed cytoplasmic organelles in the epithelioid and giant cells present in Kveim biopsies. As indicated in earlier studies these lesions are morphologically similar to those of naturally occurring sarcoidosis.

The cytologic structures observed suggest that these cells are active in phagocytosis and pinocytosis as evidenced by the numerous lysomome-like structures. In addition, as indicated previously by Hirsch et al.[1], some of these cells also have well-developed rough-surfaced endoplasmic reticulum indicating active protein synthesis, and numerous mitochondria indicating active respiration. The possible relationship between these cytoarchitectural observations and Kveim antigen remain unknown.

REFERENCES

1. Hirsch, J. G., Fedorko, M. E., and Dwyer, C. M. 1967. The Ultrastructure of Epithelioid and Giant Cells in Positive Kveim Sites and Sarcoid Granulomata. *La Sarcoidose.* Paris: Masson and cie, p. 59.

2. Basset, F., Turiaf, J., and Brocard, H. 1971. Ultrastructural Aspects of Pulmonary Sarcoidosis. *Proc. Fifth Int. Conf. on Sarcoidosis* Prague: Univ. Karlova, p. 110.

3. Jones Williams, W., et al. 1971. A Comparative Study of the Ultrastructure and Histochemistry of Sarcoid and Tuberculous Granulomas. *Proc. Fifth Int. Conf. on Sarcoidosis* Prague: Univ. Karlova, p. 115.

Kveim Reaction
—Disagreement in results and tentative criteria—

K. Iwai[1], R. Fukushiro[2], Y. Kobata[3], T. Izumi[3], T. Hirako[4],
O. Hongo[5] and M. Odaka[6]

The Kveim reaction is now widely used for the diagnosis of sarcoidosis. One major problem regarding this reaction is to get antigens of high enough potency and purity. Another is obtaining a high coincidence of diagnosis for the same histological slides. In some cases, however, disagreement of the diagnosis occurs even though the workers are quite familiar with the criteria of the Kveim reaction set down by several different authors[1-6].

Histological slides which were felt difficult to diagnose or thought to be equivocal or borderline cases, were collected from 5 institutions with some typical positive or negative slides. The patients' names were concealed and the slides, numbered at random, were read by 5 readers independently who also gave the reasons for the diagnosis.

Six slides were excluded from the observations due to poor processing or staining. The diagnoses of 5 readers for the remaining 66 slides showed the positive rate to range from 45.8% to 66.7%, and an almost identical positive rate was given by 4 readers, while stricter diagnosis was made by another reader. Furthermore, readers B and C diagnosed as equivocal in many cases, while readers A and D thought this was true in only a few.

The rate of coincident diagnosis on each slide is shown in Table 1. The histological slides were diagnosed twice, and the results of the first readings by each reader were made known to the other to permit a change of diagnosis for the second reading if necessary. In the first reading, there was agreement in diagnosis among 4 or 5 readers in 56.1% of the slides, and 62.1% for the second reading. The low coincidence of diagnosis may be due to the fact that the histological slides which were felt difficult to diagnose were mainly collected in this study. An additional reader joined the group

TABLE 1. Percent of consensus histological diagnosis of Kveim reaction.

Degree of consensus	First reading	Second reading
I. Agreement among 5 readers	19 } 56.1%	21 } 62.1%
II. „ 4 „	18	20
III. „ 3 „	14	11
IV. „ 2 „	15	14
Total	66 100%	66 100%

1) *Research Institute, Japan Anti-Tuberculosis Association, Tokyo, Japan*
2) *Kanazawa University, Kanazawa, Japan*
3) *Kyoto University, Kyoto, Japan*
4) *National Leprosarium, Tokyo, Japan*
5) *Komagome Hospital, Tokyo, Japan*
6) *JNR Central Health Institute, Tokyo, Japan*

TABLE 2. Degree of consensus with an additional reader.

Degree of consensus by 5 readers		Number of slides	Coincidental diagnosis by sixth reader
I.	Agreement among 5 readers	21	20 (95.2%)
II.	„ 4 „	20	14 (70.0)
III.	„ 3 „	11	5 (45.5)
IV.	„ 2 „	14	7 (50.0)

TABLE 3. Tentative criteria for Kveim reaction.

1. *Nodules consisting of epithelioid cells......POSITIVE*
   a) Nodule : A well-defined, round or oval lesion of densely arranged epithelioid cells, similar to a sarcoid granuloma.
   b) A fibrinoid-like central necrosis may present.
   c) A small abscess with a typical positive reaction.   +a
   b) Nodules of epithelioid cells, including foreing body.   +f

2. *Epithelioid cells without any nodule formation......EQUIVOCAL*

3. *No epithelioid cells......NEGATIVE*
   e) Foreign-body reaction only   −f
   f) Extensive nonspecific cell infiltration   −n
   g) Increase of collagenous fibers in cutis   −c

at this stage, and subsequent results are shown in Table 2. The slides of Group I, in which 5 readers previously gave the same diagnosis got 95.2% coincidental diagnosis from the 6th reader, while Group III or IV got around 45.5% or 50.0% coincidence respectively, demonstrating that many problematical slides had been included in the latter two.

In order to understand the reasons for this disagreement in the diagnosis of the slides, indivisual descriptions and comments offered by each reader on each slides that were noted at the time of diagnosis, were analysed, and the problems regarding the histological findings on these slides of Group III and IV were summarized as follows. 1) Whether proliferating cells in the area are epithelioid cells or large mononuclear cells. 2) What does epithelioid cell "nodule" means, and from what size can it be called a "nodule". 3) If epithelioid cells proliferate diffusely without any nodule formation, how are they to be diagnosed. 4) How can atrophic epithelioid cells be differentiated from nonspecific granulomatous changes. 5) How is the fibrinoid-like necrosis in the granulomatous lesion to be understood. 6) How should epithelioid cell granulomas accompanied with a small abscess be diagnosed. 7) Does the presence of a foreign body in the epithelioid cell granulomas preclude a positive diagnosis. 8) Does extensive infiltration by lymphoreticular cells without epithelioid cells have any signifance. Considering these problems, tentative criteria were developed for the Kveim reaction, as shown in Table 3.

According to these criteria, a final diagnosis was made on each slides in Groups III and IV, revealing one slide having +, 1 of +s, 5 of +a, 5 of ±, 5 of −n, 4 of −f and 4 of −, thus explaining the reason for the diversified diagnosis of the two groups.

A final diagnosis was made on slides of all the groups, then the patient's names were

TABLE 4.   The final diagnosis of Kveim reaction.

	Positive	Equivocal	Negative
Diagnosis of patients			
Sarcoidosis	32 (a3, f1)	5	17 (f4)
Cheilitis	2	—	—
Tuberculosis	1	—	3
Atypical mycobacteriosis	1 (a1)	—	—
Ileitis	1	—	—
Leprosy or sarcoidosis	1 (a1)	—	—
Rosacea	—	—	1 (f1)
Unknown	2	—	—
Source of antigen			
Dr Hurley's 004	20 (a5)	2	3
Dr Siltzbach's	5 (f1)	—	2 (f2)
Japanese Committee	13 (a1)	3	14 (f3)
Our own	—	—	—
Normal spleen	—	—	—
Unknown	—	—	2

revealed by uncovering each slide. The diagnosis of Kveim reaction and of the patients, and the source of antigen are shown in Table 4. Positive reactions were obtained in 32 out of 54 sarcoidosis patients, but there was also some positive reactions in the non-sarcoidosis cases such as cheilitis, tuberculosis, atypical mycobacteriosis and others. Among the antigen products used, Dr. Hurley's antigen showed a high positive rate. The presence of a small abscess or foreign bodies in these antigens indicates the need for further improvement in the preparation of the antigen.

REFERENCES

1. Rogers, F. J., and Haserich, H. J. 1954. Sarcoidosis and kveim reaction. *J. Invest. Dermat.* **23**: 389.
2. Sillzbach, L. E. 1961. Kveim test in sarcoidosis. *J.A.M.A.* **178**: 476.
3. Steigleder, G. K., Silva, A. J., and Nelson, C. T. 1961. Histopathology of the kveim test. *Arch. Derm. Syph.* **84**: 824.
4. Kenny, M., and Stone, D. J. 1963.   Objective eveluation of the Kveim test in a "double-blind" study. *Amer. Rev. Resp. Dis.* **87**: 504.
5. D'Arcy Hart, P., and Mitchel, D. M. 1964. Association between Kveim test results, previous BCG vaccination, and tuberculin sensitivity in healthy young adults. *Brit. Med. J.* **1**: 795.
6. Dornetzhuber, V. 1966. Routine investigation of the Kveim-Nickerson reaction in sarcoidosis. A pathologist's point of view. *Amer. Rev. Resp. Dis.* **93**: 459.

Observations on the Mechanism and Specificity of the Kveim Reaction

Harold L. Israel

Department of Medicine, Thomas Jefferson University, Philadelphia, U.S.A.

Numerous papers have been presented on the Kveim reaction at previous international conferences on sarcoidosis, with universal agreement that the 3 test materials which had been validated by comparative trials represented standardized antigens that responded alike everywhere. It seemed equally well-established that Kveim reactivity was related to the duration of disease, being most often positive in early cases associated with erythema nodosum and being least often positive in patients with chronic inactive disease.

At the 1969 Conference in Prague a brief communication was presented[1] reporting that several patients with long inactive stage I sarcoidosis had reacted strongly to Kveim tests. Further exploration of this unexpected observation led to the demonstration in a series of 104 patients that Kveim reactions occurred in patients with chronic lymphadenopathy of diverse causes and that patients with active sarcoidosis without lymphadenopathy frequently failed to react.[2] The present report is an analysis of the results of 270 tests performed with Commonwealth Serum Laboratory test materials. In 78 cases simultaneous tests with K12 antigen were made and in 23 cases tests were done in triplicate, the third antigen being supplied by Professor Turiaf.

RELIABILITY OF CSL ANTIGEN

Table 1 demonstrates the results of tests performed with the Commonwealth Serum Laboratory antigen, the majority made with lot 4, and a few with lots 3 and 5. No differences in the behavior of these lots has been noted and the results presented in Table 1 resemble those reported by many investigators using other materials. The sensitivity of the antigen in sarcoidosis is high. There is an obvious correlation with the presence of radiologically demonstrable lymphadenopathy, shown by the 80% reaction rate in stage I and II patients compared to a 35% reaction rate in patients without demonstrable mediastinal nodes.

Few reactions were obtained in subjects without sarcoidosis. Positive tests occurred in 1 patient with infectious mononucleosis, and in a patient who was admitted to a hospital with superior mediastinal obstruction. Radiation was instituted as a life-saving measure. A mediastinal lymph node was subsequently resected and showed epithelioid granulomas. I was reluctant to accept the diagnosis of sarcoidosis, but when the Kveim test proved unequivocally positive, I thought we had encountered the first instance in which sarcoidosis was responsible for superior mediastinal obstruction. A few months later, however, it became evident that the patient had Hodgkin's disease with a nodal sarcoid reaction.

Thanks are due Dr Thomas Chused, National Institute of Dental Research, Bethesda, Maryland, who collaborated in the study of patients with Sjogren's syndrome.

TABLE 1. Results of 270 Kveim tests with CSL antigen.

	No. tested	Positive
Sarcoidosis		
Stage I	81	67 (83%)
Stage II	34	29 (80%)
Stage III	46	18 (40%)
Stage 0	25	8 (32%)
Controls		
Sjögren's syndrome	11	0
Granulomatous hepatitis	11	0
Infectious mono.	9	1
Fungal disease	8	0
Hodgkin's disease	6	1
Wegener's granulomatosis	4	0
Hypersensitivity granulomatosis	1	0
Miscellaneous	22	0
Extrapulmonary tuberculosis	5	5
Chronic lymphatic leukemia	5	5
Nonspecific lymphadenitis	2	2

TABLE 2. Results of 76 duplicate Kveim tests.

Diagnosis	No. tested	Reactors to CSL	Reactors to K 12
Sarcoidosis, subacute, stage I	12	10	9
„ , chronic, inact. I	11	11	10
„ , with E. N.	7	7	6
„ , other	18	8	8
Sjögren's syndrome	10	0	0
Wegener's granulomatosis	4	0	0
Chr. lymph. leukemia	3	3	1
Nonspec. adenitis	2	2	1
Extrapulmonary tuberculosis	2	2	0
Regional ileitis	2	0	0
Hodgkin's disease	1	0	0
Parotitis	1	1	1
Asthma	1	0	0
Histoplasmosis	1	0	0
Hypersensitivity granulomatosis	1	0	1

The only patients without sarcoidosis in whom we have consistently found positive Kveim tests are those who have chronic lymphadenopathy due to lymphatic leukemia and tuberculosis, or of a nonspecific character.

The data in Table 1 do not support the hypothesis that lots 004 and 005 of Commonwealth Serum Laboratory antigen were improperly prepared and contained a foreign-body material. This concept[3] has been based on the report that Dr Izumi observed few "false positives" prior to use of lot 004. I should point out that Dr Izumi began large-

TABLE 3. Results of triplicate Kveim tests.

Diagnosis	No. tested	Reactors to CSL	Reactors to K 12	Reactors to Turiaf antigen
Sarcoidosis				
stage I	2	2	2	2
stage II	4	4	4	4
stage III	2	1	0	1
stage I inactive	1	1	1	1
suspected	1	1	0	F. B.
Histoplasmosis	1	0	0	0
Chronic lymph. leukemia	1	1	0	0
Hypersensitivity granulomatosis	1	0	1	1
Sjögren's syndrome	10	0	0	0

scale investigations of the Kveim reaction in patients with tuberculosis only after I spoke in Japan in the summer of 1970 and called to his attention our observations on the frequency of positive Kveim tests in patients with tuberculous lymphadenitis.

Futher support for the reliability of Commonwealth Serum Laboratory antigen is provided by a comparison of simultaneous tests done with K12 antigen (Table 2). Both antigens react with a high degree of concordance in patients with sarcoidosis and in most cases without sarcoidosis. In a group of 23 patients simultaneous tests were carried out with 3 antigens (Table 3). The results with all antigens was quite consistent and there is no evidence of foreign-body reactions to the Commonwealth Serum Laboratory preparation. The greater sensitivity of the Australian test material to tuberculosis is probably not due to chance since comparative studies in England showed that CSL antigen was more reactive than K12 in Asiatics with florid tuberculosis.[4, 5] Further investigation is necessary to assess the significance of the difference in results in patients with chronic lymphatic leukemia and hypersensitivity granulomatosis.

RESPONSE PATTERNS OF KVEIM REACTION

Lymphadenopathy and granulomatosis

On the basis of this evidence establishing the consistent behavior of the 3 preparations, the patterns of response of Kveim antigens may be considered. Table 4 shows the results of tests performed in patients with Stage I sarcoidosis. It will be noted that the percentage of positive reactions was lower in patients with subacute disease than in those

TABLE 4. Relationship of Kveim reaction to duration and activity of stage I sarcoidosis.

	No. of patients	No. positive
Subacute active	52	39*
Chronic active	6	6
inactive	31	30

* 5 subacute active cases with negative reactions, retested when chronic, became positive.

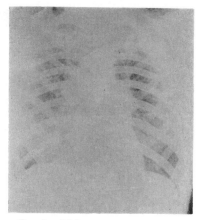 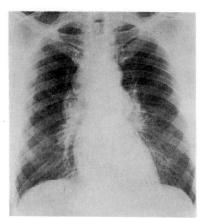

FIG. 1. This man was rejected for military service in 1943 because of hilar adenopathy. Films taken from 1947 to 1972 have shown no change in the massive lymph node enlargement. There have been no symptoms at any time. Kveim tests in 1970 and 1972 were strongly positive.

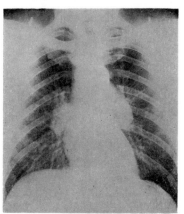 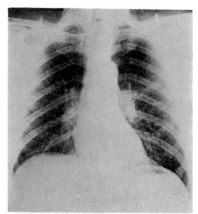

FIG. 2. This man had marked hilar adenopathy on a routine X-ray examination in July 1969. A Kveim test read on Sept. 15, 1969 was negative. The chest X-ray on Sept. 15 showed marked reduction in the nodes. A film in November 1969 was normal.

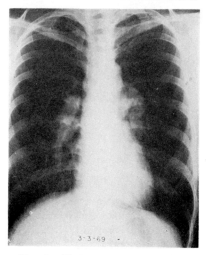 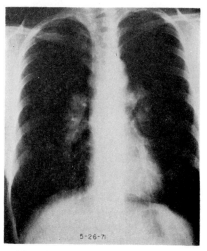

FIG. 3. This young woman was found to have hilar adenopathy on a routine examination in 1969. The Kveim test was negative at this time but was positive in 1971.

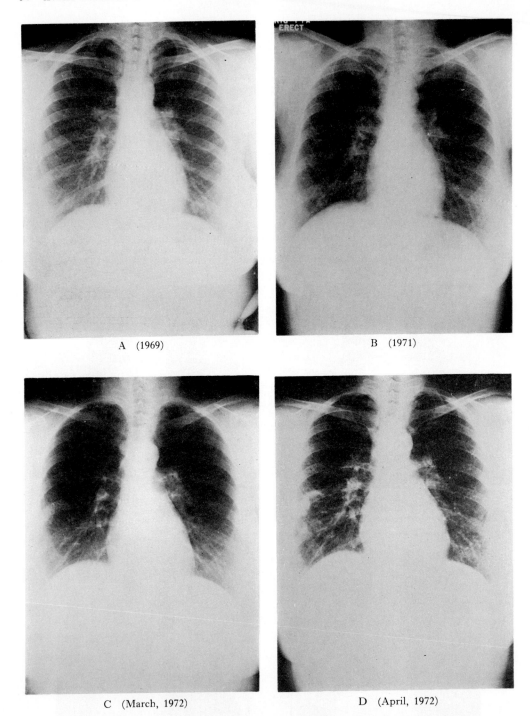

A (1969)   B (1971)

C (March, 1972)   D (April, 1972)

FIG. 4. This young woman developed uveitis following childbirth in 1967. When seen in 1969 (Fig. 4A) she was asymptomatic but had hilar adenopathy. A Kveim test was positive. Acute pulmonary dissemination developed after childbirth in 1971 (Fig. 4B), clearing after 3 months of prednisone. A film after childbirth in March 1972 was normal (Fig. 4C). In April, when disseminated pulmonary infiltration recurred (Fig. 4D), Kveim tests were negative.

with disease known to be chronic, whether activity was manifested by extrapulmonary disease, or whether the disease was clinically inactive. The period of observation extended in the chronic groups from 3 to 33 years (Fig. 1). Figure 2 demonstrates a patient with equally massive hilar adenopathy whose Kveim test was negative. This unexpected result appears related to the fact that the adenopathy had markedly reduced during the 6-week interval of the test and disappeared within 3 months. We have observed 5 instances of transient adenopathy with negative Kveim tests. On the other hand, negative Kveim tests may be obtained in patients with stage I sarcoidosis because they are tested too early. Five patients with stage I disease who had negative Kveim tests manifested persistent adenopathy. Repetition of the Kveim test was positive in each case. The roentgenograms in one such case are shown in Fig. 3. A Kveim test was negative in 1969, but strongly positive in 1971.

The relationship of the reaction to lymphadenopathy rather than granulomatosis is shown in Fig. 4. This young woman had a positive Kveim test when seen with stage I disease in 1969. There was acute pulmonary dissemination after childbirth in 1971, which cleared after 3 months of prednisone. A film taken after childbirth in March 1972 was normal. A month later there was another severe pulmonary dissemination. Kveim tests with CSL, K12 and Turiaf antigens at this time were negative.

Further evidence that sarcoidal granulomatosis is not responsible for Kveim reactivity is provided by observations in granulomatous hepatitis.[6] Kveim tests in 13 patients with well-established diagnoses of systemic sarcoidosis but normal chest roentgenograms were negative in each instance.

It is clear that we have in the past confused anatomic and temporal criteria, making the erroneous assumption that stage I sarcoidosis is early sarcoidosis. Our studies indicate that a third of patients who come under observation with hilar adenopathy remain unchanged for many years. An asymptomatic patient found to have hilar adenopathy for the first time is assumed in the absence of prior chest roentgenograms to have subacute disease, but in fact the adenopathy could have been present for decades.

In a similar misconception, erythema nodosum is often assumed to date the onset of sarcoidosis. This inference may be erroneous, as a recently studied case demonstrates. A young woman with faint but cosmetically disturbing facial sarcoids was admitted to the hospital in 1969 in order to determine whether she had systemic disease. A Kveim test was negative but a liver biopsy revealed numerous granulomas. Prednisone therapy resulted in clearing of the cutaneous manifestations and was discontinued after 6 months. In 1971, the patient developed classical erythema nodosum. Although the chest X-ray remained normal, Kveim tests performed with both CSL and K12 antigens were strongly positive.

Erythema nodosum

Further study of the relationship of erythema nodosum and the Kveim reaction reveals a striking correlation between them (Table 5). It will be noted that several patients whose thoracic abnormalities have disappeared continue to have recurrent erythema nodosum with positive Kveim reactions.

It is generally recognized that patients with erythema nodosum have a more favorable prognosis. The relationship of the Kveim reaction and the presence of erythema nodosum to the disappearance of hilar adenopathy has been examined (Table 6). All patients with erythema nodosum had positive Kveim tests, and in each case the chest roentgenograms

TABLE 5. Kveim tests in patients with erythema nodosum.

		No. tested	positive
Stage I	subacute	7	7
Stage II	subacute	1	1
Stage 0	subacute	2	2
	chronic	3	3

TABLE 6. Prognostic value of erythema nodosum and Kveim reaction in sarcoidosis (patients with stage I disease followed for a year).

	No. observed	No. recovered
Kveim-positive		
with EN	7	7
without EN	22	11
Kveim-negative	13	6

returned to normal within a year. The Kveim reaction itself has no prognostic significance. In the absence of erythema nodosum, patients with negative Kveim tests cleared no more often than those with positive Kveim tests. We have not had the opportunity of performing Kveim tests in patients whose erythema nodosum is due to infection or drug sensitivity. A study of the Kveim reaction in such cases should be of great interest.

CONCLUSIONS

1)   Many Kveim antigens uniformly produce reactions in patients with sarcoidosis. The Kveim reaction is almost invariably positive in those who have chronic hilar or peripheral adenopathy or erytheme nodosum, but tests are frequently negative in patients with active sarcoidosis and minimal or no evident lymphadenopathy.

2)   The Kveim reaction in sarcoidosis is related to the anatomic involvement and not to the duration or clinical activity of the disease. Patients with granulomatosis of the liver due to sarcoidosis in the absence of thoracic abnormalities uniformly fail to react. A positive Kveim test cannot be regarded as proof of the diagnosis of sarcoidosis although it may have corroborative value. What deserves greater emphasis is that a negative Kveim test has no value in excluding acute and active sarcoidal granulomatosis.

3)   Kveim test materials which react alike in sarcoidosis may differ in behavior in patients with regional ileitis, chronic lymphatic leukemia, disseminated lupus and chronic lymphadenitis of diverse etiology.

4)   Reactivity to Kveim antigens is related neither to a single etiologic agent nor a specific pathologic pattern. Genetic factors may cause ethnic differences in response. The Kveim test is an immunologic recognition system sensitive to multiple factors, of which chronic lymphadenopathy and erythema nodosum appear to be the most prominent.

5)   The discordant results reported by different investigators are attributable to variations in the composition of the test materials. The preparations presently available appear to include multiple antigens. Identification of the factors peculiar to sarcoidosis will be necessary before in vitro measurement of lymphocyte responses can be applied to clinical diagnosis.

ACKNOWLEDGEMENTS

Thanks are due Drs T. H. Hurley, J. Mikhail and J. Turiaf for supplies of Kveim test materials.

REFERENCE

1. Israel, H. L. 1971. Chronic lymphadenopathy and the Kveim reaction. *Proc. Fifth Int. Conf. on Sarcoidosis* Prague: Univ. Karlova, p. 391.
2. Israel, H. L., and Goldstein, R. A. 1971. Relation of Kveim antigen test to lymphadenopathy. Study of sarcoidosis and other diseases. *N. Eng. J. Med.* **284**: 345.
3. Editorial. 1972. Kveim-Siltzbach test vindicated. *Lancet* **1**: 88.
4. Mikhail, J. R., and Mitchell, D. N. 1971. Mediastinoscopy: a diagnostic procedure in hilar and peratracheal lymphadenopathy. *Postgrad. Med. J.* **47**: 698.
5. Karlish, A. J. 1971. The Kveim test in sarcoidosis. *Oxford Med. Sch. Gaz.* **23**: 26.
6. Israel, H. L., and Goldstein, R. A. 1972. Hepatic granulometosis revisited. *Presented at Sixth Int. Conf. on Sarcoidosis* Tokyo.

Experience with Our Kveim Antigen

Horst Behrend

Medizinische Hochschule Hannover, Hannover, Federal Republic of Germany

AND

Branislav Djurić and Nikola Aleksić

Institute of Tuberculosis and Chest Diseases, Novi Sad, Yugoslavia

At present the Kveim test is widely accepted in diagnostics of sarcoidosis. The greatest contribution to this diagnostic method is the international investigation of Siltzbach and Hurley, as well as a number of other studies. Besides the diagnostic specificity of this test, its etiology has remained unknown.

So far we have used Siltzbach's antigen (Goldman 1965) and Hurley's antigen (La Grasta 1969 and Giunio 1972) in Yugoslavia. Since we have obtained antigen in a relatively small amount and interest in sarcoidosis is rapidly growing in our country, we endeavoured to prepare the antigen ourselves. Thanks to professional collaboration with Professor Behrend (FRG) lasting for many years, we were able to learn and later to prepare Kveim antigen ourselves in Yugoslavia (Djurić).

A modification of Deicher's method based upon Chase's method was applied for the preparation of Kveim antigen.

Sarcoid mediastinal lymph nodes have been mostly used as material for Kveim antigen since they are rather accessible, especially following the application of parasternal biopsy in our institution.

Following standardization of Kveim antigen with previously known antigen, we injected it intradermally.

Kveim test was applied to 608 diseased persons (154 sarcoidosis, 376 other diseases and 78 did not come to biopsy).

Positive findings were obtained in 88% of 154 tested sarcoid patients (glandular stage 97%, nonfibrotic 87% and fibrotic 62%). Such high percentage is accounted for by exclusion of all diffuse shadows in lungs and mediastinal lymphadenopathies from studies, where diagnosis of sarcoidosis has not been histologically proved, as the patients refused biopsy methods and Kveim test was negative. If most of these patients were included in sarcoidosis according to their clinical course (see Table 1), the percentage would be considerably lower. In 17 extrathoracic changes, where intrathoracic were not visualized on the lung radiogram, Kveim test was found to be positive only in 59%.

Corticoids were given to 2 patients in the course of Kveim test due to severe disseminated sarcoidosis; in spite of this, positive findings were obtained in both cases.

In 376 patients ill of other diseases, Kveim test gave no positive result in any case.

Histomorphology of Kveim Test

A piece of skin extirpated from the puncture spot, irrespective of the palpability of granulomas, was serially studies in each case in 6 to 12 histologic sections.

No differences were observed on comparing both positive and negative findings in parallel applications of Siltzbach's and our antigen.

TABLE 1.   Diseases in which Kveim test was negative.

1.	Cavernous phthisis	37
2.	Miliary TB of lungs	3
3.	Inactive TB of lungs	21
4.	Mediastinal TB of lymph nodes	2
5.	Generalized TB of lymph nodes	3
6.	Silicotuberculosis	3
7.	Silicosis	8
8.	Chronic bronchitis	58
9.	Bronchial asthma	9
10.	Pulmonary emphysema	28
11.	Bronchiectasiae	38
12.	Bronchial carcinoma	21
13.	Hodgkin's disease	8
14.	Malignant lung metastasis	8
15.	Malignant lymphoma	2
16.	Bilateral bronchopneumoniae	13
17.	Chronic pneumonia	6
18.	Pleuripneumonia	2
19.	Mitral failure	6
20.	Myocardiopathy	48
21.	Neurofibroma	1
22.	Neurofibromatosis	1
23.	Mucoviscidosis	2
24.	Collagenosis	2
25.	Rheumatoid lung	1
26.	Retrosternal goiter	6
27.	Cystic lung	5
28.	Polyposis of bronchi	1
29.	Erythema nodosum (not of sarcoid etiology)	4
30.	Alveolar microlithiasis	2
31.	Visceral erythematodes	1
32.	Primary amyloidosis	1
33.	Echinococcosis of lungs	1
34.	Hilar adenopathies of unknown etiology	11
35.	Lung fibrosis of unknown etiology	10
36.	Diffuse round shadows of lungs of unknown etiology	3
	Total	376

The authors also studied necrosis in Kveim antigen. We have found necrotic central regions particularly in confluent granulomas in about 10% of cases. They seem to be acidophilic, granulated and fibrotic in the early period, but later on they are relatively without structure. In 1 case, areas of extensive necrosis contained some leucocytes, but without nucleolar detritus and they were partially surrounded with palisade-arranged epithelial cells.

Eosinophile leucocytes are found only in exceptional cases. In questionable positive

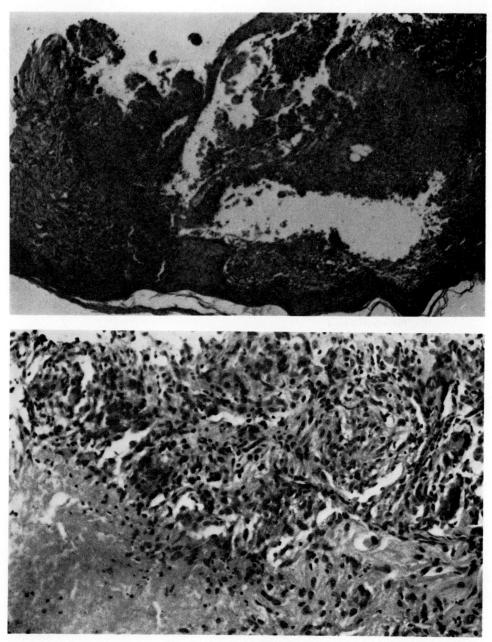

FIG. 1.   Necrosis of Kveim test.

findings the presence of histiolymphocytic granulomas accounts for probably early interrupted development of granulomas, and, probably, they might give a positive reaction
later on.

The presence of granuloma around a foreign body was observed in a number of
cases in our material. A cause of such granuloma may be a fragment of hair or horny
squama, probably introduced into the corium at the time of antigen application. In a
number of cases dark-brown to black circular irregular pieces were found to be sur-

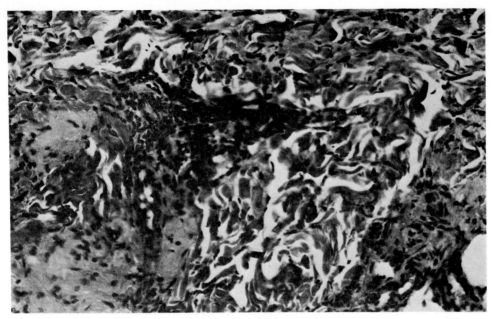

FIG. 2. Pigment in Kveim test.

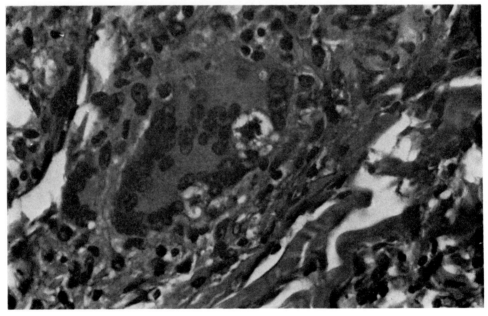

FIG. 3. Asteroid body in Kveim test.

rounded with giant cells. Such cases are anticipated as a giant-cell reaction toward probable unresorbed antigen.

In a number of specimens grey-blue inclusions of giant cells in the cytoplasm were observed, producing light bifurcation.

In a great number of our samples small granulated, powdered, dark, i.e., black, pigment was found almost predominantly in cytoplasm of histiocytes, and less frequently in giant cells. In individual cases the pigment gives positive reaction against melanin, but more frequently it is ceroid, as it stains purple-red after the method of Ziehl-Neelson. In some instances pigment particles are large often angular, brown-yellow and give positive reaction against iron, i.e., hemosiderin is considered.

With regard to the finding of inclusion bodies, literature data indicate that they are not noticed in the Kveim reaction with an explanation that a 6-week period is relatively short for their development; we may say we have found asteroid inclusions not clearly formed in 2 cases.

SUMMARY

The authors studied 608 patients to whom they applied their own Kveim antigen. Intrathoracic lymph nodes were most frequently used for antigen. Kveim test was found to be positive in 73.5% of sarcoid patients; that is 88% in intrathoracic localizations and 59% in extrathoracic localizations (sarcoid changes were not evident in the chest radiogram). The Kveim test was always negative in 376 patients ill with other diseases. In positive Kveim tests, sarcoid granulomas resembled those described in the literature. In 10%, the authors found necrotic central areas, particularly in confluent granulomas. Rare eosinophile leucocytes were exceptionally found whereas plasma cells were not observed in our material. In a great number of our speciments pigment was found which corresponded to either melanin or hemosiderin or ceroid. In 2 cases asteroid inclusions were observed which, however, were not clearly formed.

REFERENCES

1. Chase, M. 1960. The preparation and standardization of Kveim testing antigen. Sarcoidosis, Washington. *Am. Rev. Resp. Dis.* **84**: 86.
2. Siltzbach, L. 1963. An International Kveim test study, *Sarcoidosis* Stockholm. 178.
3. Hurley, T. H. and Bartholomeusz, C. L. 1969. An International Siltzbach-Kveim Test Study Using Australian /C.S.L./ Test Material /1966–1969. Prague. 343.
4. Jones Williams, W. 1969. A Histological Study of the Kveim Test Using the Australian Antigen. Prague. 349.
5. Behrend, H., Rupec, M. and Kessler, G. F. 1969. The Kveim Reaction. Prague. 352.
6. Odaka, M. et al. 1969. Kveim Test Using Japanese Antigens which Were Made from Pulmonary Hilar Lymph Nodes. Prague. 393.

Results Obtained with Australian Kveim Test Material 1966–1972

T. H. HURLEY AND J. R. SULLIVAN

The Department of Medicine, University of Melbourne, The Royal Melbourne Hospital, Melbourne, Australia

INTRODUCTION

Kveim test material has been produced at The Commonwealth Serum Laboratoires, Melbourne, since 1963 and has been distributed to investigators throughout the world since December 1966. Issue of the material was accompanied by a proforma on which details of cases tested and results obtained could be reported back to Melbourne. Between December 1966 and May 1969, 2038 completed proformas were received. Analysis of these was presented to the Fifth International Conference on Sarcoidosis in Prague in 1969. Between May 1969 and August 1972, a further 2704 reports were received. Kveim test results recorded on the proformas in these 2 periods form the basis of the present analysis.

MATERIALS AND METHODS

The test material used in all cases was derived from the same spleen obtained in Melbourne in 1963 from a patient with sarcoidosis and hypersplenism. The spleen was divided into portions of approximately 100 grams and these were stored in polythene bags at $-70°C$. Bulk tissue suspensions were prepared on 4 occasions. The ampoules of test material were dispensed from time to time from these bulk preparations which were stored at $-5°C$. Ampoules designated batch 0017–0023 were dispensed from the first bulk preparation in 1963, batch 0024–0032 from the second in 1965, batch 004 from the third in 1968 and batch 005 from the fourth in 1970. The method outlined by Chase[1] was used in the preparation of the batches prepared in 1963 and 1965. With the latter 2 preparations, 004 and 005, an additional step was introduced and the subcellular suspension, prior to diluting and ampouling, was filtered through muslin to clarify it.

Information was analysed from the proformas submitted as follows. Patients designated as having a diagnosis of sarcoidosis were those regarded by each investigator as having sarcoidosis on the basis of a compatible clinical presentation and a tissue biopsy (other than the Kveim biopsy) considered to be characteristic of sarcoidosis. Abbreviation of the information requested for the proforma after 1969 meant that it was not always possible to determine the specific diagnosis in those cases which were not thought to have sarcoidosis.

According to accepted convention, those cases of sarcoidosis with a duration of disease less than 2 years were called subacute; and those in which the disease lasted longer than 2 years were called chronic. In a number of cases the duration of disease was unknown. In the analysis these are included with the chronic group.

It was assumed that a report of a positive Kveim test was on the basis of histological examination of the test site. Many of the Kveim biopsies reported between 1966 and 1969 were read by Jones Williams. These were reported at the Fifth International Sarcoidosis Conference. After May 1969 histology was performed by the investigator in most cases.

The reports were divided into 3 groups—

Group A   Kveim tests performed between 1966–1969 with CSL batches 0017–0032*.

         * Previously reported in Prague in 1969.

Group B   Kveim tests performed between 1969–1972 with CSL batches 0017–0032.

Group C   Kveim tests performed between 1969–1972 with CSL batches 004 and 005.

This grouping permits a comparison between 2 differing batches used at the same time (groups B and C) and the same batch used at different times (groups A and B).

The number of test results in each group is shown in Table 1.

TABLE 1.

		Batches 0017–0032	Batches 004–005
Group A	(1966–1969)	2034	4
Group B	(1969–1972)	444	—
Group C	(1969–1972)	—	2260

RESULTS

In Group A, 510 cases of sarcoidosis were reported, in Group B, 129 cases and in Group C, 482 cases (Table 2). The percentages with positive Kveim tests in Groups A and B are not significantly different. The increased percentage with positive Kveim tests in Group C is significant.

If the cases reported as subacute are analysed separately, a similar percentage of positive Kveim tests is recorded in Groups A and B. The increase in positive Kveim tests in Group C is again significant.

TABLE 2.

	Total results	Positive results	% Positive
Sarcoidosis—total			
Group A	510	303	59
B	129	74	57
C	482	385	79
Sarcoidosis—subacute			
Group A	315	201	63
B	80	51	63
C	344	282	81
Sarcoidosis chronic and unknown			
Group A	195	102	52
B	49	23	46
C	138	103	74

TABLE 3.

	Total results	Positive results	% Positive
Nonsarcoids			
Group A	246	13	5*
B	41	4	9
C	363	116	31
Nonsarcoids—Tuberculosis			
Group A	48	1	2
B	1	1	—
C	112	45	40

* Cases designated " Nonsarcoid " and " Sarcoid suspect " in the 1966–1969 series reported in Prague have been in this current analysis reassessed on the basis of information submitted on the original proformas. A smaller number (246) were considered as " Non-Sarcoid " in this current analysis. This compares with 722 reported in Prague.

TABLE 4. Nonsarcoidosis diagnosis in Kveim—Positive cases.

	Group A	Group B	Group C
Tuberculosis	1	1	45
Inflammatory bowel disease	1	—	15
Carcinoma	1	—	3
Lymphoma	—	—	2
Leprosy	3	—	—
Pneumoconiosis	2	—	1
Pulmonary fibrosis	1	—	2
Agammaglobulinaemia	—	—	2
Others	4	3	46

In the cases reported as having a chronic duration of illness it is seen that a slightly lower percentage of positive Kveim test results is recorded in Group B, but this is not a significant difference. The increased number of positive Kveim tests in Group C, however, is significant.

In the cases with a disease diagnosis other than sarcoidosis it is seen that few positive Kveim tests were recorded in Groups A and B (Table 3). The slight difference in percentages is not significant. There is a marked increase in the number of positive Kveim test results in Group C. In those patients in whom a diagnosis of tuberculosis was recorded a significant increase occurred in the number of Kveim-positive cases in Group C.

Some of the other diagnoses associated with a positive Kveim test are shown in Table 4.

DISCUSSION

Group A cases and Group B cases utilised the same batches of Kveim test material. Group A cases were tested in 1966–1969 and Group B cases in 1969–1972. The results indicate no increase in the percentage of positive Kveim tests reported in these groups in patients with sarcoidosis whether they were taken in total or analysed according to disease duration. Similarly in these 2 groups there is no significant difference in the percentage of positive tests reported in patients with diseases other than sarcoidosis. The data does not permit an analysis of individual diseases other than sarcoidosis.

In Group C, a test material was used which had been prepared later and by a slightly different method. The results show significantly increased numbers of positive tests in sarcoidosis and also in patients suffering from diseases other than sarcoidosis. The change in reactivity of the Kveim test material is therefore related to use of new bulk preparations 004 and 005.

The reason for this increase in reactivity in the later prepared batches has not been established. Previous investigators[2] have recorded an alteration in reactivity of Kveim test material with time although details of storage were not recorded. The above analysis has shown that batches prepared after 1968 from the frozen spleen showed increased reactivity whereas batches prepared earlier from the same spleen but stored as ampouled test material over the same period did not.

Processing of the bulk suspension 004 and 005 after 1968 included an additional filtering step which was not included in the preparation of the earlier batches, 0017–0032. This may be significant in relation to the altered reactivity observed between these batches.

This problem is currently under investigation by in vivo testing of a further bulk preparation prepared in the same manner as was used with the batches prepared in 1963 and 1965.

ACKNOWLEDGEMENTS

The help of investigators who completed and returned the proformas, which form the basis of this survey, and of Drs L. Siltzbach and T. Izumi is gratefully acknowledged.

REFERENCES

1. Chase, Merrill W. 1961. Preparation and standardization of Kveim-Testing Antigen. *Amer. Rev. Resp. Dis.* **84**: 5, pert 2.
2. Nelson, Carl. 1957. *J. Chron. Dis.* 158.

False-Positive Reaction in the Kveim Test Using the CSL Kveim Material

TAKATERU IZUMI, YUKINOBU KOBARA, SHIGEHARU MORIOKA, ATSUHIKO SATO
AND SHUSUKE TSUJI

Chest Diseases Research Institute, Kyoto University, Kyoto, Japan

Using several lots of the CSL Kveim material from January, 1967 to June, 1971, 583 Kveim tests were done on patients with sarcoidosis and other diseases and on healthy Japanese and the results are discussed in terms of the difference in Kveim specificity among the batches.

MATERIAL AND METHODS

Ten batches of the Kveim material; 002 (0024, 0025, 0028), 003 (0030, 0031), and 004 (004–2, 004–3, 004–4, 004–5), supplied from the Commonwealth Serum Laboratories, Australia, through the courtesy of Dr T. H. Hurley, were used in our investigation.

Batches 002 and 003 were manufactured in June, 1965 and 004 in June, 1968. Following the indication, 0.15 ml of material was injected intracutaneously on the volar aspect of the forearm. Four weeks later, 6 weeks in some cases, a nodule and surrounded by erythema was measured and biopsy was done for microscopic examination. In a small numbers of cases inspection and palpation did not show any nodule and or erythema where a biopsy was omitted and the result was considered to be negative. The existence of epithelioid tubercle was diagnosed as positive, epithelioid cells without any tubercle formation as equivocal and other findings as negative.

In some cases, especially with lot 004, micronecrosis was observed macroscopically and microscopically but these were not related to the formation of epithelioid tubercles.

RESULTS AND DISCUSSION

1. In patients with pulmonary sarcoidosis showing abnormal chest X-ray findings, and within 1 year after presentation, the frequency of positive reaction was 78% (36 of 46)

TABLE 1. The Kveim Test using CSL Kveim material.

Lot number	002 and 003		004	
I. Pulmonary Sarcoidosis				
1. Active stage				
biopsy confirmed	24/30 (80%)	36/46 (78%)	32/37 (86%)	55/64 (88%)
suspected	12/16 (75%)		23/27 (85%)	
2. The stage after				
complete Regression		7/26 (27%)	25/35 (71%)	
II. Suspected Ocular Sarcoid		3/41 (7%)	44/71 (62%)	
III. Other diseases		0/25 (0%)	71/135 (53%)	
IV. Healthy		2/11 (18%)	13/29 (45%)	

Positive/tested (positive percentage).

in lot 002 and 003 and 88% (55 of 64) in lot 004.

No significant difference was observed between 2 batches in the biopsy-confirmed and suspected cases.

Where chest X-ray findings later showed complete regression, the difference in Kveim material potency between the 2 batch groups was remarkable, i.e., 002 and 003 batches showed a positive reaction in 27% (7 of 26) and 004 batches in 71% (25 of 35).

2.   Similar results observed at the regressed stage of sarcoidosis were obtained from patients with suspected ocular sarcoid lesions without abnormal findings on chest X-ray films. The Kveim-positive ratio in 002 and 003 batches was 7% (3 of 41) and 004 batches was 62% (44 of 71).

3.   In tests on patients with diseases other than sarcoid diseases, mainly composed of pulmonary diseases; pulmonary tuberculosis, chronic obstructive lung diseases, silicosis, carcinoma, etc., 004 batches showed a high percentage of positive reaction. In spite of no positive reactor out of 25 with 002 and 003 batches, 53% (71 of 135) were positive with 004 batch group.

4.   In normal individuals, 002 and 003 batches showed 2 positive of 11 and 004 batches resulted a high frequency of positive, 13 of 29.

Using 002 and 003 batches manufactured on June, 1965, false-positive results were few and the specificity of the Kveim test in sarcoidosis was confirmed as in past reports by Siltzbach and many other investigators. However, on 004 batch group, the specificity was not confirmed since there was a frequency of false-positive results, that is, 53% of diseases other than sarcoid diseases and 45% of healthy individuals.

In spite of the same sarcoid spleen origin, the specificity observed in 002 and 003 group has been lost in 004 batches. Recently, Hurley and Lane reported that the manufacturing procedure of 004 and 005 batches could possibly have resulted in the introduction into the material of small particles of cotton at the stage of final filtration (1971, Lancet **ii**: 1373) and the report is concordant with the results in our Kveim tests.

It is thought that this report re-emphasizes the recent comments on CSL antigen. It is suggested that recent false-positive reactions in nonsarcoid diseases containing Crohn' disease may be caused by inadequate antigen used for the tests.

SUMMARY

Many cases of false-positive reaction in the Kveim test were given by nonsarcoid patients and healthy individuals when tested using the CSL antigen, but it was shown by analysis of the results that false-positive results had been mainly introduced with batches of 004 manufactured on June, 1968.

Surveillance of Kveim Test Results

LOUIS E. SILTZBACH

The Mount Sinai School of Medicine, City University of New York, New York, U.S.A.

In the past 2 years, a myth seems to be developing that the Kveim reaction, which for 30 years has been considered around the world to be a valuable diagnostic tool in sarcoidosis, is no longer that, but is, in fact, a nonspecific response encountered in lymphadenopathy of all causes[1] and certain disorders of the gut.[2, 3] The investigators whose reports have been fostering this myth of Kveim nonspecificity have not, in my judgment, followed some basic rules for setting up a scientific hypothesis. Their aberrant Kveim test results have simply been a matter of failure to employ proper controls each step of the way leading toward their proposed new hypothesis.

Did it not strike these investigators as odd that for 30 years the Kveim test, which had easily withstood the few periodic challenges to its specificity, had suddenly been transformed into an almost meaningless diagnostic exercise? As one scrutinizes the published reports of those investigators reporting a high frequency of false-positive Kveim reactions in nonsarcoid conditions, one soon becomes aware of the puzzling absence of concurrent injection of the same Kveim test material (CSL 004–005) they were using in their patients with lymphadenopathy and gut diseases, into other nonsarcoid subjects who did not present lymphadenopathy or gut diseases. If they had also injected their batches of test suspensions into patients with pneumonia, asthma, chronic bronchitis, silicosis, Hodgkin's disease, collagen disorders, or into healthy controls, they would have become aware as Drs Izumi et al. from whom you have already heard, and Dr Chretien[4] and Drs Bringel and Loefgren[5] had become aware, that these batches of Kveim test material were eliciting frequent false-positive Kveim reactions in every category of subject tested and that the Kveim test results they were obtaining in their patients with lymphadenopathy of all causes and in certain gut diseases were, in fact, not specific Kveim responses at all. They would have realized that something had gone drastically wrong with those batches of Kveim test material (see Hurley et al. above) and they might have tried to obtain Kveim test material of *known* specificity and sensitivity as did Bringel and Loefgren.[5] The latter had observed positive Kveim reactions with the now-withdrawn CSL 004 batches in 9 of 12 patients with various collagen disorders; but when they retested these patients with another continually validated Kveim suspension (spleen J) they found no falsely positive reactions. In other words, monitoring of Kveim test suspensions is a continuing process but, in my experience, once validation of a bulk batch of Kveim material is established, that batch almost invariably will maintain its specificity throughout its shelf life.

A typical example of a previous challenge to the specificity of the Kveim reaction was a report of frequent false-positive reactions in nonsarcoid conditions, tuberculosis, histo-

This work was supported by a research grant from the National Heart and Lung Institute, Public Health Service (HE–13853–14).

TABLE 1. Kveim test results with 2 different sarcoidal spleen suspensions in 11 patients with active tuberculosis and 5 cass with nonsarcoid neurological disorders.

	Kveim nodule size at 4–6 weeks			Microscopic Kveim readings								
				Assessor I			Assessor II			Assessor III		
	>3 mm	3 mm or less	No nodule	+	−	±	+	−	±	+	−	±
Spleen A	9	2	5	5	9	2	8	4	4	1	8	7
Lot 8-type I (Chase-Siltzbach)	0	1	15	0	16	0	0	16	0	0	16	0

plasmosis etc. by Daniel and Schneider[6] in 1962. These authors used a sarcoidal splenic preparation processed by Dr M. Perlich of Cleveland (spleen A). I obtained some of this material and injected it in parallel with lot 8 of spleen J suspension into 11 patients with active tuberculosis and 5 patients with nonsarcoid neurologic disorders. Biopsies of all Kveim sites were made at 6 weeks and were read blind by 3 assessors, 2 being the pathologists who read the slides originally for Daniel and Schneider, the third (III) being myself (Table 1). Both papule size and microscopic assessments are shown.

Spleen A is "Perlich spleen" used by Daniel and Schneider and lot 8—type I (Chase-Siltzbach) is our standardized spleen J preparation. The 2 test materials yielded vastly different results in the 16 nonsarcoid patients. As Table 1 shows, with lot 8 only 1 insignificant Kveim papule less than 3 mm in size could be recognized with the naked eye. With Perlich's spleen A, on the other hand, 9 of the 16 patients exhibited papules larger than 3 mm at 6 weeks. More important, Assessor I read blindly 5 sites as showing positive Kveim reactions and Assessor II read 8 positive Kveim reactions out of the 16. In addition, these 2 readers found, respectively, 2 and 4 sites to be equivocal Kveim reactions. My own blind readings (Assessor III) of the Perlich spleen A results were 1 positive Kveim reaction and 7 equivocal reactions. Contrast these results obtained with Perlich's spleen A and those of the concurrently injected Lot 8 suspensions below. All 3 readers, on independent assessment, found the 16 Kveim sites uniformly negative, microscopically. Here, then, it would seem, we have an instance of conclusions concerning Kveim specificity drawn on the basis of results observed with the use of a relatively nonspecific sarcoidal test suspension (spleen A) along with a degree of over-reading of microscopic changes present at the biopsy site.

A Comparison of Two Commonwealth Serum Laboratory Kveim Batches

Doctors Hurley and Sullivan (see above) have already presented their analysis of the Kveim tests made with the Australian test suspension (CSL) from 1966–1972. (At the time the present paper was being written these results had not yet become available.) In the next 2 tables, Tables 2 and 3, are presented in a preliminary fashion some data based on published reports and on data kindly made available to me early this year by Dr T. Izumi (see above for more exact figures), by Dr Chretien[4] and by Drs Bringel and Loefgren.[5]

While CSL test material made before 1968 elicited only 10 positive Kveim reactions among 976 nonsarcoid subjects, i.e., about 1%, CSL batches 004–005 (Table 3) made in 1968 and distributed until 1971 when it was withdrawn, provoked, according to pre-

TABLE 2. Kveim test results with CSL batches 0019–0031 in nonsarcoid subjects excluding Crohn's disease.

Author	No. of tests	No. positive
Hurley et al (1963–66)	135	2
Hurley Internat (1966–69)	722	6
Izumi (1967–69)	37	2
Jaroszewicz et al (1966–69)	41	0
Siltzbach (1964, 1971)	20	0
Brodthagen et al (1966–69)	21	0
Total	976	10 (1%)

TABLE 3. Kveim tests with CSL batches 004 and 005 in nonsarcoid subjects incl. Crohn's Disease.

Author	No. of tests	No. positive	Dis. incl.
Izumi	166	84	TB, other dis., healthy
Karlish	78	33	Crohn's ulc. col., coeliac
Chretien	34	22	Assorted dis.
Israel	22	8	Adenopathy
Bringel	12	9	Collagen dis.
Bartnik	8	7	Crohn's dis.
Fitzgerald	5	2	Liver granul.
Total	325	165 (51%)	

liminary figures, cross-reactivity in 51% of 325 subjects who presented with a wide variety of nonsarcoid disorders and also included healthy controls (see Izumi et al. above).

There is no need here to dwell upon some of the causes of this sudden loss of Kveim specificity of those batches of CSL test suspensions made in 1968 since Drs Hurley and Sullivan have already presented their views (see above).

Kveim Reactivity in Crohn's Disease and Other Disorders of the Gut

There still remains the puzzle of the positive Kveim reactions reported by Mitchell et al. in Crohn's diseases, ulcerative colitis and adult coeliac disease[7, 8] using a K12 spleen suspension, lots 5 and 14. These findings have not been confirmed by other workers employing suspensions *other* than the now-withdrawn CSL lots 004–005 series. Thus, cumulative Kveim test results in Crohn's disease reported by Jones Williams[9, 10] of Cardiff, Wales, Chapman et al.[11] of Manchester and Karlish et al.[12] of Reading, England, Hannuksela et al.[13] of Helsinki, Behrend[14] of Hanover, West Germany and the present author and colleagues[15, 16] show Kveim cross-reactivity in only 3 of 130 patients with Crohn's disease, a satisfactory level of only 2.3%. (Some of these investigators used the Kveim test products from the same K12 spleen employed by Mitchell et al. but not the same lots.)

Why Mitchell and colleagues continue to observe positive Kveim reactions in Crohn's disease and other diseases of the gut remains unexplained since Mitchell has stated that the K12 Kveim lots he had used in patients with diseases of the gut were continuously monitored in nonsarcoid subjects with normal gastrointestinal systems.

Criteria to be met by Satisfactory Kveim Suspensions

In Stockholm in 1963 at our Third International Conference of Sarcoidosis[17] I outlined the properties possessed by a satisfactory Kveim test suspension to be employed as a diagnostic agent in sarcoidosis.

First, the test suspension must contain a high enough concentration of the granuloma-producing factor or factors to evoke positive Kveim reactions in a majority of patients with *active* sarcoidosis—6 or more of every 10 patients tested.

Second, a properly screened suspension elicits in a responsive patient a histologically characteristic cutaneous papule within 4 to 6 weeks. The papule is composed of compact and discrete masses of epithelioid cells and occasional giant cells, exhibiting only a minor degree of fibrinoid necrosis and nonspecific inflammatory cellular reaction. Birefringent bodies may occasionally be present in small numbers.

Third, the Kveim papule grows slowly and in about 1/3 of responsive subject measures 5 mm. or more in diameter after 4 to 6 weeks. The tissue particles in a satisfactory test suspension are fine and are evenly dispersible on shaking the vial. Simultaneous injection of an equal volume and concentration of a satisfactory test suspension yields, in a responsive subject, like-sized papules in 4 to 6 weeks.

Fourth, and most important, a diagnostically effective Kveim suspension is bland, producing in nonsarcoid subjects no sizable papules and no true sarcoidal reaction histologically. Cross-reactivity of false-positive Kveim reactions should not exceed a level of 3% and when such aberrant reactions are present at all, they are characterized by small papules at 6 weeks which histologically exhibit few granulomas, poor in epithelioid cells and less compactly arranged than in the classically positive Kveim reaction elicietd in patients with sarcoidosis.

It is to be stressed that no Kveim test suspension can qualify for diagnostic use in sarcoidosis unless its nonreactivity has been conclusively demonstrated in a sizable group of a variety of nonsarcoid subjects. As stated above, should some particular nonsarcoid disorder be under investigation with respect to Kveim reactivity, it is of paramount importance that the same Kveim test material be *concurrently* studied in nonsarcoid disorders unrelated to the condition being focused upon. Obviously, the level of Kveim sensitivity of the test material when used in patients with active sarcoidosis must also be ascertained and monitored during such investigations. But it is not enough for the particular batch being used to provoke positive Kveim reactions with regularity in patients with active sarcoidosis as did CSL batches 004–005. To repeat, the crux of the matter with respect to Kveim specificity is how the Kveim suspension behaves in nonsarcoid subjects.

Monitoring bulk batches of Kveim suspensions need not be too onerous a task from a practical standpoint, provided the volume of the Kveim batches are made up in quantities sufficient for several hundred or more test doses, preferably prepared from a sarcoid spleen. A Kveim monitoring panel has recently been convened in New York City where the Department of Health and Hospitals has undertaken to distribute a Kveim suspension to several municipal hospital centers where sarcoidosis is under study. The Kveim test material has been processed in the Bureau of Laboratories using a portion of a sarcoidal spleen which has yielded highly specific Kveim test material in the past. Successive bulk batches of Kveim material are now being monitored for specificity and sensitivity by a local panel of investigators in several sarcoidosis clinics before their general distribution. Such Kveim-monitoring panels can be established on a national or international basis. Investigators thorughout the world should be encouraged to process, validate, and monitor their own Kveim suspensions.

To help reduce the discrepancies in the microscopic reading of biopsied Kveim injection sites by assessors in various countries, I have undertaken to prepare during the next year an atlas of colored phototransparencies containing 20 to 30 histologic Kveim-site patterns encountered in positive, equivocal and negative Kveim reactions. The hope is that with a wide enough spectrum of colored photomicrographs of Kveim biopsies before him, the assessor will be able to choose a pattern closest to the slide he happens to be reading.

In my view, the intracutaneous Kveim test as currently used will continue to be employed with profit in the diagnosis of sarcoidosis so long as recognized procedures for preparation of satisfactory Kveim suspensions are followed and accurate assessments of the microscopic responses at the injection site are made. From my own recent experience, the devising of a really specific *in vitro* Kveim test as a substitute for the intracutaneous test is still some way off. A specific *in vitro* test will, in any event, require the purest and most concentrated active fractions of Kveim material obtainable. We are continuing our long-standing effort to achieve this goal.

ACKNOWLEDGEMENTS

The author wishes to acknowledge the kindness of Dr T. Hurley and his colleagues for keeping me informed during their recent Kveim investigations and to thank Dr T. Izumi, Dr J. Chretien, and Drs C. Bringel and S. Loefgren for making available to me their prepublication data.

REFERENCES

1. Israel, H. L., and Goldstein, R. A. 1971. *N. Engl. J. Med.* **284**: 345.
2. Karlish, A. J. et al. 1970. *Lancet* **2**: 977.
3. Bartnik, W., and Zych, D. 1972. *Lancet* **1**: 154.
4. Chretien, J. 1971. *Proc. of European Conf. on Sarcoidosis*, Geneva. (in press).
5. Bringel, C., and Loefgren, S. 1971. *Proc. European Conf. on Sarcoidosis*. Geneva. (in press).
6. Daniel, T. M., and Schneider, G. W. 1962. *Am. Rev. Resp. Dis.* **86**: 98.
7. Mitchell, D. N. et al. 1969. *Lancet* **2**: 571.
8. Mitchell, D. N. et al. 1970. *Lancet* **2**: 496.
9. Williams, W. J. 1965. *Gut* **6**: 503.
10. Williams, W. J. 1971. *Lancet* **2**: 926.
11. Chapman, J. A. et al. 1972. *Lancet* **1**: 1097.
12. Karlish, A. J. et al. 1971. *Lancet* **2**: 438.
13. Hannuksela, M. et al. 1971. *Lancet* **2**: 974.
14. Behrend, H. 1971. *Proc. of European Conf. on Sarcoidosis*. Geneva. (in press).
15. Siltzbach, L. E. et al. 1971. *Lancet* **2**: 634.
16. Siltzbach, L. E. Unpublished data.
17. Siltzbach, L. E. 1964. *Acta Med. Scand.* **176** (suppl. 425): 74.

Absence of Relation Between Kveim Test and Adenopathies in Sarcoidosis and Other Diseases with Lymph Node Localizations

J. Turiaf, M. Menault, F. Basset, Y. Jeanjean and J. P. Battesti

Bichat Hospital, University of Paris, Paris, France

Since 1969, at the last international conference on sarcoidosis, various authors have repeated criticisms made against the specificity of the Kveim test. Some think that it gives erroneous answers in 64.7% of conditions distinct from sarcoidosis, and propose its subdivision. Others admit that its positivity is linked essentially to the presence and duration of adenopathies during the course of sarcoidosis. Underlining the occurrence of positive tests in nonsarcoidic lymphadenites they introduce a hypothesis that the Kveim test represents a particular immunological reaction of an unknown nature, linked to the presence of chronic lymph-node alterations of various origins, independent of the presence or absence of specific granulomas.

Our short note intends, by recalling with some clear, simple and easily controliable data, to discredit the notion of the unreliability of the Kveim test for a diagnosis of sarcoidosis and to prevent tish view being used as a step towards undermining this disease nosological entity. Sarcoidosis is in fact an autonomous disease. It is frequently very easily recognizable because most of the clinical and radiological characteristics are so significant: lupuspernio and cutaneous nodular sarcoids, Heerfordt syndrome, mediastinal and mediastino-pulmonary sarcoidosis stage I and II, etc . . . The nonspecificity of the pathological characteristics does not lessen its originality and does not prevent a differentiation from other conditions in which it is observed, especially in noncaseating epithelioid tuberculosis, which differs absolutely from it in its aspect, clinical evolution, bacteriological and humoral tests, and also by a negative Kveim test in all cases.

Sharp controversies in the past, about Frei test specificity for diagnosing benign inguinal lymphogranulomatosis, and about the autonomy of this lymphadeny, before its responsible agent was identified, strongly remind one of those who today oppose the Kveim test specificity or the differenciation of sarcoidosis as a definite disease, with whom we absolutely disagree. We are strongly convinced that the Kveim test is specific for sarcoidosis, which has a well-defined autonomy of still unrecognized origin. Other very different conditions have exceptionally or accidentally the same histological characters, but, for most of them, a cause is easily identifiable.

Kveim test specificity for sarcoidosis diagnosis

Large international investigations on Kveim test specificity agree in granting it a remarkable reliability for diagnosis of sarcoidosis[3]. Disagreements usually come from comments made after research on a limited number of cases, with reactogens which do not always offer sufficient garantees, and sometimes come from hasty reading of histological preparations, especially interpreting a plain foreign-body reaction as a positive answer.

We have tested 722 cases with 2 reactogens: 1 derived from large peripheric sarcoidal adenopathies of a patient of ours, the other coming from a voluminous splenomegaly of 850 g removed in 1968 from a Prench West Indian with severe multivisceral sarcoidosis. These reactogens were prepared according to Chase and Siltzbach[4, 5]. Results obtained for specificity of sarcoidosis diagnosis were equal to those recorded by Siltzbach after an international investigation, whose conclusions were published at the Paris Conference in 1966[3].

TABLE 1.   Investigation on Kveim test results in 722 cases.

	No. of cases	Kveim test		
		Positive	Negative	Equivocal
Histologically confirmed sarcoidosis	205	162 (79%)	35 (17%)	8 (4%)
Clinically presumed sarcoidosis without histological evidence	269	108 (42%)	115 (43%)	36 (14%)
Nonsarcoidic control diseases	258	0 (0%)	247 (96%)	11 (4%)

For the 722 cases having had a Kveim test (Table 1) analysis of collected data points out two notions:

1)   Unequivocal and frankly positive Kveim test in conditions different from sarcoidosis remains an exception. We did not record it in any of the 258 controls we tested, agreeing in this way with data established by Siltzbach, who estimates at 0.7%, the percentage of falsely positive tests, as a conclusion of his large international investigation.

2)   The total number of equivocal tests is 55 out of 722 tested cases, i.e., 7.6%. But one should notice that it is very small when sarcoidosis shows, as well as clinical signs, histological evidence: it reaches 8 out of 205 cases (4%). In control diseases obviously different from sarcoidosis, a rate of 4% was also found: 11 out of 258 cases. A higher percentage, 14% (36 cases out of 258) is noted in conditions not clinically incompatible with sarcoidosis but for which this diagnosis is still debatable. Such are the 36 doubtful tests obtained in 259 patients where clinical evidence was not clear, with no histological proof and no etiological label. This relatively small figure (7.6%) of Kveim tests difficult to interpret, most of which belong to an ill-identified pathology, cannot in all fairness, be used as an argument to lessen the reliability and specificity of the test, nor to disrupt the clinical entity of sarcoidosis.

Kveim test result during the course of sarcoidosis is not linked to the presence of adenopathy
Unlike L. H. Israel and R. A. Goldstein, we think that during sarcoidosis, the Kveim test is not linked to the presence of adenopathies, nor duration or persistance of these manifestations (Table 2). In 114 cases of histologically proved mediastino-pulmonary sarcoidosis stage II, i.e., with pulmonary involvement and associated mediastinal adenopathies, the Kveim test was positive in 84 cases (73.5%). In 46 cases of pulmonary sarcoidosis at the same stage, with histological signs but with neither peripheric nor mediastinal adenopathy, nor associated splenomegaly, the Kveim test was positive in 32 cases, i.e., 70%. In 10 cases of extrathoracic histologically evident sarcoidosis, where there was no pulmonary involvement, mediastinal or peripheric adenopathies, or radio-

TABLE 2. Ineffectiveness of lymph-node involvement on Kveim test reactions.

	No. of cases	Positive Kveim tests
Mediastino-pulmonary sarcoidosis stage II	114	84 (73%)
Pulmonary sarcoidosis stage II (no adenopathy or splenomegaly)	46	32 (70%)
Extrathoracic sarcoidosis (no adenopathy or splenomegaly)	10	8 (80%)

logically or clinically identifiable splenomegaly, the Kveim test was positive in 8 cases, i.e., 80%.

Examination of these results clearly shows that the presence or absence of adenopathy or splenomegaly has no influence over the Kveim test response, during the course of sarcoidosis. Positive percentages obtained in the 3 categories, distinguished according to whether they have or not identifiable lymph-node changes, do not give stastically significant differences.

Positivity of Kveim test is closely linked with sarcoidosis activity

One of the factors involved in provoking epithelioid granulomas formation, i.e., positivity of the Kveim test in the dermal area after reactogen injection, is correlated, as is usually admitted, to the degree of activity of recorded sarcoid lesions. Most of them are more active if the onset is recent, and changes young and fresh. This is what underlines the great difference 91%–73% (Table 3) of percentages of answers obtained by Kveim tests, done on 2 series of patients all having mediastinal adenopathies but at different stages of sarcoidosis evolution.

TABLE 3. Mediastinal and mediastino-pulmonary sarcoidosis.
(No. of cases: 215, Kveim test responses)

	No. of cases	Positive Kveim tests
Lymphomediastinal sarcoidosis stage I	101	91 (91%)
Lymphomediastinal and pulmonary sarcoidosis stage II	114	84 (73%)

TABLE 4. Kveim test reaction in lymph-node diseases distinct from sarcoidosis.

	No. of cases	Kveim test response		
		Positive	Negative	Equivocal
Toxoplasmosis	1	0	1	0
Silica adenopathies	2	0	2	0
Hodgkin's disease	3	0	3	0
Tuberculous lymphadenitis	12	0	12	0
Lymphosarcoma	2	0	1	1
Adenopathies of lymphoepithelioma	2	0	1	1
Malignant reticulosis	1	0	1	0
Brill-Symmer's disease	1	0	1	0
Chronic lymphoid leukemia	1	0	1	0

Kveim test is negative during the course of adenopathies with nonsarcoidal etiology.

Using a reliable reactogen and reading histological slides carefully in order to discard inflammatory foreign-body reactions, which should be looked for and recognized, Kveim test gives no positive answer in the case of adenopathy which does not belong to the pathology of sarcoidosis. We subjected 25 cases of such adenopathies to Kveim test. In 24 cases the reaction was frankly negative. In 1 case of lymphosarcoma it was doubtful (Table 4). This is one reason among others, why we do not subscribe to Israel and Goldstein's hypothesis.

SUMMARY

We studied Kveim test reactions in patients with lymph-node sarcoidosis, in other patients with sarcoidosis without lymph-node involvement, and in patients with nonsarcoidic lymph-node diseases. Results of these studies show clearly that these reactions are linked to the sarcoidal nature of the disease, and that they have no relation with the presence or absence of lymphadenopathies.

BIBLIOGRAPHY

1. Saltiel, J. C., Hirsch, A., George, C., and Chretien, J. 1972. Etude de 182 tests de Kveim utilisant l'antigène CSL. La *nouvelle Presse méd.* **1**: 1483.
2. Israel, H. L., and Goldstein, R. A. 1971. Reaction of Kveim antigen to lymphadenopathy —Study of sarcoidosis and other diseases. *New Eng. M. Med.* **284**: 345.
3. Siltzbach, L. E. 1967. An international Kveim test study. Rapports de la IVe Conf. intern. sur la Sarcoîdose, un vol. Paris: Masson et cie. p. 201.
4. Chase, M. W. 1961. The preparation and standardization of Kveim testing antigen. *Amer. Rev. Resp. Dis.* **84**: 86.
5. Chase, M. W., and Siltzbach, L. E. 1961. Further studies on the fractionation of material used in intracutaneous diagnostic test for sarcoidosis. *Experta Med. Amst.* séries **42**: 76.
6. Turiaf, J., and Battesti, J. P. 1971. A propos de la spécificité du test de Kveim. *La Presse méd.* **79**: 2211.
7. Siltzbach, L. E. 1967. Aspects cliniques et expérimentaux du test de Kveim dans la sarcoîdose. *Le Poumon et le Cœur,* **23**: 49.

Kveim Reactivity and Patterns of Organ Involvement in Sarcoidosis

LOUIS E. SILTZBACH AND TAPAN K. SARKAR

The Mount Sinai School of Medicine, City University of New York,
New York, U.S.A.

Recently it has been suggested by Israel and Goldstein[1] that Kveim reactivity in sarcoidosis is almost completely dependent upon the presence of lymphadenopathy in this disease. It was further maintained by the authors that even with active extrathoracic or pulmonary lesions, the Kveim reaction will be negative unless lymph node involvement coexists.

A more recent study by Turiaf and Battesti[2], however, maintains that the presence or absence of lymphadenopathy *per se* does not influence the frequency of positive Kveim reactions in sarcoidosis.

In view of this disparity in the findings in these 2 reports, we undertook an analysis of the Kveim test results of 596 patients with tissue-confirmed sarcoidosis observed at the Sarcoidosis Clinic of the Mount Sinai Hospital, New York over the past quarter century. We employed our standardized and continuously monitored spleen J test suspensions in the majority of the subjects tested. Kveim biopsy test results were assessed by the usual microscopic criteria and by papule size at 4 to 6 weeks.

Out aim was to determine possible correlations between any given organ involvement present at the time of Kveim testing and the microscopic results of the Kveim test as well as the size of the Kveim papule at biopsy.

RESULTS

In Table 1 are listed microscopic Kveim test results and papule size (5 mm or larger) according to extrathoracic organ involvement present at the time of testing. In all, less than one-third of the patients manifested 1 or more extrathoracic localizations. The table shows a remarkable uniformity in percentages of positive Kveim reactions and of papules 5 mm or larger. Positive Kveim reactions ranged between 77% and 100%. Kveim papules 5 mm or larger were present in 34% to 80% of patients with the listed organ involvement. The percentages were no higher in patients who had peripheral adenopathy or positive scalene-node biopsies than they were in patients with other organ localizations.

In Table 2, the same correlation has been made between Kveim test results, papule size, and the radiographic chest X-ray stage. What is to be especially noted in this table is that even among patients with a normal chest X-ray (stage 0) or a chest X-ray with mottling only (stage III), 67% and 79% still showed positive Kveim tests. Furthermore, about 2 of every 5 of these stage 0 and stage III patients exhibited papules 5 mm or larger

This work has been supported by a research grant from the National Heart and Lung Institute, Public Health Service (HE–13853–14).

TABLE 1. Results of Kveim reaction and size of specific Kveim papules according to organ involvement among 596 patients with sarcoidosis.

Organ involv.	No. of pts tested	No. Kveim-positive	% Kveim-positive	% of pos with 5mm or larger Kveim papules
Periph. LN	171	154	90	54
Skin	107	97	91	56
Eye	98	89	91	56
Liver	92	84	91	45
E. N.	78	72	92	58
Spleen	71	60	85	34
Scalene LN	57	50	88	52
Salivary gl.	41	37	90	60
Resp. Mucos.	41	36	88	61
Lacrimal gl.	40	40	100	80
Others	62	48	77	42

TABLE 2. Results of Kveim reaction and size of specific Kveim papules according to chest X-ray patterns among 596 patients with sarcoidosis.

Chest X-ray Pattern	No. of pts Kveim tested	No. Kveim-positive	% Kveim-positive	% of Kveim pos. with 5 mm or larger papules
Stage I BHL	281	265	95	62
Stage II BHL and lung mottling	190	176	93	48
Stage III Lung mottling only	83	66	79	39
Stage 0 Normal lung pattern	42	28	67	43

at 6 weeks. The earlier stages, stages I and II, shared the highest percentage of positive Kveim reactions, but in stage II, the percentage of papules 5 mm or larger fell off significantly.

Our findings agree with those of Turiaf and Battesti[2] who could not detect any significant correlation between lymphadenopathy in sarcoidosis and positive Kveim reactions. As we have previously shown[3] the progressive loss of Kveim reactivity noted on retesting patients with sarcoidosis is governed by the subsidence of disease activity and by its duration. But even patients with no detectable activity of disease may retain their Kveim reactivity for a decade or longer.

REFERENCES

1. Israel, H. L., and Goldstein, R. A. 1971. Relation of Kveim-antigen reaction to lymphadenopathy. *New Engl. J. Med.* **284**: 345.
2. Turiaf, J., and Battesti, J. P. 1971. A propos de la specificité du Test de Kveim. *La Presse Medicale* **79**: 2211.
3. Siltzbach, L. E. 1964. Significance and Specificity of the Kveim reaction. *Acta Med. Scand.* (suppl. 425) **176**: 74.

Some Recent Observations on the Kveim Reaction

D. N. MITCHELL

MRC Tuberculosis and Chest Diseases Unit, Brompton Hospital, London, Great Britain

K. F. W. HINSON

Brompton Hospital, London, Great Britain

N. H. DYER

Queen Elizabeth Hospital, Birmingham, Great Britain

J. M. T. WILLOUGHBY

St Bartholomew's Hospital, London, Great Britain

AND

P. CANNON

Harold Wood Hospital, Essex, Great Britain

INTRODUCTION

In 1969, we reported[1] the results of Kveim tests made with a single lot (lot 5) of a carefully validated sarcoid spleen suspension (K12) and more recently[2] the results of Kveim tests with lot 5 and lot 14 of K12 and with Hurley sarcoid spleen suspension in patients with Crohn's disease. We describe here our further observations on the Kveim test in Crohn's disease and ulcerative colitis together with the results of Kveim tests in a preliminary study in patients with coeliac disease and primary biliary cirrhosis following tests with lot 5 of K12 and with early lots of Hurley Kveim test suspension.

PATIENTS AND METHODS

We aimed to do Kveim tests in patients with active or recently active disease who were not receiving corticosteroids during the period of Kveim testing. The Kveim tests were given intracutaneously (0.15 ml) on the ulnar aspect of the forearm; each test site was marked with ' Pelikan ' ink. The maximum diameter of any papule present was recorded in millimetres at the time of full-thickness skin-punch (4 mm) biopsy 4–6 weeks after injection. Serial sections of each biopsy were read ' blind ' (KFWH) according to the criteria of Siltzbach and Ehrlich[3] without knowledge of the nature of the subjects tested or the identity of the test suspension.

RESULTS

Crohn's disease: Tables 1 and 2 give the results of single tests with lot 5. Of 117 patients 52 (44%) had positive Kveim tests (Fig. 1). Of 50 patients who had positive tests 8 had papules of 5 mm or more; 17, 4–5 mm; 24, 1–3 mm and only 1 had no papule at the test site. Tables 3, 4 and 5 give the results following simultaneous tests with lot 5

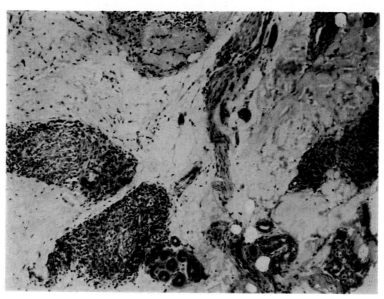

FIG. 1.

TABLE 1.   Results of microscopic reading of Kveim test biopsies
in patients tested with lot 5 of spleen K 12.

Diagnosis	Positive	Equivocal	Negative	Total
Definite Crohn's disease *with* histological confirmation	24 (5)	6 (1)	23 (5)	53
Definite Crohn's disease *without* histological confirmation	18 (1)	3 (1)	12 (3)	33
Probable Crohn's disease	7	1	5	13
Doubtful Crohn's disease	3	7	8 (1)	18
Total	52 (44%)	17	48 (41%)	117

( ): Patients receiving steroids during the period of Kveim testing.

TABLE 2.   Diameter of Kveim papules in patients with Crohn's disease tested
with lot 5 of Spleen K 12 related to microscopic reading of Kveim test.

Diameter of Kveim papule (mm)	Microscopic reading of K 12 tests			Total
	Positive	Equivocal	Negative	
5	8	0	0	8
4–5	17	0	1	18
1–3	24	8	16	48
0	1	7	30	38
Total	50	15	47	112

and Hurley (lots 0025 and 0042). No fewer than 12 of 23 patients showed a micro-scopically positive response to both tests (Table 3); results among patients previously tested with lot 5 and amongst those tested initially with lot 5 and lot 0025 or 0042, were closely similar.

TABLE 3. Results of microscopic readings of Kveim test biopsies in patients with Crohn's disease tested simultaneously with lot 5 of spleen K 12 and early Hurley spleen suspensions; lots 0025 and 0042.

Microscopic reading of K 12 suspension	Microscopic reading of Hurley suspension			Total
	Positive	Equivocal	Negative	
Positive	12	2	0	14
Equivocal	2	3	1	6
Negative	0	0	3	3
Total	14	5	4	23

TABLE 4. Results of microscopic readings of Kveim test biopsies in patients with Crohn's disease previously tested with lot 5 of spleen K 12 and subsequently tested simultaneously with lot 5 of K 12 and with Hurley spleen suspension; lot 0025.

Microscopic reading of K 12 suspension	Microscopic reading of Hurley suspension			Total
	Positive	Equivocal	Negative	
Positive	8*	1	0	9
Equivocal	2	1	1	4
Negative	0	0	3	3
Total	10	2	4	16

* Including 1 patient tested with lot 0042 Hurley.

TABLE 5. Results of microscopic readings of Kveim test biopsies in patients with Crohn's disease tested initially and simultaneously with lot 5 of spleen K 12 and Hurley spleen suspension; lot 0042.

Microscopic reading of K 12 suspension	Microscopic reading of Hurley suspension			Total
	Positive	Equivocal	Negative	
Positive	4	1	0	5
Equivocal	0	2	0	2
Negative	0	0	0	0
Total	4	3	0	7

TABLE 6. Results of microscopic readings of Kveim test biopsies in patients tested with lot 5 of spleen K 12.

Diagnosis	All patients				Patients having rectal biopsy			
	Kveim test result			Total	Kveim test result			Total
	P	E	N		P	E	N	
Definite Ulcerative Colitis	2	1	26	29	2	1	22	25
Probable Ulcerative Colitis	3	0	1	4	1	0	1	2
Doubtful Ulcerative Colitis	0	0	1	1	0	0	1	1
Total	5 (15%)	1	28 (83%)	34	3 (11%)	1	24 (86%)	28

TABLE 7. Diameter of Kveim papules in patients with ulcerative colitis tested with lot 5 of spleen 12 related to microscopic reading of Kveim test.

Diameter of Kveim papule (mm)	Microscopic reading of K 12 tests			Total
	Positive	Equivocal	Negative	
5	0	0	0	0
4–5	4	0	1	5
1–3	1	1	15	17
0	0	0	12	12
Total	5	1	28	34

TABLE 8. Results of microscopic readings of Kveim test biopsies in patients with ulcerative colitis previously tested with lot 5 of spleen K 12 and subsequently tested simultaneously with lot 5 of spleen K 12 and Hurley spleen suspension—lot 0042.

Microscopic reading of K 12 suspension	Microscopic reading of Hurley suspension			Total
	Positive	Equivocal	Negative	
Positive	0	0	0	0
Equivocal	1	0	1	2
Negative	0	1	5	6
Total	1	1	6	8

TABLE 9. Results of microscopic readings of Kveim test biopsies in patients with coeliac disease tested simultaneously with lot 5 of spleen K 12 and Hurley suspension; lot 004–4.

Microscopic reading of K 12 suspension	Microscopic reading of Hurley suspension			Total
	Positive	Equivocal	Negative	
Positive	4	1	0	5
Equivocal	0	0	0	0
Negative	4	0	1	5
Total	8	1	1	10

TABLE 10. Results of microscopic reading of Kveim test biopsies in patients tested with lot 5 of spleen K 12.

Diagnosis	Kveim test results			Total
	Positive	Equivocal	Negative	
Crohn's disease	52	17	48	115
	3	0	2	5*
Ulcerative colitis	5	1	28	34
Coeliac disease	5	0	5	10
PBC	0	1	5	6

* Lot 14; spleen K 12.

Ulcerative Colitis: Tables 6 and 7 give the results of single tests with lot 5. Of 34 patients 5 (15%) had positive Kveim tests; 4 had papules of 4–5 mm and 1 a 3 mm papule. Table 8 gives the results following simultaneous tests with lot 5 and Hurley (0042) among 8 patients previously tested with lot 5; 4 were reactive, all 4 showed a microscopically positive result at both test sites.

Coeliac disease: Table 9 gives the results in 10 patients tested initially and simultaneously with lot 5 and Hurley (lot 004–4). 4 showed a microscopically positive response to both tests but a discordance of response is indicated by the 4 patients who were positive with Hurley (lot 004–4) and negative with lot 5 (K12).

Crohn's disease, ulcerative colitis; coeliac disease and PBC: Table 10 summarises our findings in patients with Crohn's disease, ulcerative colitis, coeliac disease and primary biliary cirrhosis following initial and single tests with lots 5 or 14 of spleen K12. Of 5 patients with Crohn's disease tested with lot 14, 3 were positive. Of the 6 patients with primary biliary cirrhosis tested with lot 5, 1 was equivocal and 5 were negative.

SUMMARY AND CONCLUSION

The rate of Kveim reactivity of 50% following single tests with lot 5 in patients with definite or probable Crohn's disease is closely similar to that found in our earlier reports,[1,2] in which a similar rate of reactivity was obtained in patients with Crohn's disease following simultaneous tests with lot 5 and Hurley spleen suspension. Among patients with ulcerative colitis in the present study only 5 (15%) positive Kveim tests were encountered among 33 patients with definite or probable ulcerative colitis and there was a similar and close concordance of results following tests with lot 5 and with Hurley (lot 0042) suspensions both yielding a similar low rate of reactivity.

These findings are similar to those reported following in vitro tests. Thus, Brostoff and Walker[4] found that 47% of patients with Crohn's disease showed inhibition of leucocyte migration in the presence of lot 14 (K12) used as antigen, but found no inhibition of migration in patients with idiopathic proctocolitis. Similarly, Willoughby and Mitchell[5] found inhibition of migration of leucocytes in 12 of 18 patients with Crohn's disease using a suspension derived from yet another sarcoid spleen (K19) as antigen, but no comparable effect on leucocytes from patients with ulcerative colitis.

Lot 5 of spleen K12 has been the subject of careful validation.[6] Following simultaneous tests with lot 10 of spleen J (kindly made available by Dr Siltzbach) and lot 5, 70% of patients with active sarcoidosis gave a positive reaction whereas only 2 (1.6%) positive reactions were encountered in nonsarcoid subjects, 1 in a patient with quiescent pulmonary tuberculosis and 1 in an apparently healthy subject. Thus, the findings for lot 5 (K12) compare favourably with those for the International Kveim Test Study reported by Siltzbach in 1966.[7] The early lots of Hurley suspension were likewise found acceptable when validated alongside Siltzbach's spleen J[8] and showed only 12 (1.7%) positive Kveim tests following the routine biopsy of test sites in 722 patients with a wide variety of diseases other than sarcoidosis and Crohn's disease in the course of the continued International Kveim Test Study (1966–69).[9] Conversely, a later lot of Hurley suspension (004–2) used in our present studies showed more positive results than lot 5 (K12) following initial and simultaneous tests among patients with coeliac disease and it may be therefore, that this or other later batches of Hurley material, might be less discriminate than the earlier lots. Although lot 5 (K12) has consistently yielded positive reactions among patients with Crohn's disease, this lot (lot 5) did not yield positive Kveim tests among patients who were apparently healthy; hence, although concurrent tests in healthy subjects might be helpful in establishing the continued validity of Kveim suspensions during future prospective studies, the results in healthy subjects would be unrelated to relative selectivity in other conditions.

Suspensions derived from spleen K12 and from Hurley spleen have yielded acceptable results in Great Britain and internationally for several years. We conclude that lot 5 and lot 14 of spleen K12 and the early lots (0025 and 0042) of Hurley suspension are highly selective for sarcoidosis, but show a relative selectivity of response in certain other conditions as described in this report.

REFERENCES

1. Mitchell, D. N., Cannon, P., Dyer, N. H., Hinson, K. F. W., and Willoughby, J. M. T. 1969. *Lancet* **2**: 571.
2. Mitchell, D. N., Cannon, P., Dyer, N. H., Hinson, K. F. W., and Willoughby, J. M. T. 1970. *Lancet* **2**: 496.
3. Siltzbach, L. E., and Ehrlich, J. C. 1954. *Amer. J. Med.* **16**: 790.
4. Brostoff, J., and Walker, J. G. 1971. *Clin. Exp. Immunol.* **9**: 707.
5. Willoughby, J. M. T., and Mitchell, D. N. 1971. *Brit. Med. J.* **3**: 155.
6. Mitchell, D. N., Bradstreet, C. P. M., and Sutherland, I. 1971. *Proc. Fifth Int. Conf. on Sarcoidosis.* Prague: Univ. Karlova. p. 375.
7. Siltzbach, L. E. 1967. *La Sarcoidose* (Paris). p. 201.
8. Hurley, T. H., and Barthomeusz, C. L. 1967. *La Sarcoidose* (Paris). p. 194.
9. Hurley, T. H., and Bartholmeusz, C. L. *Proc. Fifth Int. Conf. on Sarcoidosis.* Prague: Univ. Karlova. p. 343.

The Kveim Test in Brucellosis

Eirian Williams

Pembroke County Hospital, Pembrokeshire, Great Britain

Bovine brucellosis is common in Britain, recent pre-eradication surveys in certain areas showing infection in more than 25% of herds. Human disease, especially in farm workers, is also relatively common and in West Wales 110 patients have recently been studied. In these the diagnosis was beyond reasonable doubt and in others in whom it was less certain, sarcoidosis was rarely included in the clinical differential diagnosis.

Erythema nodosum, claimed as a manifestation of brucellosis[1] was not seen in this series and chest X-rays were normal in all but 1 patient who had a transient shadow in the left lung. The occurrence of " pulmonary brucellosis " therefore, with generalised snowflake mottling and hilar adenopathy, was not confirmed and furthermore it is likely that early described examples of this supposed complication were due to unrecognised intercurrent sarcoidosis.[2] Eye changes in 1 patient caused real diagnostic difficulty. Five years after presenting with acute brucellosis he returned with uveitis. Antibody tests were no longer positive and sarcoidosis had now been diagnosed elsewhere but liver biopsy was inconclusive. Granulomas demonstrated in 37 patients with brucellosis had no special diagnostic features, except that even when numerous they were consistently smaller than some of the lesions common in sarcoidosis; and none showed hyalinisation.

In areas where brucellosis is enzootic and sarcoidosis also occurs it would seem important to know the value of the Kveim test in differential diagnosis.

MATERIALS AND METHODS

The Kveim test was performed on 58 patients. Antigen K.12, batches 16 to 18, was used, up to 0.2 ml. being injected intradermally on the left forearm. An ink marker was not employed and conventional dissection biopsy was performed at the end of six weeks.

The series was divided into 4 groups. Thirty-two patients in group I attended a brucellosis follow-up clinic. One had presented with pulmonary embolism and influenza and at the same time his blood had contained brucella antibodies in high titre. Another, a symptomless farm worker, also had strongly positive serological tests. In the remainder a clinical diagnosis of brucellosis had been made, although 1 had an associated iron deficiency anaemia and 1 was an alcoholic. All patients in this group had positive brucella antibody tests when the Kveim test was performed.

Eleven patients, in group 2, at some stage had shown serological evidence of brucellosis. In the majority antibody tests were no longer positive and it is arguable whether their persisting symptoms were due to the disease.

Group 3 comprised 8 patients with sarcoidosis, histologically confirmed in 5. Seven had presented with bilateral hilar lymphadenopathy associated in 4 with erythema nodosum. In group 4 there were 7 patients with a variety of disorders. In one, who had cholelithiasis, chest X-rays had shown prominent hilar shadows, but in none of the remainder had a diagnosis of sarcoidosis or brucellosis been entertained. Brucella

96

TABLE 1. The Kveim test in 58 patients using antigen K 12.

		Positive	Negative	Equivocal
Brucellosis	32	7	23	2
? Brucellosis	11	1	6	4
Sarcoidosis	8	5	3	0
Others	7	0	7/6	0/1

antibody tests on the patients in groups 3 and 4 were consistently negative.

RESULTS

Biopsies were evaluated ' blind ' and independently by 2 observers, Dr D. N. Mitchell and Dr K. F. W. Hinson at the Brompton Hospital, London. After reassessment when the clinical diagnoses were known their readings were unchanged (see accompanying table). One observer reported that all the Kveim tests in group 4 were negative, and the other observer reported that 6 were negative and 1 was equivocal. Their findings otherwise were identical. Six of the positive results in group 1 were obtained using K12 batch 18 and 1 using batch 17. The 1 positive result in group 2 was obtained using K12 batch 18. Six patients in group 1 had positive results 10 months to 12 years after the onset of symptoms, the test being positive also in the symptomless farm worker who had serological evidence of infection. In 5 patients the Kveim test was performed 6 months to 5 years after antibiotic treatment was first prescribed, 3 were still complaining of symptoms but 4 were symptom-free.

The patient in group 2 with a positive Kveim test was a farmer whose herd was heavily infected with brucella abortus. His wife was undergoing treatment for brucellosis and his own symptoms of two and a half years duration also suggested this diagnosis. His spleen was enlarged and after antibiotic treatment he recovered and his spleen was no longer palpable, but serological confirmation was confined to a weakly positive phenol saline agglutination test on 1 occasion, and the test was negative when the Kveim test was performed.

All patients with positive Kveim tests in groups 1 and 2 were seen by a consultant ophthalmologist. Slit-lamp examinations were normal and no evidence of sarcoidosis was found. X-rays of chest and hands were also normal.

DISCUSSION

Hitherto the Kveim test has not been tried in any large number of patients suffering from brucellosis. Test suspensions inadvertently prepared from patients suffering from brucellosis as well as sarcoidosis might be expected to contain brucella antigen but it is unlikely that the positive results in the present series are due to a late Mitsuda-like response. Spleen K12 was obtained from a patient who had always lived in an urban community. She had never been known to suffer from brucellosis and a serological test for brucella antibodies 4 years before splenectomy was negative.

These findings therefore are unexplained, and while the Kveim test using a validated antigen would appear to be unhelpful in the differential diagnosis of brucellosis from sarcoidosis, the study is now being continued using other test suspensions. Meanwhile in rural areas, especially in Britain where K12 is the antigen in routine use, when the Kveim test is unaccountably positive the possibility of past infection with brucella abortus should be considered, although serological tests for brucella antibodies may no longer provide confirmatory evidence.

ACKNOWLEDGEMENTS

I wish to thank Dr D. N. Mitchell and Dr K. F. W. Hinson for their evaluation of the Kveim biopsies, and Mr A. H. Haley, Consultant Ophthalmologist, for help with the clinical assessment of patients.

I also thank Mr D. A. Woolley for technical assistance.

REFERENCES

1. Harris, H. J. 1950. Brucellosis. New York.
2. Harvey, W. A. 1948. *Ann. intern. Med.* **28**: 768.

Preliminary Results in Testing a Commercial Kveim Antigen in Sarcoid and Nonsarcoid Patients

H. Behrend

Department of Rheumatology, Medizinische Hochschule Hannover, Hannover, Federal Republic of Germany

M. Rupec

Department of Dermatology, Phillips University, Marburg, France

AND

W. Jones Williams

Welsh National School of Medicine, Cardiff, Great Britain

We would like to present our assessment of a commercially prepared Kveim-Siltzbach, type 1, antigen and a comparison of its activity with that of a similar noncommercial antigen previously reported by Behrend, Rupec and Kessler.[1] The demand for a sufficient supply of an effective antigen is urgent and our preliminary findings are very encouraging.

The antigen was prepared from 30G of pooled mediastinal lymph nodes from 1 patient with proven sarcoidosis. The preparation was based on that of Chase[2] modified by ultrasonic homogenisation. The final product was proven free of bacteria, including tuberculosis and fungi and was tested at various concentrations.

Twenty-two patients with active sarcoidosis, not on steroids (Table 1) and 18 nonsarcoid subjects were tested (Table 2). The sarcoid patients were all injected with 2.5 mg dry weight of antigen and some also tested with 1.25, 5.0 and 7.5 mg (Table 3). The effective concentration was found to be 5.0 mg and was the dose used in testing the nonsarcoid group.

In the sarcoid group all test sites were biopsied and 11 of 18 in the nonsarcoid cases. All biopsies were adequate and included subcutaneous tissue. The slides were read independently by 2 authors (M.R. and W.J.W.) and the second author (W.J.W.) concurred with the original reading in 99% of the cases.

Our results demonstrate that the commercial antigen, in sarcoid patients, gave a positive rate of 73%, doubtful 18% and negative 9%, and no clinical or biopsy positive

TABLE 1. Kveim test with a commercial antigen—Sarcoidosis.

Sarcoidosis	Number	Diameter of the reaction papule, mms								Histology		
		0	1	2	3	4	5	6	7	Positive	Doubtful	Negative
Stage I	12			1	3	5	2		1	10	2	0
Stage II	7				2	4	1			6	1	0
Stage III	2	1		1						0	1	1
Orbital only	1			1						0		1
Total	22	1		3	5	9	3		1	16 (73%)	4 (18%)	2 (9%)

99

TABLE 2. Kveim test with a commercial antigen — Nonsarcoid.

	Diagnosis	n	Clinically		Excision	Histology negative
			Positive	Negative		
1.	Tuberculosis	7	0	7	3	3
2.	Lung abscess	1	0	1	1	1
3.	Lung mycosis	1	0	1	1	1
4.	Idiopathic lung fibrosis	1	0	1	1	1
5.	Erythema nodosum	1	0	1	1	1
6.	Idiopathic Optic neuritis	1	0	1	1	1
7.	Crohn's disease	1	0	1	1	1
8.	Polyarthritis	2	0	2	1	1
9.	Hodgkins disease	1	0	1	1	1
10.	Healthy persons 1 normal 1 gastric ulcer	2	0	2	0	0
	Total	18		18	11	11

TABLE 3. Diameter reaction papule of Kveim test using a commercial antigen.

Antigendose (dry weight in mg)	Number of patients	Diameter of the reaction papule
1.25	7	0–2 mm
2.5	22	0–5 mm
5.0	8	4–7 mm
7.5	5	4–8 mm

tests in the nonsarcoid group. In comparison, the previous report (Behrend et al.) showed 87% positive, 4% doubtful and 9% negative tests in sarcoidosis and 1 doubtful positive (tuberculosis patient) in 70 nonsarcoid subjects. The doubtful readings include biopsies which show foreign-body reaction and/or collections of epithelioid-like cells. This finding high-lights the importance of further testing before the antigen is fully evaluated.

The optimal concentration of the commercial antigen appears to be 5.0 mg as compared with 2.5 mg of the previously tested noncommercial antigen. This is likely to reflect the potency of the antigen as they were both similarly prepared from mediastinal lymph nodes.

In conclusion, our preliminary results are encouraging, as this antigen appears to be specific for sarcoidosis, though further testing is required to complete the evaluation. It has been arranged that additional sarcoid tissue will be available for the preparation of more antigen, but as is generally agreed, each batch will have to be carefully tested for specificity and potency before use.

ACKNOWLEDGEMENTS

We wish to thank Hermal-Chemie, Hamburg, for the antigen preparation and for their generous support of this investigation.

REFERENCES

1. Behrend, H., Rupec, M., and Kessler, G. F. 1971. *Fifth Int. Conf. on Sarcoidosis* (ed. L. Levinsky and F. Macholda). Prague. p. 352.
2. Chase, M. W. 1961. *Amer. Rev. Resp. Dis.* **84**: 86.

DISCUSSION

1

Chairmen: T. Hurley and T. Izumi

Dr Kataoka: Can you tell me, Dr Kalden and Dr Jones-Williams, the nature of the active principle for the MIF test, especialy the molecular size. In Dr Izumi's paper he said a rather large molecular size is needed to induce the Kveim skin reaction. In the case of the in vitro test is a macromolecular size needed or not?

Dr Kalden: We didn't look at the molecular size of the Kveim antigen and as long as even the real nature of Kveim antigen is not known. You can not expect data regarding the molecular weight. All we did was to measure the protein content of the antigen, which we put in the culture chambers. We found that we got the best results with a protein content of 70 mg per culture, measured by Lawry's method.

Dr Jones Williams: This is something that obviously needs to be done, something we are trying to do and I am sorry that at the moment, we have no information on it.

Dr Kataoka: Is there any difference, particularly in molecular size, between the in vitro test and the in vivo skin test of the Kveim reaction? If there is some difference between these factors, can you explain the discrepancy between the skin reaction and KMIF test?

Dr Jones Williams: No, there was no difference. This is the difficulty. I have no explanation for these discordant results in that it was the same preparation. The only difference was that the antigen for skin test was phenolised and that for the Kmif test, the in vitro test, was nonphenolised. Otherwise, there was the same protein concentration. I am glad you brought this up. Ours was 250 micrograms protein concentration. This was very much higher than that used

and reported by Dr Topilsky and Dr Siltzbach when they found negative results. Our protein content is also higher than that used by Dr Kalden. This is important I think, and it may reflect an excess antigen-antibody reaction, again like a PHA test. We don't really know whether this Kmif test and the PHA-type lymphocyte transformation are realy measuring delayed hypersensitivity.

Dr Izumi: I have questions to Dr Kalden and Dr Jones Williams with regard to the cells producing migration inhibition factor. I understand that in sarcoidosis and in Hodgkin's disease we can commonly find depressed T-lymphocyte function and B-lymphocyte function is normal or elevated. So, in general I would not expect the production of any substance from depressed T-lymphocytes. I suppose you get production of MIF from B-lymphocytes.

Dr Kalden: I do think that the evidence for a depressed T-cell function in sarcoidosis is not very good. Results in the literature are very conflicting. Furthermore, one simply does not know yet how much the T cell needs to be suppressed to stop producing mediators. You know that peripheral lymphocytes from patients suffering from sarcoidosis and being under steroid treatment can still produce MIF. I don't think there is at present any evidence of MIF-production by B cells.

Dr Izumi: My question to Dr Jones-Williams is whether a Kveim reaction is an immunological reaction or not. If the Kveim reaction is an immunological reaction, I think it is a very delayed reaction, and the T-lymphocytes relate to the Kveim reaction.

Dr Jones Williams: It would be nice to know whether the circulating lymphocytes used for these tests are T or B cells. In fact, of course, they are mixture of both.

The other thing that is important to remember is that though in theory we divide lymphocytes into T and B cells, in practice. I am sure that they transform one into the other and I can say that without fear of contradiction. I suspect very strongly that one type of lymphocyte T cell may be changed directly to a B, and a B can change to a T and there is no doubt at all that a B can affect a T and a T can affect a B.

DR HANNGREN: May I try to complicate it still more? When doing the MIF test or the Kmif test, we don't know what kind of cells we are dealing with, B or T. It is a mixture. And we have assumed before that the MIF was coming from the T cells: but is this sure? All these tests made in the past has been made on this mixture which may contain both T and B cells. Maybe MIF comes from B cells?

DR JONES WILLIAMS: We all presume that they are T-cells. One piece of evidence for T-cells is that the B-cell secretion of immunogloblins is very different as far as is known. There is not very much known chemically about the MIF factors, about the nature of lymphokines, but they don't appear to be ordinary globulins. They have a much lower molecular weight, and there are a number of physicochemical characteristics which distinguish them from ordinary immunoglobulins. However, we still don't really know from which of the 2 cell types they are produced. I was very happy to read Drs Douglas's and Siltzbach's paper on EM of the Kveim test, in that I have reported on the same sort of material myself. I was delighted to see that they had found the same type of vesicles, which we consider in our group is the hallmark of the epithelioid cell. He also showed many pictures of what he calls lysosomes, in that he found what some people could call dense bodies or residual bodies. There is no doubt that in the Kveim test you get these more often than you do in the sarcoid biopsy itself in sarcoidosis. Therefore I think there is some difference between the type and the nature of epithelioid

cells in the Kveim test, and in sarcoidosis: in a paper I gave in Geneva, I showed pictures of the EM of the Kveim test and like Dr Siltzbach. I did find in some cells, quite a lot of probable lysosomes but I will say more about this in a paper later in the conference.

DR NOGUCHI: Dr Kalden has employed the leucocyte migration inhibition technique, which is more popular in the northern Europe. Dr Jones Williams, however, has employed the MIF test. I would like to ask which is more reliable for evaluating the T-cell function or a delayed-type response. I would also like to ask Dr Kalden about population of leucocytes in the assay system.

DR KALDEN: I think your first question was which test is more suitable, the type of indirect leucocyte migration test as used by Dr. Jones Williams and others, or the direct leucocyte migration technique as described by Søberg and Bendiesen. Not in sarcoidosis but in other clinical hypersensitivity states both tests have been applied simultaneously giving nearly identical results. However I would think that the indirect test may be more sensitive and furthermore the indirect test has the advantage that one could try to quantitate the percentage of migration by diluting the supernatant of the antigen incubated human lymphocytes used in the migration inhibition test with guinea pig macrophages. Regarding the second question the ratio of leucocytes to lymphocytes in our test was about 60%, 70% leucocytes to 40%, 30% lymphocytes.

DR JONES WILLIAMS: I really agree with the previous answer that the macrophage, indirect method, which we have used is a cleaner, possibly more specific method. Therefore it is the one I would advocate. We obtained macrophages from guinea pig peritoneal cells which were not stimulated with oil. They were just washed with tissue culture medium and then the fluid extracted. But we find now as we are extending this test and doing it in a number of other conditions, that we get such a large bill for laboratory animals that we have to put oil into the peritoneal cavity to get enough macrophages. But, of the 2 techniques, I think possibly the indirect macrophage migration test is slightly more accurate.

2

Chairmen: A. C. DOUGLAS, R. FUKUSHIRO AND M. RUPEC

DR JOHNS: I would like to speak of my experiences with the Kveim test, using a splenic preparation from a patient at the Johns Hopkins Hospital which was validated and compared with Dr Siltzbach's preparation. It has behaved in a reliable fashion and had not seemed to give us problems of "false positives." I was aware as long as 4 years ago, having done several hundred Kveim tests, that there seemed to be a clinical correlation with the presence of sarcoid lymphadenopathy whether it be mediastinal or peripheral. To try and document this in some numerical fashion, I counted 100 consecutive Kveim tests that I had done. Selection of the patients was confined to those who had good documentation, both a compatible clinical picture and histologic confirmation of the diagnosis of sarcoidosis. It is impressive and of interest that of the positive ones in this total of 48, there were 42 who had definite adenopathy. Of the 40 who were negative, there was only 1 who had definite adenopathy. The suppressive influence of steroids on the Kveim test is something of which we are all aware. In the 44 patients who had an adenopathy and were not on steroids, 42 of those were Kveim-positive. It is certainly my impression that there is some correlation with the adenopathy, but with the adenopathy of sarcoid.

DR SATO: For our Kveim test we used lot number 0062 of the Hurley antigen. This batch was manufactured this year after discussion on 004 and 005 batches. In tests of sarcoidosis, all of the sarcoidosis patients were confirmed histologically by mediastinoscopy or other biopsy and within 2 years after presentation; 6 of 9 cases showed a positive reaction. As control cases we did the Kveim test on patients with pulmonary tuberculosis showing tuberculous bacillus and 4 suspected cases of pulmonary tuberculosis. In addition, we had healthy young people. All 16 tests showed negative results. In conclusion, the Kveim test using lot 0062 of Hurley antigen can be thought to be specific for sarcoidosis.

DR TAKAHASHI: I wish to present a couple of slides showing quite interesting granulomatous lesions in the Kveim test. The presence of fibrinoid necrosis is quite troublesome for diagnosis, and some pathologists may not accept it as positive. One side of the arm was injected only with Kveim antigen, and the other side was injected using Kveim antigen and lymphocytes collected from the patient's own peripheral blood. While typical granuloma was seen in the former case, inoculation with lymphocytes caused quite widespread fibrinoid necrosis. This inoculation was done in both arms of the patient at the same time. The presence of fibrinoid necrosis appears to be due to different hypersensitivity. I would like to hear an opinion about the criteria for Kveim reaction with fibrinoid necrosis.

DR IWAI: I think that in the case of necrosis in the Kveim reaction, we have to think about whether there are any typical granulomatous changes besides this necrosis. If there is typical change, this is positive. However, such necrosis may be seen in sarcoid lesions and if these necrotic regions in the Kveim reaction are similar to necrotic regions in sarcoid lesions, it may be judged as positive, but accompanied by necrosis, I think.

DR JONES WILLIAMS: In a previous series of 1000 cases of Kveim biopsies which I reviewed, there were 40 cases with so-called necrosis out of the 1000 biopsies. A little later, I could demonstrate fibrin in this area, and also found collagen. I demonstrated this at both the light microscopy and electron microscopy levels, and I could also demonstrate that the collagen fibrils were not always fully formed. They were sometimes deformed and did not show the correct 650 Å banding which they would normally do. Now I do not agree that finding so-called "necrosis" means the biopsy is necessarily negative. Dr Mitchell referred to the fact that I am at the moment reviewing another 500 cases of Kveim tests which come from a number of authors. One group comes from Dr Izumi, one from Professor Behrend, a number from Jaroszeicz, and from Dr Bringel and 50 cases from Dr Mitchell, making a total of 450 cases. Dr Seal at Sully Hospital in Cardiff and myself are reviewing these at the moment. Professor John Chapman, from Houston, Texas, has all the clinical information. What we are trying to do is to compare the detailed histological features with a number of different antigens, a number of different batches of antigen and in a variety of different diseases. I cannot analyze them at the moment because I have not yet been told what the antigen is or the disease in any particular case. I hope, within the next 6 months, to present this for publication. Now, we may be able to show that with one antigen there are more lymphocytes than with another. This is an impression I am getting already. But I don't know at the moment which that antigen is.

DR JOHNS: With regard to necrosis, when I was initially standardizing the spleen that we used for our Kveim suspension at Johns Hopkins, I used different dilutions. In some patients who were strongly reactive with dilute material, necrosis would occur with the more concentrated suspension, but with a more dilute suspension, I got only granulomatous change. It is my impression that the patients who are the most reactive may produce the necrosis, though the picture is fully compatible with sarcoidosis.

DR TAKAHASHI: I would like to mention the importance of lymphocytes given with the antigen in this case (JSC antigen). There may be some factor from lymphocytes, causing some damage to tissues or cells, such as lymphotoxin, but some other explanation such as accelerated hypersensitivity may be possible.

DR REFVEM: I should like to know whether pathologists studying sections from the Kveim reaction use the polarising microscope routinely. Giant cells are considered a feature of sarcoid tissue, but often they are caused by foreign bodies in the suspension and then of course they have nothing to do with a specific Kveim reaction. I was able to demonstrate this in several cases of Kveim tests carried out earlier. They are often crystalline and do not appear unless using the polarising microscope, which can visualize noncrystalline particles as well.

DR JAMES: It is worth restating the following elementary points and principles, which are important in practice:-
1) Good antigens stay good, whereas poor antigens which provoke nonspecific sarcoid responses stay poor. I would regard the reagent as a poor and nonspecific one if it provokes positive reactions in 50% of patients with Crohn's regional ileitis or indiscriminately in patients with lymphadenopathy from various causes. I found the test to be negative in a series of 30 patients with Crohn's disease, nor have I found it positive in glandular tuberculosis or toxoplasmosis. The Mount Sinai Hospital must have had unique experience over the years on this point since both L. E. Siltzbach and Burrill Crohn work there. Under the same roof, then, is a wealth of clinical material and a good Kveim antigen, but they do not find positive skin test responses.
2) It was mentioned earlier that the Kveim test could be done too soon. This is not true. It can be done too late but never too early. Indeed, the earlier you do the Kveim test the better.
3) It is most important to monitor the Kveim-Siltzbach test and the best way to do so is in a large and busy weekly Sarcoidosis Clinic to which patients with many different types of granulomatous disorders are referred. These patients with other granulomatous diseases form our inbuilt control group in

which the test is negative. If an antigen does become sour and nonspecific, then this will be recognised early because the clinic is held regularly every week. This weekly routine is far more likely to monitor adverse reactions early than some international panel sitting in lofty isolation. I distrust sarcoidologists who do not have such a weekly routine.

4) Finally, somebody stated that sarcoid granulomas in the liver constitute an indication for systemic steroids. This is, of course, quite untrue. Steroids may be given because of systemic involvement but not just because granulomas happened to be found in the liver.

DR TURIAF: J'ai été étonné par les chiffres que nous a donnés le Docteur Mitchell, 52% de tests de Kveim positifs au cours de la maladie de Crohn. J'avais déjà lu les publications du Docteur Mitchell et j'étais persuadé que ces resultats sont liés à la qualité de l'antigène qu'il utilise. Je vous ai cité les chiffres que j'ai obtenus en faisant systematiquemant des tests de Kveim avec mon propre antigène, et vous avouerez qu'ils sont en loin puisque il y en a 2 sur 35 cas. Or il y a un an j'ai eu la bonne fortune d'observer un malade atteint de maladie de Crohn en activìte. Il a été opéré d'une adénopathie ilíale, qui a été prélevée. A partir de cette adénopathie qui était assez volumineuse, j'ai fait, preparer dans mon laboratoire un antigène, et, selon les méthodes que nous employons habituelle-ment, et de cet antigène, il a été testé une douzaine de sarcoïdoses et également une douzaine et une quinzaine de sujets atteints de maladie de Crohn, comparativement avec un test de Kveim : experiénce forte interessante. Dans tous les cas, les reactions obtenues chez les malades atteints de sarcoïdose et de maladie de Crohn, se sont révélées négatives. Cette experiénce est concluante.

Elle démontre notament, que la maladie de Crohn et la sarcoïdose sont deux maladies différentes.

Elle suggère aussi que la réponse positive du test de Kveim, pratiqué dans la maladie de Crohn, est probablement la conséquence de la mauvaise qualité de l'antigène utilisé.

C'est ce que tendent aussi à prouver, en accord avec mes conclusions, les notions établies dans ce domaine par Siltzbach et par James en faisant appel à des antigènes dont la spécificité est rigoureusement éta_blie.

DR ISRAEL: I do not think the Kveim test is rubbish. I have great faith that its behavior is not wild, and that it is a specific recognition system. The factors it recognizes are most commonly found in sarcoidosis which is why everybody's results are the same in sarcoidosis. Two points I'd like to make. One is that if Hurley withdrew his antigen because of the frequency of positive reactions in other diseases, it would seem to me that British K12 antigen should be withdrawn also. It shown an almost equally high frequency of positive tests in a variety of other diseases, brucellosis, glandular tuberculosis, etc. I should like to emphasize that Dr James has been unfair in comparing my studies with some earlier Kveim studies because our studies have been carried out with the only two antigens (CSL and K12) that have been validated by controlled comparisons with Chase-Siltzbach antigen. As of our last conference in 1969, they were regarded as validated and equal. Hence we can't really dismiss those 2 antigens that easily. The final point I should like to make concerns what should be done to bring some order out of this chaos. I think I know what the International Committee, or what this Conference should recommend. An organization should be set up to which the various antigens should be sent in amounts permitting 500 tests, i.e., enough material to allow "double-blind" testing to be done. Interpretation should be done in a similarly controlled fashion. I think this will settle what differences there are. It also ought to be clear from the discussion this afternoon that there is no sense in wasting this material on healthy controls or in patients with miscellaneous pulmonary diseases. I would suggest that the control groups be confined to those patients in whom positives have been reported, namely to disseminated lupus, chronic lymphadenopathy, chronic lymphocytic leukemia, brucellosis, florid tuberculosis and regional ileitis.

DR HURLEY: I whole-heartedly agree with the suggestion which Dr Israel has made. In reply to a previous comment I would point out that in its initial validation our test material was used in 56 cases of tuberculosis and that 1 case gave a positive reaction. A nodule was also produced in a second patient in this series but biopsy was declined. Thus positive or possibly positive results were encountered in 2 of the 56 cases of tuberculosis tested. I do not know why it is that our test material now appears to react so differently. Our reason for withdrawing it, as a diagnostic agent, was that it was giving positive reactions in an unacceptably large number of patients with diseases other than sarcoidosis such as lymphoma and glandular tuberculosis, which could be confused clini_ cally with sarcoidosis. The reason for this apparent change in behaviour of our test material is still not clear but at the time we withdrew it one possible explanation for some of these positive results appeared to be that small particles of cotton may have been included in certain batches of test material during its manufacture. We thought we should alert investigators to this possibility and we did so. Since then we have not obtained any evidence that this in fact was the cause and today I personally doubt that foreign-body reactions are responsible. It seems more likely that with the passage of time some change has occurred in the test material which has altered the 'reactivity'. Early in 1971 we amended the literature accompanying our test material, indicating that positive reactions had occurred in patients not suffering from sarcoidosis.

DR ISRAEL: I must call attention to a contradiction in Dr James' remarks. He tells us that a good antigen never deteriorates, in which case there should be no need for constant surveillance. How does one tell a "good" antigen that can't deteriorate from a "bad" one that will? The CSL antigen is not producing foreign-body reactions due to some trivial change in preparation; it is producing typical sarcoid reactions in a variety of diseases. If this antigen had specificity when first prepared, it has undeniably lost it.

III GRANULOMATOUS DISEASES

Experimental Production of Sarcoidosis in the Lung

Kimio Yasuhira

*Department of Pathology, Chest Disease Research Institute,
Kyoto University, Kyoto, Japan*

It has been established that tuberculous lesions in animals can be induced by immune tissue responses to chemical factors of the tubercle bacillus. The pulmonary test which has been used in our laboratory for examination of biological activity of bacteria or their components is carried out as follows: 2 weeks after a subcutaneous injection of Freund's complete adjuvant (FCA) containing 5 mg of heat-killed tubercle bacilli ($H_{37}Rv$), 0.1 ml of the adjuvant containing usually 0.5 mg of the bacilli is instilled into the bronchial tree of sensitized and control rabbits through a fine plastic tube connected to a syringe. The animals are sacrificed at adequate intervals and the treated lung lobe is removed for histological examination. Biological activity of chemical fractions from tubercle bacilli is demonstrable by substituting 1 of the fractions for the bacteria as the challenging antigen.

Data obtained in these experiments are tabulated in Table 1. The bacterial cells caused extensive necrotizing lesions in tuberculo-sensitized animals. Bacterial polysaccharide fractions induced an Arthus type of necrotizing inflammation. Tuberculo-protein or -polypeptide fractions produced granulomas without histological specificity. Many lipoid fractions, such as fatty acids, acetone-soluble fat, and wax A, B, and C, were inactive in inducing immune tissue response. Only phosphatide fraction occasionally and wax D always could induce epithelioid cell granulomas which were specific for tuberculous lesions in histological appearance. The activity of wax D vanished after saponi-

TABLE 1. Chemical fractions of tubercle bacilli ($H_{37}Rv$) and their biological activities on tissue.

	Relative amount extracted (percent)	Immune tissue response		
		Necrotizing inflammation	Nonspecific granuloma	Epithelioid cell granuloma
Heat-killed tubercle bacilli	100.0	‖‖	‖‖	+
Tuberculopolysaccharide		‖	+	—
Tuberculoprotein		+	‖	—
Fatty acids (C_{6-27})		—	—	—
Acetone-soluble fat	9.3	—	—	—
Phosphatide	2.5	—	—	+
Wax A	3.5	—	—	—
Wax B	2.6	—	—	—
Wax C	1.5	—	—	—
Wax D	5.5	—	—	‖‖
Lipid moiety (mycolic acid)		—	—	—
Hydrosoluble moiety		‖‖	‖‖	—

fication. The lipid moiety of the saponified wax D, mycolic acid, is quite innocuous. On the other hand, the hydrosoluble part was markedly active in producing Arthus-type necrotizing lesions.

Although slight leucocytic infiltration due to bronchitis after the instillation of the oil mixture was inevitable, the granulomas induced by wax D were of epithelioid cells in appearance and regressed into fibrous tissue without any treatment within several weeks. On the basis of this evidence, we may call such lesions sarcoid. However, it should be noted that the occurrence of small necrotizing foci in the granulomas cannot be excluded on occasion. In addition, it may be difficult to consider that bacterial lipoids such as wax D are freed into tissue without concomitant liberation of the Arthus antigens of the bacteria. Therefore, a special immune condition which makes animals inactive to the Arthus antigens should be brought about. Desensitization of tuberculosensitized animals by repeated subcutaneous injections of old tuberculin until the skin reaction turns negative can change the wax D-inducing granulomas into typical sarcoid lesions without any sign of necrosis. The desensitizing treatment does not completely reduce the necrotizing inflamation in lesions caused by tubercle bacilli, although it is successful on occasion in inducing epithelioid cell-predominant lesions. On the other hand, treatment of animals with a small amount of FCA in utero or at birth can change the necrotizing lesions into sarcoid granulomas which may occur in partial immune tolerance to Arthus antigens of the bacteria.

It is well known that *Nocardia* is classified near the tubercle bacillus in microbiology and is very commonly distributed in the human environment. *Nocardia* organisms (*N. asteroides* strain No. 126) were propagated on a nonprotein liquid medium and subjected to chemical fractionation by the old methods of Anderson and Lederer after autoclave sterilization. The relative amounts of wax components of *Nocardia* cells were found to be considerably less than in tubercle bacilli. This is coincidental with the weak acid-fastness of *Nocardia*. In activity tests, the chemical fractions of this organism are very similar in activity to those of tubercle bacilli, as shown in Table 2. Epithelioid cell granulomas are induced only by the application of *Nocardia* wax D and phosphatide fractions into *Nocardia*-sensitized animals, although granulomas induced by the latter fraction consist in part of necrotizing foci due to Arthus antigens contaminating the fraction. No marked lesion is induced by the other lipoid fractions.

When heat-killed *Nocardia* organisms are introduced into *Nocardia*-sensitized animals,

TABLE 2. Chemical fractions of *Nocardia asteroides* and their biological activities on tissue.

	Relative amount extracted (percent)	Immune tissue response		
		Necrotizing inflammation	Nonspecific granuloma	Epithelioid cell granuloma
Heat-killed *Nocardia* cells	100.0	⧻	╫	╫
Acetone-soluble fat		—	—	—
Phosphatide	18.4	╫	+	╫
Wax A		—	—	—
Wax B	0.7	—	—	—
Wax C	0.06	—	—	—
Wax D	0.13	—	—	⧻

TABLE 3. Cross-reactivity between tubercle bacilli and *Nocardia* organisms.

Challenged with	Tuberculo-sensitized			*Nocardia*-sensitized		
	N*	G*	E*	N	G	E
Tubercle bacilli	+++	+++	+	+	+	++
Tuberculo-wax D	+	+	+++	−	−	++
Nocardia cells	−	−	+++	+++	++	++
Nocardia-wax D	−	−	++	−	−	+++

* cf. N stands for necrotizing inflammation, G for nonspecific granuloma, and E for epithelioid cell granuloma.

necrotizing foci surrounded by nonspecific granulomas are induced. This is quite comparable to the hypersensitive tissue response of tuberculosensitized animals to heat-killed tubercle bacilli. The epithelioid cell characteristics of these granulomas are negligible or scanty. On the other hand, when *Nocardia* organisms are injected into tuberculo-sensitized animals, epithelioid cell granulomas without a tendency toward necrosis can be induced. Similar lesions appear after injection of *Nocardia* wax D into tuberculo-sensitized animals. These data (Table 3) indicate that sarcoid lesions can be induced by cross-reactivity of *Nocardia* wax D to tuberculolipopolysaccharides. Arthus antigens of these bacteria are thought not to be cross-reactive at present. When tubercle bacilli were injected into *Nocardia*-sensitized animals, the treatment results also in epithelioid cell granulomas sometimes with necrotizing foci. Cross-reactivity between antigens from these 2 bacterial species is also recognizable in the skin test. Animals sensitized with tubercle bacilli or *Nocardia* cells reveal an evident skin reaction on intracutaneous injection of old tuberculin or of *Nocardia* culture filtrate. The reactions are typical of delayed hypersensitivity and appear less extensively at the site of the cross-reactive antigen than of the specific antigen.

In conclusion, the present author would like to present again the *Nocardia* hypothesis for the etiology of sarcoidosis as proposed by him since 1969 and supported at least in part by the successful cultivation of *Nocardia* organisms from the lymph nodes of patients with sarcoidosis (Uesaka, I. et al., 1970). Most cases of sarcoidosis may be induced by the invasion of *Nocardia* organisms into persons previously infected with tubercle bacilli or other related bacteria. This *Nocardia* hypothesis does not exclude other etiological assumptions for sarcoidosis. In addition, it may be said that sarcoid lesions can result from a delayed type of hypersensitive tissue response to any kind of antigenic lypopolysaccharides from bacteria or tissue components in animals under immune conditions avoiding the Arthus-type tissue response.

Experimental Attempts to Produce Sarcoidosis in Guinea Pigs

Takashi Matsuoka

Nihon University, Tokyo, Japan

Sabin and others injected each component of mycobacterium tuberculosis into the peritoneal cavity of guinea pigs and succeeded in producing epithelioid cell nodules in the peritoneum with protein or phospholipid. However, experimental studies have rarely been made on polysaccharide. The author tried the following experiment: Maruyama vaccine, which is a polysaccharide of tubercle bacilli, was injected subcutaneously into the right sole of guinea pigs, and histopathological studies were carried out on its influence upon the distinctly swollen right iliac lymph nodes and other organs. Maruyama vaccine is mainly composed of polysaccharide separated and extracted from the human strain of tubercle bacilli, H-37, of some free nucleic acid and rudimentary protein.

MATERIALS AND METHODS

PPD-negative normal guinea pigs weighing 300 to 400 g were divided into four groups, A, B, C, and D. 0.1 ml of Maruyama vaccine was injected 10 times in group A; 0.2 ml 10 times, 20 times and 30 times in group B; 0.3 ml 30 times in group C, and 0.2 ml 40 times in group D, in the right sole every other day. Five days after the final injection, the skin, right iliac lymph node and other organs were routinely examined histologically with hematoxylin-eosin and reticulum fiber staining. The results obtained are shown in Tables 1 and 2.

TABLE 1.   Histological findings.

No. of guinea pigs	Each dose (ml)	Times of injection	Results
Group A 5	0.1	10	Epithelioid cell (卅)
Group B 10 (2 died)	0.2	10	Epithelioid cell (卅) Reticulumfiber (卅) Giant cell (卅)
Group B 15 (2 died)	0.2	20	Epithelioid cell (卅) Giant cell (卅) Epithelioid cell tubercle (卅)

TABLE 2.   Histological findings.

No. of guinea pigs	Each dose (ml)	Times of injection	Results
Group B 5	0.2	30	Epithelioid cell (+) Leucocyte (卅)
Group C 5	0.3	30	Epithelioid cell (+) Leucocyte (卅)
Group D 5 (1 died)	0.2	40	Epithelioid cell (+) Leucocyte (卅)

CONCLUSION

Maruyama vaccine was injected repeatedly into the sole of guinea pigs intracutaneously, and histological studies were made on the iliac lymph nodes.

1. In the cases in which the injection of 0.2 ml was repeated 10 times and 20 times, sarcoid reaction was recognized histologically in the cortex and medulla, partly in the follicles.

2. No sarcoid changes were observed in the remaining cases.

The factor that sarcoid change developed in the iliac lymph node as a result of Maruyama vaccine injection into the sole of guinea pigs, led the author to the conclusion that polysaccharide, which is a component of tubercle bacilli, may play some role in the pathogenesis of epithelioid cell nodules.

Induction of Granulomas in Guinea Pigs

N. Shigematsu, T. Ishibashi, K. Matsuba, K. Emori,
T. Shirakusa, S. Ishimaru and K. Sugiyama

Research Institute for Diseases of the Chest, Faculty of Medicine,
Kyushu University, Fukuoka, Japan

Attempts to produce epithelioid granulomas have been performed by many investigaters[1-7]. An intradermal injection of Freund's complete adjuvant (FCA) has been

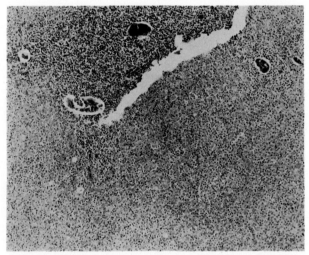

FIG. 1.   PAS-positive substances among granulomatous changes at injected site (2 weeks after FCA injection).   Mag. ×76.

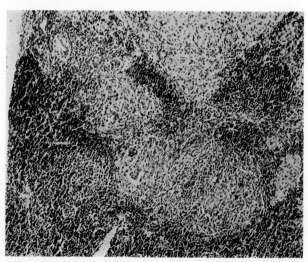

FIG. 2.   Epithelioid grnulomas in the inguinal lymph nodes at 3 weeks after FCA injection.   Mag. ×76.

shown to produce sarcoid-like granulomas in the focal lymph nodes, the lung and the liver.

In our experiments, 0.2 ml of FCA, 5 mg M. butyricum of wax D, 3 mg of acetylated wax D_6[8], 3 mg of D_6 with 1 mg of egg albumin were used. Each of the agents was injected into the footpads of 24 guinea pigs, which were sacrificed at weekly intervals. The tissues obtained from the footpads, the lymph nodes, the lungs, the liver and the spleen were stained with HE and PAS and also prepared for an electron-microscopic study.

At the site where FCA was injected, it was detected as PAS-positive substances in subcutaneous tissues a day after injection and in the granulomatous changes after 2 weeks (Fig. 1), but these substances were not clearly detected after 3 weeks.

In the inguinal lymph nodes PAS-positive substances were found in the peripheral sinuses a day after injection and epithelioid granulomas were seen predominantly at

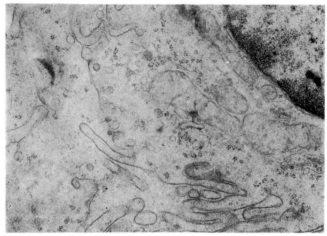

FIG. 3.   Interdigitation of cells in the epithelioid granulomas shown in Fig. 2. Mag. × 17,000.

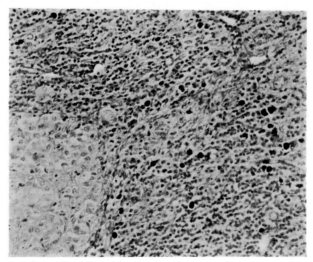

FIG. 4.   A number of PAS-positive bodies in macrophages around the epithelioid granulomas shown in Fig. 2.   Mag. × 200.

3 weeks after the injection (Fig. 2). The interdigitation of cells in the epithelioid granulomas were detected electron-microscopically (Fig. 3), and PAS-positive bodies were observed in macrophages around the epithelioid granulomas (Fig. 4). PAS-positive bodies were not found at 9 weeks after the injection.

Epithelioid granulomas in the lung were clearly found at the third week (Fig. 5). A few PAS-positive bodies were found in macrophages around the epithelioid granulomas (Fig. 6), especially in macrophage granulomas.

These findings, after intracutaneous injection of FCA are summarized in Table 1. In comparison with another experiment using wax D, FCA was shown to a similar ability to wax D for the production of such specific granuloma.

AD_6, a subfraction of acetylated wax D induced by Tanaka[8] at our institute, is known to be potent in adjuvant activity. The difference in findings induced by AD_6 and FCA

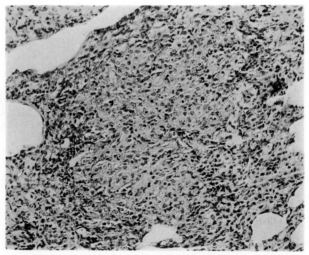

FIG. 5.   Epithelioid granulomas in the lung at 3 weeks after FCA injection. Mag. ×156.

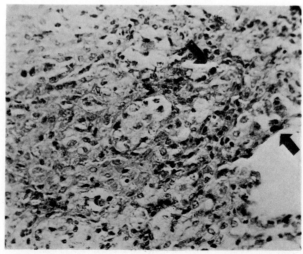

FIG. 6.   PAS-positive bodies in macrophages (arrows) around epithelioid granulomas shown in Fig. 5.   Mag. ×310.

TABLE 1. Findings after intracutaneous injection of FCA.

		2 weeks	3 weeks	4–6 weeks	9 weeks
Footpad	Epithelioid cells	±	++	++	+
	PAS bodies	+	+	±	−
Inguinal node	Epithelioid cells	±	++	+	+
	PAS bodies	+	+	±	−
Lung	Epithelioid cells	±	+	+	±
	PAS bodies	+	++	+	+

TABLE 2. Findings after intracutaneous injection of FCA and AD_6.

		AD_6 3 mg 3 weeks	FCA 0.2 ml 3 weeks	AD_6 3 mg 5 weeks	FCA 0.2 ml 5 weeks
Footpad	Epithelioid cells	±	++	±	++
	PAS bodies	±	+	−	±
Inguinal node	Epithelioid cells	±	++	±	+
	PAS bodies	±	+	±	±
Lung	Epithelioid cells	−	+	−	+
	PAS bodies	−	++	++	+

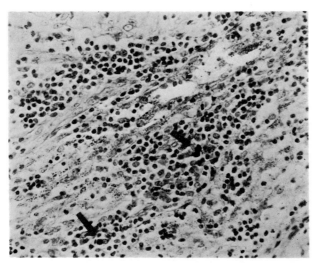

FIG. 7. A few PAS-positive bodies in macrophages (arrows) around epithelioid granuloma (upper part) in biopsied lumph node of human sarcoidosis. Mag. × 340.

injection is shown in Table 2. PAS-positive bodies were also found in the granulomas and in the alveolar septa of the lungs in guinea pigs injected with AD_6, but the cells in the granulomas were not mature epithelioid cells. As for AD_6 with egg albumin, we were unable to find a significant difference between AD_6 with albumin and AD_6 by itself.

According to the report by Carter[9], PAS-positive bodies were seen in the tissue sections in 22 of 200 human sarcoidosis cases. We have also detected PAS-positive bodies in the areas around epithelioid granulomas in human sarcoid tissue (Fig. 7). The characteristics and significance of these PAS-positive bodies in the human tissues still remains under study.

These experiments have been attempted through the need to elucidate the following problem relating to our clinical experience: In 8 of 58 cases of sarcoidosis, we have observed cloudy shadows localized in the upper or other part of the lung field in association with BHL and in the peripheral zones of the lung in distribution. The scalene node biopsies revealed sarcoid granulomas. The shadows showed spontaneous resolution in 3 months.

REFERENCES

1. White, R. G. et al. 1955. *J. Exp. Med.* **102**: 83.
2. Chase, M. W. 1959. Disseminated granulomata in the guinea pig (ed. Shaffer, Logrippe and Chase). Boston: 673.
3. Lauffer, A. et al. 1959. *Brit. J. Exp. Path.* **40**: 1.
4. Waksman, B. H. et al. 1960. *J. Immunol.* **85**: 403.
5. Waksman, B. H. et al. 1960. *Arch. Ophthal.* **64**: 751. N.Y.
6. Steiner, J. W. et al. 1960. *Arch. Path.* **70**: 424.
7. Pearson, C. M. et al. 1961. *J. Exp. Med.* **113**: 485.
8. Tanaka, A. et al. 1963. *Biochem. Biophys. Acta* **70**: 483.
9. Carter, C. J. et al. 1969. *Stain Technology* **44**: 1.

Pulmonary Sarcoid-Like Granulomatosis Provoked by Injecting Freund's Complete Adjuvant Intravenously in the Rat

F. Basset, P. Soler, L. Wyllie and J. Turiaf

Bichat Hospital, University of Paris, Paris, France

While improving a model for a physiological preparation, we checked morphologically pulmonary lesions induced in rats by intravenous injections of Freund's complete adjuvant (FCA). We were struck on the one hand by the high yield of pulmonary infiltrations and granulomas and on the other by the striking analogy of these lesions with specific noncaseating inflammatory lesions.

EXPERIMENTAL PROCEDURES

Two groups of rats were used:

1) The first group was composed of 57 male Wistar rats weighing from 300 to 500 g, of which 20 were without preparation as controls. Thirty-seven received 2 injections of 0.15 ml of CFA (Difco products Co., Chicago) at 24 hr intervals, in the femoral vein under slight ether anesthesia. All animals were killed after a variable time by lung and heart evisceration done under nembutal anesthesia, most at the end of a physiological experiment on an isolated heart-lung system.

2) In the second group 29 female rats weighing 80 g were used, 9 for control, the 20 others having survived 2 injections of 0.05 ml of FCA at 24 hr interval, in the tail dorsal vein. The total number of injected animals was 30 but 10 of them died sometime between the 2 injections or immediately after the second.

Aureomycin was given to both series of injected animals for a week.

The high mortality rate can probably be explained by the great youth of these animals. The rats had not been subjected to any physiological experiments before being killed. This allowed us to process them, for light and electron microscopy, much more carefully than in the first group, using the technique of Burri created in E. R. Weibel's laboratory[1], in the hope of obtaining suitable preparations for morphometry.

The total number of animals treated with FCA was 56 and there were 29 controls of corresponding age. It should be noted that the weights of treated animals was not significantly different from the controls.

RESULTS

A few abnormalities were irregularly found in all animals (FCA treated or not—with or without preparation) such as: diffuse cellular infiltration, macrophagic alveolitis, localized septal thickening.

They raise the question of latent or passing affections, of breeding contamination without clinical signs, or even morphological peculiarities or technical artefacts, without any specific significance.

Other modifications are exclusively observed in lungs of FCA-treated animals: they are essentially the presence of large vacuolated cells encased in alveolar walls or in connective septa, and also the presence of epithelioid cells and follicles with occasional giant cells. They are sometimes scattered all over 1 or several lobes and irregularly from 1 lobe to another in the same animal. These alterations usually predominate in subpleural and peribronchovascular areas, with a pleural cellular reaction about infiltrative and granulomatous lesions.

a)   Vacuolated cells are seen without exception in all lungs of FCA-treated animals. They contribute to the alveolar wall thickening and are often associated with mononucleated cells, mostly of the lymphocytic type. They are characterized in usual techniques by a huge vacuole or several small ones, empty-looking by usual techniques, rich in lipids stained by Sudan Black on frozen sections.

b)   Follicular structures are mostly composed of large elements with a faintly acidophilic cytoplasm, and oval- or kidney-shaped nucleus, delicately reticulated. These cells sometimes form compact groups or are arranged radially or concentrically round a central loose zone, occasionally occupied by a small necrotic or excavated area. One can also notice some giant cells amidst these follicular structures. They do not contain any cytoplasmic inclusion of a conchoid or asteroid type.

The nodule periphery is made of a crown of mononucleated inflammatory cells, predominantly lymphocytic. A discrete sclerous reaction is occasionally observed, of fibroblastic, collagenous and sometimes elastic type (later stages).

In 3 animals we also noted islets of bony metaplasia, incased in alveolar parenchyma.

QUANTITATIVE ESTIMATION

Following P. Burri's advice, a morphometric study was not undertaken: according to him, such a study, creating a large amount of work, could only bring few interpretable results, at least because of the irregular distribution of lesions from one lobe to another. Therefore an attempt to count follicular structures was made for both groups of prepared animals, particularly on the second group, where one could estimate an average number of nodules per slice of right middle pulmonary lobe. Twelve to 15 serial slices were examined for each animal according to Weibel's method.

Results are shown in tables and graph below.

TABLE 1.   FCA-treated animals of the first group.

	Time after FCA injections (T)					
	27	36	49	67	91	(days)
Approximate average number of nodules per slice of lobe ($\bar{N}$)	10	23	54	64	130	

TABLE 2.   FCA-treated animals of the second group.

	Time after FCA injections (T)										
	31	38	45	52	59	66	73	79	86	114	(days)
Average number of nodules per slice of right middle lobe ($\bar{N}$)	14	32	31	37	122	17	76	48	42	24	

Evolution of specific modifications provoked by FCA can be summarized in 3 steps:

1)   Early stage (2–4 weeks): numerous vacuolated cells are present in alveolar walls, as well as small epithelioid nodules scattered in subpleural regions.

2)   Medium stage (5–6 weeks): vacuolated cells remain while there is an increase in number of epithelioid nodules, which are predominant in peribronchovascular and subpleural regions, sometime joining into large areas.

3)   Later stage (10 to 15 weeks): lesions regress irregularly, sometimes leaving fibrosed residual granulomas. Later, bronchi are dilated, with a pus-like content amidst extensive fibrosis, in which there are vascular sections with thick walls and small lumen, alveolar gland-like remains and a few residual epithelioid nodules.

ELECTRON MICROSCOPY

Results of electron microscopy will be discussed later in a separate paper.

COMMENTS

FCA given subcutaneously[2–4] provokes an accumulation of histocytes at the injection site and a proliferation of reticular cells in regional lymph nodes.

Injected intravenously, it produces a diffuse proliferation of reticular cells and fibroblasts in many organs. This reaction is particularly marked in spleen, lung, liver, heart and lymph nodes[2–9].

Concerning the pulmonary system, the ability of dead mycobacteria to produce a tissue reaction similar to that of tuberculosis, has been known for a long time: mycobacteria killed by heat, kept in lipids, provoke pulmonary lesions in guinea pigs, rabbits, rats and also monkeys (Casals and Freund, 1939).

During sensitization of rabbits with FCA, mesenchymal cells react by forming a sensitized pulmonary substrate capable of a secondary reaction[10,11].

Detailed studies of intravenous FCA action on lung were made[5,12,13], some showing ultrastructural features. Experiments were done on rabbits and it seems that in this species, induced cellular reactions regress in 4 to 6 weeks. After 15 weeks, lungs show practically no remaining lesion, and it seems there is no residual fibrosis.

In a recent work, Strauss, Caldwell and Fritts[14] showed a model of proliferative pulmonary disease in the dog by intravenous FCA injections. They pointed out the resemblance of these granulomas with those of human sarcoidosis. Their morphometric study shows that 56% of of pulmonary tissue present granulomatous lesions and 2% have microabscesses. There were necrotic lesions only in 3 animals out of 6. Antibiotics were not given after FCA injections. Lesions were well tolerated: dogs remained apparently in good health in spite of the severeness of pulmonary lesions.

Description of these lesions was similar to the aspects we observed in rats, except that, with antibiotics, microabcesses were less frequent in our rats than in dogs studied by Strauss et al.

Results of our experiment confirm those of numerous authors previously mentioned, to which we can add some complementary remarks[15].

1)   Though reactions are roughly similar in various animal species, there may be some differences since previous authors, Strauss et al excepted, never mentioned the sarcoid-like aspect of induced granulomatous lesions. In rats as in dogs, the resemblance

of the lesions with noncaseating epithelioid granulomas of human sarcoidosis and hypersensitivity granulomatosis is striking, both in their cellular formation and their localizations, predominantly subpleural and peribronchovascular.

2) Different evolutions can also correspond to species differences. Particularly it appears from our experiments that rats keep their lesions for a much longer period than rabbits, as reported by Moore, Schoenberg et al.[6-8]. Indeed, animals killed after day 78 in the first series, showed granulomatous lesions, which were among the most numerous and the largest in this whole series. Likewise, in opposition to what Moore and Schoenberg observed in rabbits, rats seem to develop a certain residual fibrosis, that should be estimated after more prolonged experiments.

3) It appears that we can underline the high percentage of infiltrative lesions of lung tissue and noncaseating epithelioid granulomas with this method.

Such an experimental model shows 3 interesting points:—for physiological study of modified lung tissue—for a detailed morphological ultrastructural comparison of induced lesions with those of human affections of a similar histological type—from a clinical point of view: comparison of infiltrative processes and their physiological consequences, betewen experimental affections and human granulomatosis, can be bring new elements towards understanding the latter.

SUMMARY

Intravenous injection of FCA in the rat induces infiltrative and follicular pulmonary lesions, resembling human noncaseating granulomatoses of specific type in their localization and cellular pattern. They can be compared in particular to sarcoidal and hypersensitivity granulomatous lesions.

This simple method gives an experimental model with a high yield, convenient for physiological experiments. The rat appears particularly suitable because its pulmonary lesions, in spite of an excellent tolerance, regress more slowly than those of dogs and rabbits used by other authors.

Besides its physiological interest such a model allows detailed morphological studies and can bring fresh elements to the knowledge of histologically related human diseases.

REFERENCES

1. Weible, E. R. 1963. Morphometry of the human lung. Weibel-Springer. p. 49.
2. Freund, J. 1947. Some aspects of active immunization. *Am. Rev. Microbiol.* **1**: 291.
3. Freund, J., and Walter, A. W. 1944. Saprophytic acid-fast bacilli and paraffin oil as adjuvants in immunization. *Proc. Soc. Exp. Biol. Med.* **56**: 47.
4. Laufer, A., Tal, C., and Behar, A. J. 1959. Effect of adjuvant (Freund's type) and its components on the organs of various animal species; A comparative study. *Brit. J. Exp. Path.* **40**: 1.
5. Rupp, J. C., Moore, R. D., and Schoenberg, M. D. 1960. Stimulation of the reticuloendothelial system in the rabbit by Freund's adjuvant. *Arch. Path.* **70**: 43.
6. Moore, R. D., Rupp, J. C., Muhaw, and Schoenberg, M. D. 1961. The reticuloendothelial system in the rabbit. *Arch. Path.* **72**: 51.
7. Moore, R. D., and Schoenberg, M. D. 1963. Modification of cellular proliferation of the reticuloendothelial system in the rabbit. *Exp. Cell. Res.* **30**: 301–310.

8. Moore, R. D., and Schoenberg, M. D. 1964. The response of the histiocytes and macro phages in the lungs of rabbits injected with Freund's adjuvant. *Brit. J. Exp. Path.* **45**: 488.

9. Steiner, J. W., Langer, B., and Schatz, D. L. 1970. The local and systemic effects of Freund's adjuvant and its fractions. *Arch. Path. Chic.* **70**: 124.

10. Eskenasy, A., and Galbenu, P. 1966. Tuberculoprotein-induced reaction of the lung under different sensitization conditions. *Z. Immunitactsforsch* **131**: 94.

11. Eskenasy, A., Stoian, M., and Galbenu, P. 1967. Contributions to the immunomor-phology of sensitization. *Rev. Imm. Paris* **31**: pp. 75–88.

12. Bhagwat, A. G., and Conen, F. E. 1969. Characterization of " free alveolar cells " in experimental adjuvants induced pneumonia. *Arch. Path. Chic.* **88**: 21.

13. Faulkner, C. S., and Esterly, J. R. 1971. Ultrastructural changes in the alveolar epithelium in response to Freund's adjuvant. *Am. J. Path.* **64**: 559.

14. Strauss, B., Caldwell, P. R. B., and Fritts, H. W. 1970. Observations on a model of proliferation lung diseases. I and II. *J. Clin. Invest.* **49**: 1305–1310 and 1311–1315.

15. Basset, F., Soler, P., Fiez-Vandal, P. Y., Basset, G., and Turiaf, J. 1972. Granulomatose diffuse des poumons induite expérimentalement chez le rat par l'Adjuvant de Freund. *Ann. Med. Intern.* **123**: 1, 71.

Measure of Pulmonary Extravascular Water in Experimental Pulmonary Sarcoid-Like Granulomatosis in the Rat

G. Basset, P. Y. Fiez-Vandal, G. Lecouvez (Mle) and J. Turiaf

Bichat Hospital, University of Paris, Paris, France

Measuring pulmonary extravascular water by the multiple indicator method[1] was essentially applied on humans to assess pulmonary edema and secondarily in obstructive bronchopathies and emphysema. To our knowledge it was never studied in pulmonary granulomatosis. Because tritiated water can be equilibrated with extracellular and intracellular water, one can measure water in granulomatous process situated in perfused areas; unless this type of lesion invalidates the method (diffusion distance too large, transit times too widespread).

To check the possible value of measurements of this parameter during diffuse pulmonary infiltration, we studied it in pulmonary granulomatosis induced by Freund's adjuvant in rats.

METHOD

This work was done on male Wistar rats of 400–500 g. They were divided into a control group and a group receiving an intravenous injection of Frenud's complete adjuvant (FCA) at a dose of 0.45 ml/kg, during 2 consecutive days.

Measuring pulmonary extravascular water was done 1, 3 and 4 months after adjuvant injection and it was performed alternately on normal and pathological rats.

Dilution curves were obtained by a single injection of ^{131}I-labeled albumin and tritiated water, on an experimental preparation used to delay recirculation, and to obtain a better exponential decrease of the dilution curves. It is composed of a shunt made of 3 batteries of coiled glass tubing; 1 representing the arterial system, the 2 others the venous system, and the 2 systems were joined together by a collapsible tube. The whole system was kept thermostatically at 38°C (Fig. 1). A constant amount of blood in the preparation during blood sampling was ensured by perfusing homologous blood at the same rate as sampling.

From these data and using the Hamilton extrapolation method; we measured blood flow and mean transit times for each indicator. Any experiment where the flows for tritiated water and ^{131}I-labeled albumin have over 5% difference was discarded.

Pulmonary extravascular water expressed in ml per kg of animal weight is calculated with the following formula:

$$\text{Pulmonary extravascular water (ml/kg)} = \frac{\dot{Q} \times f\,(\bar{t}\,3H - \bar{t}\,Alb)}{\text{animal weight}}$$

f being the water contained in the whole blood; it is measured by weighing before and after dessication.

$\bar{t}\,3H$ = mean transit time for tritiated water

$\bar{t}\,Alb$ = mean transit time for ^{131}I-labeled Albumin

Q = cardiac output.

Schéma de la préparation

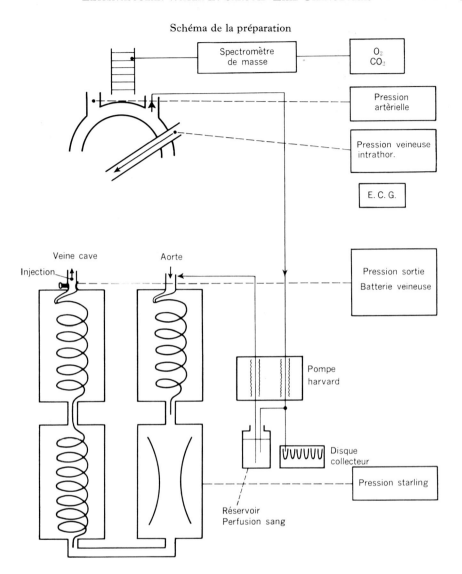

For each experiment the value of pulmonary extravascular water (PEV) is compared to the blood volume between the injection site and the sampling site (CBV).

In this experiment the whole pulmonary water was measured by weighing before and after dessication of blood-drained organs.

RESULTS

a) Pulmonary extravascular water in normal rats (PEV ml/kg) (Table 1).

Out of 41 measurements, the mean value of pulmonary extravascular water is 2.07 ± 0.509 ml/kg and the ratio DEV/CBV is 0.38 ± 0.109. These data are comparable to the values obtained on a group of animals of the same origin, studied previously, for which we found values of 2.2 ml/kg ± 0.873 for pulmonary extravascular water. and a ratio PEV/CBV of 0.39 ± 0.144.

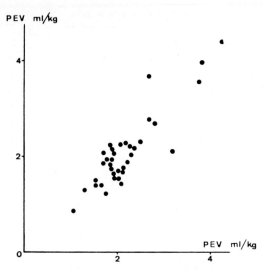

FIG. 1.   Correlations between 2 measures of PEV in the same preparation.

TABLE 1.   Pulmonary extravascular water in the rat.

	Group 1 n=53	Group 2 n=41
PEV (ml/kg)	2.2 SE=.115	2.07 SE=.0889
PEV/CBV	.39 SE=.021	.34 SE=.0169

CBV=Central blood volume.

TABLE 2.   Proliferative lung disease in the rat.
(Pulmonary extravascular water one month after Freund's adjuvant)

	Intensity of the lesions			
	Control n=41	Slight n=15	Moderate n=15	Marked n=17
PEV (ml/kg)	2.07 SE=.115	1.87 SE=.111 NS	2.11 SE=.0717 NS	2.4 SE=.136 *
PEV/CBV	.38 SE=.0169	.36 SE=.0288 NS	.49 SE=.0188 *	.58 SE=.0477 **

TABLE 3.   Proliferative lung disease in the rat.
(Pulmonary extravascular water 3 and 4 months after Freund's adjuvant)

	Control n=41	Adjuvant	
		3 Months n=18	4 Months n=9
PEV (ml/kg)	2.07 SE=.0889	4 SE=.22**	3.3 SE=.176**
PEV/CBV	.38 SE=.0169	.71 SE=.0281**	.52 SE=.042**

b)   Pulmonary extravascular water in rats treated with Freund's Adjuvant (Tables 2 and 3).

For all measurements done after 1 month's evolution of the granulomatous process, the average value of extravascular water was 2.14 ml/kg±0.493 with a ratio PEV/CBV of 0.44, Pratically, these results are close to that of the control group. Kf these data are studied in relation to a pseudo-guantitative evaluation of histological lesions the mean value of extravascular water is 1.87, 2.11 and 2.4 ml/kg for groups showing slight moderate or severe alterations; in the third group alone, data are significantly different from normal. For this group we have a ratio PEV/CBV of 0.58±0.194, very different from values seen in normal rats.

After 3 months' evolution, the increase of pulmonary extravascular water is very marked, 4 ml/kg±0.938, and with a ratio PEV/CBV of 0.71±0.115.

After 4 months' evolution the average value for 9 measurements was lower than at the third month, but was still clearly above the normal: 3.3 ml/kg±0.598 and a ratio PEV/CBV of 0.52±0.176.

DISCUSSION

Results for pulmonary extravascular water observed in rats are clearly inferior to those obtained in other animal species and in man. This fact can be correlated to a smaller amount of pulmonary parenchyma in the rat or to age, because, for technical reasons, we used big animals more than 6 months old, and extracellular water decreases with age. It should be noted that pulmonary extravascular water represents an unusual portion (69%) of the total intrapulmonary water measured by dessication of blood-drained organs, that is under conditions which overestimate the intrapulmonary water content of the quantity of water contained in the trapped blood.

In an experiment in process, where blood trapped in the lung is measured by an isotopic method, we notice that in rats, one can measure nearly the whole amount of intrapulmonary water; this can be explained by the fact that in this small animal, gradients of perfusion dependent on gravity are negligable.

To be interesting, measurements of this parameter during the granulomatuous process must fulfil 3 contitions: the multiple indicator technique must remain valid; pulmonary extravascular water must indicate correctly the granulomatous process and the method must be sensitive.

Concerning the first point one might fear that an increase of the diffusion distance linked with the pathological developement impairs complete diffusion and back diffusion of the tritiated water.   In these conditions a fraction of the diffusible indicator would be lost and the flows measured by tritiated water would be higher than those obtained with the vascular indicator. However, this is not so and the 2 measured flows are equal.

As for the second point, pulmonary extravascular water increases with the developement of pulmonary granulomatous lesions, and this increase is very significant in groups stutied 3 and 4 months after induction of the granulomatous process. Also, we noted a true correlation between the increase of pulmonary extravascular water and that of lung weight (Fig. 2). However, this method only measures water in perfused areas, and we know that in normal rats, it represents nearly the whole of the exchange. Does this also happen during granulomatous processes induced by FCA? We are not able to answer this question due to insufficient data; but we can remark that pulmonary extra-

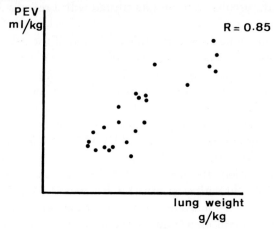

FIG. 2.   Proliferative lung disease.
(Variation of pulmonary extravascular water with lung weight)

TABLE 4.   Pulmonary extravascular water.
(Measured fraction of total pulmonary water)

Control	Adjuvant	
	3 Months	4 Months
0.69	0.72	0.72
S.E. 0.049	S.E. 0.039	S.E. 0.039

vascular water (Table 4) represents 72% of intrapulmonary water in animals studied at the third and fourth month; that is, a fraction identical to that measured in normal rats; note, however, that our reference, intrapulmonary water measured on drained organs, is an overestimation of the total intrapulmonary water.

Concerning the sensitivity, results observed after 1 month's evolution of the granulomatous process, are not very encouraging. Nevertheless, because of its importance, this point is worth investigating again using a statistically valid method for assessing histological lesions and in conditions of homogenous measurement of pulmonary extravascular water.

SUMMARY

Pulmonary extravascular water was measured by the double indicator method (Chinard) with albumin labelled by ^{131}I as a vascular indicator and tritiated water as a diffusible indicator. For the rat (400–500 g) the average was 2.07 ml/kg S.E. $\pm$0.0889.

Granulomatosis in the lung was produced by 2 intravenous injections on consecutive days of Freund's complete adjuvant.

Pulmonary extravascular water was measured 1, 3 and 4 months after induction of the granulomatous process.

After 1 month, pulmonary extravascular water increased significantly only for rats with most severe lesions, a mean value of 2.41 ml/kg, S. E. $\pm$0.136 (*).

On the third month the mean value was 4.02 ml/kg, S.E. $\pm$0.220 (**), definitely above that of the controls.

On the fourth month, while pulmonary lesions regress, pulmonary vascular water is still notably increased in comparison with the controls: 3.3 ml/kg, S. E. ± 0.176 (**).

The significance of this parameter in experimental conditions, and its importance for the evaluation of a granulomatous process are considered and discussed.

BIBLIOGRAPHIES

1. Chinard, F. P. 1966. The permeability characteristics of the pulmonary blood-gas barrier. Advances in respiratory physiology (ed. C. Caro) Baltimore: Williams and Wilkins.
2. Goresky, C. A., Cronin, R. F. P., and Wangel, B. E. 1969. Indicator dilution measurements of extravascular water in the lungs. *J. Clin. Invest* **48**, 487–501.
3. Pearce, M. L., Yamasthta, J., and Beazell, J. 1965. Measurement of pulmonary edema. *Circulation Res.* **16**: 482–488.
4. Ramsey, L. H., Puckett, W., Jose, A., and Lacy, W. W. 1964. Pericapillary gas and water distribution volumes of the lung calculated from multiple indicator dilution curves. *Circulation Res.* **15**: 275–286.
5. Turino, G. M., Edelman, N. H., Senior, R. M., Richards, E. C., and Fishman, A. P. 1968. Extravascular lung water in cor pulmonaire. *Bull. Physiol. Path. Res.* **4**: 47–64.
6. Turino, G. M., Pine, M. B., Shubrooks, S. V., and Cary, J. P. 1971. The volume of extravascular water of the lung in normal man and in disease. *Bull. Physiopath. Res.* **7**: 1161–1179.
7. Yu, P. N. 1971. Lung water in congestive heart failure. Modern Concepts of Cardiovasc. Dis **40**: 27–32.

Granulomatous Disorders Which Mimic Sarcoidosis

D. GERAINT JAMES

Royal Northern Hospital, London, Great Britain

A granulomatous reaction is the battlefield created by indigestible antigen and the responding macrophages, cellular lymphocytes and humoral antibodies, with the lymphocytes progressing to epithelioid cells and giant cells. There are many different causes for such a reaction, so a classification of granulomatous disorders (Table 1) comprises infections, neoplasms, chemicals, immunological deficiencies, a leucocyte oxidase defect, and extrinsic allergic alveolitis. These diseases may have clear-cut clinical and radiological features but the histology is the same as sarcoidosis and in this respect they may be confusingly similar.

It is, therefore, important to lay down the following criteria for interpreting a sarcoid granuloma:—

1. Is the granulomatous reaction localised to one system or is it multisystem (Table 2)?
2. The environment of the patient (Table 3).
3. The age of the patient (Table 4).
4. Kveim-Siltzbach test.

Sarcoidosis or a local sarcoid-tissue reaction (Table 2)

A sarcoid tissue reaction is usually localised to one system. Despite a careful assessment of other systems, no abnormality is found. The Kveim-Siltzbach test is negative, and is helpful in distinguishing the multisystem disorder from a localised reaction. Delayed-type hypersensitivity is usually intact, but this is not invariable.

The hallmark of sarcoidosis is the fact that it is multisystem. The frequency of involvement of various organs and systems has been analysed in 537 patients with histologically confirmed sarcoidosis so that the percentage frequency of involvement of any system can be predicted in an individual patient. The data accumulated from a personal series of 1000 patients with sarcoidosis are now being computerised so that a diagnostic index of system frequency may be adopted.

The environment of the patient (Table 3)

The interpretation of the granulomatous disorder must depend upon the country in which it is observed. It would be foolish to diagnose sarcoidosis of the skin in Africa until leprosy has been ruled out, or in India until tuberculosis has been excluded, or in Asia until cutaneous leishmaniasis has been discounted.

The pathologist in his own environment will be well aware of these local factors but in this shrinking world of jet travel, we must remind ourselves of the granulomas of other continents.

TABLE 1. A classification of granulomatous disorders.

Infections	Chemicals
Fungi	Beryllium
Histoplasma	Zirconium
Coccidioides	Silica
Blastomyces	Starch
Sporotrichum	
	Immunological deficiency
Protozoa	Sarcoidosis
	Crohn's disease
Metazoa	Primary biliary cirrhosis
Toxoplasma	Wegener's granulomatosis
Leishmania	Giant cell arteritis
Toxocara	Peyronie's disease
Schistosoma	Hypogammaglobulinaemia
	Systemic lupus erythematosus
Spirochaetes	
T. pallidum	Leucocyte oxidase defect
T. pertenue	Chronic granulomatous disease of
T. carateum	childhood
Mycobacteria	
M. tuberculosis	Extrinsic allergic alveolitis
M. leprae	Farmer's lung
Anonymous	Bird fancier's
B.C.G.	Mushroom worker's
	Suberosis (cork dust)
Bacteria	Bagassosis
Brucella	Maple bark stripper's
	Paprika splitter's
Other infections	Coffee bean
Cat scratch	
Lymphogranuloma	
	Other
Neoplasia	Pyrexia of unknown origin
Carcinoma	Radiotherapy
Reticulosis	Cancer chemotherapy
Pinealoma	Panniculitis
Dysgerminoma	Chalazion
Seminoma	Sebaceous cyst
Reticulum cell sarcoma	Dermoid
Malignant nasal granuloma	

Age of the patient (Table 4)

Sarcoidosis is a disorder of the child-bearing years of life. It is extremely uncommon in children and in the elderly. When sarcoid tissue is observed in a child, consider an infection such as tuberculosis, toxocara infestation or helminths generally, cat scratch disease, swimming pool granuloma due to *Mycobacterium balnei*, or chronic granulomatous disease of childhood.

In the older age groups, sarcoid tissue in a lymph node may reflect an underlying neoplasm of the lung, stomach, uterus or elsewhere, particularly if the patient is receiving radiotherapy or cytotoxic chemotherapy.

TABLE 2.   Differences between the multisystem disorder, sarcoidosis, and
a nonspecific local sarcoid tissue reaction.

	Sarcoidosis	Sarcoid reaction
No. of systems involved	Several	Usually one
Age group	20–50 years	Any
Chest radiography	Abnormal in 84%	Normal
Slit-lamp examination of eyes	Abnormal in 25%	Normal
Tuberculin test	Negative in 66%	Variable
Kveim-Siltzbach test	Positive in 84%	Negative
Calcium metabolism	Abnormal in 20%	Normal
Response to corticosteroids	Good	Variable
Other treatments	Oxyphenbutazone Chloroquine p-Aminobenzoate	Depends on cause :— —Anti-infective —Immunosuppressive

TABLE 3.   Significance of a granulomatous reaction : Environment.

Region	Disorder	Due to	Skin test	Serum antibody test	Other tests
Asia	Leishmaniasis	Leishmania		Formol gel	Giemsa-stained lymph node aspirate
Brazil Egypt	Bilharziasis	Schistosoma	Yes		Eind ova embedded in granuloma
Burma	Melioidosis	Pseudomonas pseudomallei	Yes	Yes	Culture organism
California	Coccidioidomy-cosis	Coccidioides immitis	Yes	Yes	Culture in Sabouraud's medium
India	Tuberculosis	Mycobacterium tuberculosis	Yes		Isolate organism. Chest radiography
Africa	Leprosy	Mycobacterium leprae	Yes		Scrapings
Ohio	Histoplasmosis	Histoplasma capsulatum	Yes	Yes	Culture in Sabouraud's medium

TABLE 4.   Significance of a granulomatous reaction : age of patient.

Age (years)	Description	Due to	Further tests
0–5	Fundus oculi suspicious of retinoblastoma	Toxocara choroiditis	Check for eosinophilia anaemia, lung, infiltration.
0–5	Eczema ; Sinuses ; Miliary Mottling	Chronic granulomatous disease	Nitroblue Tetrazolium test
0–10	Cervical lymphadenitis draining sinus in the neck	Cat-scratch disease	Cat-scratch skin test and complement-fixation test for psittacosis group
0–15	Ulceration of legs	Swimming-pool granuloma	Isolate Mycobacterium balnei
20–40	Check all systems for multisystem sarcoidosis		
40–50	Obstructive jaundice	Primary biliary cirrhosis	Antimitochondrial serologic antibodies
Over 50	Sarcoid lymph nodes	Draining carcinomas, especially in patient receiving treatment	Think of cancer ; more likely than sarcoidosis

Kveim-Siltzbach Test

This test is invaluable in distinguishing multisystem sarcoidosis from these many other granulomatous disorders. It is positive in the majority of patients with sarcoidosis and negative in all patients with other granulomatous disorders, if carried out properly with good antigen.

Potent antigen is essential, and this means that it must be obtained from the spleen of a patient with active sarcoidosis. The histologist's interpretation of the biopsy material is important, for an inexperienced observer could confuse sarcoid tissue with a non-specific foreign-body giant-cell reaction, particularly if doubly refractile crystals are not sought by polarised light. Finally, it should be remembered that the Kveim-Siltzbach test is suppressed by oral corticosteroids, just like any other sarcoid tissue.

Diseases of the Lung due to Inhaled Particles with Sarcoid-Like Histology—Similarities and differences in relation to sarcoidosis—

T. G. Villar and Ramiro Àvila

Faculty of Medicine, Lisbon University, Lisbon, Portugal

Diseases of the lungs caused by inhaled particles in which granulomatous lesions closely resembling the granulomas of sarcoidosis are seen in the lungs and elsewhere, are being recognized more frequently as industrialization and pollution increase.

The main difference between these diseases and sarcoidosis is that the foreign particles which cause them are seen within the granulomas and can generally be identified by appropriate pathologic techniques.

In this report we attempt to compare various parameters in a group of 95 patients with diseases of this group, whose common feature was the presence of sarcoid-like histology in lung biopsies, with a group of 68 patients with confirmed sarcoidosis.

MATERIAL AND METHODS

The group of 95 patients with sarcoid-like granulomas caused by inhaled particles was made up of all patients with the required histology on lung biopsy of a total of 150 such patients with lung biopsies from the following disease groups: baker's lung, bird fancier's lung, cement lung, detergent lung, DDT lung, fish-meal lung, furrier's lung, gas-oil lung, hair-spray lung, nylon lung, painter's lung, wood-worker's lung, suberosis, vineyard sprayer's lung, welder's lung and a group of this type of disease in which it was impossible to determine the nature of the foreign substance seen within the lesions. The patients in the sarcoid group were distributed as follows: 23% stage I, 42% stage II, 16% stage III and 6% stage IV.

The sarcoidosis group and this granuloma group where compared as to age and sex distribution, clinical and radiologic features, other localizations of the granulomas besides the lung, tuberculin sensitivity, Kveim reaction, blood calcium, protein fraction pattern, immunoglobulins, lung function, course and prognosis.

RESULTS

The difference in incidence in favour of the male sex was only slightly more marked (1.9/1) in the granuloma than in the sarcoidosis group (1.4/1) and was not significant. However, there was a marked difference in the age distribution of the two groups, although some overlapping occurs (Fig. 1). While the highest incidence of sarcoidosis was in the second and third decade, that of the granuloma group was in the fifth and sixth decades.

Clinically the onset was found to be abrupt or insidious in both groups and practically the same proportion were asymptomatic. While erythema nodosum was a pre-

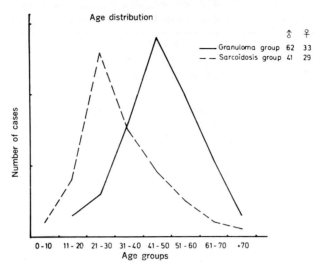

FIG. 1. Age distribution of sarcoidosis group and sarcoid-like group.

TABLE 1. Radiological aspects compared.

Groups	Normal	Enlarged mediastinal glands	Miliary	Reticulo-nodular	Infiltrates
Sarcoidosis	10%	63% (90% B.H.L.)	10%	39%	13%
Other granulomatoses	3%	14% (3% B.H.L.)	3%	80%	11%

senting feature in 7% of the sarcoidosis group it was never seen in the granuloma group.

Although the X-rays of the chest showed all aspects from normal through to pulmonary infiltrates in both groups, the incidence of the various radiological aspects was somewhat different. The dominant picture in both groups was a diffuse reticular nodular mottling but, while hilar gland involvement was seen in 63% of the sarcoidosis group, it was only seen in 14% of the granuloma group. Normal chest X-rays and fine miliary nodulation were also more frequent in the sarcoidosis group (Table 1).

The granulomas of sarcoidosis can be found in the bronchial mucosa, lymph glands, liver, etc., and constitute the basis for the biopsies used for the diagnosis of this disease. Granulomas containing the foreign substance responsible for the disease were found in random biopsies of the bronchi in 4 cases of bird fancier's lung, 5 cases of suberosis and 2 cases of furrier's lung; in scalene node biopsies on 2 cases of vineyard sprayer's lung and 9 cases of suberosis; in liver biopsies in a case of DDT lung, another of hair-spray lung and 5 cases of suberosis. This systemic distribution of the granulomatous diseases due to inhaled particles was, however, less common than in sarcoidosis.

Tuberculin tests with 10 I.U. PPD were negative in 86% of the cases of sarcoidosis and in 70% of the patients in the granuloma group. In 2 patients of this group, a positive tuberculin reaction reverted to negative as a bird fancier's lung and a cement lung developed (Table 2).

While the Kveim test was positive in 58% of the tested cases of sarcoidosis it was consistently negative in 11 patients of the granuloma group tested, although in 1 case

TABLE 2. Tuberculin and Kveim tests in sarcoidosis and other granulomatoses.

	Tuberculin tests			Kveim reactions		
	No. tested	No. negative	% negative	No. tested	No. positive	% positive
Sarcoidosis	64	55	86	36	21	58
Other granulomatoses	33	23	70	11	0	0

TABLE 3. Serum protein changes in sarcoidosis and other granulomatoses.

	Total cases	Total proteins		Albumin		α_2-globulin		Gammaglobulin	
		Normal	Low	Normal	Low	Normal	Elevated	Normal	Elevated
Sarcoidosis	33	31 (94%)	2 (6%)	15 (45%)	15 (45%)	19 (58%)	11 (33%)	7 (21%)	26 (78%)
Other granulomatoses	58	53 (91%)	5 (9%)	12 (21%)	45 (78%)	17 (29%)	40 (69%)	17 (29%)	40 (69%)

TABLE 4. The immunoglobulins in sarcoidosis and the granulomatoses.

		Sarcoidosis	Granulomatoses	Controls	Variance analysis
IgG	N	21	72	40	No significant difference between sarcoidosis and controls (p>0.05).
	AM	1321,9 mg%	2057,22 mg%	1622,5 mg%	Granulomatoses>controls (p<0.01)
	R	880–1980 mg%	720–5800 mg%	760–3200 mg%	
IgA	N	21	73	38	Sarcoidosis<controls (p<(0.01)
	AM	162,29 mg%	385,2 mg%	281 mg%	Granulomatoses>controls (p<0.01)
	R	0–384 mg%	0–912 mg%	48–760 mg%	
IgM	N	21	73	39	Sarcoidosis<controls (p<0.05)
	AM	117,38 mg%	206 mg%	176,62 mg%	No Significant difference between granulomatoses and controls (p>0.05)
	R	0–488 mg%	48–716 mg%	36–384 mg%	

N=Number of cases.
AM=Arithmetic mean.
R=Range.

a lovely nodule developed at 4 weeks that on histology proved to be merely fibrous tissue.

Blood calcium was found to be elevated in 39% of the patients with sarcoidosis and only in 23% of the other granulomas.

The changes in the serum proteins and their fractions in the 2 groups were as follows (Table 3): the total protein values were within normal values in 94% of the patients with sarcoidosis and in 91% of those of the granuloma group; the albumin fraction showed low values in 45% of the cases of sarcoidosis and in 78% of the grauloma group; the α_2-globulin fraction was elevated in 33% of the patients with sarcoidosis and in 69% of the granuloma group; the gammaglobulin fraction was significantly elevated in 78% of the sarcoidosis group and in 69% of the granuloma group.

All immunoglobulin values were lower in sarcoidosis than in the other granulomatoses (Table 4).

Ventilatory function was normal in 47% of the sarcoidosis group and in 26% of the granuloma group. Ventilatory restriction was the predominant defect in both groups.

TABLE 5. Ventilation studies in sarcoidosis and other granulomatoses.

Groups	No. of cases studied	Normal	Restrictive	Mixed
Sarcoidosis	17	8 (47%)	9 (53%)	0
Other granulomatoses	76	26 (34%)	31 (41%)	19 (25%)

TABLE 6. Blood gases in sarcoidosis and other granulomatoses.

Groups	No. of cases studied	Normal	PaO_2 Normal	PaO_2 Low	$PaCO_2$ Normal	$PaCO_2$ Low	$PaCO_2$ High
Sarcoidosis	9	5 (55%)	3 (33%)	1 (11%)	1 (11%)	3 (33%)	—
Other granulomatoses	73	15 (21%)	31 (42%)	26 (36%)	5 (7%)	49 (67%)	3 (4%)

TABLE 7. Diffusion (Dco) values in sarcoidosis and other granulomatoses.

	No. of Cases studied	Normal values (Above 10 ml/min/mmHg)	Low values (Below 10 ml/min/mmHg)
Sarcoidosis	11	7 (64%)	4 (36%)
Other granulomatoses	64	29 (45%)	34 (53%)

Blood gases were normal in 55% of the patients with sarcoidosis and in 21% of the other granulomas. In both groups the syndrome of hypoxemia and hypocapnia was most common. In the granuloma group there were 3 cases of CO_2 retention due to bronchial involvement. Low diffusion values were found in 36% of the sarcoidosis group and in 53% of the granuloma group (Tables 5, 6, 7).

As in sarcoidosis, spontaneous remission was frequent in the recent and acute cases and rare in the chronic cases of the granuloma group, provided the patients avoided specific exposure.

Prognosis was equally good in both groups in the acute or relatively recent cases, and poor in those patients in which irreversible interstitial fibrosis had developed.

DISCUSSION

The main difference between sarcoidosis and the other granulomatous diseases under consideration seems to be the possibility of demonstrating by immunologic and pathologic techniques the causes of these diseases.

Most of the parameters compared were present and showed the same trend in patients in both groups, only varying in degree. We will discuss the most outstanding differences in the 2 groups.

The age distribution of the granuloma group showed a marked shift to the older age groups in relation to sarcoidosis, probably because a longer period of exposure to the aggressive agent is needed for these patients to develop the sarcoid-like histologic features that define this group (Fig. 1).

The fact that no case of erythema nodosum was seen in the granuloma group as compared with the sarcoidosis group is somewhat unexpected in view of other signs of hypersensitivity found in this group.

The main difference between the 2 groups on chest X-ray was the much higher incidence of hilar gland involvement in sarcoidosis, although in 1 patient of the granuloma group the only X-ray changes were bilateral hilar lymphadenitis.

Multiple organ involvement, a defining feature of sarcoidosis, was also found in the granuloma group although considerably less frequently.

The finding of a 70% negative tuberculin reaction in the granuloma group, in age groups in which the general population of Portugal has an expected 70% positive reaction, together with the reversion from positive to negative of the tuberculin reaction in 2 patients, with a bird fanciers' and a cement lung, lead us to postulate that in these granulomatous diseases caused by inhaled particles there may be immunological changes very similar to those found in sarcoidosis. The study of the serum protein fractions seems to bear this out.

In our experience, the Kveim test has proved completely specific for sarcoidosis and was always negative in the granuloma group.

The differences between the 2 groups as to lung function seem to show a more diffuse involvement of the gas-exchanging structures in the granuloma group than in sarcoidosis.

The course and prognosis of the 2 groups is very similar except that in the granuloma group they depend fundamentally on the continuance or suspension of exposure.

Cutaneous and Pulmonary Manifestations of Chronic Beryllium Disease

W. Jones Williams and G. S. Kilpatrick

Departments of Pathology, and Tuberculosis and Chest Diseases,
The Welsh National School of Medicine, Cardiff, Great Britain

INTRODUCTION

The cutaneous and pulmonary manifestations of beryllium disease are of continuing interest due to the widespread usage of beryllium and its compounds in modern technology[1,2]. The chronic form of the disease is characterised by the presence of granulomas which are indistinguishable from those of sarcoidosis[3].

Detailed studies have been made on a man over a period of 9 years who originally had an injury to his hand contaminated with beryllium oxide. A chronic ulcer developed and amputation of the finger was eventually necessary. This was followed by extension of the disease process into the arm with subsequent involvement of the lungs (Fig. 1). The various clinical, pathological and radiological studies are described.

D.T. Male, aet 58

1963, Sept.	Laceration right index finger by BeO contaminated grinding wheel.
↓	
1964, April.	Positve skin biopsy.
↓	
1965, Jan.	Amputation of finger.
↓	
1965, June.	Two lymphatic nodules, right forearm.
↓	
1967.	Increasing dyspnoea.
↓	
1968.	Multiple lymphatic nodules right forearm.
↓	
1970.	Skin and lung positive biopsies.
↓	
1972.	Controlled by steroids.
↓	
?	

Fig. 1. Clinical course.

CASE HISTORY

The earlier details of this patient have been described in detail[4] and the following is a summary of the findings with the subsequent events.

The patient was aged 50 and employed in light engineering when he was first seen in September 1963. He had accidentally cut his right index finger on the sharp edge of a grinding stone with which he was working beryllium alloy. The cut was sutured on the day of the injury, appeared to heal initially, but subsequently broke down and dis-

141

charged pus. Various antibiotics were tried without effect and a biopsy in October 1963, showed nonspecific chronic inflammation. Over the next 6 months the ulcer became indolent and because healing had still not occurred, a further biopsy was performed in April 1964, which showed scattered, noncaseating epithelioid granulomata consistent with beryllium disease. Culture for tubercle bacilli was negative. At that time he was clinically well, had no respiratory symptoms, the chest X-ray was normal and detailed lung function tests were within normal range. A beryllium patch test was positive and he was negative to both Mantoux (10 TU) and Kveim tests.

Because of the delay in healing, a course of prednisone was initiated and while some healing took place by January 1965, the original injury again broke down and amputation of the finger was carried out. Histological section showed extensive epithelioid cell granulomas with 15 μg of beryllium per 100 g wet tissue.

Six months after the amputation in June 1965, he presented with 2 ulcerative nodules on the right forearm which were excised. On microscopy, similar granulomas were found in the dermis and within lymphatic channels, and again beryllium was detected (10.4 μg/100 g wet tissue). The patient remained clinically well, his chest X-ray was normal and he returned to work. He was not again exposed to beryllium.

In 1967, although clinically well, he complained for the first time of slight shortness of breath but the chest X-ray and lung function tests were normal. In 1968 the patient himself noticed further nodules in the right arm but did not seek medical advice until 1970 by which time the nodules had become more marked and he was significantly more dyspnoeic.

He was admitted to Sully Hospital for full assessment in October 1970. He looked well but there were numerous small nodules on the right arm in the subcutaneous tissues from the base of the index finger to the axilla together with some axillary nodes. Biopsy

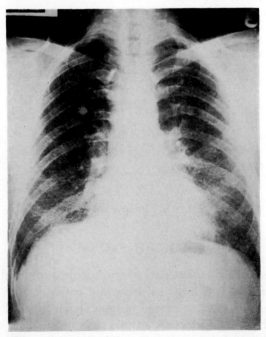

FIG. 2.   Chest radiograph (1970).   Seven years after original injury.   Diffuse fibrosis and small nodular opacities, mainly lower lobes.

of the arm nodule showed numerous sarcoid-type granulomas around a central fibrous zone with 0.08 μg beryllium per 100 g wet tissue. A chest X-ray at this time revealed quite considerable change with diffuse, largely basal small opacities the appearances being consistent with berylliosis and interstitial pulmonary fibrosis (Fig. 2). The lung function tests too had shown a marked change and in particular, the transfer factor which in 1967 had been 21.3 ml/min had fallen to 12.9 ml/min mmHG (Fig. 3). A lung biopsy was done which showed sarcoid-type granulomas, Schaumann bodies and interstitial fibrosis (Fig. 4).

Electron microscopic examination of the arm and lung lesions showed granulomas with features indistinguishable from those of sarcoidosis[5].

In 1970 further investigations were performed. A 24-hour specimen of urine showed 0.06 μg of beryllium per/1500 ml (control, 0.01 μg/150 ml).

Beryllium was not found in a 500 ml sample of whole blood nor in the separated

Lung function tests. (D.T.)

Test/Date	1964 May	1966 Sept.:	1967 May	1970 Sept.:	1971 Oct.:
FEV₁ L.	3.98	3.67	3.53	3.10	3.47
Transfer factor (ml/min/mm Hg.)	20.90	20.50	21.30	12.90	20.50
Chest X-ray		Normal		Diffuse Shadowing	Improvement

Steroid therapy (continuing).

Fig. 3. Lung function tests.

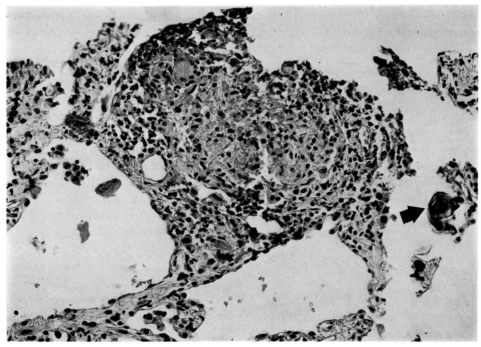

FIG. 4. Lung biopsy (1970). Sarcoid-type granuloma, interstitial fibrosis and Schaumann body (arrow). Haematosylin and eosin, Mag. ×105.

white cell fraction. Granulocyte function tests were normal (90% Staph. aureus and E. coli killed within 2 hours).

A macrophage migration inhibition test was positive, (beryllium sulphate/patients lymphocytes., migration index <0.34, controls >0.8), Jones Williams, Grey,and Pioli, unpublished.

In view of the clinical, radiological and physiological deterioration the patient was again started on a high-dose course of corticosteroids in December 1970. Clinically, he improved quite considerably and by February 1971, the nodules on the forearm had become barely palpable, and the chest X-ray, while not returning to normal, had considerably improved. The clinical improvement was maintained through 1971 and by May of that year the improvement was reflected in the respiratory function tests particularly as demonstrated by an elevation of the transfer factor to 20.5 ml/min mm Hg.

At the present time he is well and working though still somewhat dyspnoeic. The previous noted nodules in the arm have completely disappeared, and the X-ray remains improved when compared with films in 1970.

COMMENT

This case demonstrates the serious consequences of local beryllium implantation. The disease process from the beginning has been a progressive one necessitating the amputation of a finger and treatment with large doses and subsequently maintenance doses of corticosteroids to control the process which had extended into the affected arm and subsequently to the lungs. The fact that the nodules in the arm have disappeared and that the X-ray has cleared very considerably suggests that the response to treatment probably means a reversible situation with granuloma formation rather than permanent fibrosis. However, our investigations demonstrate the widespread presence of beryllium in the tissue and urine with systemic sensitisation as shown by the positive patch tests and beryllium-induced macrophage migration factor.

There has been a suggestion in the past that generalised disease does not follow local implantation, but the course of the condition in this patient suggests that there had been extension from the finger to the arm and subsequently to involve the lungs. Presumably this would be by lymphatic flow. While it is true that there was no further exposure to beryllium after the original injury one cannot deny the fact that inevitably there may have been some inhalation of beryllium oxide during the time when he was working before the injury. The exhaust ventilation in the factory concerned was particularly satisfactory, but there were occasions when it did not work as efficiently as it might have done. It is recognised that there may have been an inhalation of the beryllium at that time with a latent period before the pulmonary lesions occured and there is no method of knowing whether this or the previous hypothesis is the correct one.

ACKNOWLEDGEMENTS

We wish to thank Mr E. J. Marsh, Aldermaston, for the spectroscopic beryllium analysis and Dr Eileen Thompson, Welsh National School of Medicine, for the granulocyte function testing.

Our especial thanks are due to the late Dr C. B. McKerrow, M. R. C. Pneumoconiosis Unit, Cardiff, for the respiratory function tests.

REFERENCES

1. Tepper, L. B., Hardy, H. L., and Chamberlin, R. I. 1961. Toxicity of Beryllium Compounds. Amsterdam: Elsvier Press.
2. Raymond Parkes, W. Occupational Lung Disorders. London: Butterworth. In preparation.
3. Jones Williams, W. 1958. *Brit. J. Ind. Med.* **15**: 84.
4. Jones Williams, W., Lawrie, J. H., and Davies, H. J. 1967. *Brit. J. Surg.* **54**: 292.
5. Jones Williams, W. 1972. *Acta. Path. Microbiol. Scand.* Section A80, Suppl. 233, 195.
6. Jones Williams, W., Grey, Jennifer, and Pioli, Elizabeth 1972. *Brit. Med. J.* **ii**: 175.

Pathological Study of Sarcoid-Like Lesions Associated with Malignant Neoplasms

Yoshio Murata[1], Teruo Tachibana[1], Eiyo Yugawa[2],
Ryuhei Tateishi[3], Yoshiyuki Morimura[4],Shunichi Sakai[5],
Tsuneaki Seno[6], Shintatsu Kyo[6],
and Shunzo Onishi[7]

Regarding the etiology and pathogenesis of granuloma formation in systemic sarcoidosis, the problem of the association of sarcoid-like lesions induced by other diseases had been attracting much attention. Among these associated diseases, a relationship between malignant tumors and sarcoid-like lesions in draining lymph nodes is less well-known. During the past 10 years in Osaka Prefectural Hospital, we have experienced 2 malignant tumor cases presenting sarcoid-like lesions in the regional lymph nodes. In addition to these cases, 6 more cases encountered in other hospitals are included in this study. The purpose of the present report is to investigate pathological changes in these cases.

PATIENTS AND METHODS

The cases in this report fall into 2 groups, 4 stomach cancer cases and 4 malignant neoplasia cases other than stomach cancer. The cases with stomach cancer were studied separately from the other cases since gastrectomy permitted more systematic examination of the affected lymph nodes as well as the primary lesion. None of the cases showed clinical evidence of multisystem manifestations characteristic of genuine sarcoidosis, and chest radiographs revealed no abnormality. Surgically resected specimens were obtained from all cases, except 1 (case 6). Only 1 was autopsied.

Tissues from both the primary lesions of malignant tumors and the regional lymph nodes were fixed in a formalin solution, and stained with hematoxylin-eosin, Azan-Mallory, Van Gieson, reticulum fiber stain, PAS stain for fungi and Ziehl-Neelsen stain for acid-fast bacilli. When necessary, a polarizing microscope was employed.

The diagnosis of sarcoid-like lesions in this report was based upon the following histological findings; several or many nodules of epithelioid cell granulomas were more or less diffusely present in the local lymph nodes, particularly in the related regional nodes.

The clinical and pathological data of the cases are summarised in Table 1. All the patients with stomach cancer in group 1 underwent total and subtotal gastrectomy together with lymphoadenectomy, and all the resected specimens were histologically con-

1) *Osaka Prefectural Hospital, Osaka, Japan*
2) *Yugawa Hospital, Osaka, Japan*
3) *Center for Adult Diseases, Osaka, Japan*
4) *Kansai Rosai Hospital, Osaka, Japan*
5) *Kaisei Hospital, Osaka, Japan*
6) *Osaka University Hospital, Osaka, Japan*
7) *Osaka University Medical School, Osaka, Japan*

firmed to be tubular adenocarcinoma of gastric origin. These cases had common findings in that the primary lesions, located along the lesser curvature, had been more or less ulcerated and that the interstitium of tumor tissue showed a moderate to marked lymphocytic infiltration, sometimes with lymphoid follicles. These changes were conspicuous in case 1. None of the cases showed an appearance of sarcoid-like lesions within and around the neoplastic tissue of the stomach. The number of resected lymph nodes showing metastases or sarcoid-like lesions or both, is summarized in Table 1. Some of the resected lymph nodes were slightly enlarged and a histological investigation revealed granulomatous lesions resembling those in systemic sarcoidosis. The lesions were composed of miliary epithelioid cell granulomas diffusely distributed throughout the medullary tissue of the lymph node. Sometimes, a few granulomatous foci are conglomerated together but these lesions showed no caseation. Frequently, the enlarged cytoplasm of epithelioid cells is multinucleated, containing small vacuoles. Giant cells of Langhans' and foreign-body types dominated in some cases. Inclusions of the asteroid body were detected within the giant cells in all cases of this group. The granulomas were generally poorly demarcated from the surrounding tissues, and only infrequently were the lesions well defined in cases where the lesions might be confused with genuine sarcoidosis. All the granulomas were surrounded by reticulin strands, and the reticulum fibers passed radially into the granulomas while enclosing each epithelioid cell in a single strand. In most cases, there was pronounced evidence for "sinus catarrh" or histiocytosis around

TABLE 1.

		Age	Sex	Primary tumor	No. of lymph nodes examined	No. of lymph nodes with			Origin of specimen
						Both metastases and sarcoid-like lesions	Sarcoid-like lesion alone	Metastases alone	
Group 1	Case 1	69	male	Gasric carcinoma, Adenocarcinoma tubulare	22	2	6	0	Yugawa Hospital, Osaka
	Case 2	56	female	Gastric carcinoma, Adenocarcinoma tubulare	4	3	1	0	Kansai Rosai Hospital
	Case 3	50	male	Gastric carcinoma, Adenocarcinoma tubulare	1	0	1	0	Center for adult diseases, Osaka
	Case 4	73	male	Gastric carcinoma, Adenocarcinoma tubulare	7	0	3	0	Our case
Group 2	Case 5	64	male	Tongue, Squamous Cell Carcinoma	1 cervical	0	1	0	Kaisei Hospital, Osaka
	Case 6	57	male	Lung, Squamous Cell Carcinoma	1 mediastinal	1	0	0	Osaka University Hospital
	Case 7	64	male	Orbita, Adenocarcinoma	1 cervical	1	0	0	Our case
	Case 8	52	female	Breast, Noninfiltrating duct carcinoma (Paget' disease)	1 axillary	0	1	0	Osaka University Hospital

the granulomatous tissue in the nodal tissues. There was focal fibrosis or hyalinization in the nodules or perinodular regions. The lymph nodes of case 4, in which both meta-static and tuberculoid nodules were found, show granulomata, composed of loosely packed epithelioid cells and associated with diffuse plasmacytic proliferations through-out the medullary tissue of the nodes. Histologically these lesions resembled those found in tuberculosis. The latter, however, was precluded as a result of negative acid-fast bacilli staining in the histological sections concerned and also by the subsequent clinical course.

The topographic distribution of the 22 resected lymph nodes, normal or diseased, is shown in Fig. 1 (case 1). It is apparent from this figure that the related regional lymph nodes draining the primary tumor were inclined to be affected by sarcoid-like lesions and that the lymph nodes involving sarcoid-like lesions were more extensive in distribution than those, by metastases.

The group of malignant tumors other than stomach cancer included carcinomas of the tongue, lung, orbita and breast. The number of resected lymph nodes in this group was too small to evaluate pathologically. However, in 2 of these cases, the lymph nodes showed the coexistence of metastases and sarcoid-like lesions in the same nodal tissue, and the lymph nodes in the other 2 cases shows only sarcoid-like lesions. The histological

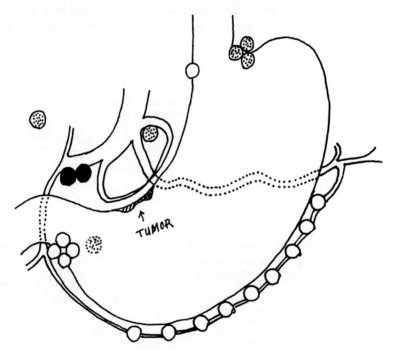

O : Normal or reactive hyperplastic lymph node (1 right cardiac, 9 left and right inferior gastric and 4 subpyloric lymph nodes)

⊛ : Lymph node with sarcoid-like lesions alone (3 left cardiac, 1 superior coeliac, 1 hepatic and 1 posterior pancreaticoduodenal lymph nodes)

● : Lymph node with both neoplastic metastases and sarcoid-like lesions (2 retropyloric lymph nodes)

FIG. 1.   Topographic distribution of 22 regional lymph nodes involved by neoplastic metastases and sarcoid-like lesions in a patient of gastric carcinoma (case 1).

appearance of these granulomas was essentially similar to that in the stomach cancer group. Of 4, only 1 case (case 5) revealed asteroid body-like structures in the cytoplasm of giant cells.

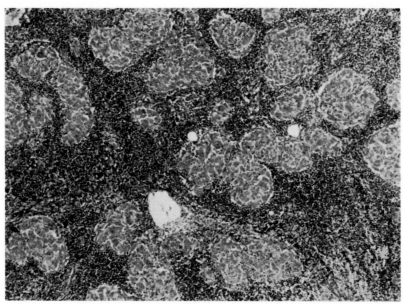

(Hematoxylin-eosin, Mag. ×130)

Fig. 2.   Coeliac lymph node in a stomach cancer patient containing sarcoid-like lesions which are composed of well circumscribed granulomas of epithelioid cells, resembling sarcoidosis (case 1).

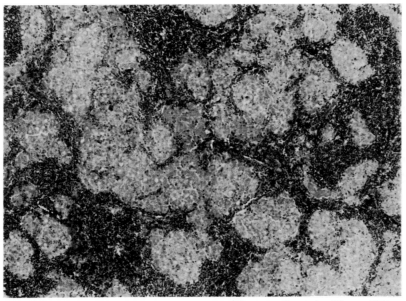

(Hematoxylin-eosin, Mag. ×130)

Fig. 3.   Cervical lymph node in a patient with carcinoma of the tongue showing many granulomas of epithelioid cells which are poorly limited to the surrounding hyperplastic lymphoid tissue (case 5).

DISCUSSION

It has generally been accepted that local sarcoid-like lesions arise in response to a variety of conditions, including infections, neoplasms, chemicals, immunological deficiency and others. It is postulated that the sarcoid-like lesions found in the regional lymph node in the cases with malignant neoplasma, might be due to the by-products of tumor disintegration. All of our cases, except 1 (case 8), had progressive malignant tumors, and the group of stomach cancers in particular showed a destructive tendency to produce ulcers in the tumor tissue. These characteristics of the tumor tissue and the distribution of lymph nodes involving sarcoid-like lesions as shown in the figure suggest the possibility that an agent, released from the tumor tissue in the stomach, spreads through the lymphatics into the regional lymph nodes, producing a granulomatous reaction in these nodes. Alternatively, it is proposed that radiation and chemotherapy in cancer patients may play a role in producing sarcoid-like lesions in the lymph nodes. We could draw no definite conclusion about this problem, because unfortunately insufficient information concerning treatment in each patient was available.

Some authors recognized histological differences between genuine sarcoidosis and sarcoid-like lesions. Symmers observed that sarcoid-like lesions could be histologically differentiated from true sarcoidosis by poor demarcation from the surrounding lymphoid tissue, by a loose packing of component cells and by a generalized marked infiltration by lymphoid cells. This observation is true for some findings, but not for others. From the pathological findings in this report, it seems likely that the histological appearance of sarcoid-like lesions in a lymph node are indistinguishable from that of sarcoidosis, and that the epithelioid cell granulomas are a nonspecific reaction caused by a variety of diseases, and are not pathognomonic for true sarcoidosis, as reported previously.

CONCLUSION

Eight cases of patients with malignant tumors coexistent with sarcoid-like lesions in the related regional lymph nodes were histopathologically studied.

An analysis of the lymph nodes involved by sarcoid-like lesions among patients with stomach cancers, provided suggestive evidence that an agent released from the tumor tissue provokes the regional lymph nodes into producing sarcoid-like lesions.

As for the histology of sarcoid-like lesions, we would agree with the opinion expressed by many authors that there is no way to differentiate it from the lesion occuring in genuine sarcoidosis.

REFERENCES

1. Nadel, E. M., and Ackerman, L. V. 1950. Lesions resembling Boeck's sarcoid in lymph nodes draining an area containing a malignant neoplasm. *Amer. J. Cl. Path.* **20**: 952.
2. Barrie, H. J., and Bococh, A. 1951. The natural history of the sarcoid granuloma. *Amer. J. Path.* **27**: 451.
3. Symmers, W. Sr. 1951. Localized tuberculoid granulomas associated with carcinoma. Their relationship to sarcoidosis. *Amer. J. Path.* **27**: 493.
4. Engle, R. 1953. Sarcoid and sarcoid-like granulomas. A study of twenty-seven postmortem

examinations. *Amer. J. Path.* **29**: 53.

5. Gorton, S., and Linell, F. 1957. Malignant tumors and sarcoid reactions in regional lymph nodes. *Act. Radiol.* **47**: 381.

6. Gresham, G. A., and Ackerley, A. G. 1958. Giant cell granulomata in regional lymph nodes of carcinoma. *J. Clin. Path.* **11**: 244.

7. Raben, A. S. 1962. Sarcoidosis and so-called sarcoid reactions. *Postgrad. Med.* **31**: 232.

8. Gregorie, H. B., Othersen H. B. Jr., and Moore, M. P. 1962. The significance of sarcoid-like lesions associated with malignant neoplasms. *Amer. J. Surg.* **104**: 577.

9. Anderson, R., James, D. G., Peters, P. M., and Thomson, A. D. 1962. Local sarcoid-tissue reactions. *Lancet* **7241**: 1211.

Hepatic Granulomatosis Revisited

Harold L. Israel

Jefferson Medical College, Thomas Jefferson University, Philadelphia, U.S.A.

AND

Robert A. Goldstein

VA-George Washington University Medical Center, Washington, D. C., U.S.A.

SUMMARY

Twenty-three patients with hepatic granulomatosis and normal chest roentgenograms have been studied. In 10 evidence of epithelioid granulomas was confined to percutaneous liver biopsies; in many of tbse cases it was impossible to determine whether the patients had systemic granulomatosis or local hepatic disease. In 13 patients, granulomas were demonstrated in multiple organs or tissues; exclusion of infectious causes made sarcoidosis the most likely diagnosis. Kveim tests were performed in 19 of the patients with uniformly negative results.

When investigation of liver diseases and unexplained fever or when the staging of Hodgkin's disease reveals hepatic granulomatosis, additional biopsies (including mediastinoscopy or laparatomy) are essential in order to determine whether involvement is systemic. The Kveim test cannot be relied upon for the exclusion of hepatic sarcoidosis. Our observations support recent reports indicating that hepatic granulomatosis is at present more often associated with sarcoidosis and Hodgkin's disease than infections.

INTRODUCTION

The growing use of liver biopsy in the study of hepatic disorders, in the staging of Hodgkin's disease, in the diagnosis of sarcoidosis, and in the investigation of unexplained fevers has resulted in the frequent demonstration of granulomatous inflammation. The result, in many instances is a difficult and controversial problem in diagnosis. Viral, bacterial, protozoan or fungal infections, as well as sarcoidosis, Hodgkin's disease, and drug hypersensitivity may produce granulomas which are indistinguishable. Often the lesions are attributed to tuberculosis because of the belief that this is the most common cause of cryptogenic hepatic granulomas. This view requires reexamination as a consequence of the rapid decline in tuberculosis, the recent demonstration of the frequency of hepatic granulomas in Hodgkin's disease[1,2], and recognition that sarcoidosis has become the most common cause of hepatic granulomas[3,4].

Since patients with demonstrable thoracic disease were excluded from our study, our series is not biased by referral of patients thought to have sarcoidosis. The principles of diagnosis which we have developed represent a logical approach to the diagnosis of all hepatic granulomas unaccompanied by abnormalities which identify the cause of the lesions.

A preliminary report[5] which included 9 of these cases led to the conclusion that sarcoidosis was not a cause because Kveim tests were uniformly negative. This view has been reexamined in the light of new evidence regarding the behavior of the Kveim reaction[6], which indicates that this test cannot be relied upon for the exclusion of hepatic sarcoidosis.

Observations

Table 1 summarizes data on cases 1–10, representing patients who had percutaneous biopsies of the liver because of unexplained fever or abnormal liver-function tests. The demonstration of epithelioid granulomas led to antituberculous treatment in 3 instances (despite negative second strength tuberculin reactions) without effect on the fever. One patient in whom Q fever was suspected had subsidence of fever after treatment with tetracycline, but serologic studies for rickettsial infection proved negative. In 3 instances fever subsided spontaneously while in 3 cases fever subsided only after corticosteroid therapy.

TABLE 1. Patients with hepatic granulomatosis (percutaneous biopsy).

Case	Tuberculin	Kveim	Outcome	Final diagnosis
1	0/250 TU	N. D.	Recovery with steroids	Hepatitis or sarcoidosis
2	,,	N. D.	Spontaneous recovery	,, ,, ,,
3	,,	Negative	Recovery with steroids	,, ,, ,,
4	,,	,,	,, ,, ,,	,, ,, ,,
5	,,	,,	Spontaneous recovery	,, ,, ,,
6	,,	N. D.	Death	Hodgkin's disease
7	,,	Negative	Spontaneous recovery	Hepatitis or sarcoidosis
8	,,	,,	Recovery with tetracycline	,, ,, ,,
9	,,	,,	(Evidence of prior mediastinal adenopathy)	Sarcoidosis
10	,,	,,	Undetermined	Hepatitis or sarcoidosis

In only 2 of these cases was a definite etiology subsequently demonstrated. A 75-year-old man (case 6) gravely ill with high fever was found to have numerous epithelioid hepatic granulomas and was treated for acute miliary tuberculosis. Necropsy demonstrated Hodgkin's disease. Case 7 was studied in 1970 because of fever of undetermined origin, and percutaneous biopsy showed numerous granulomas. A chest X-ray and Kveim test were negative. Chest roentgenograms taken in 1966 were obtained and demonstrated mediastinal adenopathy which had disappeared without therapy. Fever declined on steroid therapy but recurred and in 1971 the patient was found to have metastatic melanosarcoma. The recovery of the other patients was unrelated to antituberculous chemotherapy, and it is impossible in retrospect to distinguish those who had sarcoidosis from those who had hepatic infections or hypersensitivity reactions.

The diagnostic problem differs when granulomatosis is demonstrated in other organs or tissues (Table 2). In 8 cases laparotomy demonstrated additional evidence of granulomatosis in mesenteric or retroperitoneal lymph nodes or in the spleen. In 2 patients (cases 17–18), mediastinoscopy was utilized in order to determine whether granulomatosis was systemic or confined to the liver. In both instances, despite normal chest roentgenograms, small mediastinal nodes were obtained which showed granulomas.

Table 2 also presents data on 3 additional patients (cases 20–22) who were studied because of other manifestations (cutaneous lesion, hypercalcemia, dyspnea), had granulo-

TABLE 2. Patients with systemic granulomatosis.

Case	Tuberculin	Kveim	Extrahepatic involvement	Outcome	Final diagnosis
11	0/250 TU	Negative	Retroperitoneal nodes	Improvement with steroids	Sarcoidosis
12	,,	,,	Spleen, myocardium	Improvement with steroids	,,
13	,,	,,	Skull, hypercalcemia	Improvement with steroids	,,
14	,,	,,	Skin	Improvement with steroids	,,
15	+/5 TU	,,	Mesenteric nodes	Recovery with steroids	,,
16	+/250 TU	,,	Mediastinal nodes	Recovery with steroids	,,
17	0/250 TU	,,	Spleen	Improvement with chemotherapy	Hodgkin's disease
18	+/5 TU	,,	Marrow	Improvement with steroids	Tuberculosis, recovered ; sarcoidosis
19	0/250 TU	,,	Lung	Improvement with steroids	Sarcoidosis
20	,,	,,	Mesenteric nodes	Improvement with steroids	,,
21	,,	,,	Mediastinal nodes	Improvement with steroids	,,
22	,,	,,	Spleen	Undetermined	,,

mas demonstrated in skin, bone or lung, and had liver biopsies performed to document systemic involvement. These cases clearly represent sarcoidosis and resemble the cases previously described in that each had a normal chest roentgenogram and a negative Kveim test at the time diffuse hepatic granulomatosis was present.

In the group of 13 patients in which multiple sites of granulomatous involvement was demonstrated, 1 recovered spontaneously, 2 recovered after 6 to 12 months of corticosteroid therapy and 9 have required continuation of treatment for longer periods. In none did evidence of infection become manifest. It appears that with the exception of case 13, currently under treatment for Hodgkin's disease, all of thse patients had sarcoidosis.

DISCUSSION

Twenty-three patients with multiple hepatic granulomas identical with those commonly seen in sarcoidosis have been described. The granulomas in 2 were associated with Hodgkin's disease. In no case did tuberculosis or fungal disease develop. The cases fall into 2 groups, those with evidence of granulomatosis confined to the liver, and those in whom systemic granulomatosis was demonstrated. In most cases in the first group the diagnosis is speculative: it is impossible to determine whether the patients had viral infections, drug hypersensitivity reactions or other types of primary hepatic disease. It is quite possible, on the other hand, that they had sarcoidosis since the clinical course, laboratory abnormalities and histologic changes were identical with the cases in which multiple foci of granulomatosis were demonstrated and in which the diagnosis of sar-

coidosis seems established. The negative Kveim tests in patients with unequivocal sarcoidosis indicates that the Kveim reaction cannot be relied upon for the exclusion of
this disease.

Klatskin[7] has emphasized that a diagnosis of sarcoidosis cannot be established by
liver biopsy alone and that systemic involvement must be demonstrated by radiologic
or histologic evidence of sarcoidosis elsewhere or by a Kveim test. Although it has been
generally accepted that the Kveim reaction should serve to differentiate the hepatic
granulomatosis of sarcoidosis from that of other diseases, no evidence to support this
belief has been published. The uniformly negative Kveim tests in patients in the present
study originally led to the conclusion[5] that most of the patients in the group had some
disease other than sarcoidosis. However, further study revealed unequivocal evidence
of sarcoidosis in many of the patients. At the same time, evidence has been accumulated[6]
that the Kveim reaction is frequently negative in the absence of persistent hilar and mediastinal lymphadenopathy: patients with active sarcoidosis involving lung, skin and liver
may fail to react to Kveim antigen. As the cases in the present study demonstrate, the
Kveim test has been of little use in identification of the etiology of granulomatosis when
the chest roentgenogram is normal. Substantiation of this observation is available in the
data of Maddrey et al.[8] who performed Kveim tests in 13 patients with clinical or laboratory evidence of hepatic sarcoidosis. Tests were positive in 7 who had hilar adenopathy,
but were equivocal or negative in 5 of 6 patients without hilar adenopathy. Fitzgerald
et al.[9], on the other hand, have recently reported positive Kveim tests in 2 patients with
granulomatous hepatitis, but were skeptical of the specificity of the reactions since no
other evidence of sarcoidosis could be demonstrated. The Kveim test materials employed in most of the patients in the present study was Commonwealth Serum Laboratory lots 003 and 004. It has been suggested that the latter lot has produced false-positive reactions, but there is no evidence that this material is less potent than other preparations.

Mikhail and Mitchell[10] found that in typical sarcoidosis mediastinoscopy yielded
granulomas in 98% while the Kveim reaction was positive in 70.5%. It is evident that
in cases of unidentified hepatic granulomatosis mediastinoscopy is the procedure most
likely to establish systemic involvement. Patients with both hepatic and mediastinal
granulomas, after appropriate clinical and laboratory investigation has excluded infectious and hypersensitivity causes, are best classified and treated as sarcoidosis.

Similar considerations apply to the demonstration at laparotomy of diffuse granulomatous involvement of spleen or abdominal lymph nodes in addition to the liver. As in
the mediastinum, tuberculosis and fungal infection require exclusion before a diagnosis
of sarcoidosis is acceptable, but in most cases these infections can be excluded by skin
tests, serologic studies and cultures.

The pathogenesis of the diffuse hepatic granulomatosis which has been demonstrated[1]
in 5% of patients having laparotomies for staging of Hodgkin's disease is uncertain.
Brinker[1] has suggested that a primary abnormality of delayed hypersensitivity makes
these patients more susceptible both to sarcoidosis and Hodgkin's disease, but evidence
is lacking that anergy antedates the development of sarcoidosis. It is possible that patients with sarcoidosis have an increased risk of Hodgkin's disease. It is difficult to con-
ceive that the disseminated granulomatosis observed in 5 of Brinker's cases could represent a sarcoid reaction to Hodgkin's disease. As a result of these observations and the
2 patients described in the present study, it is clear that Hodgkin's disease can present

with a typical sarcoid reaction of the liver, and this possibility requires serious consideration if a history of pruritis or intermittent fever can be elicited.

It should be emphasized that a similar diagnostic approach is appropriate when sarcoid reactions are discovered in other organs, such as kidney, central nervous system, upper respiratory tract, etc. The essential step is to determine by biopsies of other tissues or organs whether the granulomatous reaction is systemic.

The observations we have reported are of considerably immunologic importance, providing strong support for the hypothesis that the Kveim reaction is not a test for sarcoidosis but rather a response to certain anatomic features frequent in sarcoidosis, namely chronic lymphadenopathy and erythema nodosum.

REFERENCES

1. Brincker, H. 1972. Sarcoid reactions and sarcoidosis in Hodgkin's disease and other malignant lymphomata. *Brit. J. Cancer* **26**: 120.
2. Kadin, M. E., Donaldson, S. S., and Dorfman, R. F. 1970. Isolated granulomas in Hodgkin's disease, *New Engl. J. Med.* **283**: 859.
3. Terplan, M. 1971. Hepatic granulomas of unknown cause presenting with fever. *Amer. J. Gastroent.* **55**: 43.
4. Iversen, K., Christoffersen, P., and Poulsen, H. 1970. Epithelioid cell granulomas in liver biopsies. *Scand. J. Gastroent. Suppl.* **7**: 67.
5. Israel, H. L. 1971. Granulomatous hepatitis: relationship to sarcoidosis. *Proc. Fifth Int. Conf. on Sarcoidosis* Prague: Univ. Karlova. p. 563.
6. Israel, H. L., and Goldstein, R. A. 1971. Relationship of Kveim antigen reaction to lymphadenopathy. *New Engl. J. Med.* **284**: 345.
7. Klatskin, G. 1962. The syndrome of sarcoidosis, psoriasis and gout. *Ann. Int. Med.* **57**: 1018.
8. Maddrey, W. C., Johns, C. J., Boitnott, J. K. et al. 1970. Sarcoidosis and chronic hepatic disease: a clinical and pathologic study of 20 patients. *Medicine.* **49**: 375.
9. Fitzgerald, M. X., Fitzgerald, O., and Towers, R. P. 1971. Granulomatous hepatitis of obscure etiology. Diagnostic contribution of Kveim testing and antituberculous therapy. *Quart. J. Med.* **40**: 374.
10. Mikhail J. R., and Mitchell, D. N. 1971. Mediastinoscopy: a diagnostic procedure in hilar and paratracheal lymphadenopathy. *Postgrad. Med. J.* **47**: 698.

A Comparison of Sarcoidosis and Primary Biliary Cirrhosis

D. Geraint James, A. N. Walker and K. H. G. Piyasena

Royal Northern Hospital, London, Great Britain

AND

Sheila Sherlock

Royal Free Hospital, London, Great Britain

Sarcoidosis and primary biliary cirrhosis (PBC) are 2 chronic granulomatous disorders characterised by hepatic granulomas and depression of delayed-type hypersensitivity, as shown by in vivo skin tests and in vitro lymphocyte transformation. Granuloma formation is adjacent to the cholangioles in the liver in primary biliary cirrhosis but it may

TABLE 1. Features distinguishing sarcoidosis from primary bilary cirrhosis.

Features	Sarcoidosis	Primary biliary cirrhosis
Sex F : M	Equal	8 : 1
Decade of onset onset over 40 years	3, 4 rare	5 Frequent
Erythema nodosum	Yes	No
Uveitis	Yes	No
Respiratory	Yes	No
Pruritus	No	Yes, Nearly always
Jaundice	No	Yes
Xanthomas	No	Yes
Clubbing	No	Yes (in 25%)
Hepatomegaly	No	Yes (in 100%)
Splenomegaly	Yes (in 12%)	Yes (in 50%)
Skin pigmentation	No	Yes (in 71%)
Steatorrhoea	No	Yes
Bilateral hilar lymphadenopathy	Yes	No
Kveim-Siltzbach test	Positive in 66%	Always negative
Depression of delayedtype hypersensitivity	Yes	Yes
Circulating antimitochondrial antibodies	No	Yes (in 99%)
Calcium metabolism	Hypercalcaemia vit. D Sensitivity	Hypocalcaemia (Steatorrhoea)
Raised		
—alkaline phosphatase	Yes, minority	Yes, majority
—serum cholesterol	No	Yes, majority
Liver granulomas	Yes	Yes
Corticosteroids	Helpful	Contraindicated
Vitamin D	Contraindicated	Helpful
Cholestyramine	Not necessary	Helpful
Prognosis	Very good	Poor, dead in 5 years

also extend to the abdominal lymph nodes, to the spleen, and even be present in the lungs. This multisystem granulomatous disorder may, therefore, provide superficial confusion with sarcoidosis, but there are also striking differences (Table 1).

Age and sex
Primary biliary cirrhosis almost always presents in menopausal women whereas sarcoidosis is commonly seen in both sexes and in the age group 20–40 years. Primary biliary cirrhosis commonly declares itself whereas sarcoidosis rarely does so for the first time in those aged over 40 years.

Clinical presentation
The cardinal clinical features of PBC are pruritus, jaundice, xanthomas, hepatomegaly, clubbing, steatorrhoea and pigmentation, none of which occur in sarcoidosis. Conversely, sarcoidosis usually presents with a chest X-ray abnormality, which is not a feature of PBC.

Delayed-type hypersensitivity
We have compared skin test responses using tuberculin, candida albicans and dinitrochlorobenzene (DNCB) in a series of 60 patients with sarcoidosis and 41 PBC patients; depression of delayed-type hypersensitivity is of a similar magnitude (Table 2). In addition to this cutaneous anergy, both disorders also show a similar depression of in vitro lymphocyte transformation in response to phytohaemagglutinin.

Epstein-Barr virus (EBV) antibodies
EBV antibody titres of 1:640 and over were 7 times commoner in sarcoidosis pa-

TABLE 2. A comparison of in vivo and in vitro tests in 60 patients with sarcoidosis and 41 patients with primary biliary cirrhosis.

	Sarcoidosis		Primary biliary cirrhosis	
	No.	%	No.	%
Granuloma formation	60	100	29	70
Positive Kveim-Siltzbach test	40	66	0/29	0
Negative				
—tuberculin	42	70	28	68
—candida	40	67	18/22	81
—DNCB	33	55	9/17	53
Depressed lymphocyte transformation	19/21	90	24/30	80

TABLE 3. Comparison of EBV antibody titres in sarcoidosis, primary biliary cirrhosis and control subjects.

EBV titre	Sarcoidosis		PBC		Control	
	No.	%	No.	%	No.	%
1:320 and under	58	78	35	92	58	97
1:640 and over	17	22	3	8	2	3
Total	75	100	38	100	60	100

tients than in controls and twice as common in PBC patients compared with controls
(Table 3).

Biochemical differences

Hypercalcaemia, hypercalciuria and hypersensitivity to Vitamin D are well-known
features of sarcoidosis whereas hypocalcaemia due to steatorrhoea complicates the course
of PBC. Thus PBC is further complicated by thin bones and a raised alkaline phosphatase in the majority of such patients. By way of contrast, a raised alkaline phosphatase
level is seen in the minority of patients with sarcoidosis, reflecting intrahepatic space-
occupying granulomas.

Treatment

There are vitally important differences in management. Whereas steroids are helpful
in sarcoidosis, they can but make the osteoporosis of PBC worse. Whereas vitamin D
is helpful in strengthening the bones in PBC, it magnifies the abnormal calcium metabolism and contributes to eventual nephrocalcinosis in sarcoidosis. Finally, cholestyra-
mine is useful in PBC and useless in sarcoidosis.

Prognosis

The outlook in PBC is considerably worse than in sarcoidosis. Patients with PBC
have a prognosis of only about 5 years.

Morphological Study of Granulomatous Hepatitis

Goichi Kiyonaga and Kenzo Matsuoka

Center for Adult Diseases, Osaka, Japan

AND

Teruo Tachibana, Kazuhiko Aratake and Yoshio Murata

Osaka Prefectural Hospital, Osaka, Japan

Cases of granulomatous hepatitis were examined by laparoscopy with needle biopsy, in which biopsy specimens were studied with a light microscope and, when necessary, with an electron microscope. The materials in this series were obtained in 3 ways: first, in routine morphological study on various liver disorders, the incidence of granulomatous hepatitis in Japan (about 2% of 2,000 cases in our series) being rather rare in comparison with that reported in other countries; second, in a study of patients with sarcoidosis, who were mainly detected by mass chest radiographies (33 cases); and, third, from materials offered by other hospitals.

In cases of sarcoidosis, laparoscopic changes of the liver were mildest, the liver surface being smooth and scattered with round spots (Fig. 1a and b). The granulomas were always noncaseating and the fibrous alteration in the liver tissue was minimal. There were some cases which showed a closer distribution of spots on the surface and granulomas in the tissue.

There were 3 cases of hepatic tuberculosis in this series. In general, fibrous changes were more prominent than in other kinds of granulomatous hepatitis, either in gross appearance (Figs. 2a and b) or in microscopic structure. All 3 had tubercles with giant cells and central caseation, indicating a tuberculous nature. A problem arises concerning morphological differentiation, particularly when the tubercle was noncaseating and free of microorganism. Tubercles in the tissue seemed to be distributed more sparsely than other diseases and to be larger in size even if they were not confluent.

In our series, 3 out of 12 phospholipidosis cases, induced by 4, 4′-diethylaminoethoxyl dichloride, had granulomas in the biopsy specimen. The liver in this disorder was often enormously enlarged with a hard consistency and had mostly a smooth surface, but sometimes a granulating (Figs. 3a and b) or nodular surface. The biopsy specimens showed swollen hepatic cells with foamy cytoplasma, where an electron microscope revealed characteristic myelin-like structures. No specific spotted figures were observed on the liver surface in these granulomatous cases, when the histological study revealed many granulomas were closely distributed and varied in size from small to large. All 3 were reexamined several months later, when granulomas were fewer in number and the surviving ones had enlarged during the clinical improvement of the illness.

No obvious granulomas were found in 4 cases of Hodgkin's disease. However, a recent case, who was in remission, had focal lesions composed of connective tissue with round cell infiltration in the liver tissue. Laparoscopy in this case disclosed a dotted surface pattern consisting of pink and violetish-brown areas (Fig. 4a). Moreover, there were scattered light-colored round spots, 1 of which was especially large and raised

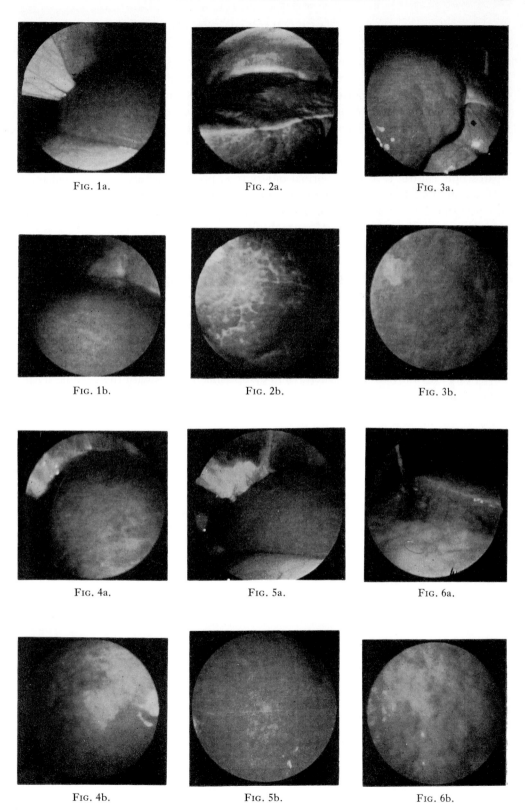

FIG. 1a.   FIG. 2a.   FIG. 3a.

FIG. 1b.   FIG. 2b.   FIG. 3b.

FIG. 4a.   FIG. 5a.   FIG. 6a.

FIG. 4b.   FIG. 5b.   FIG. 6b.

over above from the surface level (Fig. 4b). Such a peculiar appearance of the liver is likely to indicate Hodgkin's disease, as it has never been experienced in other diseases and a similar surface pattern was encountered in another case of the disease in another hospital. The remaining 3 cases had a uniformly colored red-brown liver,. In one case of them the liver had a spotted surface pattern (Figs. 5a and b) and the biopsy specimen had an accumulation of inflammatory cells in the expanded portal tracts, mingled with large cells resembling epitheloid cells. The patient developed a deep jaundice 3 months later and was reexamined by laparoscopy, in which the liver remained almost unchanged in color and appearance and direct cholecysto-cholangiography under laparoscopic control revealed a normal biliary tree, proving the absence of mechanical obstruction. The direct visualizing method accompanying laparoscopy with biopsy was also performed in another of the 3 cases because of a high titer of serum alkaline phosphatase activity, visualizing a normal biliary tree.

There were 2 cases of granulomatous hepatitis of unknown etiology. A small granuloma was unexpectedly found in the biopsy specimen in 1 case, in which the liver had a somewhat nodular surface without any spotted pattern (Figs. 6a and b): In the other case with a spotted, smooth liver surface granulomas were revealed, as was expected but after making many serial sections on the biopsy specimen.

In conclusion, laparoscopy and biopsy can prove the presence of granulomatous hepatitis with a high degree of accuracy, but as for determination of its etiology they are of little help except for a few occasions such as cases with central caseation in granulomas, cases with myelin-like structures in cytoplasma or cases with the peculiar dotted surface pattern.

DISCUSSION

1

Chairmen: D.N. Mitchell and O. Refvem

Dr Mitchell: Dr Israel drew attention to the transient nature and to the maturity of these lesions, which I think was reflected in the earlier work of Chase and Sheffer, and exemplified in Professor Turiaf's paper. Apart from that, one would wonder if there is any information with regard to the development of arthritic lesions in these animals: whether the granulomatous reaction can be transferred to other animals by leucocyte transfer, whether for instance, rat adjuvant disease is more easily transferable than that induced in guinea pigs.

Dr Yasuhira: It is well-known that after sensitization of animals with Freund's complete adjuvant, epithelioid lesions appear in the lung some weeks later. When the rabbit is used, the lesions turn into necrotizing foci frequently. This is the case in the guinea pig, but not in the rat and mouse. Human beings seem to belong to the former group of animals. The occurrence of necrotizing inflammation in epithelioid cell granulomas is important, I think, to differentiate sarcoidosis or sarcoid lesions from the other infectious diseases or lesions of an epithelioid cell character. Therefore, an attempt to induce sarcoidosis in animals experimentally should be carried out in the rabbit, guinea pig, or some other animal species not resistant to necrotizing inflammation.

Dr Turiaf: Je suppose que sur les diapositives que j'ai montrées vous n'avez pas vu de lésions nécrotiques. Il n'y a aucune nécrose. Ce que l'on voit, ce sont des vacuoles et de temps à autre de petites zones de nécrose fibrinoide, mais qui n'appartiennent pas à la nécrose caséeuse.

Dr Young: The choice of experimental laboratory animal for a model may be important. If one is going to mimic a disease in man, one probably ought to use an animal such as the horse with the same morphologic type of the lung, although it might be difficult getting a horse into many of the laboratories. Secondly I might suggest that some of these reactions may occur through inhaled enviromental substances. It may be worthwhile becoming a bit more sophisticated and aerosolizing some of the antigens that may be implicated in some of these type III immunologic lung reactions which, I suspect, is what we are seeing.

Dr Mitchell: There are epizootics of equine sarcoid in the States. I understand these are, in fact, really fibroblastic tumors largely limited to cutaneous tissues. It is a very interesting point and it leads to questions raised by Byron Waksman some years earlier of the development of these lesions, in particular arthritic lesions, in germ-free animals by the injection of adjuvant.

Dr Jones Williams: I was very interested to listen to the paper describing PAS granules and the questions as to the significance of this. Some years ago I reported the presence of 1 micron diameter PAS granules in epithelioid cells by light microscopy. In fact, from later work which I shall be reporting in this meeting, we were really demonstrating secretary granules of epithelioid cells. These are quite different and I would guess may be 4 or 5 micron diameter particles, in macrophages and not in the epithelioid cells. I don't really know the significance of the finding of 40 out of 200 cases.

Dr N. Shigematsun: In both experimental and human tissues, I can account only for PAS positive bodies found in macropheges around epithelioid cell gramulomas, not in the epithelioid cells. Dr Jones Williams can also find PAS positive granules in the epithelioid cell. Is the difference only the size between the PAS positive body or granule in epithelioid cells and in macrophages? Not being able to find PAS granules in epithelioid cells by myself I can not understand his findings in detail.

DR FUSE: I saw the PAS-positive bodies in epithelioid cells, indicated by Dr Johns. They are very tiny granules and I think correspond to cytoplasmic focal derivation, or residual bodies.

2

Chairmen: K. WURM AND R. C. JR. YOUNG

DR. YASUHIRA: In connection with the first presentation by Dr Jones Williams, I would like to call attention to the fact that an antigenic lipopolysaccharide component, wax D, of the tubercle bacillus has been established in our laboratory to be the only member of the bacterial fractions capable of inducing epithelioid cell lesions in tuberculo-sensitized animals. Generally speaking, the occurrence of sarcoid lesions depends, I think, on the amount and intensity of such antigenic lipopolysaccharides which may arise from bacteria or tissue elements. The amount of antigen necessary for the induction of epithelioid cell granulomas is very small, as in our experiments wax D less than 1 gamma could induce widespread sarcoid lesions in the lung. Dr Epstein in California pointed out in his personal communication that beryllium in as small an amount as 1 nanogamma or so may act as a potent antigen for inducing beryllium granulomas. In contrast, a large amount of the antigen may cause necrotizing foci at the site of application. This might be the case with this presentation. Therefore, I would like to ask Dr Jones Williams what amount of beryllium, at a guess, was applied to the primary focus in the patient?

DR JONES WILLIAMS: The amount of beryllium in the finger was 20.5 micrograms per gram wet weight of tissue. Of 2 separate biopsies from the lymphatic nodules, one showed 7.5 and the other, I forget the exact amount, but it was about 10. In a lung the biopsy was too small to make an analysis.

I agree with Dr Epstein that you need very little because this is obviously a hypersensitivity disease. There is no doubt that you can produce it experimentally with very minute amounts. I have done a few experiments with intratracheal inhalation in rats, with very disappointing results. I put in varying amounts, and biopsy of the lung over a period of a year, failed to produce any granulomas. I did the experiment again and gave repeated doses at monthly intervals. Again I could not produce granulomas. However, other people have done this and produced beautiful granulomas by inhalation.

DR YOUNG: I was wondering if Dr Jones Williams had examined the possibility that the beryllium disease may have been contracted perhaps years before the finger innoculation and that the finger innoculation was inconsequential in the genesis of his patient's pulmonary disease.

DR JONES WILLIAMS: I don't think that this man had previous disease. I cannot prove that but, at time of his original injury, he had no pulmonary dysfunction, his lung X-ray changes were normal, he had no symptoms and was in good general health. He was Mantoux-positive, Kveim-negative, and had normal granulocyte function. I don't think the problem is whether the absorption of beryllium from his finger went through lymphatics to his lung, or whether he may possibly have inhaled beryllium at various times. Careful control was done in this factory to make sure that the limit of beryllium in the air was never exceeded.

DR MITCHELL: There is a latent period of sometimes 15 or 20 years before the development of beryllium disease.

DR JOHNS: How long had your patient worked in the beryllium factory prior to the skin lesions and did he continue to work in the beryllium factory after the skin lesions? What dose of steroids was required to control the disease in his lung?

DR JONES WILLIAMS: He had worked in the beryllium factory for 5 years before the onset of the disease. We stopped his work at once. The dose of steroids to start with was 25 mg and he has been maintained on 10 mg.

DR JOHNS: I was interested in the dose of steroids as it compares with what it seems to take to control some of the sarcoidosis patients. I also wanted to comment on the hepatic granulomas. This is certainly a puzzling problem. I would like to mention one patient that I have encountered. This was a young, black female in her twenties whom I saw in 1963. She had been admitted to the hospital with a fever of unknown origin and as part of her work-up, a needle liver biopsy was done and hepatic granulomas of indiscriminate type were identified. She had no other stigmata of sarcoidosis. Her Kveim test was negative; her tuberculin was negative. In about 2 weeks she was entirely well and was discharged. I concluded she had insufficient evidence for sarcoidosis. I was very startled to have the same patient return 8 years later to our clinic. This time she had perfectly typical bilateral hilar adenopathy, diffuse pulmonary infiltration, characteristic skin lesions at the base of the hair line and a positive Kveim test. In this case, the hepatic granulomas long antedated the mere typical sarcoidosis manifestations and more the only initial findings.

DR ISRAEL: Most American physicians recognize primary biliary cirrhosis and the question of sarcoidosis rarely arises even when a few hepatic granulomas are encountered. Such cases have not been referred to us as a problem in diagnosis. I should like to emphasize that Klatskin and others who have written on this subject have not distinguished between patients in whom a liver biopsy was done in order to confirm a diagnosis of sarcoidosis suspected because of thoracic manifestations and cases in which liver biopsy was done because of unexplained fever or fatigue. Obviously many patients in the first category will have positive Kveim reactions because they have hilar adenopathy. Our analysis is confined to patients without clinical or roentgenologic evidence of sarcoidosis elsewhere. The problem in these cases is whether we are dealing with primary hepatic disease or systemic sarcoidosis. Our experience is that the Kveim test is rarely helpful in the diagnosis of hepatic granulomatosis in patients with normal chest X-rays.

In answer to Dr Johns' question about the mode of onset, the majority presented with fever. Often liver function test were abnormal which influenced the decision to look to the liver as a cause of the fever. There were a few patients in whom the presenting symptome was fatigue. There was 1 case which I referred to yesterday in which we did needle biopsy of the liver simply to demonstrate, that systemic involvement was present. Here too, even though there was active granuloma formation both in skin and liver, the Kveim test was negative.

It is clear that the Kveim test cannot be relied upon for diagnosis in these atypical cases of sarcoidosis. Multiple biopsies must be performed to determine whether or not several organ systems are involved. If multisystem involvement is demonstrated and infectious causes excluded, one must accept the diagnosis of sarcoidosis.

DR YOUNG: One would therefore perhaps like to utilize a double-biopsy technique to determine whether or not several organ systems are involved. If one does find this in the absence of other causes, one can fairly well rely on the diagnosis of sarcoidosis.

DR TACHIBANA: We ordinarily performed peritoneoscopy with a liver biopsy. In same cases using this technique, peritoneoscopical finding on the liver's surface, as described Dr Kiyonaga, have been able to differentiate hepatic granulomas.

DR JAMES: Can Dr Villar explain why one-quarter of his patients with extrinsic allergic alveolitis have abnormally high serum calcium levels?

Could the other speaker please explain why he used diethylaminoisoxy-hydrochloride?

Finally, I would like to exmphasise that primary biliary cirrhosis (PBC) is not just a liver disease but a chronic granulomatous disorder which involves liver, lymph nodes and even the lung (see New Engl. J. Med. 1972. 287: 1282).

DR VILLAR: I don't know why the blood calcium was raised in 23% of our pulmonary granulomas other than sarcoidosis. It is only a fact we have noted. I believe all the diseases I have shown you have essentially similar problems. For instance, in a cork factory with many workers, something like 35% will get suberosis.

IV   IMMUNOLOGY

Immunology of Sarcoidosis

D. Geraint James, A. N. Walker and A. N. Hamlyn

Royal Northern Hospital, London, Great Britain

The cardinal immunological abnormalities in sarcoidosis are 4-fold:—
1. Depression of delayed-type hypersensitivity
    (a) in vivo
    (b) in vitro
2. Lymphoproliferation
3. Granuloma formation
4. Positive Kveim-Siltzbach test

1. *Depression of Delayed-type Hypersensitivity*
This is a feature not only of sarcoidosis but also many other disorders (Table 1). It indicates impairment of cell-mediated immunity due to some defect of thymus-mediated (T) lymphocytes. We can now assess the efficiency of these T cells by means of in vivo bedside skin tests and by in vitro lymphocyte function tests.

(a) *In vivo skin tests.* Skin test antigens commonly used are tuberculin, mumps, dinitrochlorobenzene (DNCB) and Californian keyhole limpet haemocyanin (KLH). All such tests reveal cutaneous anergy in sarcoidosis (Table 2).

(b) *In vitro lymphocyte transformation.* The cultured lymphocytes from patients

Table 1. Disorders associated with depression of delayed-type hypersensitivity.

1. Physiological states	4. Thymic hypoplasia
—Newborn	Thymectomy
—Elderly	Runt disease
2. Drugs	5. Sarcoidosis
—Corticosteroids	Reticulosis
—Cytotoxic	Lymphoblastoma
—Antilymphocytic serum	6. Uraemia
—Viral vaccines	Cachexia
3. Radiotherapy	7. Hypnosis

Table 2. Correlation of various skin tests in sarcoidosis and control subjects.

Test	Sarcoidosis		Controls	
	No.	%	No.	%
Positive Kveim	15/17	88	0/12	
Negative Tuberculin	16/19	84	1/12	8
Negative DNCB	8/9	89	1/12	8
Negative KLH	16/19	84	1/12	8

TABLE 3. Correlation of in vivo DNCB skin tests with in vitro lymphocyte transformation in 21 patients with sarcoidosis and 17 control subjects.

DNCB Sensitivity Lymphocyte transformation	No.	Positive Positive		Negative Negative		Positive Negative		Negative Positive	
		No.	%	No.	%	No.	%	No.	%
Sarcoidosis	21	2	10	15	71	4	19	0	
Controls	17	13	76	0		1	6	3	18

with sarcoidosis react poorly to phytohaemagglutinin which stimulates normal lymphocytes to undergo mitotic and blastic transformation. This in vitro cellular anergy correlates accurately with in vivo cutaneous anergy. These twin defects do not occur in normal individuals but feature in the majority of patients with sarcoidosis (Table 3).

Migration inhibition factor (MIF). Another in vitro lymphocyte function test is to assess the ability of sensitised lymphocytes to respond to an antigen, which provokes the production of various soluble factors including MIF. Suspensions of sarcoid tissue have been shown to produce MIF. It is hoped that this technique may be perfected with cleaner antigens to provide an "in vitro Kveim test".

2. *Lymphoproliferation*

Whereas cellular immunity is impaired, humoral immunity is normal and the bursa-dependent (B) cells are functioning adequately or perhaps even better than normal. It should not be overlooked that an eclipse of T cells occurs at a time when there is vigorous lymphoproliferation with raised immunoglobulin levels (Table 4) and increased circulating antibodies to a variety of antigens, including mismatched blood. Circulating antibodies to Epstein-Barr virus (EBV) in titers of 1:640 and over were observed 7 times more commonly in sarcoidosis than in control subjects in our recent series (Table 5).

More work needs to be done in sarcoidosis to assess whether T and B cell functions behave in seesaw fashion towards each other. It would appear that T cell eclipse coincides with B cell proliferation.

TABLE 4. Immunoglobulin levels in 71 patients with sarcoidosis.

Increased immunoglobulin	No.	%
IgG	40	56
IgA	19	27
IgM	9	13
Total abnormal	57/71	80

TABLE 5. Epstein-barr virus (EBV) antibody titres in sarcoidosis and controls.

EBV titre	Sarcoidosis		Controls	
	No.	%	No.	%
1:320 and under	58	78	58	97
1:640 and over	17	22	2	3
Total	75	100	60	100

3. *Granuloma Formation*

The granulomatous reaction in sarcoidosis involves a battle between indigestible antigen and macrophages, cellular lymphocytes and humoral antibodies. The phagocytic cells aggregate into epithelioid and giant cells, which are the hallmarks of a sarcoid granuloma. Within these epithelioid and giant cells may be found 3 types of inclusion bodies—Schaumann, asteroid and residual bodies—all of which are nonspecific (Fig. 1). Also within the granuloma are the immunoglobulins IgG, IgA, IgM and IgD, which can be identified in variable amounts by immunofluorescence.

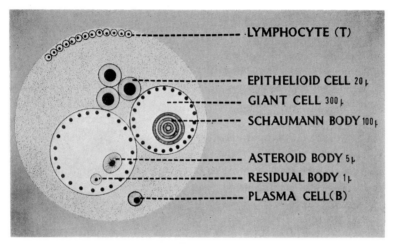

Fig. 1.

4. *Kveim-Siltzbach Test*

This is the remaining immunological abnormality and it continues to be a phenomenon unique to sarcoidosis. It is positive in three-quarters of patients with this multisystem disorder and negative in other diseases.

Other skin test reactions (Table 6) produce long-delayed granulomatous responses, which are individually specific for the diseases in question. The beryllium skin test is only positive in a patient sensitised to beryllium and likewise the zirconium skin test is only positive in an individual previously sensitised and affected by zirconium. Herein lies an indicator which may prove important in unravelling the enigma of the Kveim-Siltzbach test. By analogy, it would appear that the Kveim-Siltzbach skin test would only be positive in a patient previously exposed to and sensitised by the antigen in sarcoid and Kveim tissue. This hypothesis receives support in recent work on the "in vitro Kveim test".

TABLE 6.   Skin tests producing long-delayed granulomatous responses.
Each one is individually specific.

Disorder	Skin test
Sarcoidosis	Sarcoid suspension
Beryllium disease	Beryllium nitrate
Deodorant granuloma	Zirconium
Tuberculoid leprosy	Lepromin

In Vitro Function of Lymphocytes Tested by Micromethod of Whole-Blood Culture in Patients with Intrathoracic Sarcoidosis

Yasutaka Niitu, Masahiro Horikawa, Sumio Hasegawa, Shigeo Komatsu, Hideo Kubota and Tomiko Suetake

Department of Pediatrics, The Research Institute for Tuberculosis, Leprosy, and Cancer, Tohoku University, Sendai, Japan

Alterations in the in vitro function of cultured lymphocytes have been reported in sarcoidosis[1-6]. They may have some relation to the alterations in cell-mediated immunity, as indicated in the depression of the tuberculin reaction. The technique which has been used for the function test of cultured lymphocytes requires a large amount of blood for preparation of the lymphocytes, and so is not practicable as a routine test, especially in children.

Using the Hungerford microtechnique of peripheral blood culture[7], as we[6] reported at the Fifth Conference, we observed morphologically and biochemically the in vitro function of lymphocytes in sarcoidosis.

MATERIALS AND METHODS

Patients with intrathoracic sarcoidosis—both children and adults—showing in almost all cases bilateral hilar lymphadenopathy on chest X-ray were tested. Patients with tuberculosis and other diseases and healthy children and adults served as controls.

Heparinized peripheral blood (0.2 ml) was added to 4 pairs of culture bottles, each containing 5 ml of culture medium. After addition of 3 pairs of stimulants, PHA, PPD, and Kveim antigen, i.e., 10% saline suspension of the removed sarcoid lymph node, and without addition of any stimulant to 1 pair, the culture bottles were incubated at 37°C in a CO_2 incubator for 3 and 7 days.

For morphological study, after the cultures were harvested, some manipulations were carried out, and the smear was prepared and stained. In this method, red blood cells and cytoplasma of leukocytes were destroyed and only round nuclei remained. With the use of a square eyepiece micrometer, the sizes of 500 to 1,000 nuclei were classified. The percentage of nuclei of 7μ or more in diameter and nuclei with mitosis was given as the rate of large cells. The number of nuclei in mitosis per mill was given as the rate of mitosis.

For biochemical studies, 24 hours prior to harvesting, 2.5 μCi of ³H-thymidine and 10 μg of carrier thymidine were added to each of the above cultures. Kveim antigen was not tested. Several manipulations were made after harvesting, and the samples were counted in a liquid scintillation counter, corrected for quenching, and the incorporations were expressed as cpm per million lymphocytes counted at the beginning of the culture.

RESULTS AND DISCUSSION

In most cases, the rate of large cells and the cpm were higher in the 3-day culture than in the 7-day culture for the culture with PHA, while it was higher in the 7-day culture for cultures with other stimulants or without stimulant.

The results of morphological studies are summarized in Table 1. The rate of large cells in the 7-day culture showed higher mean values in sarcoidosis than in the control, especially in cases other than tuberculosis. This corresponds to reports[1,3,5,6] that the spontaneous transformation of lymphocytes was increased in sarcoidosis.

The rate of stimulant-induced large cells was calculated by subtracting the percentage of large cells in the control culture without stimulant from the percentage of large cells in the culture with stimulant. The degree of stimulation of lymphocytes by the stimulant was compared in terms of the rate of stimulant-induced large cells showing a higher figure between the 3-day and 7-day cultures. The rate of PHA-induced large cells and the rate of PHA-induced mitosis was lower in sarcoidosis than in the control, showing that cultured lymphocytes responded poorly to PHA in sarcoidosis, as reported by some authors[1-3,5,6]. The rate of PPD-induced large cells was clearly lower in sarcoidosis than in tuberculosis, showing that lymphocytes do not respond to PPD in sarcoidosis, as reported by Hirschhorn, Siltzbach, and associates[1,5] and by the present authers[6]. This reflected the fact that patients with sarcoidosis showed negative to intradermal

TABLE 1. Rate of large cells and rate of mitosis in whole-blood culture with or without stimulant in sarcoidosis.

Stimulant		Sarcoidosis	Controls	
			Tuberculosis	Others
None	No. of cases tested	23	24	17
	Rate of large cells (mean)	28.4%	26.5%	24.7%
PHA	No. of cases tested	23	19	15
	Rate of PHA-induced large cells (mean)	29.0%	53.0%	58.2%
	Rate of mitosis (mean)	6 ‰	17 ‰	26 ‰
PPD	No. of cases tested	21	22	10
	Rate of PPD-induced large cells (mean)	2.3%	15.9%	8.4%

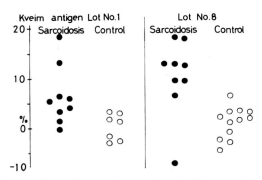

Fig. 1. Rate of large cells stimulated by Kveim antigen.

tuberculin test in most cases, while patients with tuberculosis showed strongly positive.

With Kveim antigen, the antigen from 8 samples of the lymph node did not stimulate lymphocytes in sarcoidosis or in the controls. However, the antigen from 2 samples of the lymph node stimulated lymphocytes specifically in sarcoidosis (Fig. 1), similar to the results reported by Hirschhorn, Siltzbach and associates[1, 5] and to our preliminary report[6]. The test for the specific stimulation of lymphocytes by an adequate Kveim

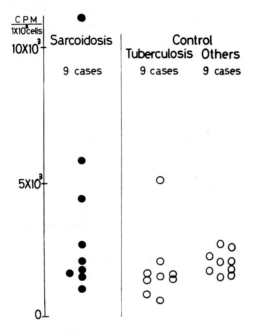

FIG. 2.   Incorporation of ³H-thymidine in 7-day culture without stimulant.

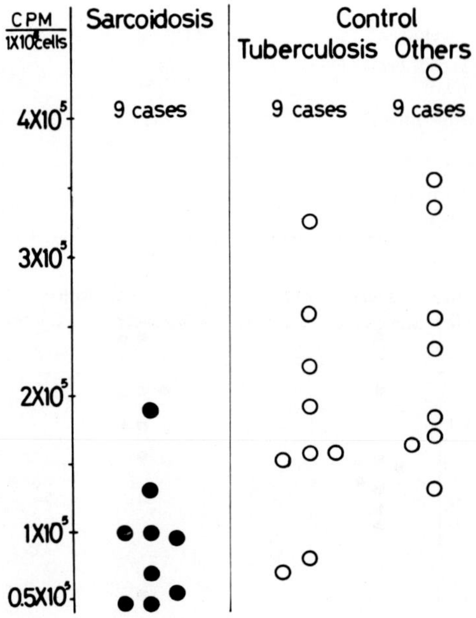

FIG. 3.   Incorporation of ³H-thymidine in 3-day culture with PHA.

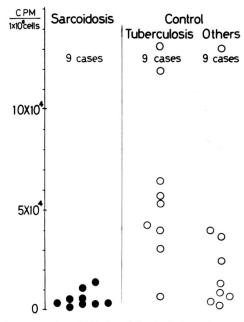

FIG. 4. Incorporation of ³H-thymidine in 7-day culture with PPD.

antigen, as well as the poor response of lymphocytes to PHA with this practicable micromethod, may be helpful for the in vitro diagnosis of sarcoidosis.

The results of incorporations of ³H-thymidine are shown in Figs. 2, 3, and 4. With cultures without stimulant, the cpm in the 7-day culture was higher on average in 3 of 9 cases of sarcoidosis than in the controls (Fig. 2). With cultures with PHA, the cpm in the 3-day culture showed lower mean values in sarcoidosis than in the controls (Fig. 3), and the cpm in the 7-day culture showed no clear difference between sarcoidosis and the controls. With cultures with PPD, the cpm in the 7-day culture showed lower values in sarcoidosis (Fig. 4). These results were similar to the results obtained in the morphological study.

SUMMARY

Morphological and biochemical studies on the in vitro function of lymphocytes with the micromethod using whole-blood culture revealed an increased spontaneous transformation of lymphocytes, a poor response of lymphocytes to PHA and PPD, and a specific stimulation of lymphocytes by an adequate Kveim antigen in sarcoidosis. The micromethod used is rather simple and practicable and may be helpful in the study of altered cell-immunity in sarcoidosis and for in vitro diagnosis of sarcoidosis.

REFERENCES

1. Hirschhorn, K., Schreibman, P. R., Bach, F. H., and Siltzbach, L. E. 1964. In vitro studies of lymphocytes from patients with sarcoidosis and lymphoproliferative disease. *Lancet* **2**: 842.
2. Buckley, C. E., Nagaya, H., and Sieker, H. D. 1966. Altered immunologic activity in

sarcoidosis. *Annals of Internal Med.* **64**: 508.

3. Selroos, O. 1967. In vitro cultured lymphocytes in sarcoidosis. *La Sarcoidose*, Rapp. Conf. Int. Paris: Masson et Cie. p. 275.

4. Girard, J. P., Press, P., and Poupon, M. 1971. Culture of peripheral lymphocytes from sarcoidosis. *Fifth Int. Conf. on Sarcoidosis*. Prague: Univ. Karlova. p. 212.

5. Siltzbach, L. E., Glade, P. R., Hirshaut, Y., Vieira, L. O. B. D., Celikoglu, I. S., and Hirschhorn, K. 1971. In vitro stimulation of peripheral lymphocytes in sarcoidosis. *Fifth Int. Conf. on Sarcoidosis*. Prague: Univ. Karlova. p. 217.

6. Niitu, Y., Horikawa, M., Hasegawa, S., Suetake, T., Kubota, H., and Komatsu, S. 1971. An attempt to diagnose sarcoidosis in vitro. *Fifth Int. Conf. on Sarcoidosis*. Prague: Univ. Karlova. p. 451.

7. Hungerford, D. A. 1965. Leukocytes cultured from small inocula of whole blood and the preparation of metaphase chromosomes by treatment with hypotonic KCl. *Stain Technology* **40**: 333.

Phytohaemagglutinin-, tuberculin- and Kveim-Induced Blast Transformation in Sarcoidosis

Maija Horsmanheimo

III Department of Pathology, University of Helsinki and the Department of Dermatology, University Central Hospital, Helsinki, Finland

INTRODUCTION

Immunological mechanisms in sarcoidosis are characterized by a normal or an increased ability to develop humoral immunological responses, and by a depression of delayed hypersensitivity.

Contradictory findings have been reported regarding the ability of sarcoid lymphocytes to respond to different stimuli[1-9,11]. The aim of the present study was to investigate the transformation of sarcoid lymphocytes by phytohaemagglutinin (PHA), by PPD of tuberculin and by Kveim reagents, and to correlate the findings with the clinical symptoms of the patients.

MATERIAL AND METHODS

Sarcoid diagnosis was confirmed in all of the patients by biopsy. An intradermal tuberculin test (Mantoux) was performed in all cases with 0.1, 1, 10 and 100 tuberculin units (TU) of purified protein derivative (PPD, Statens Seruminstitute, Copenhagen) or until a positive skin test was obtained. In a routine intradermal Kveim test Finnish Kveim material, lot 110, was used[10]. Controls were healthy volunteers and patients with various mild dermatological symptoms. Cord blood was obtained from the umbilical cord in connection with normal deliveries.

After sedimentation the buffy coat was collected, and the cell density was adjusted to 4×10^6 white blood cells per ml. Cultures (2.5 ml) were started in 35 mm plastic Petri dishes with medium RPMI 1640 and 20% newborn calf serum. PHA-P (Difco) was used in a final dilution of 1:250, and PPD in a concentration of 10 μg/ml. Kveim suspensions, lot 110, type I spleen suspension of Siltzbach-Chase (S-Ch), and Australian spleen test material (CSL), and as a control, an inactive Finnish Kveim suspension, lot 114, were used in a concentration of 8 μg/ml. The potency of all Kveim suspensions was tested in vivo before and after the period of in vitro experiments.

Cell cultures stimulated by PHA were harvested on the third day. PPD-stimulated cultures and their controls were harvested on the sixth day, and the response as well as that of the corresponding control ("spontaneous" blast transformation) are presented. The effect of Kveim suspensions was measured on the sixth and eighth days. One hour before harvesting the cultures, 1 μCi 3H-TdR was added per ml of culture fluid. Blast transformation was determined as counts per minute (cpm) of 3H-TdR uptake using liquid scintillation counting. Cell preparations for May-Gruenwald-Giemsa staining were made by using a Shandon cytocentrifuge.

RESULTS

PHA-induced blast transformation

The PHA-induced responses in 90 sarcoid patients, in 40 controls and in 73 cord blood cultures are shown in Fig. 1. There were no significant differences in the median responses between the groups. In sarcoid patients the PHA response was correlated with sex, age ($\leq 40 / > 40$ years), Mantoux sensitivity, duration of the disease ($<3/3-24/>24$ months), activity of the disease, pulmonary changes (stage I/II/III/no changes), erythema nodosum, and skin changes. PHA-induced 3H-TdR incorporation was significantly decreased in patients with hilar adenopathy and parenchymal pulmonary changes ($p < 0.05$), when compared with the controls. The PHA response was somewhat higher in 26 sarcoid patients with active erythema nodosum. The difference was significant ($p < 0.05$) when compared with patients without erythema nodosum, but neither group differed significantly from the controls. There was no significant correlation of PHA-induced blast transformation with other clinical symptoms or with Mantoux reactivity.

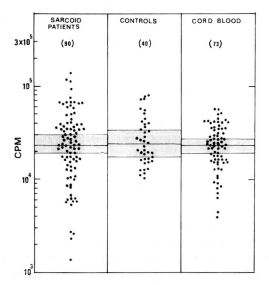

FIG. 1. PHA-induced blast transformation. The results are presented as 3H-TdR incorporation per culture. The medians of cpm and 95% confidence limits for the medians are shown. Number of cases in parentheses.

PPD-induced blast transformation

A good correlation was obtained in PPD-induced blast transformation and Mantoux sensitivity both in sarcoid patients and in controls (Fig. 2). No significant difference in reactivity in vitro was found between lymphocytes from tuberculin-sensitive sarcoid patients and from controls with the same degree of Mantoux reactivity. The tuberculin-induced blast transformation was higher ($p < 0.05$) in the younger age group and in patients with active erythema nodosum (< 0.02). The Mantoux sensitivity was significantly higher in the same groups.

A skin test negative to 100 TU was observed in 24 out of 87 sarcoid patients. When a 2-fold increase in the cpm as compared with the control cultures was regarded as a

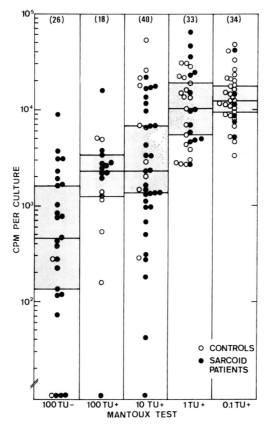

FIG. 2. Correlation of Mantoux sensitivity and PPD-induced blast transformation. For explanation, see Fig. 1.

significant response to PPD, 13 out of the 24 sarcoid patients and only 2 out of 13 comparison subjects negative to 100 TU showed an in vitro response to PPD. The difference between these groups is significant (p<0.025).

Spontaneous blast transformation

No significant difference was detected in spontaneous blast transformation between the sarcoid and control groups taken as a whole. It was, however, significantly higher in males, in the younger age group and in patients with acute sarcoidosis or erythema nodosum.

Kveim-induced blast transformation

No significant Kveim-induced blast transformation was observed with any of the Kveim suspensions (Fig. 3). Type I spleen suspension of Siltzbach-Chase caused a somewhat higher 3H-TdR incorporation in the cultures on the eighth day, but the difference was not significant. Nine different concentrations of all Kveim suspensions ranging from 0.75 to 100 μg/ml were used in the cultures from 5 sarcoid patients. No response was observed in these cultures either.

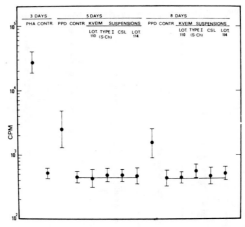

FIG. 3.   Effect of Kveim suspensions on WBC cultures from 31 sarcoid patients.   The results are presented as geometric mean of cpm per culture.   The bars indicate 95% confidence limits.

DISCUSSION

No significant difference was detected in PHA-induced blast transformation between the sarcoid and control groups, when Student's t test was applied. Some of the sarcoid patients, however, showed rather low PHA responses, and this group contained relatively more patients with stage II pulmonary changes. These results may explain some of the contradictory findings in PHA response in sarcoidosis[2-9].

Sarcoid patients with active erythema nodosum had an increased spontaneous blast transformation and a higher in vivo and in vitro tuberculin sensitivity. These findings suggest that in sarcoidosis erythema nodosum may represent a hyperactive immunological state. PPD-induced lymphocyte transformation was more sensitive than the Mantoux test in sarcoid patients, indicating that the anergy to tuberculin in the skin test is only quantitative.

The different types of Kveim test material did not cause any significant in vitro response. This is in accordance with the results of other reports, in which both blast transformation[5,9] and inhibition of macrophage migration[9,11] have been applied, whereas positive findings have been reported by others.

SUMMARY

Blast transformation of sarcoid lymphocytes by PHA, by tuberculin and by Kveim reagents was studied, and the findings were correlated with the clinical symptoms of the patients. The PHA response was significantly decreased only in patients with pulmonary stage II. A good correlation was obtained between PPD-induced lymphocyte transformation and the Mantoux sensitivity, both in sarcoid patients and in controls. Both in vivo and in vitro, tuberculin sensitivity was higher in younger patients and in patients with active erythema nodosum. The PPD-induced lymphocyte transformation as an in vitro test was more sensitive than the Mantoux test in sarcoid patients. The spontaneous blast transformation was increased in acute sarcoidosis, and in patients with active erythema nodosum. Three different types of Kveim material did not cause any significant in vitro response.

ACKNOWLEDGEMENTS

This work was supported by grants from the Finnish Anti-Tuberculosis Association, Orion Scientific Research Foundation, and Schering Corporation, U.S.A. I am grateful for the excellent technical assistance of Mrs. Hilkka Sokura, and I wish to thank Dr M. Virolainen, M.D., for valuable advice during the experiments and in the preparation of the manuscript.

REFERENCES

1. Cowling, D. C., Quaglino, D., and Barrett, P. K. M. 1964. *Brit. Med. J.* **1**: 1481.
2. Hirschhorn, K., Schreibman, R. R., Bach, F. H., and Siltzbach, L. E. 1964. *Lancet* **2**: 842.
3. Buckley, C. E., Nagaya, H., and Sieker, H. O. 1966. *Ann. intern. Med.* **64**: 508.
4. Selroos, O. 1967. *La Sarcoïdose*. Masson et cie. Paris p. 275.
5. Siltzbach, L. E., Glade, P. R., Hirshaut, Y., Vieira, L.O.B.D., Celikoglu I. S., and Hirschhorn, K. 1971. *Fifth International Conference on Sorcoidosis* (ed. Levinsky, L., and Macholda, F.) Prague, p. 217.
6. Langner, A., Moskalewska, K., and Proniewska, M. 1969. *Brit. J. Derm.* **81**: 829.
7. Girard, J. P., Poupon, M-F., and Press, P. 1971. *Int. Arch. Allergy* **41**: 604.
8. Mankiewicz, E., Kurti, V., and Béland, J. 1971. C. M. A. J. **104**: 684.
9. Topilsky, M., Williams, M., Siltzbach, L. E., and Glade, P. R. 1972. *Lancet* **15**: 117.
10. Putkonen, T. 1964. *Acta Med. scand.* **176**, Suppl. 425: 83.
11. Rocklin, R. E., Sheffer, A. L., and David, J. R. 1972. *Sixth Leucocyte Culture Conf.* (ed. Schwarz, R. S.). New York p. 743.

In Vitro Induced Tuberculin Sensitivity in Sarcoid Patients with a Negative Skin Test to 100 TU

Maija Horsmanheimo

III Department of Pathology, University of Helsinki, and the Department of Dermatology, University Central Hospital, Helsinki, Finland

INTRODUCTION

Supernatants from tuberculin (PPD)-stimulated lymphocyte cultures prepared from tuberculin-sensitive donors contain a nondialysable factor which, in the presence of PPD, causes stimulation of nonsensitive lymphocytes in vitro[1] This factor is called the lymphocyte transforming factor (LTF)[2]. In these experiments LTF was used to study the ability of non-tuberculin-sensitive cord blood and sarcoid lymphocytes to transform into blasts in vitro.

MATERIAL AND METHODS

The patient material and culture methods are presented elsewhere.[3] LTF was prepared using the method described by Valentine and Lawrence,[1] and was used in a final dilution of 1 : 4.

RESULTS

The effect of supernatants from lymphocyte cultures prepared from tuberculin-sensitive donors on cord blood lymphocytes is shown in Fig. 1. The PPD supernatant was taken from cultures where lymphocytes were cultured with PPD, and the control supernatant from cultures without PPD. These supernatants were tested both with and without added PPD. The PPD supernatant without added PPD also contained PPD, but less than the optimal concentration. PPD did not cause any response in cord blood-derived lymphocytes. Neither did control supernatants with or without PPD cause any response. The factor from PPD-stimulated cultures caused a 3.5-fold increase in the 3H-TdR uptake in cord blood cultures.

Lymphocytes from sarcoid patients and controls, negative to tuberculin both in vivo and in vitro, did not release any active factor in the presence of PPD.

The effect of supernatants from lymphocyte cultures prepared from tuberculin-sensitive donors on sarcoid lymphocytes is shown in Fig. 2. Out of 14 sarcoid patients, 8 responded in vitro to PPD in spite of a skin test negative to 100 TU. A significant, average 8-fold, response was obtained with the active supernatants in cultures from sarcoid patients negative in the in vitro tuberculin test. An increase was also obtained in those cultures in which PPD alone already induced slight transformation.

The ability of PPD-sensitive sarcoid lymphocytes to produce LTF was tested using cord blood lymphocytes as responding tuberculin non-sensitive cells (Fig. 3). PPD-stimulated lymphocytes from tuberculin-sensitive sarcoid patients released significantly

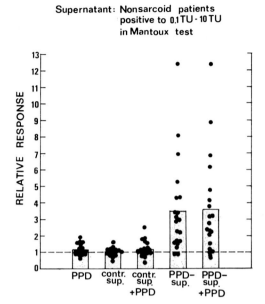

FIG. 1. Effect of supernatants from lymphocyte cultures prepared from tuberculin-sensitive donors on cord blood lymphocytes.   The total 3H-TdR incorporation in control cultures is taken as 1, and the responses are given as relative responses compared with the control cultures.

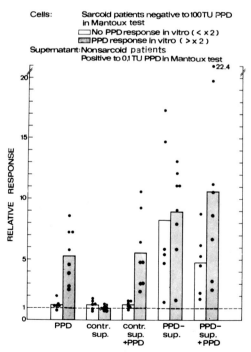

FIG. 2. Effect of supernatants from lymphocyte cultures prepared from tuberculin-sensitive donors on sarcoid lymphocytes.

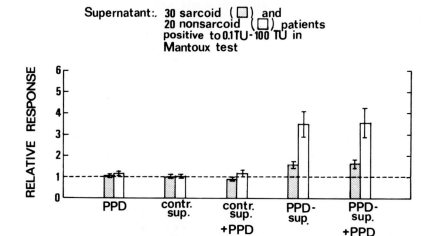

FIG. 3.   Production of active supernatant by PPD-sensitive sarcoid and control lymphocytes.   The mean±SE of relative responses are shown.

less (p<0.02) of this active factor than did control lymphocytes.

DISCUSSION

It has not yet been established whether LTF-induced blast transformation is immunologically specific or whether LTF could be a nonspecific mitogen.[2] The former
possibility is supported by the finding that the activity of LTF is dependent on the
antigen dose.[1] It has been reported that antigen-stimulated sarcoid lymphocytes were
in some cases unable to produce migration inhibition factor (MIF), although the
lymphocytes were capable of transforming into blasts with the antigen.[4] PPD-stimulated
lymphocytes from tuberculin-sensitive sarcoid patients released significantly less LTF
than did tuberculin-sensitive control lymphocytes, suggesting that the ability of sarcoid
lymphocytes to produce a second mediator, LTF, is also decreased.

SUMMARY

The effect of the lymphocyte transforming factor (LTF) on tuberculin-negative cord
blood and sarcoid lymphocytes was studied. Non-sensitive sarcoid lymphocytes responded to LTF as well as nonsensitive control lymphocytes. Sensitive sarcoid lymphocytes produced significantly less active LTF than did control lymphocytes. The results
suggest that the impairment of delayed hypersensitivity in sarcoidosis is not caused by
a primary response defect of the lymphocytes, but may be caused by a defect in, or a lack
of, some mediators of delayed hypersensitivity.

ACKNOWLEDGEMENTS

This work was supported by grants from the Finnish Anti-Tuberculosis Association, Orion Scientific Research Foundation, and Schering Corporation, U.S.A. I am

grateful for the excellent technical assistance of Mrs Hilkka Sokura, and I wish to thank Dr M. Virolainen M.D., for his valuable advice during the experiments and in the preparation of the manuscript.

REFERENCES

1. Valentine, F. T., and Lawrence, H. S. 1969. *Science* **165**: 1014.
2. Lawrence, H. S., and Valentine, F. T. 1970. *Amer. J. Path.* **60**: 437.
3. Horsmanheimo, M. (in these proceedings).
4. Rocklin, R. E., Sheffer, A. L., and David, J. R. 1972. *Sixth Leucocyte Culture Conf.* (ed. Schwarz, R. S.). New York. p. 743.

Peripheral Blood Monocyte IgG and C3 Membrane Receptor Activity in Patients with Sarcoidosis

S. D. Douglas, M. E. Schmidt and L. E. Siltzbach

The Mount Sinai School of Medicine, City University of New York, New York, U.S.A.

The abnormal immunologic findings described in sarcoidosis have been related to impaired cell-mediated immunity. They include a negative skin reaction to a variety of antigens, a high spontaneous rate of blast transformation of lymphocytes in vitro, and a diminished response of cultivated lymphocytes to tuberculin or PHA. These findings, however, are inconsistent and normal reactivity of lymphocytes has been reported by some investigators.

Although the interaction between macrophages and lymphocytes has been considered to be of major importance in the immune response there are but few investigations of monocyte-macrophage metabolism and function in human diseases. These studies are of special interest in sarcoidosis, because granulomas are formed and maintained by emigration and turnover of circulating mononuclear phagocytes. Furthermore, monocytosis and a higher phagocytic activity of peripheral monocytes has been reported in active stages of this disease.

Monocytes and macrophages have membrane receptor activity for IgG and the third component of complement, as demonstrated in previous studies from this laboratory and by others.[1–6] These membrane receptor sites have been studied on monocytes from patients with sarcoidosis.

Monocytes were obtained from 22 healthy donors and 26 patients with sarcoidosis (8 subacute, 16 chronic, 2 in an inactive stage of the disease). The diagnosis had been confirmed by a positive Kveim reaction (22) or the demonstration of characteristic granulomas in lymph node, liver or spleen. The PPD skin reaction was negative in 24 patients, transiently negative in 1, and positive in 1 patient.

Monocytes were isolated from peripheral blood by centrifugation in 27% bovine serum albumin gradient modified from the technique of Bennett and Cohn[1, 7] and were allowed to attach to cover slips contained in Leighton tubes. The attached cells were washed free of serum proteins and contaminating nonadherent lymphocytes. They were then incubated with sheep erythrocytes coated with rabbit antibody against Forssman antigen or the purified IgG or IgM immunoglobulins from these antisera. Fresh human serum served as a complement source. In parallel, human red cells from an O Rh+ donor coated with anti-CD Ripley or Heyman antisera were used.

Monocytes (200–400) were counted on each slide. Latex particles were used to evaluate the percentage of phagocytic cells and the rate of nonspecific phagocytosis. Rosette formation around monocytes, ingestion of specifically coated red cells by monocytes, or a combination of these phenomena, "combined" were evaluated. In some experiments

Supported by USPHS NIH Grants, AI-09338, 1 KO 4 HL 42575, HL 13853 and the Max Kade Foundation.

the inhibitory effect of different IgG subclasses added to the fluid phase was investigated.

The cells were evaluated using the following criteria: negative—monocytes surrounded by fewer than 3 erythrocytes; rosettes—circumferential binding of 3 or more erythrocytes; phagocytosis—engulfment of 1 or more erythrocytes; "combined" rosette formation plus phagocytosis.

Uncoated sheep or human red cells were bound to or were engulfed by less than 1% of the attached monocytes in all experiments. More than 90% of the monocytes from both normal individuals and patients with sarcoidosis engulfed latex particles after separation in BSA, which indicates well-maintained cell function in the in vitro assay system (Table 1).

The percentage of phagocytic cells using latex or EA 1:3200 (in contrast to higher

TABLE 1. Phagocytosis.

Nonspecific latex particles (0.81 μ)	Normal (n=21)	Sarcoidosis (n=18)	
% phagocytic cells	93.9± 9.9	94.4± 6.9	
Latex particles/monocyte	14.0± 6.0	24.0±11.0	p<0.005
Coated Red Cells (EA 1:3200)	Normal (n=14)	Sarcoidosis (n=16)	
% phagocytic cells	43.6±24.0	49.3±26.0	
RBC/monocyte	1.6± 0.4	2.6± 0.6	p<0.005

TABLE 2. Studies of various dilutions of anti-Forssman antibody coated RBC.

A. Rabbit anti-Forssman antibody 1:800

Percentage	Normal (n=16)	Sarcoidosis (n=19)	
Rosettes only	10.9±12.5	12.1±18.6	
Phagocytosis only	51.6±20.1	39.5±29.2	
Combined	23.8±20.5	43.9±26.2	p<0.0125
Total	84.6±14.4	96.0± 4.5	p<0.0025

B. Rabbit anti-Forssman antibody 1:3200

Percentage	Normal (n=17)	Sarcoidosis (n=20)	
Rosettes only	11.5±12.6	13.8±12.3	
Phagocytosis only	43.7±24.1	49.3±26.0	
Combined	5.9± 7.0	23.3±24.0	p<0.005
Total	61.1±23.9	87.0±14.0	p<0.0005

C. Rabbit anti-Forssman antibody 1:6400

Percentage	Normal (n=10)	Sarcoidosis (n=13)	
Rosettes only	4.7± 6.1	6.4± 5.7	
Phagocytosis only	25.3±20.6	47.1±21.0	p<0.025
Combined	3.4± 5.8	9.8±11.2	p<0.10
Total	33.4±28.3	55.4±29.1	p<0.05

antibody dilution (see Table 2) was approximately the same for normal and sarcoid patients. The phagocytic index, however, was significantly higher in sarcoidosis (almost 2-fold) than in the controls, indicating a greater phagocytic activity for antigen-antibody (Ag-Ab) complexes as well as inert material (latex).

Monocytes incubated with erythrocytes coated with antibody at different concentrations revealed differences in the extent of attachment or engulfment by normal and sarcoid monocytes. The results are illustrated in Table 2. The findings are characterized by: 1. A higher percentage of total reactive monocytes from sarcoid patients at lower antibody concentrations. 2. An increase in the number of sarcoid monocytes which have red cells engulfed and bound to their membrane, designated as "combined", at nearly all dilutions of Forssman antibody. 3. An increase in sarcoid monocytes which exhibit erythrophagocytosis at antibody dilutions where normal cells show a diminished rate of red cell ingestion.

The IgG subclass specificity of human monocyte receptors for IgG_1 and IgG_3 but not for IgG_2 and IgG_4 has previously been demonstrated.[8] This specificity could also be shown by the effect of IgG_1 and IgG_3 added to the fluid phase which resulted in an inhibition of coated red cell binding. The data confirm previous findings that higher concentrations of IgG_2 and IgG_4 in the fluid phase caused some nonspecific reduction of RBC binding. IgG_1 at .01 times the concentration of IgG_2 and IgG_4, however, specifically inhibited the attachment and phagocytosis of coated erythrocytes. Normal monocytes were affected more than cells from sarcoid patients, a finding consistent with increased receptor activity in this disease.

The biological significance of our findings remains uncertain since the function of IgG and C3 receptors in mononuclear phagocytes in vivo remains to be established. They may be involved in plasma membrane attachment and engulfment of antigen-antibody complexes. Whether a higher receptor activity or greater number of binding sites on the plasma membrane in sarcoid monocytes contributes to the findings of increased phagocytic and membrane receptor function in sarcoidosis remains to be elucidated. In summary, the observation of increased receptor activity in monocytes from patients with sarcoidosis represents the first disease in which altered receptor function has been conclusively demonstrated. Whether this reflects an increased number of binding sites or altered membrane dynamics remains to be proven.

REFERENCES

1. LoBuglio, A. F., Cotran, R. S., and Jandl, J. H. 1967. *Science* **158**: 1582.
2. Huber, H., and Fudenberg, H. H. 1968. Int. Arch. Allergy Appl. *Immunol.* **34**: 18.
3. Huber, H., Polley, M. J., Linscott, W. D., Fudenberg, H. H., and Müller-Eberhard, H. J. 1968. *Science* **162**: 1281.
4. Huber, H., Douglas, S. D., and Fudenberg, H. H. 1969 *Immunology* **17**: 7.
5. Huber, H., and Douglas, S. D. 1970. *Brit. J. Haematol.* **19**: 19.
6. Abramson, N., LoBuglio, A. F., Jandl, J. H., and Cotran, R. S. 1970. J. Exp. Med. **132**: 1191, 1970, and *J. Exp. Med.* **132**: 1207.
7. Bennett, W. E., and Cohn, Z. A. 1966. *J. Exp. Med.* **123**: 145.
8. Huber, H., Douglas, S. D., Nusbacher, J., Kochwa, S., and Rosenfield, R. E. 1971. *Nature* **229**: 419.

Diverse Immunological and Serological Studies of Sera from Sarcoidosis Patients

KARL WURM

University of Freiburg, Freiburg, Federal Republic of Germany

PRECIPITATING ANTIBODIES AGAINST ANONYMOUS MYCOBACTERIA
(Speer*, Wurm)

The findings of Chapman[1] are of interest concerning the etiology, immunology and epidemiology of sarcoidosis. Together with Speer and Bickhardt[2,3] we have examined sarcoidosis patients and control persons in exact the same manner as Chapman, using 2-dimensional Agar gel precipitation after Ouchterlony,[4] with micromodification after Crowle.[5] We used 6 original antigens, kindly placed at our disposal by Chapman.

Parallel examinations were carried out with several other antigens of atypical mycobacteria of the Behring-Werke Marburg, of the Statens Serum Institutes at Kopenhagen, and antigens obtained by the same method as purified tuberculin, placed at our disposal by Mankiewicz.

We have examined the sera of 54 sarcoidosis patients of all 3 stages, of 20 patients with active tuberculosis and of 40 dermatologic patients without TB and without sarcoidosis.

Results
From 54 sarcoidosis patients, 52 (96%) showed positive sera reactions to mycobacterial antigens, to photochromogenic mycobacteria (96%), and to nonchromogenic mycobacteria (52%). There were no reactions to antigens of the scoto-chromogenic group.

There were positive reactions to almost all sera of the control groups and of these the highest percentage was to the photochromogenic, and to a lesser degree to the nonchromogenic group. In no case was there reaction to the scotochromogenic antigen.

The results of these examinations show that no conclusions can be drawn regarding the role of atypical mycobacteria in the etiology of sarcoidosis. Chapman already has identified very striking geographic differences in his control groups. The obvious geographic peculiarity of the total population concerning their reactions to atypical mycobacteria makes a proper evaluation very difficult.

Based on our findings, the conclusion can be drawn that the German population has a high degree of sensitization to atypical mycobacteria as Meissner[6] has already mentioned. As far as the hypothesis of Mankiewicz[7] of an atypic mycobacterial etiology is concerned, no arguments—either pro or contra,—can be derived from our findings. However, the findings of other authors are confirmed, that capability to form antibodies in sarcoidosis shows no significant difference from the norm.

With the above antigens, (however, not with those from Chapman) we received only negative reactions. It is supposed that a special technique in the production of antigens is mandatory for ensuring the quality of the antigens and the comparability of such examinations with different mycobacteria.

* Speer A., Dermatological Clinic, University Freiburg, Fed. Rep. of Germany.

EPSTEIN-BARR VIRUS AND SARCOIDOSIS
(Fleckenstein*, Thomssen**, Wurm)

Hirshaut and co-workers[8] first referred to a relationship between Epstein-Barr virus and sarcoidosis.

Epstein-Barr virus (EB virus) is a member of the herpes virus group which has been detected in tissue cultures derived from Burkitt lymphomas and other human malignant tumors.[9] It is universally propagated and suspected of being responsible for infectious mononucleosis.[10]

They detected fluorescent antibodies to EB virus capsid antigens (VCA) in all of 131 sera from sarcoidosis patients. In their control group, only 75% of the sera had these antibodies, in lower titers. The authors discussed whether the EB virus could be the etiological agent of sarcoidosis. Therefore, we tested the sera of 38 patients in different stages of sarcoidosis in comparison to 42 sera of healthy persons with the method developed by Henle.

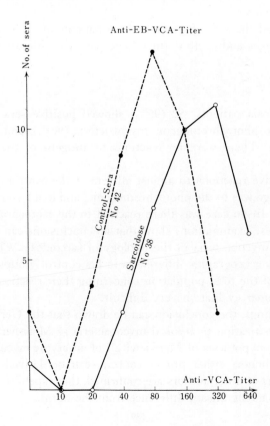

The EB virus containing HRIK and EB-3 cell lines were grown in suspension culture. Cell smears were fixed by acetone, overlayered with the serum dilutions, washed 3 times with phosphate-buffered saline and stained with a fluorescein—conjugated anti-human IgG rabbit antiserum.

Further we prepared a complement-fixing antigen from arginine-deprived cell cultures by extraction with an alkaline glycine buffer. The mean titer in the patient sera was about 4-fold higher than in the controls. This is in coincidence with the findings of Henle's and Loefgren's groups who detected a greater percentage of light EB virus antibodies in sarcoidosis sera.[11]

However, the demonstration of fluorescent or complement-fixing antibodies to EB virus is not of diagnostic significance, since the anti-VCA titers of patients and controls overlap in a broad range, and we have even seen a serum-negative case of histologically proved severe chronical sarcoidosis.

The serology will not contribute to the elucidation of the etiology of this disease. For this purpose, the presence of EB virus in the sarcoidosis granulomas should be proved.

Zur Hausen and his co-workers[12] purified the DNA of EB virus and transcribed it to a highly tritiated c-RNA[13, 14] appropriate for nucleic acid hybridization experiments.

This biochemical method is the most sensitive one for the detection of latent viral infections. If the EB virus is a causal factor in the pathogenesis of sarcoidosis, growing in the sarcoid granuloma, virus-specific c-RNA will hybridize with the DNA extracted from granuloma biopsies. These investigations are now in preparation.

* Fleckenstein B., Institut of the clin. Virology, Loschgestr. 7, Erlangen Fed. Rep. of Germany.
** Thomssen R., Hyg. Institut, University Göttingen, Fed. Rep. of Germany.

IMMUNOLOGICAL INVESTIGATIONS
(Tolk*, Müller**, Stojan, Wurm)

The reaction of the lymphocytes is of interest for questions concerning cellular immunity (Table 1). Therefore we determined their transformation ratio after stimulation with phytohaemagglutinin (PHA).

The ratio of lymphoblasts in the nonstimulated control group of normal persons was less than 10% and increased significantly to 36% after addition of PHA. In the cultures of sarcoidosis donors the rate of lymphoblasts was 12%, but did not further increase after stimulation with PHA. Thus, the tendency to spontaneous transformation in sarcoidosis is somewhat higher than in normal persons though the reason is unknown. After stimulation with PHA, however, the transformation rate did not increase. Hence it follows, that cellular immunity in sarcoidosis is reduced.

On the contrary, an increase of humoral antibodies was reported in sarcoidosis. In this way we examined the sera of 137 sarcoidosis patients for different specific and non-specific organic antibodies, namely for the rheumatism factor in the latex test and in the Waaler-Rose test, thyreoglobulin antibodies, mitochondrial thyreoid antibodies, stomach-fundus antibodies, vessel-wall antibodies and antinuclear factors. All these examinations showed no distinct difference in findings compared with a control group and did not indicate any autoimmunization.

However, examinations of the γ-globulins, that is of the immunee globulins IgA, IgG and IgM by serum electrophoresis or by the method of agar gel diffusion according to

TABLE 1.   Stimulation of lymphocyte transformation with phytohaemagglutinin (PHA).

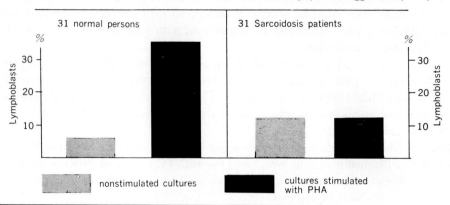

Donors	Number	Transformation rate	
		Before	After
Normal persons	31	10%	36%
Sarcoidosis pat	31	12%	12%

In sarcoidosis the spontaneous transformation is a little higher than in normal persons, but after stimulation with PHA there is no increase of lymphoblasts.

Mancini demonstrated significant differences of the 284 examined sarcoidosis sera compared with the control test group of 124 normal persons.

Whereas the albumins drop continuously during the course of the disease, the α_1-, α_2-, β-and γ-globulins show a slight increase in the first and second stages, and in the third stage they show such a high increase that significant differences compared to healthy test persons can be confirmed. The increase of γ-globulins in the third stage is due to the increased formation of IgA and even more of IgG, even if IgM is decreased. As IgM is significantly decreased in all stages of the disease, possibly because of the frequently existing lymphopenia, since circulating lymphocytes, as is well-known, are suitale for an IgM synthesis.

According to our findings the number of the circulating lymphocytes on average amounted to 1316 ($\pm$425) in sarcoidosis against 1787 ($\pm$934) in healthy persons.

On the contrary, IgA and IgG show a significant increase during the course of the disease.

Compared with controls differences are found, but they are not significant. However you can notice a characteristic increase of sarcoidosis within the stages.

These findings which are so characteristic for sarcoidosis do not become evident on examination of undifferentiated patients, but they become clearly evident on separating the cases into the different stages.

In consideration of the findings reported by Favez and his co-workers[15] about circulating Kveim antibodies, we sensitized rabbits with Kveim antigen and Freund's adjuvant. In the following examinations by the capillary precipitation test, with agar gel diffusion after Ouchterlony, as well as immune electrophoresis we were not able to demonstrate specific antibodies. The reason could be that the sensitization of the animals was not quantitatively sufficient, or that the Kveim antigen is not capable of effecting the formation of humoral antibodies and therefore has no antigenic qualities.

* Tolk J., Diesterwegstr. 15, Kiel, Fed. Rep. of Germany.
** Müller W., Rheumatological Clinic, Burgfelder Str. 101, University Basel, Switzerland.

COLLAGEN METABOLISM IN SARCOIDOSIS
(Stojan*, Müller, Wurm, Tariverdian**)

Sarcoidosis is characterized histopathologically by granuloma of the epitheloid cells with extraordinary formation of collagen fibrils. The further development of the collagen is evidently connected with the outcome of the sarcoidosis. For that reason, we started investigations on collagen metabolism. Partial results were reported in another paper.[16] An extended report concerning our further results with descriptions of the technique employed is presently in press.[17]

On this occasion I wish to report only some of our most important results. We know that every inflammation is connected with a change of enzymes, mostly of the various

TABLE. 2.   Emzyme activity and course of disease.

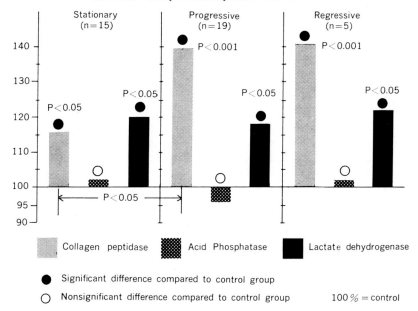

lysosomal enzymes. We know further that in every inflammation disease the nature of the enzymes differs quantitatively as well as qualitatively, i.e., is specific to each disease, and may even show a typical course of progress.

In our investigations we carried out preliminary tests for the determination of collagen peptidase. We also tested the activity of the acid phosphatase and the lactate dehydrogenase (LDH).

The most striking and new result was the fact that in all cases of sarcoidosis, collagen peptidase was significantly higher when compared with control persons. This enzyme activity is particularly high in the dynamic forms of sarcoidosis, i.e., in those with a progressive or regressive course. (Table 2, 3) There was, however, no difference between the latter. Evidently there exists a strict relationship between the synthesis and decomposition of collagen and the collagen peptidase activity.

TABLE 3.   Collagen peptidase and course of disease.

Control	Stationary	Progressive	Regressive
24,4 ± 5,0 (n = 24)	28,2 ± 7,2 (n = 15)	34,2 ± 8,3 (n = 19)	34,6 ± 5,5 (n = 5)

← P<0,05 → ← P<0,05 → ←→
← P<0,001→
← P<0,001

TABLE 4.   Influence of medicaments on enzyme activity (Corticosteroids, Azapropazone).

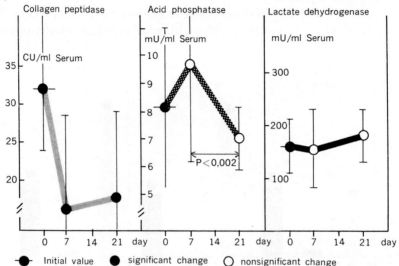

—●— Initial value   ● significant change   ○ nonsignificant change

The degree of activity was demonstrated to be dependent on the course of the disease, i.e., the dynamics of the disease. However it showed no distinct difference between the various stages of the sarcoidosis. On the other hand, we had so far no occasion to examine the enzyme activity in the initial phase of the acute course of the disease.

The collagen peptidase activity is indeed not a specific parameter for sarcoidosis, as it is widespread also in other diseases and even in healthy persons. It is, on the other hand, always so much increased in untreated cases of sarcoidosis that this represents a peculiarity of sarcoidosis such as has been the object of our investigations for some time.

We could not observe similar conditions in the case of acid phosphatase and lactate dehydrogenase. The LDA activity is in fact significantly increased in all cases of sarcoidosis, however, without any correlation of the course of the disease and the therapeutical effect. The acid phosphatase was not found to be increased, and it is noteworthy that it shows only a temporary increase under influence of therapy.

The question of whether the activity of the collagen peptidase is the only enzymatic peculiarity or the most effective enzyme activity, is still remaining unsolved.

The observation of a clear correlation between the therapeutic effect and the change in activity of collagen peptidase is of special interest. The higher the initial value of the collagen peptidase (and the steeper the decline with a lasting decrease until it is beyond the values of the control group), the greater is the therapeutic effect.

The clinical evaluation of these enzymatic findings is as follows:

The determination of collagen peptidase activity gives us some hints for the recognition of the progress, in the sense of a stationary or dynamic course, and moreover hints at a more differentiated therapeutic indication. This is evident especially in cases in which, during the first examination, we do not know the previous phases of the disease.

Furthermore, the determination of collagen peptidase activity allows a certain prediction of the therapeutic effect. A highly significant increase of the activity is a sign of a prospective good therapeutic effect. A somewhat lesser increase suggests stationary sarcoidosis which, according to our experience,[18] reacts less under drugs.

Finally, the determination of collagen peptidase activity could, on one hand, be suitable as an activity test in correlation with a complete cure of the disease and, on the other hand, as a test in clinical investigation of new research substances. (Table 4) This must be verified by future investigations.

* Stojan B., Rheumatological Clinic, Burgfelder Str. 101, University Basle, Switzerland.
** Tariverdian M. T., Höchenschwand, Sonnenhof, Fed. Rep. of Germany.

REFERENCES

1. Chapman, I. S., and Speight, M. 1964. *Acta Scand. Suppl.* **425**: 61.
2. Speer A. Inaug. Diss. Freiburg/Brsg.
3. Bickhardt, R., and Speer, A. 1966. *Prax. Pneumol.* **20**: 601.
4. Schmidt, N. J., and Lenette, E. H. 1962. *J. Immunol.* **89**: 85.
5. Schwick, G. 1958. *Laboratoriumsblätter Jg* **8**: 11.
6. Meissner, G. 1963. *Ergebn. d. Inn. Med. u. Kdhkol* **20**: 37.
7. Mankiewicz, E. 1963. *Can. Me. Ass. J.* **88**: 593.
8. Hirshaut Y. et al. 1970. *New Engl. J. Med.* **283**: 502.
9. Epstein, M. A., and Barr, Y. M. 1964. *Lancet* **1**: 702.
10. Henle et al. 1971. *J. Infect. Dis.*, **124**: 58.
11. Warren, B. et al. 1971. *J. Nat. Cancer Inst.* **47**: 747.
12. Schulte-Holthausen et al. 1970. *Virology* **40**: 776.
13. Schulte-Holthausen et al. 1971. Symp. Oncogenesis and Herpes-type Viruses. Cambridge.
14. Schulte-Holthausen et al. 1970. *Nature* **228**: 1056.
15. Favez G., and Leuenberger Ph. 1971. *Amer. Rev. Resp. Dis.* **104**: 599.
16. Stojan, B., Müller, W., Wurm, K., and Tariverdian, M. T. 1972. Schweiz. *Rundschau Med.* (Praxis) **61**: 591.
17. Stojan, B., Müller, W., Wurm, K., and Tariverdian, M. T. *Schweiz. Med. Wschr.* 1973. **103**: 337.
18. Wurm K., *Mschr. Tbk. Bekpf.* **10**: 57.

Serum Immunoglobulin D Levels in Sarcoidosis

ROBERT A. GOLDSTEIN

VA-George Washington University, Medical Center, Washington, D.C., U.S.A.

HAROLD L. ISRAEL

Jefferson Medical College, Thomas Jefferson University, Philadelphia, U.S.A.

BERNARD W. JANICKI

Veterans Administration Hospital Washington, D.C., U.S.A.

AND

MITSUO YOKOYAMA

Kuakini Medical Research Institute, Honolulu, Hawaii

INTRODUCTION

At the last conference we reported that elevations of serum immunoglobulins G, A and M in sarcoidosis patients were related not only to race but also to the duration and severity of illness.[1] Unfortunately, the changes were found not to be specific for sarcoidosis nor did they appear to correlate with any immunologic characteristics of sarcoidosis. More recently, however, it has been reported that serum immunoglobulin D levels were lower than normal in sarcoidosis patients and possibly correlated with tubercluin anergy[2]. Since the specific function of IgD is unknown and, apart from IgD myeloma, few clinical reports are available, it appeared of interest to examine sarcoidosis patients to see whether changes in this immunoglobulin might be of immunopathologic importance in sarcoidosis.

MATERIALS AND METHODS

Serum samples were collected from 214 patients with sarcoidosis and 74 with tuberculosis. The concentration of IgD was estimated by a radial diffusion technique with commercially available plates and these values were compared with determinations in 101 healthy persons.

RESULTS

By this technique serum IgD levels below 3.2 mg% were undetectable. For statistical purposes, therefore, we compared the frequency distribution of IgD levels within and between all groups. Among sarcoidosis patients, 50% had undetectable serum levels; 30% had values between 3.2 and 6.3 mg%; 13% had levels between 6.4 and 9.5 mg%; and 7% had levels 9.6 mg% or greater. There were no significant differences between sarcoidosis patients and healthy controls. In the latter group, 48% had undetectable values; 32% were between 3.2 and 6.3 mg%; 12% were between 6.4 and 9.5 mg%, and 8% had values 9.6 mg% or greater. On the other hand, IgD levels were significantly higher among persons with tuberculosis; their respective frequency distribution was 16% undetectable, 45% between 3.2 and 6.3 mg%, 23% between 6.4 and 9.5 mg%, and 16% at 9.6 mg% or higher. The frequency of undetectable IgD levels among sarcoidosis patients with positive and negative tuberculin skin tests was similar; there were no significant differences related to stage or duration of disease.

DISCUSSION

IgD is normally present in very low concentrations in healthy individuals. In the present study one-half of healthy persons had undetectable levels. Although patients with subacute sarcoidosis had higher levels than inactive, there were no significant differences between sarcoidosis patients and healthy persons. There were no significant racial differences and nondetectable levels were not associated with a higher frequency of tuberculin anergy.

In striking contrast were the markedly elevated IgD levels observed in tuberculosis patients. Similarly elevated levels of serum IgD have been found by others in tuberculosis[2] and leprosy.[3] It is interesting that levels are elevated in these conditions because chronic infection has been implicated as a possible reason for increased IgD levels. Thus, children with Down's syndrome, who are known to have an increased incidence of infection, also have elevated serum IgD concentrations.[4]

It would be of interest to examine patients with atypical mycobacterial infection to see if they have similar elevations. If true, then patients with tuberculosis, leprosy and atypical mycobacterial infections, in contrast to those with sarcoidosis, might serve as study models to determine whether IgD has a specific antibody function. On the other hand, it is known that women who are pregnant or taking oral contraceptives also have elevated levels of IgD suggesting a possible hormonal influence not affecting immunoglobulin G, A or M.[5]

In conclusion, we have found that immunoglobulin D levels are essentially normal in sarcoidosis but strikingly elevated in tuberculosis. Absent or undetectable levels were not related to tuberculin anergy.

REFERENCES

1. Goldstein, R. A., Israel, H. L., and Rawnsley, H. M. 1971. Effect of race and stage of disease on the serum immunoglobulin's in sarcoidosis. *Fifth Int. Conf. on Sarcoidosis.* Prague: Univ. Karlova. pp. 178–180.
2. Buckley, C. E., and Trayer, H. R. 1972. Serum IgD concentrations in sarcoidosis and tuberculosis. *Clin. Exp. Immunol.* **10**: 257–265.
3. Sirisinha, S., Charupatana, C., and Ramasoota, T. 1972. Serum immunoglobulins in leprosy patients with different spectra of clinical manifestations. *Proc. Soc. Exp. Biol. Med.* **140**: 1060–1068.
4. Rundle, A. T., Clothier, B., and Sundell, B. 1971. Serum IgD level and infections in Down's syndrome. *Clin. Chim. Acta* **35**: 389–393.
5. Klapper, D. G., and Mendenhall, H. W. 1971. Immunoglobulin D concentration in pregnant women. *J. Immunol.* **107**: 912–915.

Serum Immunoglobulin Levels in Sarcoidosis

MINORU MATSUDA

The Center for Adult Diseases, Osaka, Japan

AND

TERUO TACHIBANA

Osaka Prefectural Hospital, Osaka, Japan

Recently, concentrations of immunoglobulin in patients with sarcoidosis have been quantified in many clinics, but studies of serum immunoglobulin levels in sarcoidosis have been conflicting. On the other hand, significant changes in immunoglobulin levels in healthy individuals with respect to age, race and sex have been demonstrated by several reports. Therefore, it is necessary that immunoglobulin levels in sarcoidosis should be compared with similar observations in healthy controls. The present authors have compared the concentrations of immunoglobulin in healthy Japanese people and Japanese cases of carcoidosis.

MATERIALS AND METHOD

The serum samples in healthy controls used in this study were obtained from blood donors and were divided into 4 age groups, that is the twenties, thirties, forties and fifties.

Sera were obtained from 68 patients with sarcoidosis, who had had no treatment prior to determination of serum immunoglobulin levels. About 70% of them did not show any abnormalities on chest X-ray 6 months previously. Sera from less than 19-year-old patients with sarcoidosis were omitted because no immunoglobulin levels in healthy controls of the same age were available.

These sera were stored in a deep-freezer before use. Concentrations of immuno-globulin were determined by a single radial immunodiffusion method.

RESULTS

Table 1 presents the values of IgG, IgA and IgM in the sera of 160 normal males and 152 normal females over 20 years of age. As the values of 3 immunoglubulins in each age group of both sexes showed a logarithmic normal distribution, the means and standard deviations of the logarithms of the values in each group were calculated. When no age-related variation was shown, the values which belonged to each age group were calculated for their means and standard deviation collectively.

There was a significant difference of IgG between the 20-year-old to 49-year-old group and the over 50-year-old group in the males. There was a significant difference of IgA among the 20-year-old to 39-year-old group, the 40-year-ld group and the 50-year-old group in the famales. There was a significant difference of IgM between the 20-year-old group and the over 30-year-old group in the males. A significant difference was also noted in IgM between the 20-year-old group and over the 50-year-old group

TABLE 1. Normal human serum immunoglobulin levels (mg/dl).

Age Group		20–29	30–39	40–49	50–59
IgG	M	1313 (789–2183) n=120			1133 (713–1800) n=40
	F	1462 (851–2072) n=152			
IgA	M	253 (120–533) n=160			
	F	221 (115–426) n=78		254 (139–466) n=37	208 (101–427) n=36
IgM	M	139 (73–263) n=40		116 (63–213) n=120	
	F	203 (100–413) n=116			159 (82–306) n=36

Remarks : Figures denote mean values.
Parathensized figures denote 95% ranges.
n expresses the number of samples.

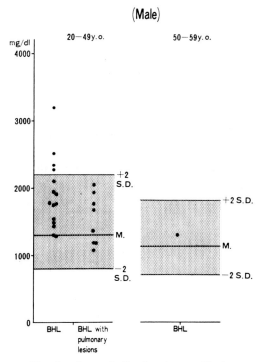

FIG. 1. Serum IgG values in sarcoidosis.

in the females. However, there was no significant difference of IgG in the females or
of IgA in the males in each age group. The authors consider that immunoglobulin levels
in the Japanese are intermediate between white and black levels.

Serum immunoglobulin concentrations in sarcoidosis were not always normally distributed in each age group. Therefore, statistical tests (such as the means or standard

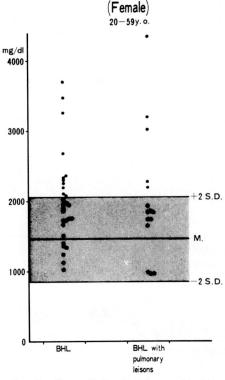

FIG. 2. Serum IgG values in sarcoidosis.

deviations) based on a normal distribution are not appropriate. When the values for the 3 immunoglobulins were over 2 S.D., the immunoglobulin levels of these patients were assumed to be increased.

In the males of the 20-year-old to 49-year-old group, increased IgG was found in 4 out of 15 cases having BHL (Fig. 1). In the females, increased IgG was found in 11 out of 29 cases having BHL and in 5 out of 15 cases having BHL with pulmonary lesions (Fig. 2).

In the males, only 1 showed an increased IgA out of 16 cases having BHL (Fig. 3). In the females of the 20-year-old to 39-year-old group, increased IgA was found in 2 out of 22 cases having BHL and in 5 out of 12 cases having BHL with pulmonary lesions. In the females of the 40-year-old group, only 1 showed increased IgA out of 2 cases having BHL with pulmonary lesions (Fig. 4). Increased IgM was not found in the males. In the females only 1 showed an increased IgM out of 14 cases having BHL with pulmonary lesions.

Immunoglobulin levels in 68 patients with sarcoidosis were quantified at intervals to assess improvement of chest X-rays. In 11 of them, immunoglobulin levels have been quantified for more than 1 year after complete disappearance of chest X-ray abnormalities. After the disappearance, IgG values decreased in some cases and increased in others (Fig. 5). IgA values remained constant during the course of sarcoidosis (Fig. 6). IgM values fluctuated within normal range and showed no definite tendency. Consequently, immunoglobulin levels did not always decrease after the disappearance of chest X-ray abnormalities.

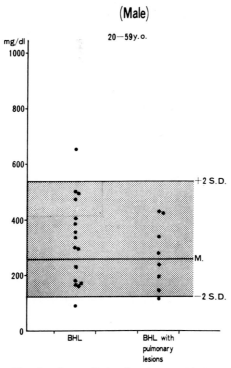

FIG. 3.   Serum IgA values in sarcoidosis.

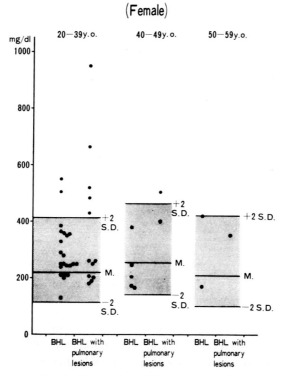

FIG. 4.   Serum IgA values in sarcoidosis.

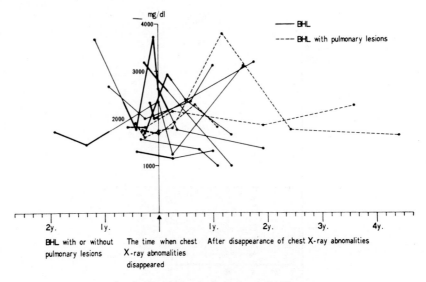

FIG. 5.   Changes in serum IgG values with course of sarcoidosis.

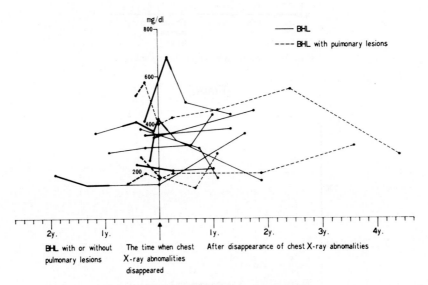

FIG. 6.   Changes in serum IgA values with the course of sarcoidosis.

SUMMARY

The serum levels of IgG, IgA and IgM were determined in 68 cases with sarcoidosis. The values were compared with those for 312 healthy individuals.

1.   In the males, increased IgG and IgA were found in some patients with sarcoidosis, while in the females, increased IgG was found in the highest incidence followed by cases with increased IgA at the time of onset.

2.   Even with the disappearance of abnormal chest X-rays, immunoglobulin levels did not always decrease. Changes in immunoglobulin levels were not associated with the morbid course of sarcoidosis.

Immunoglobulins in Serum and Bronchial Secretions in Pulmonary Sarcoidosis

A. BLASI AND D. OLIVIERI

Clinic of Tuberculosis and Respiratory Diseases, Naples University, Naples, Italy

Hypergammaglobulinaemia is frequently found in pulmonary sarcoidosis.[1, 2] This increase is usually related to the extent of lung involvement and to the amount of pulmonary fibrosis.[3, 4] Following intense treatment with corticosteroids, one often observes an amelioration of the imbalance of all serum globulins and of the immunoglobulins in particular.[5]

Using electrophoretic and immunological methods, it is possible to measure quantitatively and to evaluate individually each of the IgA, IgG and IgM immunoglobulin fractions of the serum.[6–8] In this way the behaviour of the different immunoglobulin fractions has been placed in relationship to the difference in race, to the stage of the illness, or to the degree of fibrosis already existent in the lung tissue.[9–11] With respect to hypergammaglobulinaemia IgA, many authors have pointed out that there is a prominent increase in the serum.[5, 6, 13]

In the literature to date, however, there are no data regarding the behaviour of the immunoglobulin fractions in the bronchial secretions, where the IgA assumes a particular significance.

It is known, that, in the bronchial secretions too, the immunoglobulins G, A and M are to be found and that they can be determined with ease.[14]

The presence of IgA in the bronchial secretions, however, is not due to a simple, passive, transport mechanism from the blood.[15, 16] It is bound 2:1 to a polypeptide which is produced locally by the bronchial mucosa and is called the "secretory piece" or the "secretory component". This is not present in the serum.[16–18]

In this complete form, bronchial IgA assumes a special polymeric structure, which renders it much more resistant to the action of bacterial or viral agents. For this reason it is more effective for the purposes of immunological defence locally at the bronchial mucosa.[19]

PATIENTS AND METHODS

Using electrophoretic and immunological methods, the serum and bronchial secretions of a group of patients with pulmonary sarcoidosis were studied for their immunoglobulin contents. In 18 subjects, repeated measurements of the serum immunoglobulin fractions were made, coinciding with the different evolutive phases of the illness. In 12 of these the effects of the illness were not limited only to hilar adenopathy, but there was also a marked broncho-pulmonary involvement. In these 12, therefore, the immunoglobulin fractions were also measured in the bronchial secretions. In the last 5 cases which came under our observation, a semiquantitative evaluation of the "secretory component" was made.

In every case, diagnosis was reached either after lung biopsy, or after biopsy of a peripheral lymph node. Biopsies were performed in some of the cases at varying stages in the evolution of the disease. In this way the results have been related to the observed modifications of the serum and bronchial secretion proteins.

Some of the data to be referred to have already been published.[4, 8]

For the immunoelectrophoretic analysis of the serum and the bronchial secretions, immune sera, both total and specific for each fraction (Behringwerke), were used. For the study of the bronchial secretions, several technical procedures, as previously described, were adopted.[4, 20]

Radial immunodiffusion was carried out either on normal plates (Behringwerke), or on plates adapted for biological fluids at a low concentration.[14, 21, 22]

For analysis of the "secretory component," a specific antiserum was used. This was obtained from colostrum adsorbed with normal human serum by recognized methods, which we have used previously.[16, 23]

RESULTS

The results of measurements of the immunoglobulin fractions and the relationship between IgA and IgG in the serum and bronchial secretions are shown in Table 1.

The mean values obtained, and the values considered to be normal for the serum are indicated. No values are given for the bronchial secretions, due to their great variability even under normal conditions. In the evaluation of the "secretory component" in the bronchial secretions of 5 cases, the polypeptide was always found to be present in quantities which are considered to be normal.

TABLE 1.

Pulmonary sarcoidosis	No. cases	IgG mg%	IgA mg%	IgM mg%	IgA/IgG
Serum	18	1600±234 (800–1680)	380±4.24 (140–420)	140±26.63 (50–190)	0.2
Bronchial secretion	12	24±8.63	31±8.94	7±5	1.2

COMMENTS

The first consideration relates to the behaviour of the serum immunoglobulin fractions. There is a small mean increase of IgA, and there is also some increase of IgM and IgG. This data has already been pointed out as being either an isolated hypergammaglobulinaemia,[3, 24] or corresponding to an increase of alpha-globulin with a reciprocal decrease of albumin. The latter case especially is related to the initial or acute phase of the illness.[5, 25, 26]

As far as the clinical aspects of our observations are concerned, it should be said that the degree of disequilibrium of the immunogloblins is related to the stage of the illness and is directly related to the gravity of the pulmonary pathology. By means of repeated analyses in the same patients, we have seen that the degree of this disequilibrium is greater proportionately with the evolutionary progress of the illness towards parenchymal fibrosis.[4, 5] In those cases which resolve spontaneously, however, or in those which respond to corticosteroid therapy, there is also a tendency for all the immunoglobulin fractions to return to normal.[5, 8] It is not possible to recognize the precise chronological order of the variations of the 3 fractions, because their behaviour is not uniform.

It is more difficult to comment on the data obtained from the bronchial secretions, especially because there are no normal values for comparison. As has already been stated, even under normal conditions, IgA is really abundant in the bronchial secretions.[14, 16] The total protein content of the bronchial secretions, moreover, is not constant as is that of the serum, but is very variable, because it is connected with the modality of secretion of the mucosa and with the physical characteristics of the secretions.

It is very simple to demonstrate, however, that the quantity of IgA in the bronchial secretions is greater than that in the serum. Examining the relationship between IgA and any immunoglobulin fraction, for example IgG, one can see that in the bronchial secretions the proportion of IgA to IgG is always greater than in the serum.[23, 27]

In the cases which we observed, we can only say that the IgA content in the secretions is high in every case. This is demonstrated by considering the relationship of IgA to IgG in the secretions with respect to the serum.

We must, however, also say that the values found in mediastino-pulmonary sarcoidosis do not greatly differ from those found in other broncho-pulmonary diseases, either of specific or nonspecific nature, including simple chronic bronchitis.

Finally, the completely normal behaviour of the "secretory component" should be noted, since it is important in the formation of bronchial IgA, in view of the role of protection and of local immunological defense of IgA in the bronchial tree.[16, 23]

SUMMARY

Hypergammaglobulinaemia is frequently found in pulmonary sarcoidosis, and this increase is usually related to the extent of lung involvement and to the amount of pulmonary fibrosis.

Using electrophoretic and immunological methods, the serum and bronchial secretions of a group of patients with pulmonary sarcoidosis, were studied for their immunoglobulin content. A semiquantitative evaluation of the "secretory component" in 5 cases was also made.

The serum fractions which most frequently exhibit quantitative modifications are IgA and IgM, although these changes are not always found. The bronchial secretions, however, always contain a greater increase of IgA than of the other immunoglobulins. One should not forget, though, that, even in normal subjects, the level of IgA in bronchial secretions is noticeably higher than that of the other immunoglobulins. Finally a completely normal behaviour of the "secretory component" was noted.

In every case the diagnosis was reached either after lung biopsy, or after biopsy of a peripheral lymph node. Biopsies were performed in some of the cases at varying stages in the evolution of the disease. In this way, the results have been related to the observed modifications of the serum and bronchial secretion proteins.

REFERENCES

1. Salvensen, H. A. 1935. *Acta Med. Scand.* **86**: 127.
2. Harrel, G. T. and Fisher, S. 1939. *J. Clin. Invest.* **18**: 687.

3. Turiaf, J., and Brun J. 1955. La Sarcoidose Endothoracique de B. B. S. Paris: *Expansion Scientifique Française.*
4. Blasi, A., Berti R., and Olivieri, D. 1966. *Riv. Tub. Mal. App. Resp.* **14**: 189.
5. Blasi, A., Olivieri, D., and Rabinovici, A. 1968. *Riv. Pat. Clin. Tuberc.* **41**: 339.
6. Daddi, G., and Gialdroni-Grassi, G. 1966. *Amer. Rev. Resp. Dis.* **94**: 970.
7. Daddi, G., Gialdroni-Grassi, G. 1967. *La Sarcoidose.* Rapp. IV Conf. Int. *Masson* et Cⁱᵉ.
8. Berti, R., Di Perna, A., and Olivieri, D. 1964. Giorn. *Pneumol.* **8**: 547.
9. Celikoglu, S., Vieira L. O. B. D., and Siltzbach, L. E. 1971. *Proc. Fifth Int. Conf. on Sarcoidosis.* Prague.
10. Sharma, O. P., James, D. G., Bird, R., and White E. W. 1971. *Proc. Fifth Int. Conf. on Sarcoidosis.* Prague.
11. Goldstein, R. A., Israel, H. L., and Rawnsley, H. M., 1971. *Proc. Fifth Int. Conf. on Sarcoidosis.* Prague.
12. Daddi, G., and Gialdroni-Grassi, G. 1971. *Proc. Fifth Int. Conf. on Sarcoidosis.* Prague.
13. Simecek, C., Zavazal, V., Sach, J., and Kulich, V. 1971. *Proc. Fifth Int. Conf. on Sarcoidosis.* Prague.
14. Olivieri, D. 1970. *Proc. Intern. Symposium of Inhalation Therapy.* Naples.
15. Voisin, C. 1968. *Proc. Coll. Intern. Path. Thor.* Lille.
16. Tomasi, T. B., Bienenstock, J. 1968. *Adv. Immunol.* **9**: 2.
17. Cebra, J. J., and Small, R. A. 1967. *Biochemistry* **6**: 503.
18. Havez, R., Muh, J. P., Bonte, M., and Biserte, G. 1967. *Clin. Chim. Acta* **15**: 7.
19. Smith, R. T. 1969 *Pediatrics* **48**: 317.
20. Blasi, A., Olivieri, D., and Rabinovici, A. 1967. *Poum. et Cour* **23**: 805.
21. Medici, T. C., and Buergi, H. 1971. *Am. Rev. Resp. Dis.* **103**: 784.
22. Olivieri, D., Bocchino, M., and Caputi, M. 1970. *Arch. Monaldi* **25**: 537.
23. Blasi, A., and Olivieri, D. 1971. *Les Bronches* **21**: 547.
24. Israel, H. L., and Sones, M. 1955. *Annals of Internal Med.* **43**: 1269.
25. Levitt, N. 1959. Dis. *Chest* **36**: 243.
26. Rudberg-Roos, I. 1964. *Acta Tub. Pneumol. Scand. Suppl.* **52**: 41.
27. Keimovitz, R. J. 1964. *J. Lab. Clin. Med.* **63**: 54

Antibodies to Epstein-Barr Virus in Sera from 70 Patients with Sarcoidosis

Matao Naito, Yoko Akiyama and Shiro Kato

Research Institute for Microbial Diseases, Osaka University, Osaka, Japan

AND

Teruo Tachibana

Osaka Prefectural Hospital, Osaka, Japan

This paper is concerned with the study of antibodies to Epstein-Barr virus (EBV) in in sera from patients with sarcoidosis by an indirect immunofluorescence technique. P3HR-1 cells from Burkitt's lymphoma which had been supplied by Dr Hinuma, Kumamoto University, were used for EBV antigen preparations. These samples contain 20–30% stainable cells. Sera of patients with nasopharyngeal carcinoma (NPC) which had high titers of antibodies to EBV antigen, were used for reference. Specimens were examined under ultraviolet illumination with a Tiyoda immunofluorescence microscope, type FM 200A. The positive rate of anti-EBV titers in 143 samples of sera from 70 patients with sarcoidosis and 108 sera from control groups was examined. All these sera were supplied by Dr Tachibana. As a positive control, the positive rate of anti-EBV titers of 23 sera from NPC patients in the Osaka area were also examined.

Dissociation in frequency distribution of control and sarcoidosis cases was found to become maximum when the boundary of positive reaction is set at a titer of $1:640\leq$ (Fig. 1). As shown in Table 1, 60.1% of sarcoidosis patients' sera exhibited anti-EBV titers higher than $1:640$ and the positive rate in the control group was 21.3%. Sarcoidosis and control cases were divided into groups as shown in Table 1. There was no significant correlation between the titers and groups of disease, although a group of sarcoidosis patients who became clear in X-ray changes, showed somewhat lower posi-

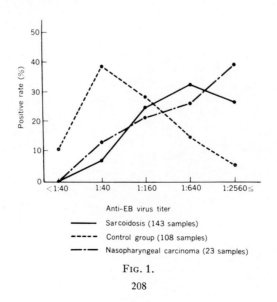

Anti-EB virus titer

——— Sarcoidosis (143 samples)

- - - - Control group (108 samples)

—·—·— Nasopharyngeal carcinoma (23 samples)

Fig. 1.

208

Table 1. Distribution of anti-EBV (VCA) titers among normal subjects and selected disease.

Group	Anti-EBV (VCA) titers					Total cases	1 : 640≤ Positive %	Ridit analysis
	<1 : 40	1 : 40	1 : 160	1 : 640	1 : 2560≤			
Sarcoidosis	0	11	36	47	39	143	60.1	0.733±0.048
Control group	12	42	31	16	7	108	21.3	0.500±0.056
Sarcoidosis								
Before treatment	0	6	17	22	19	64	64.1	0.831±0.072
Under treatment	0	1	18	17	20	56	66.1	0.867±0.077
After clearing of X-ray changes	0	4	11	8	0	23	34.8	0.722±0.120
Tuberculosis	1	6	2	3	2	14	35.7	0.591±0.154
Other diseases	3	15	10	9	3	40	30.0	0.593±0.091
Normal subjects	8	21 (2)	19 (2)	4	2 (2)	54 (6)	11.1	0.500±0.079

( ) Family of patients.

Table 2. Antibody to early antigen of EBV in sera from sarcoidosis and normal subjects.

Group	Number of tested sera	Number of EA positive	% of EA positive
Patients with sarcoidosis, before treatment	54	12	22.2
Normal subjects	12	1	8.3

$\chi^2=1.2$ $p>0.05$

tive rate in anti-EBV antibody than other groups. The data were analyzed statistically, employing the ridit method by taking the anti-EBV titers among the control group as the identified distribution. The sera of sarcoidosis patients exhibited higher average ridit as compared with those of the control.

Sera from 54 patients with sarcoidosis and 12 healthy persons were examined for antibodies to early antigens of EBV. NC-37 cell line inoculated with EBV was used as early antigen material. Twelve sera among sarcoidosis patients showed positive (Table 2). However, they showed rather low antibody titers.

Studies on the Immunological Status of Sarcoidosis
—Humoral immunity and local hyperglobulinosis—

M. Takahashi, H. Osada, K. Sasaki, A. Kawaguchi,
K. Kawamata, H. Ueda and Y. Chiba

Japanese National Railways Central Hospital, Tokyo, Japan

INTRODUCTION

It has been mentioned that there is a dichotomy in sarcoidosis whereby T cell-dependent delayed hypersensitivity is depressed while the ability to produce circulating antibodies remains. Depression of PHA-induced blastoid transformation of lymphocytes in peripheral blood did not recover to the normal range in spite of remarkable clinical improvement.[3] This study is concerned the stage of humoral immunity after influenza vaccination, variations of serum immunoglobulin levels according to the stage of the disease and local globulinosis in the epithelioid cell granulomas. Electron microscopic studies were also carried out to clarify the significance of active epithelioid cells in local globulinosis.

MATERIAL AND METHODS

Circulating antibodies by influenza vaccination

Inactivated influenza viruses containing A2 (Aichi 2/68, Fukuoka 1/70) and B (Tokyo 7/66, Kagoshima 1/68, Osaka 2/70) were injected subcutaneously twice with a 1-week interval in patients with sarcoidosis and healthy persons. Three weeks after vaccination, its effect was studied serologically by the hemagglutinin inhibition test and the complement fixation test.

Serum immunoglobulins

Serum immunoglobulins were quantified by a single radial immunodiffusion method with Ouchterlony plates. The diameters of precipitation rings, parallel to the quantity of immunoglobulins, were measured after a 4-hour incubation for IgG and a 20-hour incubation for IgM and IgA.

Phagocytosis of blood monocytes

A drop of Pelikan special black ink (Günther Wagner) in a capillary tube was added to 1 ml of heparinized blood in a small glass tube. After a 2-hour incubation at 37°C thin films of the blood were made and stained by the Giemsa method. Before use of the Pelikan ink, it was filtered twice with the same filter paper.

Immunofluorescent antibody technique for determination of local globulinosis

Rabbit antibodies against human immunoglobulins were labeled with fluorescein isothiocyanate (FITC). Tissue specimens of sarcoidosis were immediately fixed with cold acetone and embedded into paraffin of low melting point, strictly below 56°C.

Secondly, gammaglobulin from patients with productive granuloma was purified and labeled with FITC to investigate the presence of antigenic substance in epithelioid cell granuloma. Light microscopic and electron microscopic studies for granuloma were performed as a routine examination.

RESULTS

1. Titers in the hemagglutinin inhibition test were evaluated by increased dilution times of sera after vaccination regardless of the absolute dilution times. A majority of the cases with sarcoidosis revealed a remarkable response to vaccination, as is observed in healthy persons (Table 1). A complement fixation test showed no significant values in both groups and was found to be of no value for estimation of vaccination.

2. Although the time of detection in sarcoidosis determined by routine annual examination for healthy control or with physical complaints does not always represent the onset of the disease, variations in immunoglobulin values were measured according to the progress of the disease from the time of notification of the disease (Table 2). High IgG values above 1.5 g/dl were seen in half of 34 cases at the onset. Furthermore, in about 6 to 12 months, 55% of the cases showed high IgG values. It decreased in one and a half years or later, but 7 out of 17 cases were still over the normal range. IgM also gave similar results; hyper-IgM-globulinemia was seen in 59% of the case at the onset, 55% in about 6 to 12 months, and 47% in one and a half years. The increase in value of IgA was evidently less marked than IgG and IgM. Hyper-IgA-globulinemia was seen in 27% of the case at the onset, 18% in 6 to 12 months, and only 6% in one

TABLE 1. Humoral immunity by influenza vaccination.

Case	Hemagglutinin inhibition test				CFT test		Group
	A2 (Aichi)	A2 (Fukuoka)	B (Kagoshima)	B (Osaka)	A2 (Aichi)	B (Tokyo and Kagoshima)	
Y. K.	⧺ (128)	⧺ (256)	+ (64)	+ (64)	− (32)	− (32)	
H. S.	⧻ (128)	⧺ (128)	⧺ (128)	⧺ (256)	− (16)	− (8)	
T. M.	⧺ (64)	+ (64)	− (256)	+ (512)	− (32)	− (16)	
H. T.	⧻ (512)	⧻(1024)	⧻ (128)	⧻ (256)	− (16)	− (8)	Sarcoidosis
K. C.	⧻ (128)	⧻ (128)	+ (256)	+ (512)	+ (16)	+ (32)	
O. Z.	⧻ (128)	⧻ (256)	⧻ (64)	⧻ (64)	− (32)	+ (16)	
K. J.	⧻ (256)	⧻ (256)	⧻ (128)	⧺ (256)	+ (16)	− (16)	
M. Y.	− (256)	− (256)	− (128)	+ (256)	−(256)	− (64)	
K. G.	⧻ (64)	⧻ (128)	⧻ (256)	⧻ (64)	+ (32)	− (32)	
T. S.	+ (256)	+ (256)	+ (128)	+ (128)	+ (32)	− (16)	
Y. K.	− (64)	− (128)	+ (16)	+ (32)	+ (32)	− (16)	
U. B.	⧻ (128)	⧻ (256)	+ (32)	− (32)	+ (32)	− (16)	
S. M.	⧻ (64)	⧻ (64)	⧻ (64)	⧻ (64)	− (8)	− (16)	Healthy
Y. S.	⧺ (32)	⧻ (64)	+ (128)	⧺ (256)	⧺ (32)	+ (16)	
O. D.	⧺ (256)	⧺ (256)	⧻ (64)	⧻ (128)	− (16)	− (16)	
S. Z.	⧻(2048)	⧻(2048)	⧻ (128)	⧻ (256)	+ (16)	+ (64)	
O. T.	+ (128)	+ (256)	+ (256)	+ (512)	− (16)	+ (16)	

Note :   Increase in dilution times 2× +, 4× ⧺, 8× ⧻.

TABLE 2.   Immunoglobulin values according to the stage.

		Onset	6–12 months	After 18 months
IgA	above 400 mg	●●●●●● ○○○	●●● ○	●
	160–400 mg	●●●●●● ●●●● ○○○○○○○ ○○○○○○	●●●●●● ○○○	●●●●●● ●● ○
	below 160 mg	● ○○	●●	●
IgM	above 100 mg	●●●●●● ○○○○○○ ○○○○	●●●●●● ○	●●●●●● ○
	50–100 mg	●●●●● ○○○○○ ○	●●●●● ○○○	●●●●●● ●●●
	below 50 mg	● ○	●	
IgG	above 1500 mg	●●●●●● ●●●● ○○○○○○ ○	●●●●●● ●●●● ○○	●●●●●● ●
	900–1500 mg	●●●●● ○○○○○○ ○○○	●●●●● ○○	●●●●●● ●●● ○
	below 900 mg	● ○○	●● ○	

○ Single quantification.
● Followup quantification available.

and a half years or later.

3.   Phagocytosis of Pelikan black ink particles by blood monocytes was observed throughout the entire field of the slides and evaluated in terms of the phagocytosis rate (Table 3). The rates in sarcoidosis ranged from 0.461 to 0.952 (mean$\pm$1SD: 0.756$\pm$ 0.168), the same as in healthy persons (0.734$\pm$0.158). In a control group, however, 2 cases of malignant lymphoma disclosed decreased phagocytic activity; 0.366 and 0.315, apparently lower than normal.

4.   The immunofluorescent antibody technique revealed accumulation of immuno-globulins, particularly IgM and IgG, within the epithelioid cell granulomas (Fig. 1, Table 4). The intensity of the immunofluorescence was more marked in productive granuloma than fibrotic granuloma. IgA deposition was seen in a few cases and was less marked in intensity than IgM or IgG. It was proved that epithelioid cells as well as Langhans giant cells were fluorescent. Secondly, a direct immunofluorescence method using the patient's own gammaglobulin, which was purified and labeled with FITC, disclosed intracellular fluorescence scattered within the epithelioid cell granuloma. Electron microscopically, epithelioid cells in productive granulomas disclosed well-developed cytoplasmic organelles. There were marked increases in the numbers of mito-chondria, rough endoplasmic reticulum (RER), polysomes and lysosomes. Golgi com-plexes were well-developed. Cellular membranes revealed marked interdigitations in association with occasional development of desmosomes (Fig. 2). Pinocytotic vesicles were not infrequently observed. Multiple centrioles were occasionally encountered in

TABLE 3. Phagocytosis of blood monocytes.

Case	Disease	Phagocytosis	
K. C.	Sarcoidosis manifest	0.809 (34/42)	mean±1SD=
S. D.	Sarcoidosis manifest	0.806 (100/124)	0.756±0.168
I. H.	Sarcoidosis manifest	0.842 (91/108)	
T. D.	Sarcoidosis manifest	0.461 (12/26)	
M. M.	Sarcoidosis persistent	0.923 (36/39)	
T. M.	Sarcoidosis persistent	0.724 (42/58)	
T. Y.	Sarcoidosis persistent	0.468 (15/32)	
N. T.	Sarcoidosis recovered	0.820 (32/39)	
H. T.	Sarcoidosis persistent	0.952 (60/63)	
O. K.	Lymphoma	0.366 (11/30)	
S. W.	Lymphoma	0.315 (6/19)	
K. M.	Lung cancer	0.608 (56/92)	
T. G.	Lung cancer	0.400 (18/45)	
S. Z.	Multiple myeloma	0.513 (19/37)	
T. G.	Tuberculosis	0.680 (51/75)	
I. T.	Tuberculosis	0.758 (66/87)	
O. A.	Tuberculosis	0.703 (35/45)	
F. S.	Tuberculosis	0.440 (22/50)	
T. S.	Healthy	0.641 (25/31)	mean±1SD=
K. T.	Healthy	0.939 (31/33)	0.734±0.158
Y. K.	Healthy	0.931 (27/29)	
O. T.	Healthy	0.764 (26/35)	
O. D.	Healthy	0.600 (24/40)	
U. B.	Healthy	0.531 (17/32)	

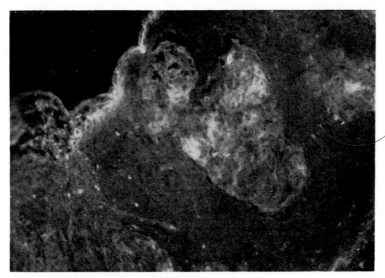

FIG. 1. Accumulation of IgG in the epithelioid cell granuloma of sarcoidosis. Immunofluorescent antibody technique.

TABLE 4. Local globulinosis in granulomatous lesions.

Case	Histology	FITC-labeled rabbit antiserum				FITC-labeled patient's gammaglobulin
		IgA	IgM	IgG	beta-1c/beta-1a	
K. T.	fibrotic	−	−	+	−	± (YD)
S. D.	fibrotic	−	+	±	±	*
S. Z.	productive	+	++	++	++	+ (YD)
H. K.	productive	±	+	+	+	± (MM)
Y. D.	productive	+	++	+++	++	+ (AI)
K. I.	productive	±	+	+	+	*
M. M.	productive	+	+	+++	+	*
H. E.	productive	+	++	+++	*	+ (MM)
H. T.	productive	+	+	+++	*	± (MM)
K. C.	productive	+	+	+++	*	++ (MM)
O. H.	productive	−	+	+++	*	− (MM)

Note :   * Not examined ; (YD), (MM), (AI) source of patient's gammaglobulin.

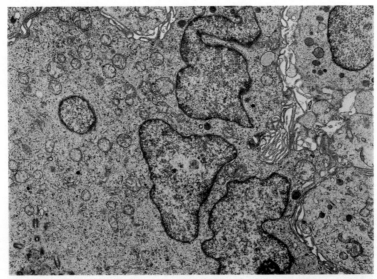

FIG. 2.   Langhans' giant cell rich in mitochondria and ribosomes shows marked inter-digitations of cellular membrane and well development of Golgi complexes.   Note centrioles at the lower left corner.   Mag. ×8,000.

Langhans' giant cells (Fig. 2). Above all, noteworthy findings in epithelioid cells were development of RER with a lamellar arrangement and cystic dilatation containing a finely granular or somewhat amorphous substance of low density (Figs. 3 and 4). The interstitial substance with a fibrillar structure and glassy, amorphous content was next to the above active epithelioid cells.

DISCUSSION

The immunological defect in delayed hypersensitivity of patients with sarcoidosis has been represented as depression for contact sensitizers,[9] diminished reactivity to a wide

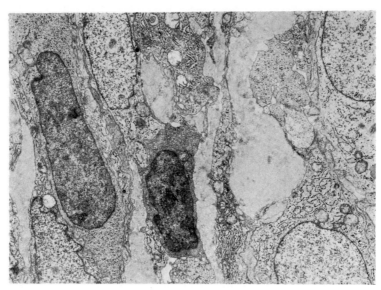

FIG. 3. Active epithelioid cells with light, broad cytoplasm show a marked increase in number of RER. Note cystic dilatation and a lamellar arrangement of RER. An interstitial substance which is fibrillar and with glassy, amorphous density is next to the above epithelioid cells with indistinct borders. Mag. ×8,000.

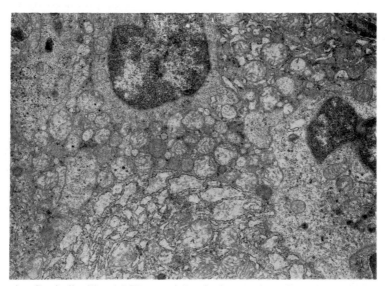

FIG. 4. Cystically dilated RER containing finely granular substance with low density. Mag. ×12,000.

spectrum of skin tests such as histoplasmin, trichophytin and mumps virus, and decrease of tuberculin sensitivity. In addition, the PHA-induced blastoid transformation of peripheral lymphocytes is markedly depressed in cases of sarcoidosis. On the other hand, humoral immunity has been considered not to be impaired, as shown by the complement fixation test to mumps or to antigens prepared from tubercle bacilli,[4] the Dubos-Middlebrook test,[2,5] etc. Increases in serum protein and gammaglobulin have long been known as a nonspecific phenomenon of sarcoidosis. Hypergammaglobulinemia is evident in the manifestation of the disease but returns to a normal range after complete regression. Concerning serum immunoglobulins, varying reports have been presented in the Fifth International Conference on Sarcoidosis and no definite results have been obtained till now. Quantification of serum immunoglobulins according to the stage or progress of the disease disclosed elevation of immunoglobulins of the polyclonal type during the manifestation (Table 2). However, elevation became less marked after 18 months or later. At any rate, increased immunoglobulins in the stage showing productive granulomas may be related to activation of B cell-dependent immunity. Telium[13] pointed out that accumulation of plasma cells around the granuloma accounted for hyper-globulinemia. He regarded the pathogenesis of amyloid-like hyalinosis around the granuloma as local globulinosis, stimulated by an immune mechanism, related to activation of reticuloendothelial cells.[13] Ober and Löfgren have come to the similar conclusion that PAS-positive pyroniophilic cells were derived from reticuloendothelial cells and were responsible for production of amyloid-like material.[7] It has long been a point of discussion whether amyloid-like substance was precipitated from plasma or produced intracellularly. Gusek emphasized the presence of ergastoplasm-rich epithelioid cells to be related to PAS-positive cells as sites of globulin synthesis. In the present report we found in productive granuloma active epithelioid cells which were rich in RER arranged in a parallel fashion (Fig. 3). In addition to increased RER, cystic dilatation full of finely granular or somewhat amorphous material of low density was a noteworthy finding. Multinucleation of the Langhans, type was thought to be produced by fusion of the epithelioid cells. However, the presence of multiple centrioles indicates active prolifera-tion of cells abundant in organelles (Fig. 2).

The immunofluorescent antibody technique proved the accumulation of immuno-globulins, particularly IgG and IgM, within the epithelioid cell granuloma.[12] Intra-cellular fluorescence and positive $\beta_1 C$ complement in epithelioid cell granuloma are sug-gestive of local hyperglobulinosis induced by an immune mechanism. This hypothesis can also be sustained by electron microscopic findings on active epithelioid cells which are rich in RER showing a plasmacytoid lamellar pattern. The origin of epithelioid cells, whether they are transformed lymphocytes[10] or proliferated reticuloendothelial cells, is an important point for further investigation. The presence of antigenic substance as suggested by the direct immunofluorescence method using the patient's gammaglobulin may indicate the formation of an antigen-antibody immune complex in the granuloma.

SUMMARY

Humoral immunity in the patient with sarcoidosis was normally elevated after in-fluenza vaccination. Serum immunoglobulin levels, particularly IgM and IgG, were elevated during the manifestation of the disease. Although PHA-induced blastoid trans-formation of lymphocytes was depressed, the function of phagocytosis of blood mono-cytes was not impaired. Accumulation of immunoglobulins in the productive epithelioid cell granuloma was proved by the immunofluorescent antibody technique. Good de-velopment in the rough endoplasmic reticulum and its cystic dilatation with a content of finely granular substance of low density were suggestive of local globulinosis as an immune mechanism. The presence of an antigenic substance was also suggested.

REFERENCES

1. Carnes, W. H., and Raffel, S. A. 1949 A comparison of sarcoidosis and tuberculosis with respect to complement fixation with antigens derived from the tubercle bacillus. *Bull. J. Hopkins Hosp.* **85**: 204.

2. Fleming, J. W., Runyon, E. H., and Cummings, M. M. 1951. An evaluation of the hemagglutination test for tuberculosis. *Amer. J. Med.* **10**: 704.

3. Gusek, W. 1968. Formale Pathogenese der hyalinen Transformation des Sarcoidose-granuloms. *Virchows Arch. Abt. A Path. Anat.* **345**: 264.

4. Hirschhorn, K., Schreiber, R. R., Rach, F. H., and Siltzbach, L. E. 1964. In vitro studies from patients with sarcoidosis and lymphoproliferative diseases. *Lancet* **ii**: 842.

5. Izumi, T. 1972. Immunological symptoms in sarcoidosis. *Saishin-Igaku* (in Japanese) **27**: 1317.

6. Mikata, A. 1971. Tuberculosis and sarcoidosis. *Metabolism and Disease* (in Japanese) **8** (No. 1).

7. Ober, A-L., and Löfgren, S. 1964. Pathogenesis of hyaline formation in sarcoidotic lymph nodes. *Acta Med. Scand. Suppl.* **425**: 27.

8. Osada, H., Hosoda, Y., Odaka, M., Matsumoto, M. Takahashi, M., Yanaka, M., and Chiba, Y. 1972. Impaired lymphocytes in the patients recovered from sarcoidosis. Abstract, *Sixth Int. Conf. on Sarcoidosis.* Tokyo.

9. Epstein, W. L., and Mayock, R. L. 1957. Induction of allergic contact dermatitis in patients with sarcoidosis. *Proc. Soc. Exp. Biol. Med.* **96**: 786.

10. Jones Williams, W., Fry, E., and Valerie James, E. M. 1972 A comparison of the fine structure of lymphocytes in the peripheral blood and granulomas of sarcoidosis. Abstract, *Sixth Int. Conf. on Sarcoidosis.* Tokyo.

11. Seki, K. 1972. Fine structure of epithelioid cell granuloma in liver. *Saishin-Igaku* (in Japanese **27**: 1291.

12. Takahashi, M. 1970. Histopathology of sarcoidosis and its immunological bases. *Acta Path. Jap.* **20**: 171.

13. Teilum, G. 1964. Morphogenesis and development of sarcoid lesions. *Acta Med. Scand. Suppl.* **425**: 14.

Serological Hyperreactivity to Epstein-Barr Virus and other Viral Antigens in Sarcoidosis

Earl B. Byrne, Alfred S. Evans, David W. Fouts and Harold L. Israel

Jefferson Medical College, Thomas Jefferson University, Philadelphia, U.S.A.

SUMMARY

Sera from 216 patients with sarcoidosis were examined for antibodies against Epstein-Barr virus (EBV) and 13 other viral antigens including hepes simplex, cytomegalovirus, adenovirus, rubella, respiratory syncytial, measles, mumps, influenza and parainfluenza viruses. Compared to 92 controls, significantly higher titers were found in the sarcoidosis patients against EBV, herpes simplex, rubella, measles and parainfluenza 1–3 viruses. However in a subsample of 74 matched pairs, only elevations in EBV, rubella and parainfluenza 3 antibodies remained significant. Among sarcoidosis patients, highest titers were observed in females and blacks but no correlation could be made either by stage of disease or activity. The role of these viruses, and of EBV particularly, in the etiology of sarcoidosis remains speculative.

Since sarcoidosis was first described in 1878 its etiology has remained elusive. Histopathologically, the chronic granulomatous character of sarcoidosis has led many to suspect an infectious agent, or at least an exogenous antigen as the ultimate cause. None has been identified convincingly. Most recently EB virus (EBV), the herpes virus identified by Epstein and Barr in Burkitt's lymphoma tissue, and subsequently proposed as the etiologic agent of infectious mononucleosis, has been linked to sarcoidosis. Seroepidemiological studies by Hirshaut et al.[1] and by Wahren et al.[2] have revealed that sera from persons with sarcoidosis have a significantly higher prevalence of elevated antibody titers against EBV than that from comparable normal individuals. Both groups have been cautious in ascribing any etiologic role to EBV. Additional studies to extend the observations reported seem a fertile avenue to pursue, not only in understanding sarcoidosis, but also in elucidating the full range of herpes virus infection.

MATERIALS AND METHODS

Patient and control material

The Sarcoidosis Clinic at Thomas Jefferson University Hospital carries over 700 patients with sarcoidosis on its register. Approximately 300 are seen at least once yearly.

This work was supported by research grants AI08731 from the National Institutes of Allergy and Infectious Diseases, National Institutes of Health, Bethesda, Maryland, and CC00242 from the Center for Disease Control, Atlanta, Georgia.

Table 1.   Comparison of sarcoid patients and control group.

		Sarcoid	Control
Number		216	92
Average Age		36.5	26.9
Sex	Male	35%	42%
	Female	65%	58%
Race	Black	83%	63%
	White	17%	37%

Between June 1970 and March 1971 serum specimens were obtained from 181 patients attending the clinic. Sera from 35 private patients being seen by one of the authors and obtained as long ago as 1967, were also added to the collection, making a total of 216 patients studied. Diagnoses were established at varying intervals before serum collection using a combination of generally accepted clinical, radiological and histological criteria.[3] Skin testing with Kveim antigens was not used routinely, however a small number of patients did undergo testing with Kveim material. Control sera were obtained from 92 essentially healthy persons of approximately comparable age, sex, race and socioeconomic status who were seen either as patients in the student and employee health clinics or the maternity clinic or as volunteer blood donors. As shown in Table 1, the controls averaged 10 years younger and had somewhat higher ratios of males and whites than the sarcoid group. To control these differences separate analyses of each of these variables are presented. A matched subsample has also been studied.

All specimens were stored at $-20°C$ and coded prior to being shipped frozen to the WHO Reference Serum Bank at Yale University School of Medicine where a battery of viral antibody tests (described below) were performed. Only after all tests were completed was the code broken and sera identified as to diagnosis.

Immunofluorescence test

EBV antibody was measured by the indirect immunofluorescence test developed by Henles[4] employing the EB3 cell line of Burkitt lymphoma cells as the source of antigen. In this system 1:160 is taken as the upper level of normal because only 5–7% of over 400 normal sera tested by us with this same technique and which possess antibody reach levels this high. The geometric mean titer in healthy subjects with antibody has been about 1:62. Experience has shown that, because of minor differences in cell lines, the conjugate used, the technique of the test, and the criteria of the end point, valid comparisons between titers in sera from diseased and healthy persons can be made only within the same laboratory.

Hemagglutination inhibition (HI) test

This was carried out in microtiter plates with inactivated sera according to the general method of Sever.[5] Influenza tests were done with the A2/Taiwan/1/64, A2/Hong Kong/8/68 and B/GL1739/54 antigens supplied by the Center for Disease Control (CDC). Parainfluenza 1, 2, and 3 antigens and measles antigen was also supplied by CDC. Mumps antigen was obtained commercially from Microbiological Associates, Bethesda, Md. Measles antibody was measured after the method of Black.[6] Rubella antigen obtained commercially from Flow Laboratories, Rockford, Ill. was used following the procedure of Liebhaber.[7] Positive and negative serum controls were included in all runs.

Complement fixation tests

A microtiter test based on a 50% end point tecnnique as outlined by the CDC was employed.[8] Cytomegalovirus antigen was procured commercially from Microbiological Associates, as were herpes simplex and respiratory syncytial antigen; the adenovirus type 4 antigen used in the CF tests was obtained from CDC. Positive and negative controls were included in each run.

Statistical methods

The criterion for elevation of either hemagglutination inhibition or complement fixation titer is that level exceeded by no more than 10% of normal sera tested by the same technique. Calculations of the percent of sera with elevated titers and the geometric mean titer (GMT) were based only on sera with demonstrable antibody. Differences in titers between sarcoid and control groups were measured for significance by Student's *t* test, while differences between the frequency of elevated titers were evaluated by the *chi* square test.

RESULTS

EBV antibody

Antibody to EBV was present in 97.2% of the sarcoid sera and 97.8% of the control

TABLE 2.   EBV I.F. antibody titers in sarcoid and control sera.

	Sarcoid	Controls	P value between sarcoid & controls
No. of patients tested	216	92	
Percentage with antibody at 1 : 10 or more	97.2	97.8	N.S.
Of those with antibody			
Percentage at 1 : 320 or more	33.3	7.8	< .005
Geometric mean titer	1 : 150	1 : 68	< .001

TABLE 3.   EBV antibody titers by age, sex, and race in sarcoid and control sera.

		Sarcoid		Controls	
		No.	GMT	No.	GMT
Age	15–24	18	179.6	48	61.7
	25–34	75	122.4	25	77.8
	35–44	72	163.1	12	80.0
	45–54	35	166.5	3	40.0
	55+over	10	183.8	1	160.0
		210	149.8	89	67.9
Sex	Male	74	121.9	36	63.5
	Female	136	167.5	53	71.1
		210	149.8	89	67.9
Race	White	31	87.5	33	64.8
	Black	177	165.1	56	69.8

sera. In serum with antibody, the geometric mean titer (GMT) for EBV antibody was 1 : 150 in the sarcoid and 1 : 68 in the control sera; 33.3% of sarcoid sera had titers of 1 : 320 or higher as compared to 7.9% of the control sera. Both these differences were statistically significant (Table 2).

Examination of anti-EBV titers in sarcoid patients by age revealed the highest levels in the 15–24 age group (Table 3). EBV antibody titers were consistently higher in each age group than in controls of comparable age. In the sarcoid group, females had titers impressively higher than male patients. This same sex trend was seen in the control group to a lesser extent. When analyzed by race the EBV antibody titers were much higher in black sarcoid patients than in white sarcoid patients. No significant difference existed between control sera by race (Table 3). While the titers in sera of sarcoid patients were higher than in control sera of both races, the differences were much more marked in blacks.

Other viral antibodies

The results of quantitative titers for antibodies to EBV and 13 other viral antigens are summarized in Table 4. No difference in the *presence* or *absence* of any antibody was

TABLE 4.   Comparison of viral antibody titers in sarcoid patients and controls.

Virus	Test	Tested		with		% ≥ indicated level		χ^2 p value	GMT	t test p value
				Antibody	%	Level	%			
EBV	IF	S*	216	210	97.2	320	33.3		149.8	
		C*	92	90	97.8		7.8	<.005	68.1	<.001
HS	CF	S	209	180	86.1	160	16.7		43.9	
		C	89	68	76.4		4.4	<.025	27.2	<.001
CMV	CF	S	208	118	56.7	160	11.0		19.9	
		C	89	37	41.6		5.4	N.S.	20.0	N.S.
Adeno	CF	S	209	104	49.8	160	3.8		14.5	
		C	89	45	50.6		2.2	N.S.	14.5	N.S.
RS	CF	S	107	83	40.1	40	8.4		9.4	
		C	89	30	33.7		3.3	N.S.	8.1	N.S.
Rubella	HI	S	216	192	88.9	256	15.1		60.2	
		C	92	84	91.3		4.8	<.05	38.7	<.005
Measles	HI	S	211	207	98.1	640	12.1		85.3	
		C	92	89	96.7		5.6	N.S.	54.6	<.005
Mumps	HI	S	210	113	53.8	40	8.0		13.2	
		C	92	47	51.1		0	N.S.	11.4	<.025
Inf A2/HK	HI	S	216	152	70.4	320	6.6		28.0	
		C	92	68	73.9		7.4	N.S.	29.2	N.S.
Inf A2/T	HI	S	216	213	98.6	1280	6.1		87.1	
		C	92	92	100.0		8.7	N.S.	95.9	N.S.
Inf B/GL	HI	S	216	205	94.9	320	6.3		32.7	
		C	92	87	94.6		4.6	N.S.	29.3	N.S.
Para 1	HI	S	216	180	83.3	80	11.7		21.8	
		C	92	74	80.4		2.7	<.05	15.2	<.005
Para 2	HI	S	216	206	95.4	80	17.0		24.8	
		C	92	85	92.4		3.5	<.005	17.6	<.001
Para 3	HI	S	216	207	95.8	160	16.4		42.3	
		C	92	89	96.7		2.2	<.005	22.8	<.001

GMT=Geometric mean antibody titer in sera with antibody.

N.S.=Not significant.

*S=Sarcoid.   *C=Control.

apparent between sarcoid and control sera. However, the *geometric mean titer* (GMT) in those with antibody was significantly higher than controls for herpes simplex, rubella, measles, parainfluenza 1, 2, and 3 viruses and mumps virus. The frequency of *raised titers* over controls was also higher in sarcoid patients for all antibodies except for the 2 influenza A2 antigens.

Multiple antibody analysis

Antibody levels to all 14 antigens were completed on 204 sarcoid sera and 88 control sera. Elevations of 1 or more antibodies were present in 82% of the sarcoid sera, of 2 or more in 49.7%, of 3 or more in 31.6%, of 4 or more in 12.8%, of 5 or more in 3.0%, and of 6 antibodies in 1%. In the control sera there were only 7.9% that showed elevations of 2 or more antibodies, 5.6% with 3 or more and but one serum had 4 elevated titers. Analysis by *chi* square tests of the 26 sarcoid patients with 4 or more elevated antibodies was made to determine if there were distinguishing characteristics of these "multiple hyper-reactors" as compared to those with under 4 elevations. No significant differences were found by race or age group but there were significantly more females than expected (p<.05). Of 72 males tested 5.6% had 4 or more antibodies elevated as compared to 16.7% of 132 females tested.

Matched subsample

Because of the possible introduction of bias through differences between sarcoid patients and controls a matched subsample was analyzed. This consisted of 74 sarcoid patients and 74 controls matched for age within 5 years (usually 2), sex, and race. Three tests of significance were applied for the 14 antibodies tested: the *chi* square test was

TABLE 5.   Comparison of viral antibody titers in sera from 74 sarcoid patients and 74 controls matched for age, sex, and race.

Antibody tested	Group	Percentage with elevated titers*			Geometric mean titers (GMT)*		
		Level	%	χ^2 (p value)	GMT	*t* test (p value)	paired *t* test (p value)
EBV	S	≧1 : 320	33.8		140.9		
	C		6.8	<.005	69.5	<.001	<.005
Rubella	S	≧1 : 256	21.2		67.5		
	C		5.9	<.025	40.5	<.01	<.05
Para 3	S	≧1 : 160	14.3		38.1		
	C		2.8	<.05	22.7	<.001	<.005

S=Sarcoid.   C=Controls.
* Based on sera with antibody.

TABLE 6.   Comparison of EBV antibody levels in 74 matched sarcoid and controls group by race and sex.

Sex	Race	Percentage at ≧1 : 320		Geometric mean titer	
		Sarcoid	Control	Sarcoid	Control
Female	White	40.0	16.7	198.4	89.8
	Black	41.0	5.0	162.9	66.1
Male	White	0.0	0.0	67.3	68.2
	Black	40.0	13.3	152.8	72.9

used to test differences between the frequency of elevated titers, and the t test and the paired t test were used to test differences in mean titers between the groups. The *chi* square test and the unpaired t test were based on sera with demonstrable antibody. Under these rigorous conditions only 3 of the 14 antibodies met all 3 criteria of significance: EBV, rubella, and parainfluenza type 3 (Table 5). Elevated titers were more common among females and black sarcoid patients than in male or white sarcoid patients; the lowest titers were in white male sarcoid patients (Table 6).

Relation to clinical illness

The relation of the geometric mean titer for the 6 antibodies found significantly elevated in the overall group of sarcoid sera to the activity and extent of illness was analyzed. No significant correlation between active and inactive phases of sarcoid and any of the antibodies could be observed. Likewise, in patients classified by the clinical and radiological criteria in which stage 0 indicates nonpulmonary or extrapulmonary involvement only, stage 1 represents hilar adenopathy, stage 2 the presence of hilar plus parenchymal involvements, and stage 3 reflects involvement of the pulmonary parenchyma alone, the results showed no clear cut trend.

DISCUSSION

Sera from 33.3% of 216 sarcoid patients were found to have EBV antibody titers elevated to 1:320 or higher by the indirect immunofluorescence test as compared to 7.8% in control sera (p<.005). The geometric mean titers were 1:150 and 1:68 respectively (p <.001). This compares very closely with the 35% with elevated EBV antibody titers in 90 sarcoid patients and the 7% in 90 controls found by Wahren et al.[2] using the same cell line. Using the more reactive Jijoye line and a titer of 1:640 or higher as elevated, Hirshaut et al.[1] found 75% of sera from 131 sarcoid patients with titers at this level or higher as compared to 24% at this level in 93 controls. The different frequencies may reflect differences in technique and/or antigenic differences between the EB virus in EB3 and Jijoye cell lines although both were derived from Burkitt lymphomas. The evidence from 3 laboratories and the diverse geographic, racial, and socioeconomic characteristics of the patients studied thus support the validity of the results. In our series EBV antibody titers were higher in black sarcoid patients as compared to white sarcoid patients. The titers were also higher in females than in males.

Antibody levels for 13 other viral antigens revealed a wide spectrum of raised titers in sarcoid over control patients. As judged by geometric mean antibody titers and the percentage with raised titers, in the entire group of sarcoidosis patients the increases were statistically significant for EBV, rubella, herpes simplex, and parainfluenza viruses but not for measles, mumps, influenza, CMV, adeno-, or respiratory syncytial viruses. In the subsample of 74 sarcoid and 74 controls matched by age, sex, and race where the most rigorous tests of significance were used, only EBV, rubella, and parainfluenza type 3 remained significantly elevated over controls. This however may be mostly an effect of reduced sample size. Wahren et al.[2] also tested their sarcoid sera against 9 viral antigens and *Mycoplasma pneumoniae* antigen by the complement fixation (CF) test and against 4 other viral antigens by the hemagglutination-inhibition (HI) test. Their sarcoid sera had a higher percentage of antibodies than control sera only to cytomegalo and herpes viruses. The geometric mean antibody titers for these were slightly higher than controls but due to the high frequency of sera lacking antibody, a detailed comparison was not made.

Antibody production and bacterial antibody levels in sarcoidosis previously have been described mostly as normal.[9] An exception is the investigation of Sands et al.[10] who found hyper-reactivity to the injection of small amounts of mismatched blood in 19 sarcoid patients prior to ACTH therapy as compared to normal controls or patients with tuberculosis. The present study and those of Hirshaut et al. and Wahren et al. appear to be the first demonstration of hyper-reactivity to several viral antigens in sarcoidosis. Hyper-reactivity to multiple viral antigens, namely EBV, rubella, measles and parainfluenza 1 virus, has been demonstrated by us and others in 1 additional disease of obscure etiology, systemic lupus erythematosus.[11,12] Conditions associated with raised anti-EBV titers now include infectious mononucleosis, Burkitt's lymphoma, nasopharyngeal cancer, and possibly lepromatous leprosy.[13]

The relationship of raised antibody levels to EBV and other viruses to the pathogenesis of sarcoidosis remains obscure. Raised antibody levels might precede the development of disease and be a factor in its pathogenesis or they might follow the onset of illness and be merely a consequence of the disturbed immunological state associated with it. As serum was not available prior to the onset of illness it is not known which of the possibilities is correct. However since most of the viruses involved usually produce infection early in life, and since most sarcoid cases occur in adult life, it seems somewhat more probable that the initial viral infections preceded the development of sarcoidosis. The occurrence of higher EBV antibody levels in blacks and females suggests that a genetic factor may be operating, though a wholly environmental etiology cannot be ruled out. Recently attention has been called to the association of certain genetically determined histocompatibility antigen patterns, specific immune responsiveness and susceptibility to disease, especially lymphoproliferative disorders.[14,15] In some cases, at least, the sharing of antigenic determinants between histocompatibility antigens and an exogenous viral agent appears to underly the pathogenesis. The possibility of a similar mechanism resulting in sarcoidosis is in many ways an attractive hypothesis since it offers the opportunity for planned investigation in well-defined areas. Clearly the genetic aspects of sarcoidosis need to be re-examined. Analysis of kinships for serological hyper-reactivity to viral agents and histocompatibility type are obvious avenues to be pursued. Studies of sarcoid lymphocyte mediating substances, already underway in many laboratories, should be extended. From a sero-epidemiological standpoint the prospective serial collection of sera, though difficult to achieve because of the low incidence of overt disease and presumed lengthy "incubation period", offers one of the best means of documenting the role, if any, of EBV and other viruses in sarcoidosis.

ACKNOWLEDGEMENT

The technical assistance of Miss Virgina Richards, Miss Linda Cenabre and Miss Joan Wanat is gratefully acknowledged.

REFERENCES

1. Hirshaut, Y., Glade, P., and Viera, L. O. 1970. Sarcoidosis, another disease associated with serologic evidence for herpes-like virus infection. *New Engl. J. Med.* **283**: 502–506.

2. Wahren, B., Carlens, E., Espmark, A., Lundbeck, H., Lofgren, S., Madar, E., Henle, G., and Henle, W. 1971. Antibodies to various herpes virus in sera from patients with sarcoidosis. *J. Natl. Cancer Inst.* **47**: 747–755.

3. Israel, H. L., and Sones, M. 1965. Immunologic defect in patients recovered from sarcoidosis. *New Engl. J. Med.* **273**: 1003–1006.

4. Henle, G. and Henle, W. 1966. Immunofluorescence in cells derived from Burkitt's lymphoma. *J. Bact.* **91**: 1248–1256.

5. Sever, J. 1962. Application of a microtechnique to viral serologic investigations. *J. Immunol.* **88**: 320.

6. Black, F. 1970. Manual of Clinical Microbiology (ed. Blair, J., Lennette, E., and Truant, J. P.). *Am. Soc. Microbiol.* p. 524.

7. Liebhaber, H. 1970. Measurement of rubella antibody by hemagglutination inhibition. II. Characteristics of an improved HAI test employing a new method for the removal of non-immunoglobulin HA inhibitors from serum. *J. Immunol.* **104**: 826–834.

8. CDC, Standard diagnostic complement fixation method and adaptation to microtest. *Public Health Mono.* #74.

9. Siltzbach, L. E. 1971 *Sarcoidosis in Immunological Diseases* (ed. Samter, M.). Little Brown and Co. ch. 29.

10. Sands, J. H., Palmer, P. P., Maycock, R. L., and Creger, W. P. 1955. Evidence for serologic hyper-reactivity in sarcoidosis. *Amer. J. Med.* 404–409.

11. Evans, A. S., Rothfield, N. F., and Niederman, J. C. 1971. Raised antibody titers to EB virus in systemic lupus erythematosus. *Lancet* **1**: 167–168.

12. Hurd, E. R., Dowdle, W., Casey, H. et al. Viral antibody levels in systemic lupus erythematosus (SLE). *Arth. Rheum.* **13**: 324–325.

13. Evans, A. S. 1971 The spectrum of infections with EB virus: A Hypothesis. *J. Inf. Diseases.* **124**: 330–337.

14. McDevitt, H. O., and Bodmer, W. F. 1972. Histocompatibility antigens, immune responsiveness and susceptibility to disease. *Amer. J. Med.* **52**: 1–8.

15. Fudenberg, H. H. 1971. Genetically determined immune deficiency as the predisposing cause of " autoimmunity" and lymphoid neoplasia. *Amer. J. Med.* **51**: 295–298.

Serum Immunoglobulins and EB Virus Antibody in Intrathoracic Sarcoidosis

Yasutaka Niitu, Masahiro Horikawa, Momoyo Sakaguchi, Nobuko Ikeno, Sumio Hasegawa, Shigeo Komatsu, Hideo Kubota and Tomiko Suetake

Department of Pediatrics, The Research Institute for Tuberculosis, Leprosy, and Cancer, Tohoku University, Sendai, Japan

Many authors have reported on the levels of the serum immunoglobulins, IgA, IgG, and IgM, in sarcoidosis. One, two or all of the three immunoglobulins were shown to be increased in sarcoidosis, but the results are conflicting. Hirshaut and associates[1] reported that sarcoidosis is the fourth disease to be linked serologically with EB virus infection.

We determined the levels of the three immunoglobulins and those of EB virus antibody in serial sera from patients with sarcoidosis, observed the course of the levels, and compared the values with those in healthy controls.

MATERIALS AND METHODS

Immunoglobulins were determined by means of an agar ring technique with use of the Hyland immunodiffusion plate. Sera were stored at $-20°C$ after being separated and were used without prior thawing and freezing in most samples and after being thawed once in some samples. It was confirmed that 1 or 2 cycles of freezing and thawing of sera did not result in any significant variation in the levels. The determination was carried out 8 different times. Each time, serial sera from the same patient and sera from the healthy controls were determined. Both groups of sera were examined simultaneously using the same lot of the plate in order to obtain exact information about the level changes in the individual patient and to permit comparison of the levels between the patients and the healthy controls.

Determination of the serum immunoglobulins was carried out in serial sera from 24 patients with intrathoracic sarcoidosis and from 2 patients with eye sarcoidosis. Three of them were first tested at the time of exacerbation in the lungs or eyes. Diagnosis was confirmed by biopsy or Kveim test in 18 cases. The age ranged from 8 to 38 years, being from 8 to 15 years in 13 cases. The normal levels were determined in 67 healthy teenagers and adults.

Serum antibody to EB virus was determined by the immunofluorescence technique in serial sera drawn from 26 patients with intrathoracic sarcoidosis, of whom 10 cases were from 10 to 15 years old, and 16 from 16 to 38 years old, and 2 patients with eye sarcoidosis without intrathoracic involvements. Diagnosis was confirmed by biopsy or Kveim test in 18 cases. Sera from 24 healthy early teenagers served as controls. The determination of the antibody was made at the same time in the serial sera from the same patients and in 1 or 2 samples of control sera.

RESULTS AND DISCUSSION

In 23 patients with intrathoracic sarcoidosis, the levels of the 3 immunoglobulins were compared between the first sera drawn at the time of the detection of the disease and the last sera drawn 6 months to 4 years later. Abnormal X-ray findings, bilateral hilar lymphadenopathy in most patients, were observed when the first sera were drawn, but had disappeared in 20 cases when the last sera were drawn. For the 3 immunoglobulins, IgA, IgG, and IgM, the mean levels were higher in the first sera in sarcoidosis than in sera from controls, and decreased in the last sera in sarcoidosis (Table 1). Corticosteroid hormones were given to 12 patients. The degree of decrease in levels between the first and last sera was higher in patients with steroid treatment than in patients without it.

The course of the levels of the 3 immunoglobulins in the 23 patients is shown in Figs. 1, 2, and 3. A decrease in levels with the course of the disease is frequent for IgA, IgG, and IgM. As compared with the first sera, the last sera showed a decrease in the level in 61% of the cases tested for IgA, in 70% for IgG, and 61% for IgM.

With 3 patients, whose sera were first tested at the time of exacerbation 3 to 9 years after the onset of the disease, the levels of IgA and IgG were higher, but the level of IgM was not so high, as compared with the controls (Figs. 1, 2, and 3).

Summarizing the results, it can be concluded that the levels of serum immunoglobulins in patients with sarcoidosis are higher at the early stage as compared with those in healthy controls and decrease with the course of the disease for IgA, IgG, and

TABLE 1. Serum immunoglobulin levels in sarcoidosis (M±SD).

		IgA (mg/dl)	IgG (mg/dl)	IgM (mg/dl)
Sarcoidosis	23 cases			
First serum (at detection)		288±109	1774±417	133±55
Last serum (6 months to 4 years later)		254± 91	1633±485	124±43
Controls	67 cases	240± 93	1490±508	113±62

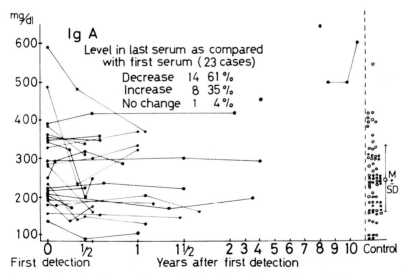

FIG. 1. Course of serum IgA level in patients with sarcoidosis.

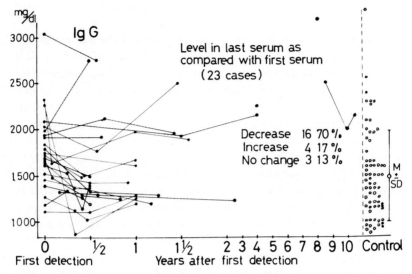

FIG. 2.   Course of serum IgG level in patients with sarcoidosis.

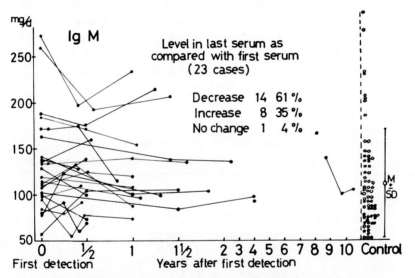

FIG. 3.   Course of serum IgM level in patients with sarcoidosis.

IgM. It seems that the immunoglobulin levels show a difference for IgM between the early stage and the time of exacerbation of the disease.

The distribution of the antibody titers to EB virus was compared between sera from the 24 controls and sera drawn from 21 patients with intrathoracic sarcoidosis at the time of the detection of the disease (Table 2). No significant difference was observed in the distribution of the antibody titer to EB virus between the 2 groups of sera. However, sera drawn from 10 patients with sarcoidosis one and a half years or more after the detection of the disease showed higher values in the distribution of the antibody titers, as compared with the sera drawn from the 21 patients with sarcoidosis at the time of detection.

Table 2. Distribution of immunofluorescence antibody titer of serum to EB virus
in patients with sarcoidosis.

	No. tested	Antibody titer to EB virus			
		<10	10	40	160
Controls	24	2 8%	10 42%	11 46%	1 4%
Sarcoidosis					
At the first detection	21	2 10%	7 33%	9 43%	3 14%
After 1½ years or more (higher figure)	10		1 10%	6 60%	3 30%

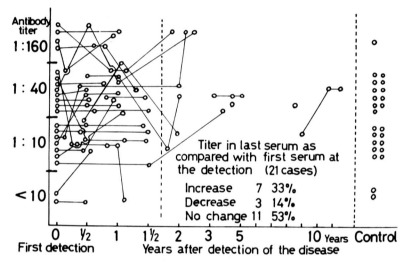

Fig. 4.   Course of serum antibody titer to EB virus in patients with sarcoidosis.

The antibody titer during the course of the disease in the 28 patients with sarcoidosis is shown in Fig. 4. The antibody titer was compared between the first sera drawn when the disease was found and the last sera in 21 patients. The antibody titer of the last sera showed a decrease in 33% of cases, an increase in 14%, and no change in 53%, as compared with that of the first sera. At the time of examination of the last sera, abnormal X-ray findings had disappeared in 16 cases and remained in 5 cases.

It seems that the results are similar to those reported by Hirshaut and associates[1] that higher serum antibody titers to EB virus were observed more frequently in chronic and inactive sarcoidosis than in subacute sarcoidosis.

SUMMARY

The levels of the immunoglobulins, IgA, IgG, and IgM, were increased at the early stage of sarcoidosis and decreased to approach normal values with the course of the disease. The serum antibody titer to EB virus in patients with sarcoidosis showed no abnormality at the early stage of the disease but showed a tendency to increase with the lapse of years after detection of the disease.

REFERENCE

1. Hirshaut, Y., Glade, P., Vieira, L. O. B. K., Ainbender, E., Dvorak, B., and Siltzbach, L. E. 1970. Sarcoidosis, another disease associated with serologic evidence for herpes-like infection. *New Engl. J. Med.* **283**: 502.

Antibodies to Epstein-Barr Virus in Sera from Patients with Sarcoidosis in Japan

T. Kataoka and T. Murohashi

National Institute of Health, Tokyo, Japan

R. Mikami

Tokyo University School of Medicine, Tokyo, Japan

Y. Hosoda and M. Odaka

Japanese National Railways Central Health Institute, Tokyo, Japan

Y. Hiraga

Japanese National Railways Sapporo Hospital, Sapporo, Japan

AND

K. Hatta

I.P.C. Clinic, Tokyo, Japan

Recently, Hirschaut and his co-workers observed that sarcoidosis patients in the U. S.A. exhibited high titers of antibodies against EB virus in their sera.[1] Last year, Wahren and his co-workers also reported moderately elevated titers of antibodies against EB virus, cytomegalovirus and herpes simplex antigens, in the sera from Swedish patients with sarcoidosis.[2] In 1970 and 1971, the Japan Sarcoidosis Committee collected sera from sarcoidosis patients and the examination of them for anti-EB virus antibody has been initiated.

Serum specimens were collected from patients with sarcoidosis at the onset of symptoms. The clinical diagnosis had been given by chest X-ray films, which showed bilateral hilar lymphadenopathy with or without parenchymal infiltration. Involvement of the eyes or skin also coexisted in some cases. Almost all of the cases were biopsied and the results of the examination were compatible with the clinical diagnosis of sarcoidosis. The geographic distribution of tested sera reflected the local incidence of sarcoidosis in Japan. Control sera were collected from age- and sex-matched healthy blood donors. These control persons were diagnosed as normal by clinical examinations, including chest X-ray findings. Serum specimens were stored at $-20°C$ until tested.

For the assay of antibody to EB virus, cell smears were prepared by the method of Henle[3] from suspension cultures of Burkitt's lymphoma cell line P3HR 1,[4] and fixed in cold acetone for 20 minutes. For the titration, cell smears were first exposed to a 4-fold dilution series of test serum and then to a fluorescein isothiocyanate-conjugated rabbit anti-human IgG preparation. Readings were made by Chiyoda fluorescent light microscope, type FM 200 A. The titers of anti-EB virus antibody were given as reciprocals of the highest serum dilution giving unequivocal staining.

The summarized results of the present examination for anti-EB virus antibody titers are shown in Table 1. In the sarcoidosis group, consisting of 29 men and 29 women, the detectable anti-EB virus antibodies for titers of more than 40 were found in 91.4%

Table 1. Anti-EB virus antibody in sarcoidosis patients and in normal persons.

	Number of subjects with indicated EB virus antibody titers					Ridit analysis
	<40	40	160	640	2560	
Sarcoidosis (total 58)	5 (8.6%)	22 (37.9%)	18 (31.0%)	10 (17.2%)	3 (5.2%)	0.799±0.076
Normal (total 50)	27 (54.0%)	17 (34.0%)	4 (8.0%)	2 (4.0%)	0	0.500±0.082

Table 2. Distribution of anti-EB virus antibodies in relation to clinical symptoms of disease.

Clinical symptoms	Number of patients with indicated EB virus antibody titers					Total No.
	<40	40	160	640	2560	
BHL only	2	10	8	5	1	26
BHL+Lung	1	8	6	2		17
BHL+Eyes	2	2	3	1	1	9
BHL+Lung+Eyes		1	1	1	1	4
BHL+Lung+Skin		1		1		2
Total	5	22	18	10	3	58

of the cases and only 5 cases (8.6%) had low titers of less than 40. On the contrary, in a healthy control group, consisting of 25 men and 25 women, the anti-EB virus antibodies of more than 40 were shown in only 46.0% of the specimens. The geometric mean titers were 109 in the sarcoidosis group and 24 in the control group. By Ridit analysis, it was revealed that the antibodies to EB virus were significantly higher in the sarcoidosis group than in the control group. The positive rates for titers of 40 and 160, respectively, were also significantly higher in the sarcoidosis group than in the control group by a χ^2 test, where P is less than 0.001. In both groups, there was very little correlation between the anti-EB virus titers and the age groups. There was also no correlation between the antibody titers and the sex groups.

The anti-EB titers of the patients are given in Table 2 in relation to their clinical findings at the onset. Patients were classified into a few groups according to the following findings: BHL only and BHL plus parenchymal infiltration, with or without involvement of the eyes or skin. Among these groups the differences were not statistically significant both with respect to their levels and the rates of positivity of anti-EB virus antibody.

Next, the correlation between the anti-EB virus titers and tuberculin hypersensitivity of sarcoidosis patiehts was investigated. According to the size of skin reaction caused by 2.5 TU of PPD they were divided into two major groups (Table 3). In this investigation, patients who showed weak tuberculin reactivity, i.e., redness in the reactions was less than 10 mm in diameter, were included in the negative group. The 14 patients who showed skin reactions of 10 mm or more were included in the positive group. The positive rates of anti-EB virus antibodies at the titer of 160 were 61% in the tuberculin-negative group and 29% in the positive group. By the χ^2-test, the difference is statistically significant, and P is less than 0.05.

Blood samples from 13 patients were examined again 6 months later for their anti-EB

TABLE 3. Distribution of anti-EB virus antibodies in relation to tuberculin-reactivity of patients.

Size of tuberculin skin test (mm)	Number of patients with indicated EB virus antibody titers					Total No.
	<40	40	160	640	2560	
(−) 0–5		10	8	5	2	25
6–9	1	4	7	2		14
(+) 10–	3	7	1	2	1	14
Total	4	21	16	9	3	53

TABLE 4. Antibody titers to EB virus in sera from sarcoidosis patients bled 2 times with an interval of 6 months.

Patient No.	Anti-EB virus titers	
	First	Second
1003*	40	<40
1022	40	<40
1024*	640	40
1028	40	<40
1038*	160	40
1066	640	40
1073	160	<40
2002	160	40
2025	40	<40
2029	40	40
2058*	40	40
2062	40	<40
2067	40	<40

virus titers (Table 4). At the time of the second examination their chest X-ray findings cleared except in the 4 cases asterisked in the table, whose findings were unchanged. In 10 cases, 4- to 16-fold titer decreases were found. However, the relation between the titer change and the course of the disease, was rather complicated. For consideration of the anti-EB virus titer change in relation to the course of sarcoidosis, a more precise time-course investigation might be necessary.

In the present study, we found that the antibody to EB virus was frequently at higher titers in sarcoidosis patients than in controls. It seems likely that there is some kind of correlation between EB virus and sarcoidosis. However, some patients had no detectable anti-EB virus antibody, and accordingly the theory of the possible etiologic role of EB virus would seem less convincing. In our results, tuberculin hypersensitivity in sarcoidosis patients appeared to be in inverse proportion to anti-EB virus titer. The evidence might indicate immunological disturbance in the disease.

We are deeply indebted to Prof. S. Kato and Dr. M. Naito, Osaka University for their kind help in this investigation. We also thank Dr. T. Tokunaga and S. Uchida, N.I.H. Tokyo, for their helpful advice.

REFERENCES

1. Hirshaut Y., et al. 1970. *New Engl. J. Med.* **283**: 502.
2. Wahren B., et al. 1971. *J. Nat. Cancer Inst.* **47**: 747.
3. Henle, G., et al 1966. *J. Bact.* **91**: 1248.
4. Hinuma Y., et al. 1967. *J. Virol.* **1**: 1045.

Histocompatibility (HL-A) Antigens in Sarcoidosis

D. Brackertz*

Basel University, Basel, Switzerland

F. Kueppers

Hamburg University, Hamburg, Federal Republic of Germany

B. Schwab, Ch. Mueller-Eckhardt,** and D. Heinrich

Giessen University, Giessen, Federal Repablic of Germany

AND

K. Wurm

Freiburg University, Freiburg, Federal Republic of Germany

During the last couple of years it has become fashionable to do histocompatibility testing in all sorts of diseases. As a result, associations of certain HL-A antigens and particular diseases were found. However, some of these associations have collapsed due to subsequent studies while others have stood the test of time. To that last group belongs the high incidence of HLA-5 and W18 (4c-complex) in Hodgkin's disease.[1-4] Other associations are of HL-Al and A8 in adult coeliac disease[5] and HL-A8 and W15 in systemic lupus erythematosus.[6]

There is good reason to assume from more theoretical considerations that the presence of certain HL-A antigens predisposes to some types of disease involving the immunological apparatus. The argument is, in brief, as follows: by analogy to the H2-system of the mouse we assume that human HL-A antigens play an important part in the immune response. In the mouse it is well-known that the possession of some H2-antigens render certain strains susceptible to some virus infections (for example, Gross and Friend leukemia virus) and resistant to others.[7] The immune response to several synthetic polypeptides is also controlled by a gene that is closely linked to the H2-system.

Although the etiology of sarcoidosis is unknown, there are features in that disease that clearly indicate an immunological disturbance, particularly of the delayed hypersensitivity response. With this in mind, we investigated the HL-A antigens in patients with sarcoidosis and normal controls. We selected a group of 132 patients, 78 men and 54 women. The mean age was 39.8 years with a S.D. of 12.5 and a range of 21 to 72 years. The diagnosis of sarcoid was based on following criteria: 1. clinical aspect and general findings. 2. X-ray findings, 3. characteristic course of the disease, 4. histology of noncaseating epitheloid cell granuloma, 5. lack or diminished reaction of delayed-type hypersensitivity to tuberculin and often positive Kveim reaction, 6. response to steroid therapy. The control group consisted of a large number of about 600 normal blood donors from the Giessen area. This group was not age-matched.

Testing of histocompatibility of HL-A antigens was performed using the lymphocyte

This work was supported in part by Schweiz. Nationalfonds zur Förderung der wissenschaftlichen Forschung, Credit No. 3.479.70* and in part by Deutsche Forschungsgemeinschaft (Mu 277/3)**.

TABLE 1. Comparison of the lymphocyte toxicity method to that
of the platelet micro-complement fixation test.

Antigen	N	PMCF/ML tox				Discordance	
		+/+	−/−	+/−	−/+	<2%	>2%
Locus 1:							
HL–A 1	125	33	92	0	0	0	
HL–A 2	121	60	61	0	0	0	
HL–A 3	127	33	92	0	2	1.57	
HL–A 9	127	23	102	1	1	1.57	
Gi–2 (W 19.5)	131	8	120	0	3*		2.29
Locus 2:							
HL–A 5	129	15	114	0	0	—	
HL–A 7	127	35	91	1	0	0.78	
HL–A 12	129	11	118	1	0	0.77	
HL–A 13	129	2	127	0	0	—	
W 5	130	11	117	2	0	1.53	
W 10	130	10	118	2	0	1.53	
W 14	131	4	126	0	1	0.76	
W 15	128	11	113	0	4		3.12
W 27	131	6	124	1	0	0.76	
SL	131	2	119	4	6		7.93

* Cross-reaction with HL–A 10.

TABLE 2. Number of test sera.

Antigen	ML tox	PMCF	Antigen	ML tox	PMCF
HL–A 1	3	4	HL–A 12	3	3
HL–A 2	4	5	HL–A 13	3	3
HL–A 3	3	3	W 5	3	3
HL–A 9	3	3	W 10	2	2
HL–A 10	2	—	W 14	4	2
HL–A 11	3	2	W 15	2	4
Gi–2 (W 19.5)	2	2	W 27	3	2
			SL	3	4
HL–A 5	3	5	W 18	2	2
HL–A 7	4	5	W 22	—	2
HL–A 8	3	—			

toxicity test described by Terasaki and McClelland[8] and the platelet micro-complement fixation test as agreed by the Third International Congress of the Transplantation
Society.[9] There was good agreement between the 2 tests as shown in Table 1. The
antisera that were used in typing are listed in Table 2.

Our results are summarized in Table 3. I believe that there is no association of any
HL-A type and the disease in question. The possible associations with HL-A1, A10,
A11 and W18 are not significant on the 5% level, especially if one corrects for the fact
that, of 20 tested characters, an association of one and the disease would be unlikely by
chance on the 5% level.

TABLE 3. HL–A types in sarcoidosis and controls.

HL–A antigen	Sarcoidosis	Controls	P
Locus 1 :			
1	39 (29.6%)	140 (23.1%)	<0.2 N. S.
2	70 (53 %)	310 (52 %)	N. S.
3	39 (29.6%)	162 (27.1%)	N. S.
9	29 (22 %)	123 (20.3%)	N. S.
10	3 (2.2%)	44 (7.1%)	<0.1 N. S.
11	5 (3.8%)	53 (8.8%)	<0.1 N. S.
W 19.5	11 (8.2%)	43 (7.1%)	N. S.
Locus 2 :			
5	17 (13 %)	82 (13.5%)	N. S.
7	40 (30.4%)	158 (26.2%)	N. S.
8	28 (21.3%)	99 (16.6%)	N. S.
12	14 (10.5%)	51 (9.4%)	N. S.
13	4 (3 %)	40 (6.5%)	N. S.
W 5	14 (10.5%)	94 (15.5%)	N. S.
W 10	13 (9.9%)	78 (12.8%)	N. S.
W 14	5 (3.8%)	35 (5.7%)	N. S.
W 15	18 (13.7%)	88 (14.4%)	N. S.
W 27	7 (5.3%)	38 (6.3%)	N. S.
SL	12 (9.2%)	70 (11.5%)	N. S.
W 18	4 (3 %)	43 (8.2%)	<0.1 N. S.
W 22	4 (3 %)	22 (3.6%)	N. S.

N. S.=Not significant.

The conclusions that can be drawn from our results are rather limited. Our initial hypothesis was that if we could find an association of certain HL-A antigens and the disease, this would point to an immunological mechanism important in the development of sarcoidosis. Now that such associations can clearly be denied, we can only make the inverse statement with extreme caution. Clearly many immunological mechanisms are conceivable that do not involve the HL-A system and the investigation of such mechanisms in sarcoidosis can hardly be emphasized enough.

SUMMARY

The frequency of HL-A antigens in a group of 132 patients with sarcoidosis was compared to that found in normal individuals from the same population. No significant difference was found.

REFERENCES

1. Amiel, J. L. 1968 Study of the leucocyte phenotypes in Hodgkin's disease. Histocompatibility Testing 1967 (ed. E. S. Curtoni, P. L. Mattiuz, R. M. Tosi). Copenhagen: Ejnar Munksgaard, pp. 79–81.
2. Zervas, J. D., Delamore, J. W., and Israels, M. C. G. 1970 Leucocyte phenotypes in Hodgkin's disease. *Lancet* **2**: 634.

3. Forbes, J. F., and Morris, P. J. 1970 Leucocyte antigens in Hodgkin's disease. *Lancet* **2**: 849.
4. Bertrams, J., Kuwert, E., Böhme, U., Reis, H. E., Gallmeier, W. M., Wetter, O., and Schmidt, C. T. 1972. HL-A-antigens in Hodgkin's disease and multiple myeloma. *Tissue Antigens* **2**: 41–46.
5. Stokes, P. L., Asquith, P., Holmes, G. K. T., Mackintosh, P., and Cooke, W. T. 1972. Histocompatibility antigens associated with adult coeliac disease. *Lancet* **2**: 162.
6. Grumet, F. C., Coukell, A., Bodmer, J. G., Bodmer, W. F., and McDevitt, H. O. 1971. Histocompatibility (HL-A) antigens associated with systemic lupus erythematosus. *New Engl. J. Med.* **285**: 193.
7. Tennant, J. R., and Snell, G. D. 1968. The H-2 locus and viral leukomogenesis as studied in congenic strains of mice. *J. Nat. Cancer Int.* **41**: 597.
8. Teraski, P. I., and McClelland, J. D. 1964. Microdroplet assay of human serum cytotoxins. *Nature* **204**: 998.
9. Colombani, J., D'Amaro, J., Gabb, B., Smith, G., and Svejgaard, A. International agreement on a microtechnique of platelet complement fixation. Transpl. Proc. In press.

Relationship of Cryptococcosis to Sarcoidosis

STEPHEN B. SULAVIK

St. Francis Hospital, Hartford, Connecticut, U.S.A.

AND

RICHARD QUINTILIANI

Hartford Hospital, Hartford, Connecticut, U.S.A.

Six patients with well-documented clinical and histological evidence of thoracic sarcoidosis who developed varied clinical manifestations of cryptococcosis form the basis of this communication. Four of these cases were personally observed by the authors during the past 4-year period. Two further cases were brought to our attention. All patients resided in Connecticut, U.S.A., a state comprising approximately 3 million people where sarcoidosis is relatively common, but where clinical cryptococcal infection is rarely seen. In all patients the cryptococcal organism was demonstrated by staining techniques of the cerebrospinal fluid (CSF.), central nervous system (CNS) tissue, lung tissue, bone or subcutaneous (SC.) abscess. In all patients culture for cryptococcus n. was positive. Cryptococcal infection was diagnosed in all patients either at the time of, but most often months or years after the initial diagnosis of thoracic sarcoidosis.

Though the association of cryptococcal infection in patients with sarcoidosis has previously been reported, it is felt that on the basis of our findings and review of the literature that more emphasis should be given this association.

Our roentgen staging of sarcoidosis is as follows: stage 0—normal chest X-ray, stage I—hilar and/or mediastinal adenopathy without obvious lung parenchymal

TABLE 1. Associated sarcoidosis and cryptococcosis (authors' series).

Patients	Age race sex	Prior DX sarcoid (mos)	Organs of involvement	
			Sarcoidosis	Cryptococcosis
1. IR	31 WM	21	lung II* liver spleen lymph nodes	CNS
2. SB	38 WF	7	lung II lymph nodes	CNS rib
3. BC	31 BF	2	lung II lymph nodes liver skin	s.c. tiss. (groin)
4. CH	25 BM	50	lung II lymph nodes	CNS
5. MA	31 WM	0	lung II lymph nodes	lung nodule (with cavitation)
6. EH	22 BM	9	lung II lymph nodes uveal tract	bone (rt. 7th rib & rt. clavible)

* Roentgen staging.

involvement, stage II—bilateral, usually symmetrical, lung lesions with or without hilar adenopathy. For stage III we have required any of the following indicating fibrosis: fibrocavitary change, honeycombing, reduction in volume of lung areas, retraction of the hilae, fissures or mediastinum. The following X-rays are from our 6 patients. All were classified roentgen stage II.

Table 1. In our series the age ranged between 22–38 years. In only 1 case was the diagnosis of cryptococcosis made simultaneously with the diagnosis of sarcoidosis. The CNS and bone were the most common organs affected by cryptococcus. Table 2. Prior corticosteroid was given in 2 cases. Amphotericin B was effective therapy for cryptococcal meningitis as was 5-fluorocytosine in 1 patient with cryptococcal meningitis. Table 3. In summary, there were 4 males and 2 females. All cases were roentgen stage II. CNS was involved in 3 cases and lytic bone lesions were observed in 2 patients. Both involved ribs. The lung, however, was involved in only 1 patient. Five patients survived their illness. The patient who died had untreated cryptococcal meningitis.

Table 4. To determine the incidence of associated sarcoidosis and cryptococcosis an exhaustive 10-year survey of cryptococcal infection in the state of Connecticut was made. Fourteen cases of cryptococcal infection were found to have occurred in the 10-year period, 1961 through 1971. Four of these cases had associated sarcoidosis repre-

TABLE 2. Authors' series continued.

Patients	Prior corticosteroids	Crypto. treatment	Course
1. IR	0	0	Died c. meningitis
2. SB	Meticorten 7 months prior crypto dx	Amph. B 0.73 gm IV	No recurrence after 14 yrs
3. BC	0	0	No recurrence after 5 yrs
4. CH	Prednisone 15 mg/qd 5 months prior crypto dx	5-Fluorocytosine	No recurrence after 14 months
5. MA	0	Amph. B 1.29 gm IV-nodule resected	No recurrence after 48 months
6. EH	Topical- for iritis	Amph. B 1.5 gm IV	No recurrence after 3 months

TABLE 3. Sarcoidosis associated C̄ cryptococcosis (Authors' series).   (6 cases)

Race & sex	Sarcoid stage	Crypto. involv.		Prior C.S.*	Course
BM 2	All II	CNS	2	2	Died 1
BF 1		Bone	1		(CNS S̄
WM 2		CNS & bone	1		treatment)
WF 1		Lung	1		Surv. 5
		S.C. & tiss.	1		

* Corticosteroid.

TABLE 4. Cryptococcosis associated with Sarcoidosis (incidence).

Cases of cryptococcosis (State of Connecticut) 1961–1971	14
No. of above cases with sarcoidosis	4 (28%)

senting a surprising incidence of 28%. These 4 cases have been described in the authors' series.

Table 5. Other associated diseases in this series of 14 cases included: Hodgkin's disease (2 cases), post-renal transplantation (2 cases), and terminal cancer (1 case). In 5 cases no associated disease was found. Of interest is the development of cryptococcal infection in patients having undergone renal transplantation (1 lung and 1 skin).

Table 6. This shows the incidence of organ involvement in 14 consecutive cases of cryptococcosis.

Table 7. In a review of the English literature, 16 isolated case reports were found of patients having well-described sarcoidosis with associated cryptococcal infection. Fifteen more cases were found in which the diagnosis of sarcoidosis and cryptococcal infection was made but complete description was lacking. Adding our own 6 cases there exists a total of 37 examples of sarcoidosis and cryptococcosis.

TABLE 5. Cryptococcosis, State of Connecticut.

1961–71 (14 cases)

Associated disease	No. of cases	%
Sarcoidosis	4	28.5
Hodgkin's	2	14.0
Post renal transplant	2	14.0
Terminal cancer	1	7.0
No associated disease of cases	5	36.0

TABLE 6. Cryptococcosis, State of Connecticut.

1961–71 (14 cases)

Cryptococcosis organ involv.	No. of cases	%
CNS	6	43
Lung	4	28
Bone	1	7
S.C.	1	7
Skin	1	7
CNS, lung and bone	1	7

TABLE 7. Reported cases of sarcoidosis and cryptococcosis.*

	Cases
Well-documented $\bar{C}$ detailed description	16
Well-documented $\bar{S}$ detailed description	15
Authors' series	6
Total	37

* 3 further cases of cryptococcosis may have had associated sarcoidosis.

Table 8. By combining our 6 cases and the 16 isolated case reports, which were well-described, we have assessed some clinical aspects of the combined diseases. The incidence of CNS involvement is quite common as one would expect. An important corollary, therefore, is that a diagnosis of CNS sarcoidosis must be made with extreme caution and every effort to rule out CNS cryptococcal infection must be made. Bone involvement (lytic bone lesions sparing the cortex) appears to be much more common (36%) in patients with sarcoidosis than in patients who do not have sarcoidosis (10%). Lung involvement by cryptococcus in sarcoidosis patients is unusual, having been found in only 2 of 22 cases in the combined series.

Table 9. Sarcoidosis roentgen stage II was the most common stage found when cryptococcal infection was diagnosed. No cases of clinical cryptococcal infection were found in patients with stage III sarcoidosis; a stage where aspergillus (esp. aspergilloma) is often diagnosed.

Table 10. Survival was most dependent upon whether or not CNS involvement was present; there were no deaths in the non-CNS cases whether treated or not. Four of 4 cases without CNS involvement survived without any form of therapy.

TABLE 8. Incidence of cryptococcal organ involvement in sarcoidosis (Combined series).

Organ	No. of cases	% (22 cases)
CNS	10	45
Bone	8	36
S.C.	4	18
Skin	4	18
Kidney	3	13. 6
Lung	2	9
Prostrate	1	4. 5
Liver	1	4. 5
Adrenal	1	4. 5

TABLE 9. Roentgen stage of thoracic sarcoidosis in 22 cases of associated sarcoidosis and cryptococcosis (Combined series).

Stage	No. of cases
0	1
I	3
II	18
III	0

TABLE 10. Clinical course in 22 patients with sarcoidosis and cryptococcosis (Combined series).

$\bar{C}$ CNS involvement		$\bar{S}$ CNS involvement	
Treated $\bar{C}$ Amph. B	Died 1 Surv. 3	Treated $\bar{C}$ Amph. B	Died 0 Surv. 7
Not Treated $\bar{C}$ Amph. B	Died 5 Surv. 1	Not Treated $\bar{C}$ Amph. B	Died 0 Surv. 4

* 2 patients were treated with 5-fluorocytosine. Both survived. One had CNS involvement.

Table 11.   The male to female incidence was 1:1. The incidence of black versus white revealed an incidence of 2:1 in favor of the black.

Table 12.   Corticosteroid therapy was being used at the time of diagnosis of cryptococcosis in 5 cases (an incidence of 22.7%).

Table 13.   Our cryptococcal serology studies were kindly carried out by Dr L. Kaufman at the C.D.C. in Georgia, U.S.A. The serological tests employed included: the tube agglutination test (TA) which tests for antibody. This test will show a 10–12% false-positive result in dilutions under 1:8 in normal controls; The indirect fluorescent antibody test (IFA). This test will show a false-positive result in 25% of normal controls; The latex agglutination test (LA) which tests the antigen. This test may be falsely positive when carried out on the serum of patients who have a positive rheumatoid factor. However, if the test is carried out on the cerebral spinal fluid a positive test indicates cryptococcal infection even if a positive rheumatoid factor of the serum is present. When carried out on the spinal fluid this test is diagnostic in 95% of cases with CNS involvement.

Table 14.   We have found that there is no increased incidence of positive antibody or antigen titer in the serum of patients with sarcoidosis as opposed to normal controls.

From the immunologic standpoint, based on animal studies, circulating antibody to cryptococcus n. has not been found to protect against infection. Also, specific antibody

TABLE 11.   Race* and sex of 22 cases of sarcoidosis
and cryptococcosis (Combined series).

Black	M	6	White	M	3
Black	F	7	White	F	3
Total		13	Total		6

* Race of 2 males and 1 female not known.

TABLE 12.   Corticosteroid therapy prior to DX of cryptococcosis
(Combined series).

Corticosteroid played a questionable role in the development of cryptococcosis in 5 of 22 patients with combined cryptococcosis and sarcoidosis (22.7%)

TABLE 13.   Percentage of normals $\bar{C}$ false positive serology
for cryptococcosis.

% False positive		
TA<1:8	IFA	LA
10–12%	25%	(Serum) only $\bar{C}$+R.F. (CSF) 0%

TABLE 14.

	Positive				Negative
	IFA	TA	IFA & TA	LA	
Sarcoidosis	0	0	1	0	37
Control	1	3	0	0	35

to cryptococcus is not detected in the majority of patients either with disseminated infections or with isolated pulmonary infections. This makes doubtful any significant role played by cryptococcal antibody as a primary host defense factor. There is increasing experimental evidence to indicate that cellular immunity against cryptococcus plays a very vital and possibly primary role as a host defense factor. Cellular immunity appears to involve interaction between macrophages and lymphocytes, neutrophils, and monocytes in the killing of cryptococcal organisms.

Of interest from the standpoint of cellular immunity and its role as a significant host defense mechanism against cryptococcosis is the increased incidence of cryptococcal infection in patients with Hodgkin's disease. Both Hodgkin's disease and sarcoidosis have impaired cellular immunity of a similar nature. Both diseases, however, appear to have intact circulating antibody formation. It is therefore logical to assume that there might be an increased incidence of cryptococcal infection in both of these diseases. The increased incidence in Hodgkin's disease is well-documented and we feel that this is also true in sarcoidosis.

Other factors which may play an important role in host defense against cryptococcus n. Which have recently been described by Igel are an inhibitory serum factor which, however, is not found in the cerebral spinal fluid and a fungicidal inhibitory substance found in saliva. Since the respiratory tract is the major initial route of infection, the saliva inhibitory factor may indeed play a vital role in the body's initial defense. The integrity of these cellular, saliva and serum factors have as yet not been studied in patients with sarcoidosis.

In summary, the following conclusions may be drawn with respect to the relationship of cryptococcosis and sarcoidosis in the State of Connecticut.

1.   There is a significant association between cryptococcal infection and sarcoidosis.

2.   Cryptococcus n. is the most common fungal infection in sarcoidosis patients other than aspergillus.

3.   Cryptococcal disease should especially be suspected in any sarcoidosis patient presenting with the following:

    A.   C.N.S. signs or symptoms

    B.   Lytic bone lesions (usually sparing the cortex especially if bones other than the hands and feet are involved.)

    C.   Skin or S.C. nodules or abscesses

4.   Defects in cellular immunity found in sarcoidosis may play a significant role in the acquisition of cryptococcal infection.

5.   The role of cellular immunity, saliva and serum inhibitory factors in sarcoidosis and Hodgkin's patients should be evaluated.

Association of Sarcoidosis with Herpes Zoster

R. Mikami

Tokyo University School of Medicine, Tokyo, Japan

AND

O. Hongo

Komagome Hospital, Tokyo, Japan

The association of sarcoidosis and herpes zoster appears not to have been reported previously. Of 82 patients in our sarcoidosis clinic, 4 patients or 4.8% suffered from herpes zoster. These cases will be briefly reviewed.

CASE REPORTS

Case 1: An 18-year-old student. BHL was found on his mass chest X-ray film in July 1961. Thirty mg of predonisolone was administered and in 5 weeks BHL disappeared. Seven weeks after the initiation of steroid therapy, erythematous lesions with vesicles appeared on his left chest along with severe pain. He also had a headache and fever. Diagnosis of herpes zoster was made by a dermatologist. In this case, it required about 14 days for recovery.

Case 2: A 33-year-old housewife. In April 1966, she noticed a blurring of vision. The following month, she noticed a swelling of the bilateral parotid glands which regressed spontaneously in a month. In June, BHL was noted on her chest X-ray film. From 29th November, she was given 30 mg of prednisolone daily. Three weeks after the initiation of steroid therapy, she noticed a severe pain in her left lower abdominal wall and skin rashes characteristic of herpes zoster. She also had fever, a headache and backache. Herpes zoster subsided 3 weeks later.

Case 3: A 32-year-old housewife. Sarcoidosis was first discovered by visual disturbance and subsequently BHL and pulmonary lesions were recognized on her chest X-ray films. She was placed on dexamethasone and prednisolone therapy. Both the BHL and pulmonary lesions regressed in 18 months. However, BHL again appeared in May, 1968. While under observation without steroid therapy, vesiculated skin rashes erupted on her right chest accompanied by intercostal neuralgia-like pain. In this case the patient suffered from herpes zoster not during the steroid therapy but 6 months after the cessation of therapy.

Case 4: A 27-year-old housewife. She visited an ophthalmologist in June 1969, complaining of visual difficulty and a diagnosis of uveitis was given. Rentgenologically, she had only a slightly enlarged right paratracheal lymph node. The Kveim test gave a positive result. Five months later uveitis recurred, and BHL and pulmonary lesions were apparent. She was placed in a placebo group in a corticosteroid therapy study and no steroid was given to her throughout the observation period. In March 1970, vesiculose eruptions appeared on her right chest wall with pain, which disappeared within a week. Chest X-ray findings cleared spontaneously in August 1970.

CLINICAL DATA OF THE 4 CASES

Table 1 summarises the clinical data for the 4 cases described above. All 4 had intra-thoracic lesions and 3 were accompanied by ocular lesions. Two of the 4 cases suffered from herpes zoster during steroid therapy, and 2 others showed the same complication independantly. Herpes zoster presented for 14 days in case 1 and 21 days in case 2, whereas it was only for 7 days in case 3 and 10 days in case 4. Thus, with the patients on steroid therapy, duration of herpes zoster was much longer than with non-steroid

TABLE 1.   Clinical data of cases.

Sex & age	Thoracic invol.		Herpes zoster					
	Intra	Extra	After sarcoid. onset	Steroid therapy	Locliza-tion	Dura-tion	Symptoms	T.R.
1. 18M	$M_2H_3P_0$	—	3 m	+	l. I.C.N. 5–8	14 days	fever headache	+
2. 33 F	$M_1H_2P_0$	ocular parotis	8 m	+	l. L. 1, 2	21 days	fever headache backache	—
3. 32 F	$M_1H_2P_0$	ocular	2 ys 1m	—	l. I.C.N. 6–8	10 days		—
4. 27 F	$M_1H_2P_{n2a}$	ocular	9 m	—	r. I.C.N. 7–9	7 days		—*

* DNCB test (+).

patients, and moreover, the steroid-treated patients had more marked accompanying symptoms, such as severe headache and fever. Tuberculin reaction was negative in 3 out of 4 cases. Other examinations relating to lymphocyte functions were not performed on these subjects.

DISCUSSION

It would seem that the association of sarcoidosis with herpes zoster has never previously been noted in the literature. In 1961, Wright and his co-workers[1] reported on the incidence of association of herpes zoster with neoplastic and other diseases (Table 2). Zoster occurred in 0.22% of patients hospitalized for non-neoplastic disease in the 5-year period, whereas in patients with various types of malignant diseases, the rate of

TABLE 2.   Herpes zoster in diseases and neoplasi (Wright et al.).

	No. of cases	No. cases with herpes zoster	
Total hospital admissions	55,279	147	0.26%
Total non-neoplastic	51,292	113	0.22%
Total neoplasms	3,987	34	0.85%
Total skin and visceral neoplasms	3,449	16	0.46%
Total lymphoma	538	18	3.34%
Hodgkin's disease	107	10	9 %
Sarcoidosis (Mikami et al.)	82	4	4.8 %

occurrence was 0.85% or 4 times that of non-neoplastic disease. The incidence of herpes zoster in skin and visceral neoplasms was 0.46%, whereas in patients with malignant lymphomas, it was 3.34%. In patients with Hodgkin's disease, the incidence was approximately 9%. In patients with sarcoidosis in our clinic, the incidence was approximately 4.8%. Recently, Hirshaut et al.[2] observed that sarcoidosis patients exhibited high titers of antibodies against Epstein-Barr virus (EBV) antigens. And also, Wahren et al.[3] reported that the rates of antibodies to herpes simplex and cytomegaloviruses were significantly higher in sarcoidosis patients than in control groups. These findings may be due to nonspecific factors such as increased reactivity to certain antigens or an increased susceptibility to infections or a higher tendency towards recurrences of latent infections. Therefore, the association of herpes zoster and sarcoidosis is a fact of special interest.

SUMMARY

As far as can be ascertained, the association of sarcoidosis and herpes zoster has not so far been reported. Eighty-two patients with sarcoidosis visited our clinic from January, 1959 to March, 1972. Of these, 4 patients (4.8%) suffered from herpes zoster infection.

Herpes zoster is a viral infection caused by the varicella-zoster virus. It is well-known that herpes zoster is more common in patients with Hodgkin's disease. An immunological defect is claimed to exist in sarcoidosis as in Hodgkin's disease.

REFERENCES

1. Wright, E. T., and Winer L. H. 1961. Herpes zoster and malignancy. *Arch. Dermat.* **84**: 242.
2. Hirshaut Y., Glade P., Viera L. O., et al. 1970. Sarcoidosis, another disease associated with serologic evidence for herpes-like virus infection. *New Engl. J. Med.* **283**: 502.
3. Wahren B., Carlens E., Espmark A. et al. 1971. Antibodies to various herpes viruses in sera from patients with sarcoidosis. *J. Nat. Cancer Inst.* **47**: 747.

Tuberculin Sensitivity in Active and Cured Sarcoidosis in Finland

OLOF SELROOS AND MARKUS NIEMISTÖ

Fourth Department of Medicine, Helsinki University Central Hospital, Helsinki, and Mjölbolsta Hospital, Finland

It is generally known that in active sarcoidosis the skin sensitivity to tuberculin is depressed. It has been indicated by series from a number of countries that about two-thirds of the patients do not react to second strength tuberculin (100–250 TU of purified protein derivate (PPD), or corresponding units of old tuberculin).[3,5,10,15] Swedish series have shown somewhat lower degree of nonreactors; 47% negative[6] and 60% negative[9] to 100 TU. However, the pattern of tuberculin sensitivity in Finnish sarcoidosis patients displays a marked difference.[1,11] At the sarcoidosis conference in Paris in 1966, Siltzbach drew attention to the atypical sensitivity of the Finnish series, which exhibited the highest frequency of positivity to all strengths of tuberculin on comparison with series from some other countries.[12]

As a consequence of large-scale BCG vaccination (almost total at birth, and with revaccination at school if tuberculin negativity is found), and the still frequent occurrence of pulmonary tuberculosis (annual incidence of new cases in 1970, 86 per 100,000 of population) the Finnish people are tuberculin-positive to a high degree (Fig. 1). Below the age of 60, only about 10% of the population does not react to intermediate strength PPD (10 TU). The figure also indicates that sarcoidosis patients, considered as a group, have a depressed tuberculin sensitivity as compared with healthy controls of the same

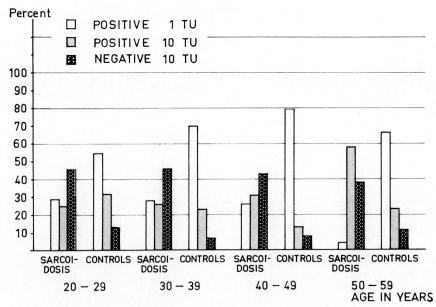

FIG. 1. Percentage distribution of tuberculin sensitivity in different age groups in sarcoidosis and in a control series.

age distribution. However, several patients display quite unchanged sensitivity, and a positivity to 0.1 TU does not exclude sarcoidosis.[1]

It has been clearly demonstrated that tuberculin negativity does not necessarily precede sarcoidosis. In the clinical vaccine trial of the British Medical Research Council (54,239 participants) 52 cases of sarcoidosis developed. Before the onset of the disease, nothing unusual was remarked about the patients' tuberculin sensitivity, but when sarcoidosis was diagnosed, a noticeable swing in sensitivity towards more negative reactions was observable.[14] Moreover, a Japanese study has shown that the sensitivity of patients prior to disease is the same as that of the healthy population.[2]

Some observations have indicated that persons who react to tuberculin before falling ill with sarcoidosis are less sensitive during the course of the disease, but react positively again on recovery.[2,7,8,13] If the disease is in progress for several years without recovery, as a rule the depressed tuberculin sensitivity remains on a depressed level, or even diminishes.[10,15] However, in 60 patients who recovered from sarcoidosis, the tuberculin anergy was persistent after the disappearance of all symptoms and signs of the disease, and 11 patients who recovered developed only weak and transient tuberculin positivity after BCG vaccination,[3] as had been shown in 1937 by Lemming.[4] These observations led to expression of the opinion that the inability to develop and maintain delayed hypersensitivity is a "constitutional defect that is prerequisite to the development of sarcoidosis."[3]

The following study was made with a view to investigation of the tuberculin sensitivity of active and cured sarcoidosis patients, derived from the generally tuberculin-positive Finnish population.

MATERIAL AND METHODS

During the years 1960–66, 115 sarcoidosis patients (stage I and II with and without erythema nodosum) were diagnosed. All the patients displayed a typical clinical picture, along with a positive biopsy specimen and/or positive Kveim test. In all, 82 patients had a known positive tuberculin reaction before the onset of sarcoidosis. The remaining 33 patients could not remember any previous testing, but 18 of them had a BCG vaccination scar. During the first hospitalization, tuberculin skin tests were made up to 10 TU of PPD (PPD-RT 23, Statens Seruminstitut, Copenhagen). In some cases, 100 TU was used. In 1971, the patients took part in a follow-up examination, including tuberculin testing. It was found that 108 patients had recovered; in 7 cases, the disease was still in progress.

RESULTS

Figure 2 indicates the tuberculin sensitivity of the patients who recovered. Of those with erythema nodosum in the active stage, 34% were positive to 0.1–1 TU, and only 18.7% were not positive to 10 TU. When the same patients had recovered, 75% were positive to 1 TU. Those without erythema nodosum displayed a higher degree of depressed tuberculin sensitivity, but in this group also, only one-third (31.6%) of the patients did not react to 10 TU in the cured stage. Table 1 summarizes the tuberculin state of the recovered patients. In the erythema nodosum group, 63% of the patients were more sensitive in the cured stage, compared with 37% in the group of those without

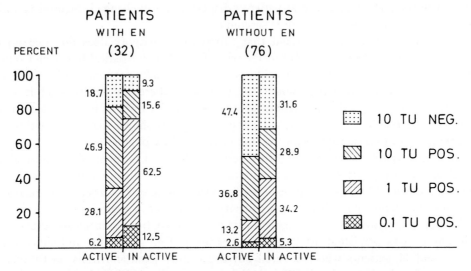

Fig. 2. Percentage distribution of tuberculin sensitivity in sarcoidosis patients with and without erythema nodosum in active and inactive stage of the disease.

Table 1. Tuberculin sensitivity of sarcoidosis patients who had recovered from the disease, compared with the sensitivity in the active stage of the disease.

Patient group	Pulmonary stage	No. of patients	Tuberculin state in cured stage, compared with the sensitivity in active stage	
			Unchanged	More sensitive
Cases with EN	Stage I	26	10	16
	Stage II	6	2	4
	Total	32	12	20 (63%)
Cases without EN	Stage I	36	20	16
	Stage II	40	28	12
	Total	76	48	28 (37%)

erythema nodosum. In no case was the tuberculin sensitivity more depressed in the cured than in the active stage. No patient had developed tuberculosis.

The 7 patients with the disease still active at the time of reexamination had not suffered from erythema nodosum. Five of them had a known tuberculin positivity before the onset of sarcoidosis. Five patients exhibited an unchanged sensitivity (2 negative to 100 TU, 2 positive to 100 TU, and 1 positive to 1 TU), 1 patient was more sensitive (10 TU positivity changed to 1 TU positivity), and 1 displayed more depressed sensitivity (10 TU positivity had changed to 100 TU positivity).

DISCUSSION

The results indicate that if the lymphocytes are sensitized to tuberculin prior to sarcoidosis (BCG vaccination, or contact with tuberculosis), the tuberculin sensitivity is depressed only moderately during the active phase of the disease. In combination with erythema nodosum, the sensitivity may often even remain unchanged. In the cured stage, in most cases the sensitivity returns to normal. In these cases, which are common in Finland, no evidence exists that an immunological defect precedes the development of sarcoidosis. It seems more probable that the depressed delayed-type hypersensitivity is induced by the disease. Even total anergy in the active stage of sarcoidosis is of little diagnostic importance if the tuberculin sensitivity prior to sarcoidosis is unknown. Serial testing of the healthy population at regular intervals would yield important information in all diseases in which tuberculin testing is applied.

In the few cases with long-standing disease, the tuberculin sensitivity was found to be more depressed; moreover, it remained on this depressed level. These few cases do not provide an adequate basis for determination of whether the immunological defect precedes the disease, or is caused by it. However, the latter alternative seems more probable, since 5 of the 7 patients had a known tuberculin positivity prior to sarcoidosis.

CONCLUSIONS

1. As a rule, sarcoidosis patients react to first or intermediate strengths of tuberculin, if they are derived from a generally tuberculin positive population.

2. Sarcoidosis patients who react to tuberculin prior to the disease reveal only moderately depressed or even unchanged tuberculin sensitivity during the active phase of the disease. If they recover, the tuberculin sensitivity often returns to normal. In long-standing disease, the depressed sensitivity usually remains on a depressed level.

3. The result of tuberculin testing is of minor diagnostic importance if the tuberculin sensitivity before the development of sarcoidosis is unknown; this particularly applies to countries with a low degree of normally occurring tuberculin positivity.

4. The behaviour of tuberculin sensitivity in patients positive to tuberculin prior to sarcoidosis, and who completely recover from the disease, does not support the view that an immunological defect precedes the disease. The results obtained seem to indicate that the depression of the skin sensitivity to tuberculin is caused by the disease.

REFERENCES

1. Hannuksela, M., and Salo, O. P. 1969. The significance of the quantitative Mantoux test in sarcoidosis. *Scand. J. Resp. Dis.* **50**: 259.

2. Hosoda, Y., Odaka, M., Hiraga, Y., Chiba, Y. and Oka, H. 1969. Tuberculin sensitivity prior to the onset of sarcoidosis. *Fifth Int. Conf. on Sarcoidosis*, Prague: Univ. Karlova. p. 156.

3. Israel, H. L., and Sones, M. 1965. Immunologic defect in patients recovered from sarcoidosis. *New Engl. J. Med.* **273**: 1003.

4. Lemming, R. 1937. Om den positiva anergien vid febris uveoparotidea och lymfogranulomatosis benigna (Schaumann). *Nord. Med. Tidskr.* **14**: 1822.

5. Longcope, W. T., and Freiman, D. G. 1952. A study of sarcoidosis. Based on a combined investigation of 160 cases including 30 autopsies from the Johns Hopkins Hospital and Massachusetts General Hospital. *Medicine* (Baltimore) **31**: 1.

6. Löfgren, S., and Lundbäck, H. 1952. The bilateral hilar lymphoma syndrome. A study of the relation to tuberculosis and sarcoidosis in 212 cases. *Acta Med. Scand.* **142**: 265.

7. Löfgren, S. 1954. Morbus Besnier-Boeck-Schaumann (sarcoidosis). *Nord. Med.* **52**: 976.

8. Nitter, L. 1953. Changes in the chest roentgenogram in Boeck's sarcoid of the lung. A

study of the course of the disease in 90 cases. *Acta Radiol.* (Stockh.) Suppl. 105.

9. Rudberg-Roos, I. 1962. The course and prognosis of sarcoidosis as observed in 296 cases. *Acta Tuberc. Pneum. Scand.* Suppl. 52.
10. Scadding, J. G. 1967 Sarcoidosis. London: Eyre & Spottiswoode.
11. Selroos, O. 1969. The frequency, clinical picture and prognosis of pulmonary sarcoidosis in Finland. *Acta Med. Scand.* Suppl. 503.
12. Siltzbach, L. E. 1967. An international Kveim test study 1960–1966. *La Sarcoïdose.* Paris: Masson et cie. p. 201.
13. Sommer, E. 1964. Primary and secondary anergy in sarcoidosis. *Acta Med. Scand.* Suppl. **425**: 195.
14. Sutherland, I., Mitchell, D. N., and D'Arcy Hart, P. 1965. Incidence of intrathoracic sarcoidosis among young adults participating in a trial of tuberculosis vaccines. *Brit. Med. J.* **2**: 497.
15. Wurm, K. 1963. Untersuchungen über das Tuberkulinverhalten bei Sarkoidose. *Beitr. Klin. Tuberk.* **127**: 195.

Impaired Lymphocytes in Patients Recovered from Sarcoidosis—Tuberculin sensitivity, lymphocyte count and PHA-induced lymphoblastic transformation—

H. Osada[1], Y. Hosoda[2], M. Odaka[2], M. Matsumoto[3], M. Takahashi[1], M. Yanaka[1] and Y. Chiba[1]

In the past International Conferences held in Stockholm, Paris and Prague, we disclosed the following 3 points based on the serial tuberculin testing records of the patients with sarcoidosis: 1. Sarcoidosis occurred regardless of the degree of prior tuberculin sensitivity. This suggests that immunological deficiency might not be a cause of the disease. 2. At the onset of the disease, prior weak reactors were more frequently converted to a negative reaction than were the prior strong reactors. This indicates that the degree of impairment in tuberculin sensitivity depended on the degree of tuberculin sensitivity prior to the disease. 3. After clinical recovery, the negatively converted cases among the prior strong reactors frequently reverted to positive, while those among the prior weak reactors frequently remained negative.

To advance our study further, the present investigation focused on what changes might be found in the lymphocyte count in peripheral blood and the PHA-induced lymphoblastic transformation in relation to tuberculin sensitivity. The subjects comprised 27 cases; 22 males and 5 females. The duration since the onset of the disease was 2 to 5 years in 14 cases, 5 to 10 years in 6 cases, and more than 10 years in 7 cases. Of these cases, 23 showed a clearing in the chest X-ray findings, leaving no other involvement.

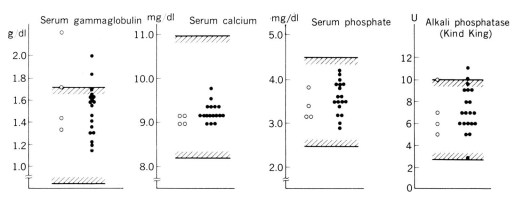

○ : Persistent involvement cases
● : Recovered cases

Fig. 1. Biochemical laboratory examination.

1) *Japanese National Railways Central Hospital, Tokyo, Japan*
2) *Japanese National Railways Central Health Institute, Tokyo, Japan*
3) *Tochigi National Sanatorium, Kawachi, Tochigi, Japan*

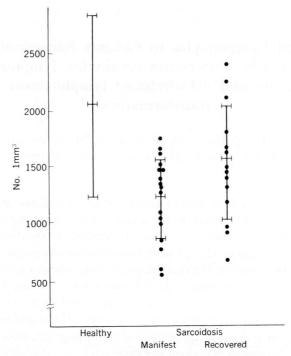

FIG. 2. Lymphocyte count in peripheral blood.

Before discussion of the lymphocyte count or tuberculin sensitivity, it would be useful to show the results of serum examinations of gammaglobulin, calcium, phosphate and alkali phosphatase as indicated in Fig. 1. Hardly any difference was found between the values during the disease and after recovery.

The lymphocyte count in peripheral blood was 1230 ± 357 in 17 patients with chest X-ray findings and 1535 ± 511 in 14 patients with cleared chest X-ray findings. The count in 211 healthy persons was 2831 ± 767. The recovered cases still showed lower rates than did healthy persons (Fig. 2). The PHA-induced lymphoblastic transformation rates were $26.4\pm11.6\%$ in 16 patients with chest X-ray findings, $47.0\pm11.9\%$ in 16 patients with cleared X-ray findings, and $62.2\pm10.1\%$ in healthy persons. Tuberculous patients showed $53.6\pm7.0\%$ in the same test. The rates in patients recovered from sarcoidosis still remained low, the difference being statistically significant between the healthy and sarcoidosis patients (Fig. 3).

As a whole, tuberculin sensitivity was not restored in 5 of the 16 cases with the previous serial records of tuberculin test (31.3%). Lymphopenia was recognized in 3 of them (18.8%) and the PHA-induced lymphoblastic transformation rates were abnormally low in 11 of them (68.8%). It can be said that the PHA-induced lymphoblastic transformation is a test the results of which are difficult to restore to a normal range in sarcoidosis. It is also note worthy that there was no definite correlation among the results of the 3 tests and that all but 3 cases had abnormally low values either in lymphocyte count or blastic transformation rates even in cases with subsequently restored tuberculin sensitivity and with cleared X-ray findings. In conclusion, 13 of 16 cases (81.3%) of the patients still showed signs of immunological deficiency when measured by these 3 methods (Table 1).

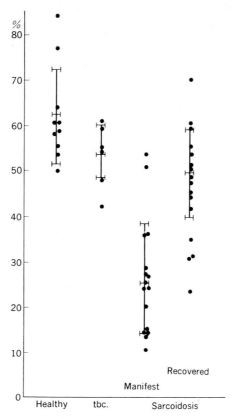

Fig. 3.   PHA-induced lymphoblastic transformation test.

Table 1.   Tuberculin sensitivity in cases recovered from sarcoidosis in relation to peripheral blood lymphocyte count and PHA-induced lymphoblastic transformation.

Before onset		After clearing			
Tuberculin sensitivity		Tuberculin sensitivity		Lymphopenia	Low lymphoblastic transformation
Strong	2	Positive	2	0/2	1/2
		Negative	0	0	0
Medium	10	Positive	8	1/8	6/8
		Negative	2	2/2	0/2
Weak	4	Positive	1	0/1	1/1
		Negative	3	0/3	3/3
Total	16	Positive	11	1/11	8/11
		Negative	5	2/5	3/5

REFERENCES

1. Hosoda, Y. 1964. *Acta Med Scand Suppl.* **425**: 202.
2. Hosoda, Y., Oka, H., Kitamura, K., and Chiba, Y. 1964. La Sarcoidose, *Rapp. IVᵉ Conf. Int.* Paris: Masson et cie. p. 308.

3. Hosoda, Y., Odaka, Y., Hiraga, Y., Chiba, Y., and Oka, H. *Proc. Fifth Int. Conf. on Sarcoidosis.* Prague: Univ. Karlova. p. 156.

Granulomatous Hypersensitivity in Sarcoidosis

Osamu Hongo

Komagome Hospital, Tokyo, Japan

Sarcoidosis may be one of the diseases associated with granulomatous hypersensitivity. Shelley and Hurley[1] reported that a trace amount of zirconium ions provoked epithelioid granulomas through a kind of allergic reaction. An intradermal injection of only $0.02\,\gamma$ of sodium zirconium lactate produced epithelioid granulomas. On the other hand a colloidal silica granuloma does not have an allergic origin, but is produced by 0.5 mg of colloidal silica, a quite considerable amount of particulate material.

Granulomatous hypersensitivity is the term designated by Epstein[2] to express the allergic reaction that causes epithelioid granulomas. Epithelioid granulomas at Kveim-tested sites might be produced by granulomatous hypersensitivity.

Zieler[3] reported epithelioid granulomas at tuberculin-tested sites using old tuberculin in tuberculous patients. Hurley and Shelley[4] reported epithelioid granulomas at tuberculin-tested sites using PPD in 5 cases out of 50 cases of normal subjects.

There are several reports concerning epithelioid granulomas in patients with sarcoidosis at the sites where BCG, killed tubercle bacilli and old tuberculin were intracutaneously injected[5-8], but it seems that there has been no report concerning epithelioid granulomas at test sites using PPD.

I have found epithelioid granulomas at intracutaneous test sites using 0.1 ml of PPD $(0.05\,\gamma)$ in 3 cases of sarcoidosis and 1 suspected case of Mikulicz's disease (Table 1). In these cases small papules (about 3 mm in diameter) developed at the tuberculin test sites about 2 weeks after the intracutaneous injections of PPD. In the first case of sarcoidosis the tuberculin sensitivity was reversed to negative at the onset of the disease, but a DNCB sensitization test using 0.02 ml of a 1% acetone solution of 2, 4-dinitro-1-chlorobenzene (an occlusive dressing technique for 24 hours) was positive. In the second case of sarcoidosis both the tuberculin test and Kveim test were positive, but a DNCB

TABLE 1.

Case No.	Sex	Age	Diagnosis (Group)	Tuberculin reaction		Kveim test antigen No.	DNCB sensitization
				48 hrs	Granuloma (days)		
1.	M	24	Sarcoidosis (III)	$\dfrac{0\times0}{0\times0}$	+ (60)	− 22	⧺*
2.	M	22	Sarcoidosis (II)	$\dfrac{0\times0}{17\times20}$	⧺ (33)	+ 23	±
3.	M	54	Sarcoidosis (IV)	$\dfrac{0\times0}{6\times6}$	+ (26)	− 23	
4.	F	29	Mikulicz's disease? (Sjögren's syndrome?)	$\dfrac{3\times3}{3\times3}$	+ (37)	− 21	

* Spontaneous flare-up was seen, but patch test was not performed.

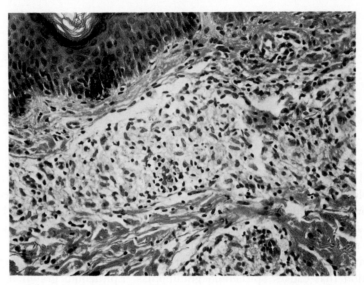

Fig. 1. Epithelioid granuloma at the tuberculin test site using PPD in the second case of sarcoidosis.

sensitization test was equivocal. In the third case of sarcoidosis, Mantoux reaction was equivocal and a Kveim test negative, but a DNCB sensitization test was not performed.

Figure 1 shows an epithelioid granuloma at the tuberculin-tested site using PPD in the second case of sarcoidosis. These epithelioid granulomas at the tuberculin-tested sites using PPD may not be caused by contamination of the test material or by secondary tissue destruction, but may well be due to granulomatous hypersensitivity to PPD.

Considering these data, no correlation between the development of these epithelioid granulomas and tuberculin sensitivity and the results of the DNCB sensitization test was observed.

REFERENCES

1. Shelley, W. B., and Hurley, H. J. 1958. The Allergic Origin of Zirconium Deodorant Granulomas, *Brit. J. Dermat.* **70**: 75.
2. Epstein, W. L. 1967. Granulomatous Hypersensitivity, *Prog. Allergy* **11**: 36. Basle/New York: Karger.
3. Zieler, K. 1926. Zur Spezifität der Tuberkulinreaktion mit besonderer Berücksichtigung ihrer histologischen Grundlage, *Beitr. Klin. Tuberk.* **64**: 94.
4. Hurley, H. J., and Shelley, W. B. 1960. Sarcoid Granulomas after Intradermal Tuberculin in Normal Human Skin, *Arch. Derm.* **82**: 65.
5. Lemming, R. 1942. Development of Boeck' Sarcoid at the Place on the Skin Where BCG Vaccination Had Been Made in a Case of Schaumann's Disease, *Acta Med. Scand.* **110**: 151.
6. Warfvinge, L. E. 1943. Boeck's Sarcoid Experimentally Produced by Virulent Human Tubercle Bacilli in a Case of Schaumann's Disease, *Acta Med. Scand.* **114**: 259.
7. Bjørnstad, R. 1948. Intracutaneous Tests with Killed Tubercle Bacilli in Patients with Boeck's Sarcoid. *Acta Dermat. Venereol.* **28**: 174.
8. Billings, F. T. and Shapiro, J. L. 1954. The Induction of Sarcoid-like Lesions by the Injection of Tuberculin, *Bull. Johns Hopkins. Hosp.* **94**: 139.

DISCUSSION

1

Chairmen: D. G. JAMES AND Y. NIITU

DR JONES WILLIAMS: If we can confirm our preliminary findings with the beryllium MIF (BeMif) test, it could be a useful tool to screen exposed workers and detect sensitisation in vitro. I would not advocate the beryllium skin patch test as a screening method because obviously this would sensitise the worker and preclude further employment.

DR MITCHELL: I merely wanted to seek a point of further clarification to the question Dr James raised about Professor Villar's paper, simply to ask, "Were these hypercalcemias transient or persistent?" The other interesting point you raised is a problem regarding the delayed cell-mediated sensitivity defect. Is this defect limited to tuberculin or is it the usual wide-spectrum defect of delayed cell-mediated sensitivity? Are the tuberculin sensitivity results based upon tests with 10 TU or were tests with 100 TU included?

DR VILLAR: Both in our cases of sarcoidosis and in 23% of the nonsarcoid granulomatoses, serum calcium was elevated and these elevations were presistent.

All the tuberculin tests were done intradermally and with 10 IU PPD. As we had decided that they would be positive anyhow, we were not going to do them, so the finding of 70% negative tests came as a great suprise. In these same age groups tuberculin tests done in these conditions are positive in 70 to 80% of the general population.

DR SOMCHAI: I would like to make a few comments on Professor Israel's paper in connection with Dr James' remarks. I fully accept Professor Israel's hepatic sarcoidosis, and have no objection to the negative Kveim test in that connection. I would rather name the cases "Kveim-negative sarcoidosis", in analogy to "tuberculin-negative tuberculosis" which we use for tuberculosis with negative tuberculin test. I positively do not agree with Dr James' criterion of positive Kveim test in the diagnosis of sarcoidosis. I am sure that many who have had enough experience with the Kveim test must have encountered typical cases of sarcoidosis with negative outcome from time to time.

As regards the relationship between sarcoidosis and Hodgkin's disease, I once came across a 30-year-old housewife who had suffered from cervical lymphadenopathy for over 6 years. In the early part of her illness some nodes broke and discharged a watery pus; at that time the tuberculin test with 1 TU dilution gave unequivocal reaction, and the chest radiographs showed only a calcified primary complex in the right middle lung field. The patient received full first-line antituberculosis regimen. A few years later more masses developed in the neck; this time tuberculin tests were repeatedly negative even at 1000 unit strength, and the chest radiograph showed bilateral hilar lymphadenopathy; a cervical lymph node specimen showed chronic granulomata consistent with sarcoidosis. The patient improved dramatically on corticosteroid therapy, but succumbed about 2 years later from Hodgkin's disease.

DR KALDEN: Firstly, I do think that one cannot speak generally of a depressed cellular immune reactivity in sarcoidosis. There are quite a few papers in the literature which question depressed delayed-type hypersensitivity including depressed tuberculin skin and in vitro reactions. These findings correspond with results presented by Dr

Horsmanheimo to this conference.

To clear the situation of delayed-type hypersensitivity in sarcoidosis I would like to see a study using a number of different in vivo and in vitro tests for delayed hypersensitivity similar to a study in Hodgkin's patients recently published by Dr Young et al. (Amer. J. Internal Med. 1972. 52: 63) Young et al demonstrated that the frequently described cutaneous anergy in Hodgkin's disease was quite uncommon in 103 patients tested with a variety of antigens. Secondly, regarding the antibody titer to EB virus in sarcoidosis, we found only a significant difference in the titers (higher in sarcoidosis patients) but not in the overall incidence of EB virus antibodies.

Lastly, regarding the discussed immune pathogenesis and especially the role of possible antibody antigen complexes, we checked bone marrow biopsies from sarcoidosis patients for the presence of capillaritis (vasculitis). In systemic lupus erythematodes—an immune complex disease—it has been shown that complex-induced capillaritis is always present in the bone marrow and the degree of the vasculitis corresponds well with the clinical stage of the disease. In sarcoidosis we so far did not find evidence for capillaritis and so I don't think that immune complexes play a major role in the pathogenesis of sarcoidosis. A last word regarding the in vitro stimulation experiments with PHA and pokeweed mitogen on lymphocytes from sarcoidosis patients, no difference was found between sarcoidosis patients in comparison to nornal and clinical controls and in respect to different stimulation of T cells (PHA) and B cells (pokeweed mitogen).

DR. HANNGREN: What is a monocyte? Maybe the monocyte is some sort of precursor to the developed B-cell? Maybe the defect B-cells are defect monocytes?

DR JONES WILLIAMS: I would like to support Professor Hanngren's remarks and will say more later in a comparison of the fine structure of circulating and granuloma lymphocytes. A monocyte with contained debris and lysosomes is a macrophage. A monocyte without the contained debris is very difficult to distinguish from what I call an activated lymphocyte. I am tired of hearing that 'epithelioid cells come from monocytes'. They develop from mononuclear cells and in our paper we will suggest that these may be modified lymphocytes.

DR MITCHELL: Dr John Mikhail, Dr David McSwiggan, Professor Margaret Turner-Warwick and I have been looking at the question of individual immunoglobulin values and EB virus titres in a series of more than 50 patients. They are all compared with controls matched for age, race and sex. A second serum sample has been examined 9–18 months later and the results compared. It would appear that there is some elevation of HLV titre amongst patients with sarcoidosis in general; we are currently relating the findings with the form and the known duration of sarcoidosis. The point about chronicity has been made earlier by Dr Louis Siltzbach's group, and a more marked elevation of HLV titres among patients with longstanding sarcoidosis was a feature of their study. It may be that the ethnic group of the patients examined is a factor relating to this finding. With regard to the individual immunoglobulins, thus far there is just a suggestion that persistence in elevation of IgM might be related in some way to the progression of sarcoidosis.

DR JAMES: Your first point was on EB virus, was it? All groups, ours, Stiltzbach's and Löfgren's groups, we all agreed that there is no difference between subacute and chronic sarcoidosis, which is very interesting of course.

DR MITCHELL: I understood that in the initial studies, the most marked elevations were noted in patients with chronic rather than subacute sarcoidosis.

2

Chairmen: H. L. ISRAEL AND T. TACHIBANA

DR ISRAEL: The reports presented at this session have often been contradictory, and appear to have little clinical application; yet I think the papers are of great importance! The central question is whether these rather inconstant alterations in the serum immunoglobulins and the rather constant elevations of EB virus and certain other viral antibody titers are of fundamental importance as Dr Hanngren earlier in this conference and Caspary and Field in England have suggested. Does increased circulating antibody production exert an influence on the impairment of delayed hypersensitivity with which we have been so long concerned in sarcoidosis? I hope the speakers will give us their impressions regarding the significance of the circulating antibody elevations in sarcoidosis.

DR YOUNG: I was rather interested in hearing Dr Wurm's comments on how collagen petidase decreases with inactive sarcoidosis and I recall a study we had done with Massaro on the excretion of 24-hour urinary hydroxyproline as an index of activity in sarcoidosis.

As you know, hydroxyproline is one of the major constituents of collagen. As the enzyme that splits it decreases, you'd expect to find the urinary hydroxyproline decreasing as well.

DR ISRAEL: May I ask Professor Hanngren to comment on his evaluation of the group of papers on the viral antibodies. Do you attach great importance to these?

DR HANNGREN: All titers maybe unspecifically increased when B-cells are stimulated by a mitogen. If you remember discussions 12 years ago concerning tuberculosis, high titers of different kinds were reported. We thought it was secondary infections. Now we find high titers of different kinds of viruses in sarcoidosis patients.

Maybe this is some sort of a Freund's effect in vivo? If we have a B-cell mitogenic effect we may have an increase of titers. I think we have to be a bit cautious when saying it depends on solely an EB virus infection.

DR HORSMANHEIMO: Drs Virolainen and Nikoskelainen and myself have studied the anti-EBV titers and the establishment of blast lines in sarcoidosis. We found that blast lines could be established significantly more often from patients with chronic sarcoidosis, and from patients who were negative in the Mantoux test with 100 TU, as compared to other patients with sarcoidosis. However, the correlation of these clinical findings to anti-EBV titers was not significant.

DR BYRNE: There is one consideration that has not been mentioned at least in publication by anybody reporting on EB virus. That is a possible relationship to Kveim testing. Theoretically administration of Kveim antigen prepared from lymphoid material offers an opportunity for concurrent administration of EB viral antigen which could provoke an elevation of EB antibody titer. We have attemped to look for that effect in our patients.

The best test of whether or not Kveim testing contributes to elevated EB titers, of course, would be examination of serial specimens collected before and after testing. Unfortunately our study did not incorporate this design. What we did do was to select patients who had been Kveim tested at least 1 month before we obtained a blood specimen, and we compared them with other patients, matched by age, sex and race, who had never been Kveim tested. There is no obvious difference.

DR BRACKERTZ: So far as I know, the surface antigens are not influenced by the degree of the disease, or by treatment with steroids or other medicaments.

DR ISRAEL: Is it possible that histocompatibility might be demonstrated in patients with sarcoidosis in different stages of the disease? Could you see differences between patients who were Kveim-positive and Kveim-negative?

DR BRACKERTZ: We have not done those studies.

DR TACHIBANA: Many papers have been presented about antibody to viral capsid antigen of EB virus. My co-worker, Dr Naito will discuss antibody to early antigen of EB virus in sera from sarcoidosis, normal subjects and others.

DR NAITO: Our paper is concerned with the study of antibodies to EB virus in sera from patients with sarcoidosis by the indirect immunofluorescence technique. P3HR-1 cells from Burkitt lymphoma were used for EB virus antigen preparation, containing 20–30% stainable cells. Sera of patients with nasopharyngeal carcinoma who had high titers of antibodies to EB virus antigen were used for reference. Specimens were examined under ultraviolet illumination with a Tiyoda immunofluorescence microscope, type FM 200 A.

The positive rate of anti-EB virus titers of sera of 143 samples from 70 patients with sarcoidosis and 108 sera from control groups were examined. All these sera were supplied by Dr Tachibana, Osaka Prefectural Hospital.

As a positive control, the positive rate of anti-EB virus titers of 23 sera from nasopharyngeal carcinoma patients in the Osaka area were also shown. Dissociation between the frequency distributions of control and sarcoidosis were found to become maximum when the boundary of positive reaction is set at a titer of $1:640\leq$. The percentage of cases with anti-EB virus titers higher than $1:640$ was 60.1% of sarcoidosis patients, and the positive rate of the control group was 21.3%. Sarcoidosis and control were subdivided in each groups (sarcoidosis: before treatment, under treatment and clear in X-ray changes. Control: tuberculosis, other diseases and normal subjects.). There is no significant correlation between the titers and groups of disease, although a group of sarcoidosis patients who became clear in X-ray changes, showed a somewhat lower positive rate in anti-EB virus activities than other groups. The data were analyzed statistically employing the Ridit method, taking the anti-EB virus titers among the control group as the identified distribution.

The sera of sarcoidosis patients exhibited a higher average as compared with those of control. Sera from 54 patients with sarcoidosis and 12 healthy persons were examined for antibody to early antigen induced by EB virus. NC-37 cell line inoculated with EB virus was used as early antigen material. Twelve sera among sarcoidosis patients showed positive. However, they showed rather low antibody titers.

3

Chairmen: J. TURIAF AND O. SELROOS

DR ISRAEL: I think Dr Sulavik's reports of very great interest. We have found 4 cases of cryptococcosis in our patients with sarcoidosis, which is not as high a percentage as he found in Connecticut but still high enough to indicate that it is not a chance association. We have long searched for some clinical consequences of the defect in delayed hypersensitivity in sarcoidosis and I think that the increased frequency of cryptococcosis is a manifestation of that.

May I comment also on Dr Selroos' paper, which is of very great interest? Dr Siltzbach recently reported his observations on recovered sarcoidosis in New York and they correspond much more closely with our own, suggesting that exogenous infection must be important in maintaining tuberculin sensitivity in Finland because both in New York as in Philadelphia most patients recovered from sarcoidosis do not regain tuberculin sensitivity. I would agree that all of the evidence that has accumulated since we proposed the hypothesis that anergy antedates the sarcoidosis has failed to support that suggestion; the evidence indicates that the defect is a result of sarcoidosis. It is a most remarkable thing that mild and transient cases of sarcoidosis result in permanent impairment of delayed hypersensitivity. My final comment is that your paper convinces me that the development of sarcoidosis is unrelated to the frequency of tuberculosis in a country. If it were related to mycobacterial infection, you should have 10 times as much sarcoidosis as they do in Denmark, where tuberculous infection is so infrequent. The difference in incidence of sarcoidosis between Northern Europe and Southern Europe must be attributed not to the influence of mycobacterial infection but to genetic factors.

Dr James: Dr Hongo should contine to study the response to intracutaneous inoculation of various antigens and note whether they provoke the torpid production of sarcoid granulomas in the course of one month or so, for we would all welcome the discovery of a synthetic equivalent to the present Kveim-Siltzbach suspensions. The granuloma-producing principle seems to lie in the lipopolysaccharide fraction of various bacterial suspensions. I have been unable to produce granulomas if the lipid element is removed and only the water-soluble polysaccharide fraction is used. I have produced intracutaneous sarcoid granulomas with Choucroun tuberculin lipoplysaccharide and with pollen, which contains lipopolysaccharide. I have been unable to do so with antigiens prepared from Salmonella typhisuis or Pasteurella pestis, nor from sarcoid tissue prepared from a cholazion. Unfortunately these granulomas are not specific for sarcoidosis and may be provoked in healthy control subjects.

Dr Sulavik: The highest incidence of cryptococcosis associated with sarcoidosis was reported in English cases. The nature of the cellular defect and how well they can combat cells can only be determined by doing studies where tests of whether various cells have killing effect, particularly on cryptococcosis, are done. I don't think we can draw a conclusion just from degrees of cellular immunity.

Dr Niitu: Dr Mikami presented sarcoidosis cases with complicating herpes zoster. Herpes zoster is caused by varicella zoster virus in persons who have immunity to it, and so herpes zoster occurs in older children and adults, while varicella occurs in younger children without immunity. I observed a case of pulmonary sarcoidosis in a 9-year-old girl who developed varicella. The course of varicella was very severe. The fever rose to 40°C and pneumonia and dyspnea developed. Varicella often worsens the course of leukemia. The severity of varicella in the patient may be related to the impairment of cell-mediated immunity in sarcoidosis. Sarcoidosis is usually not found in younger children and the chance to observe varicella complications in sarcoidosis may be rare.

Dr Hosoda: Dr James has just told us that the depression of delayed hypersensitivity in sarcoidosis is moderate. Dr Hiraga and I observed 5 cases recovered from the disease and tested them with a DNCB-sensitizing test. All of them had had a positive tuberculin reaction before the onset of the disease, a negative reaction during the disease and regained tuberculin sensitivity after clearing of the disease. After the recovery of the disease, they were all sensitized by DNCB. We can say that sarcoidosis patients usually regained the past tuberculin sensitivity after recovery from the disease, and were newly sensitized by DNCB.

V HISTOPATHOLOGY

A Case with Sarcoidosis Histologically Suggesting a Mode of Development of the Disease on the Basis of Biopsied Lung

Tzihiro Takahasi

Health Control Institute, Ajinomoto Co., Inc., Kawasaki, Japan

CASE

Mr T. S., a 31-year-old male, company employee.

Family history

His father is in good health; his mother suffered from miliary tuberculosis in Nov. 1963, and was treated with chemotherapy. Three years after treatment she was cured and thereafter has been in good health. Mr. T. S. has 5 brothers and sisters who, together with his wife and son are all in good health.

Past history

He has had a so-called " allergic " disposition from childhood and since his high school days has sometimes had supposedly bronchial asthma. No BCG vaccination was given. He had been smoking from 10 to 20 cigarettes daily and sometimes drank a small amount of sake. Born in Osaka, he has lived in the urban district of that city.

Status

A chest X-ray taken in autumn 1965 was normal. In the beginning of May 1966 he suffered from a swelling of the left submaxillar lymph nodes, with pain in the joints and chest with a fever of 37.8°C.

A chest X-ray revealed unilateral hilar adenopathy and nodular shadows and small mottlings in both lungs, especialy in the upper lobe.

He was admitted on 27th May, 1966, with an irregular type of fever (ca. 37°C in the morning and ca. 38°C in the evening), accompaied by symptoms of acute bronchitis.

The following laboratory examinations revealed no abnormality: urinalysis, blood haemoglobin concentrations, erythrocyte count, total leucocyte count (6300) and erythrocyte sedimentation rate. The following results were a little higher than normal: 8.5% of eosinophilic leucocytes in differential leucocyte count and 19.0% serum gamma-globulin. The 17 KST (Zimmerman-Miyake method) of 7.6 mg/day was a little lower than normal.

Sputum culture was negative for tubercle bacilli. A tuberculin test using 1:2000 dilution of old tuberculin showed a redness of 11×12 mm at the 48-hour reading. Suspected of having tuberculosis, he was treated with 1 g of SM twice a week, and PAS-1NH every day. In the meantime further examinations were carried out, i.e., roentgenological examination of the bones in the hands and feet. Bronchographic, bronchoscopic and, ophthalmological examinations showed nothing abnormal.

Scalene node biopsy (on 7th June 1966) revealed no specific histological findings.

267

Suspected of having tumor of the lung, a left thoracotomy and a lung biopsy were performed on 13th June, 1966. Three nodular subpleural lesions in S⁵ and S⁶ were resected. The largest was ca. 14×18 mm in size and the cut surface was of a grayish-black appearance and solid in consistency. A negative culture for tubercle bacilli, fungi and other bacteria was confirmed. After the operation the regimen of chemotherapy was changed to KM, PAS and 1NH.

On 13th August, a Kveim test was negative. The patient was discharged on 22nd Dec., 1967 and has since been in good health.

Histopathological findings in the biopsied lung

The resected nodular lesion is histologically a clump of typical sarcoid granulomas and there were many separated fresh or old granulomas in the development stage, i.e., some are proliferative and others are atrophic.

Some granulomas were located in the subepithelial layer of the bronchus or bronchiolus; giant cells were the foreign-body type and the bronchus showed a partial lack of elastic fibers and destruction of collagenous fibers in bronchial wall. Some of the bronchi showed stenosis of the bronchial lumen by the sarcoid granulomas in the bronchial wall, but no ulcerating bronchitis could be detected.

Some granulomas were located in the venous wall, and protruded into the lumen of a small pulmonary vein. The endothelium remained almost intact. However, a partial lack of elastic fibers in the venous wall was evident.

Some granulomas were found in the media and outside of a vein, resulting in stenosis of the lumen of the vessel. A partial lysis of the elastic fibers and degeneration of the endothelium was revealed.

Some granulomas had invaded the vessel wall from the outside, showing the above pathological changes in a more advanced stage. Some granulomas were located in a small pulmonary-vein wall, in a chain-like arrangement along the wall of the vessel.

CONCLUSION

The above histopathological findings and the localization of sarcoid granulomas in the wall of the bronchus and vessel suggest a mode of development of the disease, i.e., the invasion and spread of the disease could occur through the lymphatics or vasa vasorum in the wall of the bronchus or vessel, resulting in the local destruction of elastic fibers and collagenous fibers in lower degree and at a very slow pace, and sometimes resulting in bronchial or venous stenosis.

The Fine Structures of Sarcoidal and Kveim Granulomas

Yusuke Fuse and Yomei Hiraga

Japanese National Railways Sapporo Hospital, Sapporo, Japan

This report describes and compares the ultrastructure of epithelioid cells in sarcoidal and Kveim granulomas. The ultrastructures of macrophages and lymphocytic cells which appeared in those granulomas and of human splenic red pulp are also described in order to determine the origin of epithelioid cells. From our observations, transitions from blood monocytes into tissue macrophages and from tissue macrophages into epithelioid cells were suggested.

MATERIALS AND METHODS

The materials examined were obtained from 4 sarcoidal cervical lymph nodes, 1 sarcoidal parotid gland, 1 nodule in the nasal cavity and 2 Kveim granulomas. Each of these materials was obtained from different patients with sarcoidosis. For electron microscopy, small cubes of granulomas in lymph nodes were fixed in 2% osmium tetroxide buffered phosphate, pH 7.4, for 2 hours. The other materials were fixed in 5% glutaraldehyde buffered phosphate, pH 7.4, for 6 hours and then fixed in 2% osmium tetroxide solution at 4°C. The fixed materials were dehydrated and embedded in epon 812. Sections were stained with uranyl acetate and lead citrate and examined with an HU-11 electron microscope.

Scheme 1. Circulating blood monocyte.

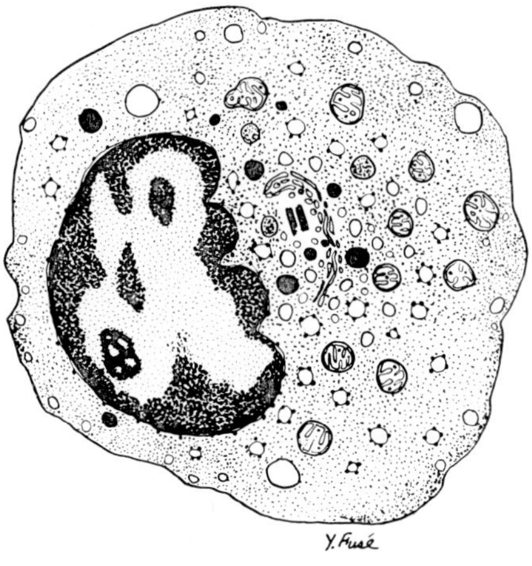

Y. Fuse

269

RESULTS

Blood monocytes and macrophages in human splenic cord

In splenic red pulp, circulating blood monocytes were observed inside venous sinuses and macrophages and fixed reticular cells were seen in the splenic cords. The monocytes were characterised by the presence of a well-developed Golgi apparatus, widely distributed vesicular rough-surfaced endoplasmic reticulum and of a moderate number of small round mitochondria and dense azurophilic granules. Cell margins were smooth. Coated vesicles, phagosomes and cytoplasmic filaments were not prominent. On the other hand, the macrophages and fixed reticular cells contained various phagosomes, coated vesicles and cytoplasmic filaments. The fixed reticular cells showed condensation of cytoplasmic filaments sticking to reticular fibers. Comparison of the ultrastructural characteristics among monocytes, macrophages and sarcoidal epithelioid cells is made in Table 1.

TABLE 1. A comparison of characteristic ultrastructural features among monocyte, macrophage and sarcoidal epithelioid cell.

		Blood monocyte	Tissue macrophage	Epithelioid cell
1.	Nuclear body	+	‖‖	‖‖
2.	Lysosome	+	‖‖	+
3.	Residual body	−	+	‖‖
4.	Mitochondria	+	‖	‖‖
5.	Cytoplasmic filament	±	‖	‖‖
6.	Coated vesicle	±	‖‖	‖‖
7.	Villous protrusion	±	‖	‖‖
8.	Phagosome	±	‖‖	+
9.	Cytoplasmic vacuole	±	‖‖	‖‖
10.	Rough-surfaced ER	+	‖	‖‖
11.	Golgi apparatus	‖	‖	‖‖

Macrophages and activated lymphocytes in sarcoidal granulomas

Macrophages and activated lymphocytes were frequently observed around sarcoidal granulomas. These cells were similar to the killer cells in cardiac transplants.[1] The macrophages showed more developed nuclear bodies, mitochondria, dense lysosomal granules, cytoplasmic filaments and villous cytoplasmic protrusions compared with the splenic cells. The transition of cells from macrophages into epithelioid cells was frequently observed. These cells showed increase of mitochondria, free ribosomes and rough-surfaced endoplasmic reticulum and decrease of lysosomal granules. Developing into epithelioid cells, the contents of the lysosomes were probably discharged. The activated lymphocytes found around the sarcoidal granulomas showed irregular nuclear outlines, increase of the euchromatinic area and increase of cytoplasms containing more abundant mitochondria and dense granules. The lymphatic cells often showed the presence of centrioles. However, these cells did not show the presence of coated vesicles, cytoplasmic filaments and phagosomes. They were not considered progenitors of sarcoidal epithelioid cells.[4]

Scheme 2.   Activated lymphocyte.

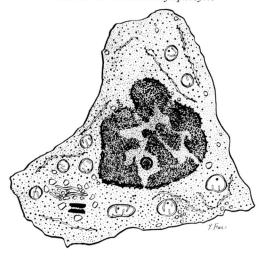

Scheme 3.   Tissue macrophage.

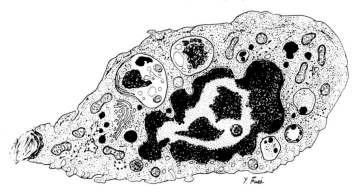

TABLE 2.   A comparison of hypertrophic and atrophic epithelioid cells.

	Hypertrophic epithelioid cell	Atrophic epithelioid cell
1. Irregularity of nuclear outline	+	⧺
2. Nuclear euchromatinic area	⧺	+
3. Nuclear heterochromatinic area	+	⧺
4. Nucleolus	⧺	±
5. Nuclear body	⧺	±
6. Mitochondria	⧺	+
7. Rough-surfaced ER	⧺	+
8. Golgi apparatus	⧺	+
9. Microvesicle	⧺	+
10. Coated vesicle	⧺	+
11. Lysosome	+	+
12. Residual body	+	⧺
13. Interdigitation of cell membrane	⧺	+
14. Ceutriole	±	—
15. Aggregates of fine particles	+	—

Sarcoidal epithelioid cells

Epithelioid cells were divided into 2 types: hypertrophic and atrophic cells.[2] The hypertrophic cells were mainly found in the central portions of fresh nodules. Atrophic cells were observed in the periphery of the aged nodules, especially those treated by steroid therapy.[3] The hypertrophic cells could be proved to develop into atrophic cells. The hypertrophic cells had various well-developed cytoplasmic organelles such as mitochondria, endoplasmic reticulum, Golgi apparatus and lysosomes. The cells showed no acceleration of phagocytosis activity and seemed to be immunologically activated. They had centrioles, indicating the possibility of their division inside the nodules. On the other hand, the atrophic epithelioid cells showed a decrease of various cytoplasmic organelles and an increase of residual bodies. The fine granules histologically identified

Scheme 4. Hypertrophic sarcoidal epithelioid cell.

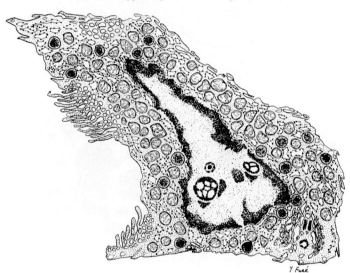

Scheme 5. Atrophic sarcoidal epithelioid cell.

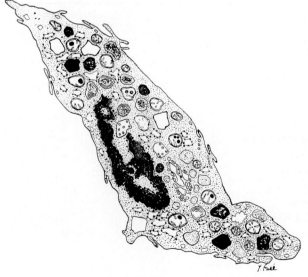

as positive in PAS reaction might correspond to these residual bodies. In the hypertrophic epithelioid cells, aggregates of fine particles about 30 Å in size were infrequently observed. The aggregates of fine particles had no limiting membrane and were arranged in a linear pattern. The significance of these particles was not known. The ultrastructural differences between the hypertrophic and atrophic epithelioid cells are summerized in Table 2.

Epithelioid cells in Kveim granulomas

The macrophages and epithelioid cells observed in the Kveim granulomas were essentially similar to those in sarcoidal granulomas. The former were more abundant in the lysosomes and phagosomes. The phagosomes were composed of various unidentified materials. However, the great majority were probably foreign materials contained in the injected solution of Kveim antigen. It was histologically presumed that Kveim granulomas contained various kinds of foreign bodies such as glass-like crystals, brown pigments and fibrillar bundles.

SUMMARY

From the electron microscopic observation of 6 sarcoidal granulomas and 2 Kveim granulomas, transition from blood monocytes into tissue macrophages and then into epithelioid cells was suggested. Activated lymphocytes observed around the granulomas were not considered to be progenitors of epithelioid cells. The epithelioid cells were divided into 2 types hypertrophic and atrophic cells. The ultrastructural differences between them were compared. In the cytoplasms of hypertrophic cells, aggregates of fine particles (30 Å size) were infrequently observed.

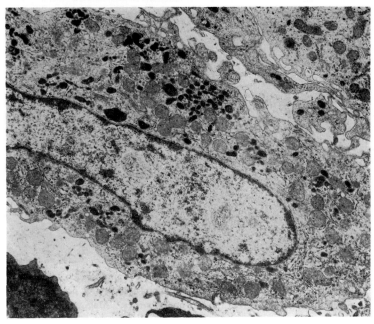

FIG. 1.   A macrophage observed in a sarcoidal granuloma shows 3 nuclear bodies and numerous dense bodies.   Mag. ×15,000.

Ultrastructural and Cytochemical Observations on Sarcoid Granulomas

Ryoichi Fukushiro, Takae Hirone and Yoshichika Eryu

Department of Dermatology, Kanazawa University School of Medicine, Kanazawa, Japan

This report presents observations of the ultrastructure and acid phosphatase activity of epithelioid cell granulomas in sarcoidosis by electron microscopy.

MATERIALS AND METHODS

Materials used for this study were as follows: 2 cutaneous nodules, 1 occurring 4 months previously and the other 2 years previously; 3 Kveim nodules, 4 weeks after the injection of Kveim antigen; and 3 enlarged cubital lymph nodes. These materials were taken from 6 patients with sarcoidosis. For electron microscopy, they were prepared by routine procedures, and in addition, some of them were prepared by the Barka-Anderson modification of the Gomori method for demonstration of acid phosphatase activity.

OBSERVATIONS

Two types of epithelioid cells (types 1 and 2) were distinguished. The cells of type 1 were predominant in early granulomas of Kveim nodules and in a 4-month-old cutaneous nodule, while the cells of type 2 predominated in advanced granulomas of a 2-year-old cutaneous nodule and enlarged cubital lymph nodes.

The cells of type 1 were characterized by a fairly well-developed endoplasmic reticulum and by variable numbers of lysosomes (Fig. 1). The endoplasmic reticulum consisted primarily of randomly disposed, rough-surfaced, tubular and cisternal elements. The ribosomes attached to the endoplasmic reticulum were not so numerous. The Golgi apparatus was fairly well-developed. Lysosomes were round or oval, membrane-limited vacuoles containing an amorphous material of moderate density. Some of them showed positive acid phosphatase reaction (Fig. 2). The reaction product was not seen in the lysosomal vacuoles after incubation of tissue in control media. The cells of type 2 were identified by variable numbers of peculiar cytoplasmic vacuoles (Fig. 3). The endoplasmic reticulum consisted predominantly of rough-surfaced cisternae, often disposed in parallel array. The attached ribosomes were more numerous. The cytoplasmic matrix usually appeared darker. The Golgi apparatus was more extensive and often multicentric. Peculiar cytoplasmic vacuoles were round or oval, varying from 0.5 to 1.5 μ in diameter. They were limited by a single unit membrane and contained a finely granular or fluffy material of low density. Smaller vacuoles, or vesicles, containing a similar material, were seen in close proximity to the Golgi apparatus. Both vesicles and vacuoles showed no positive acid phosphatase reaction. In fully matured cells, the cytoplasm was filled with peculiar vacuoles. A few vacuoles were found in the extracellular space lying near intact cells of type 2 (Fig. 4).

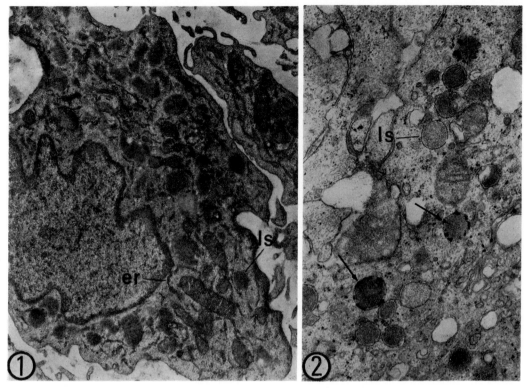

FIG. 1. Epithelioid cell of type 1 in an early sarcoid granuloma of a 4-month-old cutaneous nodule. The cytoplasm contains a fairly well-developed endoplasmic reticulum with rough-surfaced cisternae (er) and numerous lysosomes (ls) are seen. Mag. ×20,000.

FIG. 2. Epithelioid cell of type 1 in an advanced sarcoid granuloma of a cubital lymph node after incubation in Barka-Anderson modification of Gomori medium. Many lysosomes (ls) are seen. Some of them show reaction product (arrows). Mag. ×200,000.

Transitional cells with features of both types of cells were occasionally encountered both in early granulomas and in advanced granulomas.

DISCUSSION

The cells of type 1 appeared to be identical with the initially active epithelioid cells described by Gusek.[1] Our observations demonstrated that they contained a fairly well-developed endoplasmic reticulum and variable numbers of lysosomes, and that some of the lysosomes showed acid phosphatase activity. However, evidence of phagocytosis was practically nonexistent. Therefore it seemed likely that the cells of type 1 were not phagocytic but immunologically activated. The cells of type 2, similar to vacuolated epithelioid cells observed by others,[1-4] were distinguished by the cytoplasmic vacuoles containing a finely granular or fluffy material. Concerning the nature of the cytoplasmic vacuoles, opinions were divided. Some authors assumed the phagocytic or autophagocytic origin of the vacuoles,[2,3] while others supposed them to be synthesized or secretory granules.[1,4] Up to the present, however, there has been no direct evidence to support either of these hypotheses. Our observations provide evidence for the latter by demon-

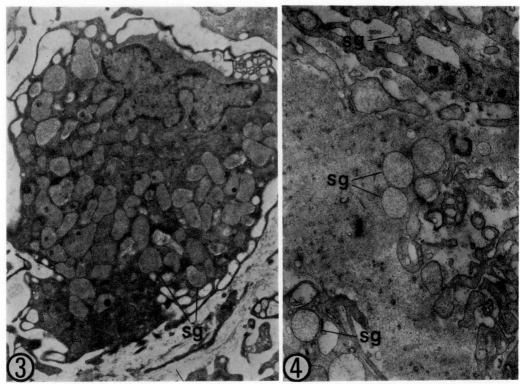

FIG. 3. Epithelioid cell of type 2 in an advanced sarcoid granuloma of a 2-year-old cutaneous nodule. The cytoplasm is filled with characteristic secretory granules (sg.) Mag. ×8,300.

FIG. 4. Part of the intercellular space in an advanced sarcoid granuloma of a cubital lymph node. A few vacuoles (sg), containing a finely granular material, are seen in the extracellular space as well as in the cytoplasm of the epithelioid cell. Mag. ×13,000.

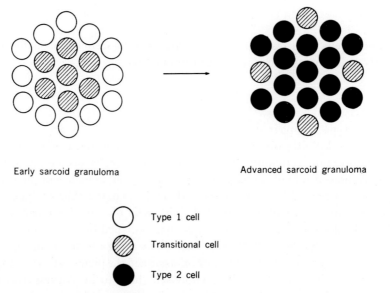

Early sarcoid granuloma   Advanced sarcoid granuloma

○ Type 1 cell

◑ Transitional cell

● Type 2 cell

FIG. 5. Schematic diagram illustrating the different cellular population in different stages of sarcoid granulomas.

strating that there are few vacuoles in the extracellular space of intact cells of type 2. Since there were only a few vacuoles in the extracellular space, the majority of them might degrade and disappear as soon as they are released. The material contained within the vacuoles seemed to be identical with the PAS-positive substance which was observed in sarcoid granulomas under the light microscope.[1] Our observations also suggest the Golgi origin of the cytoplasmic vacuoles by demonstrating the close proximity of early vacuoles to the Golgi apparatus.

The exact relationship of type 1 and 2 cells could not be determined from our static observations. It was of interest, however, that the cells of type 1 predominated in early granulomas and the cells of type 2 in advanced granulomas, and that transitional cells were present in both stages of granulomas (Fig. 5). These findings suggest that type 1 is an earlier phase of type 2, and that the former is transformed into the latter via transitional cells.

The results obtained in this study support the view that the different cellular populations of sarcoid granulomas and the different ultrastructures of their epithelioid cells represent differences in the functional stage of the cells as well as in the age of the granulomas.[5]

SUMMARY

Two types of epithelioid cells were distinguished in Kveim granulomas as well as in sarcoid granulomas of the skin and lymph nodes. Cells of type 1 were characterized by the presence of lysosomes and those of type 2 by the presence of secretory granules of unknown function. These 2 types of cells were considered to be different stages of the development of a single cell type.

REFERENCES

1. Gusek, W. 1966. *Arch. klin. exp. Derm.* **227**: 24.
2. Hirsch, J. G., Fedorko, M. E., and Dwyer, C. M. 1967. *La Sarcoïdose. Rapp. IVe Conf. Int.* Paris. p. 59.
3. Wanstrup, J. 1967. *La Sarcoïdose. Rapp. IVe Conf. Int.* Paris. p. 110.
4. Jones-Williams, W., Erasmus, D. A., Jenkins, D., Valerie James, E. M., and Davies, T. 1971. *Proc. Fifth Int. Conf. on Sarcoidosis.* Prague: Univ. Karlova. p. 115.
5. Gusek, W., and Behrend, H. 1971. *Proc. Fifth. Int. Conf. on Sarcoidosis.* Prague: Univ. Karlova. p. 124.

A Comparison of the Fine Structure of Lymphocytes in the Peripheral Blood and Granulomas of Sarcoidosis

W. Jones Williams, Elizabeth Fry and E. M. Valerie James

Pathology Department, The Welsh National School of Medicine, Cardiff, Great Britain

INTRODUCTION

In our previous studies of the fine structure of epithelioid cell granulomas in sarcoidosis, tuberculosis,[1] Kveim Test[2] and chronic beryllium disease,[3] we have been impressed by the close proximity and the intermingling of mononuclear and epithelioid cells. These mononuclear cells have lymphocytic features with no evidence of mitotic or phagocytic activity. Many appear to be classical resting lymphocytes[4]: others, although retaining a lymphocyte-like nucleus, are larger with increased amounts of cytoplasm and organelles, which we have referred to as activated lymphocytes. We have considered the possibility that activated lymphocytes may be an intermediate cell between resting lymphocytes and epithelioid cells and have suggested the possibility that epithelioid cells may originate from antigenically stimulated lymphocytes.[2,5]

Our present communication describes and compares the fine structure of peripheral lymphocytes with those found in granulomas and also with in vitro antigen stimulated lymphocytes.

MATERIALS AND METHODS

Circulating lymphocytes

Circulating lymphocytes were examined from 4 apparently normal subjects, 7 patients with sarcoidosis, 1 with chronic beryllium disease and 1 with farmer's lung disease. Lymphocytes were examined from 1 normal Mantoux-positive subject following incubation with purified protein derivative (PPD), 100 μg/ml for 72 hours. Total and differential white cell counts were within normal limits for all subjects studied.

Lymphocytes were separated by the technique of Dolby[6] from heparinised blood, using carbonyl iron and methyl cellulose to remove neutrophils and monocytes, giving a 98% pure suspension. The cells were fixed in 3% glutaraldehyde, with 0.067 M cacodylate buffer at pH 7.4 for 30 mins. The suspension was centrifuged for 5 mins at 1,000 g and the pellet was resuspended in cacodylate buffer for 12 hours prior to postfixation in osmium tetroxide, alcohol dehydration and embedding in araldite. All sections were stained with uranyl acetate and lead citrate.

Cell counts: 100 cells from each of 5 blocks of every case were examined and the different types expressed as percentages.

Granuloma lymphocytes

Tissue blocks from mediastinal lymph glands of 3 Kveim-positive sarcoid patients and a skin biopsy from 1 proven chronic beryllium case were examined. Tissues were fixed in glutaraldehyde, postfixed in osmium tetroxide and stained with uranyl acetate and lead citrate.

RESULTS

Circulating lymphocytes

In both normal and diseased subjects, 2 morphologically similar types of lymphocytes were found: those containing scanty organelles and others with numerous organelles.

The first type (Fig. 1) has an average diameter of 5–6.5 μ, with a central nucleus of 2.5–5.0 μ diameter, surrounded by a thin rim of cytoplasm. The nuclei, usually with a smooth outline, contain large quantities of densely stained heterochromatin and a few show single sometimes 2 nucleoli. The cytoplasm contains scanty organelles, including free ribosomes, very sparse rough endoplasmic reticulum, RER, 1 or 2 mitochondria and an occasional 0.1–0.8 μ diameter fat-like body. Golgi complexes and vesicles are inconspicuous. The cell outline is usually smooth, sometimes irregular but lacks microvilli.

The second type (Figs. 2 and 3) tends to be larger, average diameter 5–7.5 μ, shows a relatively smaller nucleus and greater amount of cytoplasm and number of organelles. Ribosomes are prominent, although polyribosomes are infrequent and occasional cells show a few short strands of RER. Mitochondria are well-developed and number 6–8. Golgi complexes and associated small vesicles are well-developed. Very occasionally cells contain phagolysosome-like vesicles, although the cell membrane appears smooth and

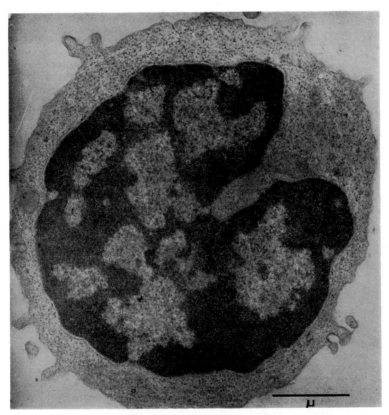

Fig. 1.   Circulating lymphocyte—Type 1, Mag. × 30,000.

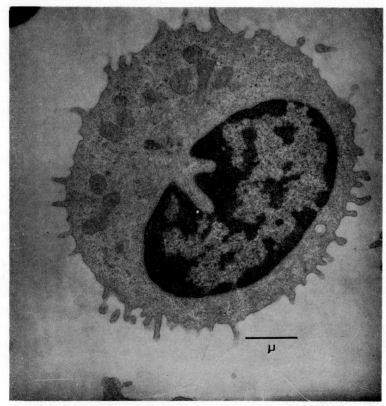

FIG. 2.   Circulating lymphocyte—Type 2, Mag. ×20,000.

evidence of phagocytosis is absent. Occasional fat-like globules are also present.

None of the diseased patients showed the ' activated ' lymphocytes as described in the granulomas (vide infra). Only 6 of the 2,500 lymphocytes examined in sarcoid patients showed somewhat paler nuclei with margination of chromatin similar to the nuclei of epithelioid cells.

A percentage count of types I and II lymphocytes showed no convincing difference between the normal and diseased subjects (Table 1).

TABLE 1.   Percentage of type 2 lymphocytes in the peripheral blood.

Normal	Sarcoidosis	Beryllium disease	Farmer's lung	
69.8	83.8	82.6	77.8	
65.7	73.5			
63.4	71.6			
60.6	74.6			
	69.7			
	75.8			
	75.4			
64.8	74.9	82.6	77.8	Aver age

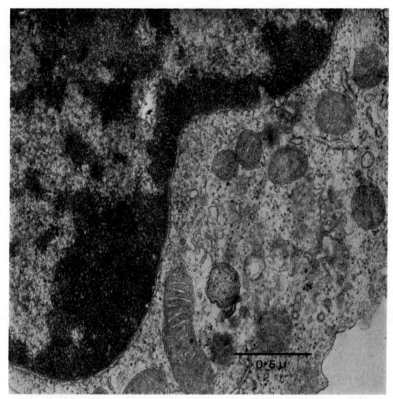

Fig. 3.   Circulating lymphocyte—Type 2, Details of organelles, Mag. ×60,000.

Granuloma lymphocytes

Intermingled with the epithelioid cells and at the periphery of the granulomas are a variety of lymphocytic cells. These include types I and II, as described above in the circulation and in addition, numerous 'activated' lymphocytes. Activated lymphocytes retain a lymphocyte-type nucleus, but are larger than type I and II cells with an average diameter of 6–11 μ, and contain more numerous organelles (Fig. 4). The cytoplasm contains many mitochondria, prominent Golgi complexes and associated small vesicles, abundant ribosomes and a few short strands of rough endoplasmic reticulum. Occasional lymphocytes contain moderate numbers of glycogen granules which stain by the Rambourg's periodic-chromic acid silver methenamine technique[7] They do not show the numerous larger, 0.4–0.7 μ. diameter vesicles characteristic of mature epithelioid cells.[1] Some cells with epithelioid-type nuclei, however, contain very scanty large vesicles and their cytoplasmic features are otherwise similar to the activated lymphocytes.

In vitro stimulated lymphocytes

The PPD-stimulated lymphocytes differed considerably from those in the above subjects. They were considerably larger, diameter 8–16 μ, with a nuclear diameter of 5–9 μ. The nuclei showed a smooth outline, conspicuous nucleoli and sparse dense chromatin, giving a 'pale' appearance. Though the amount of cytoplasm was large, intracellular organelles were sparse with a few short strands of RER but abundant polyribosomes. A few showed prominent Golgi complexes and very occasional cells showed 3 or 4 dense bodies 0.3 μ in diameter.

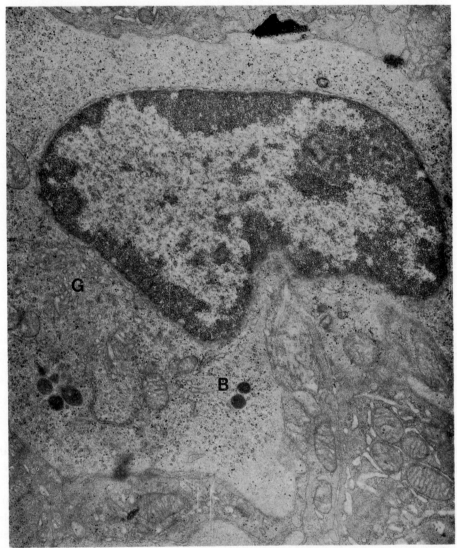

FIG. 4.   Granuloma lymphocyte—activated.

G—Golgi complex.

B—Unidentified bodies as occasionally seen in lymphocytes, Mag. ×25,000.

All sections were stained with uranyl acetate and lead citrate in this and previous figures.

Normal, sarcoid, chronic beryllium disease and farmer's lung patients all show 2 types of lymphocytes in the circulation and in the granulomas. Type I shows the features of a normal, resting, lymphocyte and type II that of a possible antigenically stimulated cell.

A third type, which is an intermediate form between lymphocytes and epithelioid cell, was not present in the circulation but is a feature of all these sarcoid type granulomas.

DISCUSSION

Light microscopy studies have shown no consistent changes in white cell population of sarcoid patients.[8]

The present observations on the fine structure of circulating white cells are confined to lymphocytes. Monocytes were not identified, or expected, as a result of the technique used for cell preparation, although occasional polymorphs were present. This study shows that there are 2 types of circulating lymphocytes present in both normal subjects and patients with granulomatous disease. Type I is a small lymphocyte with few intracellular organelles, while type II is of comparable size, but has an increased number of organelles and constitutes 70–80% of the total circulating lymphocyte population. Larger activated lymphocytes, similar to those found in the sarcoid granulomas are not present in the circulating cells examined.

Lymphocytes form an integral part of the granulomatous lesion and include cells which are morphologically intermediate between normal lymphocytes and epithelioid cells. Epithelioid cells may originate from these activated lymphocytes which have probably, at some stage, been antigenically stimulated.[2] Since sarcoid granulomas are known to occur in a wide variety of organs, it is suggestive that the responsible factor is present in the circulation. Based on these premises we expected to find activated lymphocytes in the circulation but they were only found in the granulomas. This suggests that the possible change from lymphocytes to epithelioid cells may occur within the tissues.

It appears strange that a normal lymphocyte can develop into a complicated epithelioid -like cell, but it is known that lymphocytes when antigenically stimulated, in vitro, are capable of considerable morphological change. This is seen in this study, using PPD, and Douglas,[9] using poke-weed mitogen, illustrated antigenically stimulated lymphocytes which appear remarkably similar to the activated lymphocytes in the granulomas.

It is interesting to find such a high percentage of lymphocytes in normal subjects with a more elaborate intracellular apparatus than is usually described for normal lymphocytes. Zucker-Franklin,[4] in a fine-structure study of normal subjects found that all small circulating lymphocytes were not " resting " cells, since there were always a few of similar size which had a more active appearance of cytoplasm or nucleus and she suggested that they either had a different function or origin. It seems, however, from this study that these small active-looking lymphocytes are more abundant in the normal circulation than Zucker-Franklin suggests. In view of these studies it is important to consider the possibility that morphological differences may reflect the varying functional roles of lymphocytes.

In conclusion, normal, sarcoid, chronic beryllium disease and farmer's lung patients all have types I and II lymphocytes in the circulation and the granulomas. In addition, activated cells which are morphologically intermediate between normal lymphocytes and epithelioid cells are present in sarcoid-type granulomas.

ACKNOWLEDGEMENTS

We wish to thank Dr J. R. Mikhail, London, for the specimens of sarcoid lymph glands. Mrs Fry and Mrs James are supported by the Clinical Research Fund of the Welsh Regional Board.

REFERENCES

1. Jones-Williams, W., Erasmus, D. A., James, E. M. Valerie, and Davies, T. 1970. *Postgrad. Med. J.* **46**: 496.
2. Jones-Williams, W. 1972. *Proc. First European Sarcoid Conf.* Geneva Suisse Praxis (in press).
3. Jones-Williams, W., Fry, Elizabeth, and James, E. M. Valerie 1972. *Acta. Path. Microbiol. Scand.* In press.
4. Zucker-Franklin, D. 1969. *Seminars Haemat.* **6**: 4.
5. Jones-Williams, W. 1971. *Fifth Int. Conf. on Sarcoidosis* (ed. L. Levinsky and F. Macholda). Prague. p. 644.
6. Dolby, A. E. 1969. *Immunol.* **17**: 709.
7. Rambourg, A., Hernandez, W., and Lebiond, C. P. 1969. *J. Cell. Biol.* **40**: 395.
8. Scadding, J. G. 1967. *Sarcoidosis*. London: Eyre and Spottiswoode.
9. Douglas, S. D., Hoffman, P. F., Borjeson, J., and Chessin, L. N. 1967. *J. Immunol.* **98**: 17.

A Comparison of Lysosomal Enzyme Levels in Lymphoid Tissue of Sarcoidosis and other Diseases

P. B. HOUGHTON, W. JONES WILLIAMS AND M. DAVIES

Pathology Department and Tenovus Institute, Welsh National School of Medicine, Cardiff, Great Britain

INTRODUCTION

Considerable controversy exists as to the nature of epithelioid cells in the granulomas of sarcoidosis. Epithelioid cells have been considered as modified macrophages, Spector and co-workers,[1,2] and also as synthesising cells.[2-5] We therefore considered that it would be of interest to compare, by chemical analysis, the total levels of lysosomal enzymes in lymphoid tissue of sarcoid patients with the levels found in normal, in hyperplastic and in neoplastic lymphoid tissue. The enzymes included acid phosphatase, β-glucuronidase and cathepsin D in homogenates of spleen and lymph glands.

MATERIALS AND METHODS

The material examined (Fig. 1) included tissue showing (a) normal, no evidence of disease, (b) sarcoid granulomas, (c) inflammatory and systemic hyperplasia associated with generalised reticulo-endothelial disorders and (d) neoplastic proliferation. Our previous investigations, Houghton et al. (unpublished), have shown that the lysosomal enzymes examined retain their full activity after freezing.

	Spleen	Lymph glands
Normal	9	2
Sarcoidosis	11	5
Hyperplasia	9	3
Inflammatory	1	
Hypersplenism	1	
Idiopathic Thrombocytopaenia	4	
Spherocytic Anaemia	3	
Neoplasia	2	3
Lymphosarcoma	2	2
Hodgkin's disease	0	1

FIG. 1. Case examined.

(a) *Normal tissues*

Nine spleens were examined, 7 removed incidentally during the course of other abdominal surgery, and 2 following traumatic rupture. Two inguinal glands removed during varicose vein operation. Histological examination of all these tissues showed no evidence of disease.

(b)   *Sarcoid tissues*

Due to difficulties in obtaining fresh tissues we examined portions of spleens from 11 sarcoid patients which had been frozen at $-70°C$, for periods ranging up to 3 years. Ten showed variable numbers and 1 no granulomas on histological examination. The 5 lymph glands were examined fresh after an interval, due to transportation at $0°C$, of around 6 hours. They all showed numerous granulomas.

(c)   *Inflammatory and systemic hyperplasia*

All were kept at $0°C$ and were homogenised within 2 hours of excision. The following number of hyperplastic spleens were examined: 1 from a subject with generalised peritonitis, 1 associated with panhaemocytopaenia (hypersplenic syndrome), 4 from patients with idiopathic thrombocytopoenia, and 4 from patients with congenital spherocytic anaemia. Three lymph nodes were examined. All tissues histologically showed sinusoidal and histiocytic cell hyperplasia with prominent reticulum cell centres.

(d)   *Neoplastic tissue*

The tissues were kept at $0°C$ and homogenised within 2 hours of excision. Two spleens, 1 with diffuse and 1 with nodular lymphosarcoma, and 3 lymph glands, including 2 with lymphosarcoma and 1 with Hodgkin's disease were examined.

Sampling of human spleens and lymph glands

After surgical removal, the capsule of the spleen was removed and a representative sample was placed in ice-cold 0.25 *M* sucrose. Glands were trimmed to remove associated fat before the sample was taken. Sample bottles were surrounded by ice in a vacuum flask and transported to the laboratory without delay. When large samples were available, a portion was placed in a deep-freeze immediately and stored at $-70°C$. Representative samples were taken for histological examination.

Homogenisation of human tissue

The pieces of spleens or glands were blotted dry and forced through the pores of a perforated stainless steel plate (average pore size 1 mm diameter) in a hand-operated mincer with a screw-driven plunger, which had been kept at $0°C$ before use. The brei was collected in a tared beaker containing ice-cold 0.25 *M* sucrose, and the beaker and contents were weighed. The minced tissue was homogenised with a Potter-Elvehjem-type, Teflon-on-glass homogeniser.

Determination of enzyme levels

All enzyme concentrations are expressed as units/g of brei. One unit is defined as the quantity of enzymes which will liberate 1 μmole of degradation product in one minute at $37°C$.

(a)   *Acid phosphatase*

Determined by the method of Gianetto and de Duve,[6] using β-glycerophosphate as substrate, at pH 5.0. Inorganic phosphate liberated during the reaction was measured by the method of Fiske and Subburow.[7]

(b)   *Cathepsin D*

Determined by a modification of the method of Anson[8] in which the enzyme preparation is allowed to act on denatured haemoglobin at pH 3.3, and the liberated tyrosine measured.

(c) *β-glucuronidase*

β-glucuronidase was measured by the method of Gianetto and de Duve[6] at pH 5.0, using phenolphthalein β-D-monoglucuronide as substrate.

RESULTS

Acid phosphatase (Fig. 2)

Spleen   The values in histologically normal samples ranged from 1.77–2.15 units/g of brei, mean value of 1.96 (S.D.±0.12).

In the 10 sarcoid spleens with granulomas all the enzyme values were higher than normal with a range of 2.32 to 3.85 units. In the 1 spleen with no evidence of granulomas, the enzyme level, 1.86 units, was within the normal range.

In the hyperplastic group, the idiopathic thrombocytopaenic cases showed raised levels, (2.33, 2.37, 2.43, 2.47), but the others were within the normal range. The 2 cases of lymphosarcoma showed low values, (0.88 & 1.9).

Glands   A value of 1.55 units was obtained in 1 normal gland. Results are not available in the other normal and hyperplastic glands due to insufficient amounts of tissue. The levels in 4 sarcoid lymph nodes were 1.59, 2.14, 2.92 and 3.47 units. A reliable result could not be obtained for the Hodgkin's gland, using β-glycerophosphate substrate, due to the presence of unidentified interfering substances. In the 2 glands with lymphosarcoma, values of 0.69 and 0.78 were found.

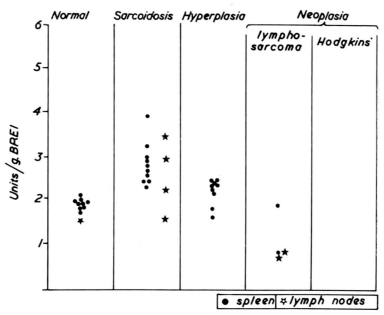

Fig. 2.   Acid phosphatase.

Cathepsin D (Fig. 3)

Spleen   The value normal spleens ranged from 2.51–3.37 units, mean value, 2.95, (S D±0.26).

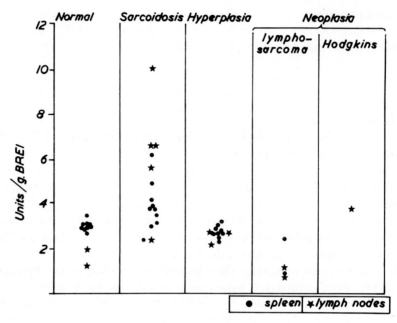

FIG. 3.   Cathepsin—D.

For sarcoid spleens the values ranged from 2.52–6.17 and 7 of 10 were higher than the upper limit of normal and all but 1 were above the normal mean. The spleen from a sarcoid patient without granulomas showed a value of 2.93 which is within the normal range.

In the hyperplastic group the values were within the normal range but both varieties of lymphosarcoma were lower than normal, 0.98 and 2.49.

Lymph gland   Values of 1.33 and 1.96 units were found in the normal glands. However, the values in the sarcoid glands were markedly raised varying from 2.35–10.03 units. The hyperplastic glands showed slightly higher levels than normal (2.17, 2.20 and 2.75 units). The Hodgkin's disease gland showed a raised value of 3.79 units and in contrast the values in lymphosarcoma were lower than normal (0.78 and 1.20).

β-glucuronidase (Fig. 4)

Spleen   In normal spleens we found a wide range of enzyme level, 0.29–0.57, mean value 0.41, (S D±0.08).

In sarcoid spleens the range was 0.13 to 0.53 and 4 of 10 samples showed lower levels than the lowest normal. In the granuloma-free spleen from a sarcoid patient a value of 0.44 units was on the high side of the normal range.

In the hyperplastic group, the 3 cases of spherocytic anaemia (0.3, 0.25 and 0.17) and 1 of hypersplenism (0.15) are lower than normal, while the other cases were within the normal range. Values in neoplastic spleens were all reduced.

Lymph glands   The 2 normal glands showed values of 0.24 and 0.17. All 5 sarcoid glands showed lower values (0.08 to 0.14). Two of the 3 inflammatory glands showed slightly raised levels, (0.29 and 0.27), while the third case showed a value of 0.2. All the neoplastic glands showed reduced activity, Hodgkin's 0.10, and lymphosarcoma, 0.06 and 0.13.

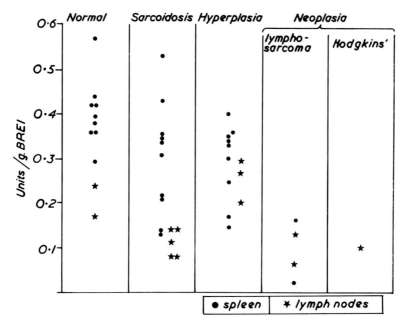

Fig. 4. β-Glucuronidase.

DISCUSSION

In the work presented in this paper, the activity of acid phosphatase, cathepsin D and β-glucuronidase has been estimated in normal, sarcoid, hyperplastic and neoplastic lymphoid tissue. These enzymes are normally associated with lysosomes and recent work from these laboratories has demonstrated a similar location in human lymphoid tissue (Houghton et al. unpublished). Acid phosphatase and cathepsin D levels were increased in the sarcoid tissue compared to normal tissue, but the levels of β-glucuronidase were lower. The raised levels of cathepsin D and acid phosphatase may suggest a special role for the lysosome in sarcoid tissue, particularly since in a number of cases the increase in enzyme activity appears to be associated with the presence of granulomas. Of particular interest are enzyme levels within the normal range recorded for a spleen tissue, devoid of granulomas, but obtained from a patient with clinical sarcoidosis. The enzyme levels in hyperplastic tissue were frequently within the normal range. Variations from normal which occurred were not as great as those observed in sarcoid tissue.

Our findings of reduced β-glucuronidase in Hodgkin's and lymphosarcoma are in agreement with the findings of Monis, et al.[9] The acid phosphatase and cathepsin D levels were also reduced in lymphosarcoma but in Hodgkin's the cathepsin D level was raised. The enzyme pattern in Hodgkin's appears to resemble that of sarcoidosis. The raised levels of acid phosphatase found biochemically are in agreement with the previous histochemical findings from these laboratories that epithelioid cells were rich in acid phosphatase.[10] Recent detailed examination by electron microscopy showed that the epithelioid cells contain numerous vesicles which stained for mucoglycoproteins (5, and James and Jones-Williams, unpublished). The presence of mucoglycoprotein in epithelioid cells could result from either increased synthesis or decreased degradation. In view of the low value of β-glucuronidase found in sarcoid tissue it could be inferred that the latter explanation is true. It will be of interest to learn the levels for other glycosidases in sarcoid tissue, since these lysosomal enzymes are believed to be concerned with the degredation of mucopolysaccharides.

ACKNOWLEDGEMENTS

We wish to thank the following for their support:
1. Welsh Hospital Board Clinical Research Fund.
2. Tenovus for valuable laboratory facilities and assistance.
3. Drs D. N. Mitchell (Medical Research Council) and P. Bradstreet (Public Health Laboratory Service) for supplying frozen sarcoid spleen material, and Dr J. R. Mikhail (Central Middlesex Hospital) for fresh sarcoid lymph glands, and clinicians of Cardiff Hospitals for other fresh tissues.

REFERENCES

1. Papadimitriou, J. M., and Spector, W. G. 1971. *J. Path.* **105**: 187.
2. Epstein, W. L. 1971. Advances in Biology Skin (ed. Montagna, W., and Billingham, R. E.). New York. p. 313.
3. Gusek, W. 1968. *Virchow. Arch.* (Path. Anat.) **345**: 264.
4. Wanstrup, J., and Christensen, H. E. 1966. *Acta. Path. Microbiol. Scand.* **66**: 169.
5. Jones-Williams, W., Erasmus, D. A., James, E. M. V., and Davies, T. 1970. *Postgrad. Med. J.* **46**: 496.
6. Gianetto, R., and de Duve, C. 1955. *Biochem J.* **59**: 533.
7. Fiske, C. H., and Subburow, Y. 1925. *J. Biol. Chem.* **66**: 375.
8. Anson, M. L. 1937. *J. Gen Physiol.* **20**: 565.
9. Monis, B., Banks, B. M., and Ruttenburg, A. M. 1960. *Cancer* **13**: 368.
10. Williams, D., Jones-Williams, W., and Williams, J. 1969. *J. Path. Bact.* **97**: 705.

DISCUSSION

Chairmen: W. JONES WILLIAMS AND K. IWAI

DR FUSE: We tried in vain to find out the difference between sarcoidal and tuberculous epithelioid cells. Dr Jones-Williams did you study the fine structure of tuberculous epithelioid cells and did they also contain many secretary vacuoles?

DR JONES WILLIAMS: Yes, we have done this in sarcoidosis, in tuberculosis, in beryllium disease, farmer's lung and we are trying at the moment to do it in Crohn's disease. In all these conditions on light microscopy and on fine structure, we get similar results. This is why I think this diagram I have put up suggests, a yet to be proven common pathway.

I thought the first paper showed beautiful photograph of the granulomas in the walls of the vessels. And as I understood what was said by the author, these were in the pulmonary veins. Occasionally one does see it in the arteries, I feel that one ought to see it, if the agent is going round systemically in a circulation. I personally think a sarcoid causative agent must be circulating. One does see this reasonable often in the lung.

DR RUPEC: I greatly enjoyed your beautiful electronmicroscopical cytochemical pictures. How long did you incubate your material? I remember very similar but not exactly the same pictures in the case of lipid droplets in parakeratotic cells. They were nonspecific.

I would ask if you tried histochemically, to differentiate the cells in the early Kveim granuloma. We call such cells, in early granuloma, lymphoid cells. We did not know if these were monocytes, or maybe lymphocytes. Did you try histochemically to separate the monocytes from the lymphocytes? After 10 days we saw cells, that were similar to fibroblasts. We suppose they were young epithelioid cells. [Rupec et al. Arch. Klin.,

exp. Derma 237, 811, (1970)]

DR JONES WILLIAMS: Optimal time of incubation was about 15 minutes. As regards the second question, I am not at all sure morphologically that one ever knows or recognizes a monocyte. You can only really recognise it when you see a moving pattern on a tissue culture stage or when you see that it has taken something in. But life gets even more complicated now of course, in that lymphocytes also may contain a few acid phosphatase vesicles. I am not at all sure which are monocytes or lymphocytes. Let's pretend they are all lymphocytes. I think it would be much more sensible.

DR JONES WILLIAMS: Dr Fuse asked in his paper, what I thought of those fine particles, those aggregates, but I don't know the answer to that. They were not membrane bound. We have on occasions seen odd unidentified particles and I have shown the pictures to Professor Epstein, who doesn't reckon that any of the particles are viruses.

DR SOMCHAI: I have 3 questions for Dr Jones-Williams. The first is: To which stage or stages of sarcoidosis did your patients for enzyme study belong? The second question: Did your enzyme study include pre- and post-treatment examinations? This is just to ascertain whether any improvement might have occurred after corticosteroids or any other medication. This last question: Have you correlated your findings regarding tissue enzymes to the enzymes circulating in the blood, such as the serum phosphatases?

DR JONES WILLIAMS: Concerning the last question, we have not looked at the serum acid phosphatase, which is an excellent idea, I nor have we looked at the cells before and after steroid treatment.

DR SHIGEMATSU: Yesterday I presented two X-rays of a patient with sarcoidosis showing small numbers of cloudy shadows on the upper field of the first X-ray. And also the patient had a positive scalene node biopsy revealing sarcoid granulomas. Spontaneous resolution occurred in three months in that case, shown on the other X-ray. Is this case called today primary sarcoidosis in the lung or not? X-ray photos presented by Dr Takahashi showed almost the same features. The exact features of his biopsied specimen seemed to be sarcoid granulomas in the bronchial wall and also in the walls of the vein. I would like to ask all participants if they have seen the same features in their patients at autopsy or in a biopsy.

DR TAKAHASHI: I have only observed these in this 1 case.

DR JAMES: Since a large number of histopathologists are present at this session, I would like to know from them whether there is lack of involvement of certain organs in multisystem sarcoidosis. It is always said that the pancreas and adrenals are spared. I realise that autopsies on sarcoidosis are infrequent, but we should be able to have a consensus of opinion from so many pathologists here now.

DR IWAI: I would like to comment briefly on the important problem of the origin of epithelioid cells, whether they come from lymphocytes or monocytes or macrophages. Concerning the diagnosis of malignant lymphoma, Japanese pathologists often diagnose reticulum cell sarcoma, but American pathologists often say lymphosarcoma. This is really a big difference. In Japan extensive research on the reticuloendothelial system has been carried out and we tend to consider the origin of epithelioid cells as relating to the reticuloendothelial system. This is perhaps, one of the reasons why we often use the term reticulosarcoma in our diagnosis. It is very difficult to elucidate the origin of epithelioid cells. We need more experimental evidence under strict conditions as to the origins of epithelioid cells.

VI   EPIDEMIOLOGY

Epidemiology of Sarcoidosis in Japan

Y. Hosoda[1], Y. Hiraga[2], M. Furuta[3], Y. Niitu[4], K. Iwai[5], M. Odaka[1],

Y. Maeda[1], T. Hashimoto[1], M. Yamamoto[6], T. Izumi[7], S. Oshima[8],

T. Tachibana[9], Y. Nishimoto[10], N. Shigematsu[11]

and N. Tateishi[12]

There is much useful information relating to the frequency of sarcoidosis in Japan. This country carried out tuberculosis prevalence surveys in 1953 and has also been enforcing mass chest X-ray surveys in accordance with the Antituberculosis Law. These procedures were very helpful in obtaining information about sarcoidosis. The purpose of this paper is to discuss the epidemiological features of the disease in this country, based on the survey results.

Deaths and autopsy cases

According to statistics in Japan, 16 deaths were notified in 1968, 13 in 1969 and 19 in 1970.[1] Besides these, there have been 32 autopsy cases, 20 of which died from myocardial involvement.[2]

Prevalence survey results

The prevalence of sarcoidosis across the country was obtained from the tuberculosis prevalence surveys which the Ministry of Health and Welfare has been making at 5-yearly intervals since 1953. No BHL cases were reported in the 1953 and 1958 surveys, but 1 case was found in 1963 and 3 in 1968. In the 1963 and 1968 surveys, 1:1,200 and 1:1,300 of the Japanese people were selected at random, the number of cases being estimated at 1,200 in 1963 and 3,900 in 1968. The prevalence rates per 100,000 were given as approximately 1.2 and 3.9 respectively for these 2 surveys.

Incidence survey results

There are 3 sources of information concerning the incidence of the disease (Table 1).

1. The Japan Sarcoidosis Committee assembled 1,752 cases with sarcoidosis through 4 enquête surveys which were performed in the 4,000 hospitals in this country in 1960,

1) JNR (Japanese National Railways) Central Health Institute, Tokyo, Japan.
2) JNR Sapporo Hospital, Sapporo, Japan.
3) Schritsu Akita Sogo Hospital, Akita, Japan.
4) Tohoku University, Sendai, Japan.
5) Japan Anti-Tuberculosis Association Research Institute, Tokyo, Japan.
6) Department of Medicine, Nagoya City University, Nagoya, Japan.
7) Kyoto University, Kyoto, Japan.
8) Japan Anti-Tuberculosis Association, Osaka Dispensary, Osaka, Japan.
9) Osaka Prefectural Hospital, Osaka, Japan.
10) Hiroshima University School of Medicine, Hiroshima, Japan.
11) Kyushu University, Fukuoka, Japan.
12) Kumamoto University Medical School, Kumamoto, Japan.

1961, 1964 and 1970 (JSC enquête source).

    2. The Japanese National Railways' Sarcoidosis Study Team assembled 66 cases in a defined working group through a 10-year study using a notification system (JNR notification source).

    3. The Joint Study Team, comprising physicians experienced in sarcoidosis, made a case-finding study among schoolchildren and students in several representative Japanese cities through annual mass chest X-rays (student source). This team assembled 110 new cases during an average observation period of 7 years (Table 2). These figures can be regarded as representing a minimum rate of incidence of the disease. The student source and the JNR notification source were compiled to compare new cases discovered in the mass chest X-rays in the corresponding cities.

    Involved sites   The JSC enquête source disclosed that 95% of the 1,752 cases had

TABLE 1. Incidence surveys in Japan.

	Materials	Observation period	New case	Total No. observed	Method	Surveyed by
1)	Hospital cases	–1969	1,972	—	Enquete	Japan Sarcoidosis Committee
2)	Adult workers	1961–1970	66	4.5 million	Notification	Japan National Railways Sarcoidosis Study Team
3)	School children and students	Average 10 years (–1970)	110*	6.1 million	Annual mass X-ray surveys	Authors of this paper

* 19 in primary school, 43 in middle school, 39 in high school, 9 in universities.

TABLE 2. New cases with sarcoidosis detected

School	Items investigated	Sapporo	Akita
Primary School (6–11 yrs)	Rate (per 100,000)	*3.7*	
	New cases	5	
	No. examined (in thousand)	134.7	
	Period	(1965 & 71)	
Lower Second School (12–14 yrs)	Rate (per 100,000)	*6.5*	
	New cases	7	
	No. examined (in thousand)	108.4	
	Period	(1965 & 71)	
Upper Second School (15–17 yrs)	Rate (per 100,000)	*7.4*	*0*
	New cases	*6*	
	No. examined (in thousand)	80.9	16.1
	Period	(1965 & 71)	(1971)
University (18–21 yrs)	Rate (per 100,000)		
	New cases		
	No. examined (in thousand)		
	Period		

Reporters : Sapporo : Hiraga, Y., Miyagi, Y.   Sendai : Niitu, Y.   Akita : Furuta, M.
             Tokyo : Iwai, K., Tsuruta, K., Shiozawa, H., Kinoshita, T., Maeda, Y., Hosoda, Y.
             Osaka : Tachibana, T., Okada, S.   Kyoto : Oshima, S., Izumi, T.,

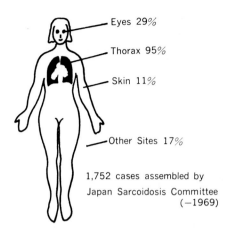

Eyes 29%

Thorax 95%

Skin 11%

Other Sites 17%

1,752 cases assembled by
Japan Sarcoidosis Committee
(−1969)

Frequency of Intra- and Extrathoracic Sarcoidosis

FIG. 1.   Involvement of sarcoidosis.

intrathoracic involvement, comprising 57% with intrathoracic involvement only and 38% with both intrathoracic and extrathoracic involvement. Of the remaining cases, 5% showed extrathoracic involvement only. Eye involvement was found in 28.5% of the cases, skin lesions in 11.1% and other extrathoracic sites in 16.7% (Fig. 1). Two other sources gave similar results.

Mode of discovery of the disease   In the JSC enquête source, 50% of the cases were discovered by annual mass X-rays, 41.2% by subjective symptoms and 15% by other

by annual mass X-rays in schools in Japan.

Sendai	Tokyo	Osaka	Kyoto	Fukuoka	Kumamoto	Total
1.3	*0*	*0.3*	*0.5*		*0*	*0.6*
7	0	6	1		0	19
528.2	556.0	1742.1	200.5		23.6	3185.0
(1960–71)	(1960–71)	(1960–71)	(1960–71)		(1960–71)	
10.1	*0.6*	*0.5*	*1.1*	*0*	*0*	*2.8*
28	2	5	1	0	0	43
277.8	316.7	729.0	90.5	29.4	11.2	1563.8
(1960–71)	(1960–71)	(1960–71)	(1969–71)	(1971)	(1971)	
	4.0	*2.1*	*16.0*	*0*	*0*	*3.3*
	15	14	4	0	0	39
	373.8	678.4	25.3	12.6	15.8	1202.8
	(1960–71)	(1968–71)	(1969–71)	(1971)	(1971)	
	5.1	*4.0*	*7.9*	*0*		*5.3*
	5	2	2	0		9
	87.6	49.0	25.5	11.1		173.0
(1963–66)	(1970–71)	(1968–71)	(1969–71)	(1971)		

Fukuoka :   Shigematsu, N., Sugiyama, K., Masuo, M., Kido, H., Matsuyama, T.
Kumamoto :   Tateishi, N., Shima, K., Fukuda, Y., Soejima, R.

methods. On the other hand, in the JNR notification source, 83.3% of the cases were detected by annual mass chest X-rays and only 16.7% by other methods. It is notewothy that 40% of the Japanese people have undergone mass chest X-ray examinations every year and that nearly 100% of schoolchildren, students and workers have been X-rayed every year. It appears that about 50% to 80% of the cases would have been overlooked had it not been for the annual mass X-rays.

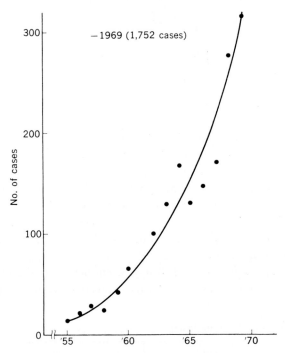

FIG. 2.   Incidence of sarcoidosis—registered cases (Japan S. Committee).

TABLE 3.   New cases with sarcoidosis detected by annual mass chest X-rays.

Rates by districts	School and age	6–11 yrs*	12–14 yrs**	15–19 yrs	20–29 yrs	30–39 yrs	40–49 yrs	50– yrs	Total (corrected rate)
Hokkaido (Sapporo)	Rate (per 100,000)	*3.7*	*6.5*	*8.0*	*10.2*	*0*	*0*	*4.1*	*4.8 (4.8)*
	New cases	5	7	7	9	0	0	2	30
Tohoku (Sendai– Akita)	Rate (per 100,000)	*1.3*	*10.1*	*4.1*	*5.3*	*0*	*0.6*	*0*	*3.1 (3.5)*
	New cases	7	28	1	3	0	1	0	40
Kanto (Tokyo)	Rate (per 100,000)	*0*	*0.6*	*3.8*	*6.4*	*0.9*	*1.5*	*1.1*	*1.6 (2.2)*
	New cases	0	2	15	12	4	4	1	38
Kinki (Kyoto– Osaka)	Rate (per 100,000)	*0.4*	*0.7*	*2.5*	*5.5*	*0*	*0.7*	*0*	*0.9 (1.5)*
	New cases	7	6	18	6	0	1	0	38
Kyushu (Fukuoka– Kumamoto)	Rate (per 100,000)	*0*	*0*	*0*	*2.6*	*0*	*0.7*	*0*	*0.5 (0.5)*
	New cases	0	0	0	2	0	1	0	3
Total districts	Rate (per 100,000)	*0.6*	*2.8*	*3.3*	*6.2*	*0.8*	*0.8*	*1.0*	*1.7*
	New cases	19	43	41	32	4	7	3	149

* Primary school.   ** Lower secondary school.

This table was synthesized from previous tables and the JNR notification source.

Chronological trends   The number of new cases showed geometrical increase in the case of the enquête source (Fig. 2) but only a slight increase in the JNR notification source. Though the incidence seems to be increasing, the sharply rising curve will be due mainly to doctors' recent interest in the disease.

Age and sex   In the JSC enquête source, the 20–29 age group had the highest incidence rate in cases with intrathoracic involvement, but no age difference was found in cases with extrathoracic involvement only. No sex difference was found in intrathoracic cases, but females were 3 times more numerous than males in cases where extrathoracic involvement only was revealed. The other sources also gave similar results.

Tuberculin reaction   In the enquête source, 31% of the histologically confirmed cases were tuberculin-positive, while 80% of Japanese people, according to the 1968 tuberculosis prevalence survey, were estimated to show positive reactions. When comparing the rates of positive reactors in the 20–29 age group, 31.3% of the cases with sarcoidosis were tuberculin-positive against 80% of the people in general.

Geographical distribution   In all 3 sources, the cases were more concentrated in the northern districts than in the southern ones. In the JSC enquête source, the incidence rate in Hokkaido, the northern most island, was 6 times as high as that in Kyushu, the southernmost island. In Table 3 and Fig. 3, synthesized from the 2 sources, the corrected incidence rate in Sapporo, a representative city of Hokkaido was 4.8 per 100,000 and in Fukuoka and Kumamoto, representative cities in Kyushu, 0.5, the former rate being about 10 times higher than the latter.

Estimated number of cases with sarcoidosis in Japan   To estimate the number of new cases detectable in the annual mass X-rays, incidence rates by age and districts, as shown in Fig. 3, were applied to the whole population. The estimated number of newly detectable cases was 1,500. As the rates of cases newly discovered through mass X-ray examinations were 50% to 80% in the above 2 sources, the estimated minimum number of new cases occurring in Japan would be from 2,000 to 3,000 a year. These figures do not show a great discrepancy if compared with the prevalence of 4,500 cases given for 1968, as shown in this paper.

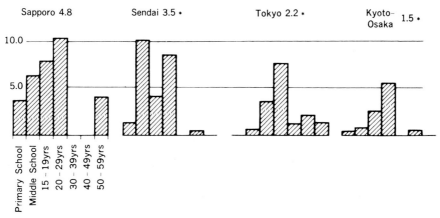

FIG. 3.   Rates of new cases with sarcoidosis detected by once-a-year mass X-rays (per 100,000).

 * Corrected to the Sapporo population.

REFERENCES

1. Tuberculosis Prevalence Survey Result. 1968. Japanese Ministry of Health and Welfare.
2. Hosoda, Y., Chiba, Y. and Nobechi, K. 1967. Incidence and prevalence of sarcoidosis in Japan. *La Sarcoidose. Rapp. IVe Int. Conf.* Masson et cie. p. 361.

Epidemiology of Sarcoidosis in a Japanese Working Group
—A ten-year study—

Y. Hiraga[1], Y. Hosoda[2], M. Odaka[2], K. Takeuchi[3], T. Takahara[2],

K. Kondo[2], T. Kurihara[2], H. Osada[4] S. Miura[5], T. Tameshige[5],

M. Kanatomi[6], I. Zenda[7], H. Ohtake[2] and Y. Chiba[4]

Even in sarcoidosis surveys by notification, it is quite difficult to collect asymptomatic cases. Mass chest X-ray surveys may fill up this omission to some extent. The best possible method of notification would require symptomatic cases to visit clinics and asymptomatic cases to be screened by mass X-rays at short intervals. The Japanese National Railways' (JNR) Sarcoidosis Study Team organized by JNR physicians, commenced in 1961 a joint study for the registration of all sarcoidosis cases occurring in workers who had been mass X-rayed at least once a year. Part of the results were reported at previous International Sarcoidosis Conferences. The workers, about 460,000 aged from 18 to 55, (3% being female) were distributed across the nation. In addition to notifying the cases to the study centre, all member physicians were requested to confirm cases occurring during the year on the year-end enquête cards.

During the observation period, 66 cases were notified. All but 3 had BHL in chest X-ray examinations. The average incidence rate was 1.5 per 100,000.

The incidence rates by age were; 4.0 in the 18–19 age group, 6.2 in the 24–25 group, 3.3 in the 26–29 group, 0.6 in the 30–34 group, 0.1 in the 35–39 group, 0.6 in the 40–44 group, 1.0 in the 45–49 group and 0.9 in the 50-and-over group. The highest rate was found in the 20–24 age group with a small peak in the 40–44 group. (Fig. 1).

Of 66 notified cases, 61 were male and only 5 female. The female incidence rate seems a little higher than the male one though no valid conclusion could be drawn from the limited numbered of cases under study.

As for the mode of discovery, 83.3% of the cases were discovered at the annual mass X-ray surveys which were enforced by the Antituberculosis Law, 10.6% by subjective symptoms and the remaining 6.1% by other means, such as promotion physical examinations (Table 1). These results offer some contrast with the Japan Sarcoidosis Committee enquête surveys, which showed about 50% of the cases to have been discovered by subjective symptoms. In other words, if mass chest X-ray surveys had not been carried out once a year, the notified cases would have been less than 20% of the actual number.

---

1) *JNR Sapporo Hospital, Sapporo, Japan.*
2) *JNR Central Health Institute, Tokyo, Japan.*
3) *JNR Osaka Health Control Institute, Osaka, Japan.*
4) *JNR Central Hospital, Tokyo, Japan.*
5) *JNR Moji Health Service, Fukuoka, Japan.*
6) *JNR Moji Railway Division, Fukuoka, Japan.*
7) *JNR Hiroshima Hospital, Hiroshima, Japan.*

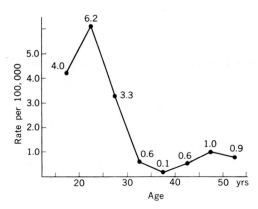

FIG. 1.   Incidence rate of newly discovered cases with sarcoidosis during 1961–70 (per 100,000), JNR.

TABLE 1.   Modes of discovery of sarcoidosis in JNR.

Modes of discovery	Cases	Percent
Mass X-ray surveys	55	83.3
Subjective symptoms	7	10.6
Others	4	6.1
Total	66	100.0

TABLE 2.

	Less than 29 yrs old						More than 30 yrs old					
	Population*	No. of cases	Incidence rate	Population	No. of cases	Incidence rate (100,000)	Population*	No. of cases	Incidence rate	Population	No. of cases	Incidence rate (100,000)
Hokkaido	95	10	10.5				392	4	1.0			
Tohoku	65	4	6.2	523	35	6.7	414	0	—	2248	16	0.7
Kanto	211	14	6.6				801	10	1.2			
Chubu	152	7	4.6				641	2	0.4			
Kinki	124	7	5.6				459	3	0.7			
Chugoku Shikoku	86	1	1.2	291	11	3.8	491	0	—	1388	4	0.3
Kyushu	81	3	3.7				438	1	0.2			

* The number (thousand) of workers in 1964 were 10-folded.

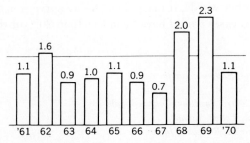

FIG. 2.   Incidence rate (per 100,000) of sarcoidosis using the 1961 population numbering 437,900.

The annual incidence rates fluctuated between 0.7 and 2.3 per 100,000 on the basis of the 1961 population; 1.1 in 1961, 1.6 in 1962, 0.9 in 1963, 1.0 in 1964, 1.1 in 1965, 0.9 in 1966, 0.7 in 1967, 2.0 in 1968, 2.3 in 1969 and 1.1 in 1970 (Fig. 2). The incidence rates were a little higher in the 1961–65 period[1,7] than in the 1966–70 period,[1,2] the difference being significant (Table 3). Such a tendency contrasted with the sharp rise of the rates in the results obtained by the JSC surveys. These 2 results suggest that the increased incidence rates were mainly caused by the greater interest of physicians in this disease.

The incidence rates by district during the whole observation period were 1.8 in the northern district and 0.9 in the southern. In an analysis of the rates for cases under the age of 29, these were 10.5 in Hokkaido, 6.6 in the Kanto area, 5.6 in the Kinki area and 3.7 in Kyushu (Table 2). Above the age of 30, the difference in incidence rates by districts could no longer be considered valid for the north and south, probably due to the small number of cases that could be statistically analysed.

When the results are considered separately for the periods 1961–65 and 1966–70, the incidence rates in the north were higher than in the south during the earlier period, and lower in the later period. As shown in Table 3, the 1961–65 incidence rate in the below-30 age group was 17.0 in the northernmost part, i.e. Hokkaido, and null in the Kinki area, where Osaka and Kyoto are located, while the 1965–70 incidence rate in the same age group was 3.2 in Hokkaido and 7.8 in the Kinki area. There was no difference in the age distribution and the involved sites among districts though the cases with persisting pulmonary parenchymal lesions were found to be slightly higher in Hokkaido than in other districts.

TABLE 3. Incidence rate of sarcoidosis by district, age and period.

North ↕ South	1961–65				1966–70			
	below-29 age group		above-30 age group		below-29 age group		above-30 age group	
	Cases/ observed persons	Rate	Cases/ observed persons	Rate	Cases/ observed persons	Rate	Cases/ observed persons	Rate
Hokkaido	8/ 47,500	17.0	2/196,000	1.0	2/620,000	3.2	2/187,000	1.0
Tohoku	2/ 32,500	6.2	0/207,000	0	2/ 50,000	4.0	0/196,000	0
Kanto	6/105,500	5.7	3/400,500	0.7	8/160,000	5.0	7/381,500	1.8
Chubu	0/ 76,000	0	3/320,500	0.6	7/108,000	6.4	0/314,500	0
Kinki	0/ 62.000	0	0/229,500	0	7/ 91,500	7.8	3/221,500	1.4
Chugoku	1/ 37,000	2.7	0/189,500	0	0/525,000	0	0/176,500	0
Shikoku	0/ 6,000	0	0/ 36,500	0	0/ 11,000	0	0/ 51,000	0
Kyushu	2/ 40,500	2.5	1/219,000	0.5	2/ 54,500	3.7	0/202,500	0
Total	18/407,000	4.5	8/1798,500	0.4	28/1620,000	4.7	12/1730,500	0.7
	26/2205,500	1.2			40/3350,000	1.7		

REFERENCES

1. Bauer, H. J., and Löfgren, S. 1964. International study of pulmonary sarcoidosis in mass chest radiography. *Acta Med. Scand.* suppl. **425**: 103.
2. Hosoda, Y., Chiba, Y., and Nobechi, K. 1967. Incidence and prevalence of sarcoidosis in Japan *La Sarcoidose. Rapp. IVe Int. Conf.* Masson ét cie. p. 361.

3. Odaka, M., Akagi, Y., Hiraga, Y., Hosoda, Y., and Chiba, Y. 1969. Incidence rate of sarcoidosis in a defined group of Japanese population. *Proc. Fifth Int. Conf. on Sarcoidosis.* p. 311.

The Search for Sarcoidosis in Korea

JAY Q. LEE AND WOONG-KU LEE
Lee Chest Clinic, Seoul, Korea

Sarcoidosis has been found in almost every country in which it was sought. The search for sarcoidosis in Korea has been stimulated by work in our neighbouring country, Japan, where they have found a considerable number of sarcoidosis cases since the early 1960's concurrent with a marked decline in tuberculosis, and we are deeply indebted to Japanese scholars for the groundwork for sarcoidosis case-finding attempts in Korea.

The nationwide survey on tuberculosis in Korea in 1970 revealed for the first time in the nation's history a decrease in the prevalence of tuberculosis to 4.2% from a rate of 5.1% in 1965. In view of the fact that the incidence of sarcoidosis has been rising in countries where tuberculosis is on the wane, we considered it worthwhile to search for sarcoidosis in Korea at the present time. So far, not a single case of sarcoidosis has been reported in Korea except for a suspected ocular involvement which was lost to follow-up.

In August, 1971, Dr Teramatsu Oshima and his colleagues of Kyoto University came to Seoul, and we reviewed a large series of chest X-rays to single out cases of bilateral hilar lymphadenopathy, a suggestive radiological sign of sarcoidosis. The results are shown in Table 1.

TABLE 1. Four cases of BHL, Lee Chest Clinic.

Name	Sex	Age	OT	Kveim	Skin biopsy	Scalene biopsy
Chung, J. I.	F	19	(−)	(−)		
Kim, Y. M.	M	21	(−)	(−)	(−)	
Chang, J. K.	M	21	(−)	(−)		
Choi, J. C.	M	47	(+)	(−)	(−)	(−)

Among the 27 radiologically identified bilateral hilar lymphadenopathy, 2 cases appeared very striking, but 1 gave a strong positive reaction to PPD and the lymphadenopathy improved with chemotherapy for tuberculosis. The other case did not respond to our call for follow-up.

Since then we have reviewed several series of mass chest X-rays and identified many more cases of bilateral hilar lymphadenopathy. I will describe each series and their characteristic features.

1. Railroad employees and their families, about 40,000 films; 4 cases of BHL. The railroad company, a government enterprise, has achieved outstanding tuberculosis control among their employees in the past 20 years, and their tuberculosis prevalence rate was less than 1.0% when the national average stood at 5.1%.

2. Ewha Women's University students, about 6,000 films; 53 cases of BHL, but all PPD-positive. The female university students were mainly from relatively well-to-do

307

families and belonged to the age range 18–23 which represented the ages yielding higher incidences of sarcoidosis in Japan.

3.   Bae-Wha Girl's High School students, 2,000 films; girls in the age range 15–17, 4 cases of BHL.

4.   Soong Jun University students, 1,000 films; men with an average age of 20 years, 3 cases of BHL.

5.   Selected cases from the outpatients of my own chest clinic; 4 cases of BHL. Kveim tests were performed on all 4, and biopsies was taken.

Kveim tests were performed on 18 cases altogether, but all turned out negative. Skin biopsy over the area of the test was taken from 4 of the 18 cases in spite of negative reactions, and parts of each biopsy specimen were sent to both the National Medical Center in Seoul and Kyoto University in Japan simultaneously for independent microscopic studies. Both reported negative findings for sarcoidosis granulomas in the examined tissues.

The above is the result of our search for sarcoidosis in Korea from August, 1971 through July, 1972. We have not been able to find any cases belonging to Groups I, II and III of the international diagnostic criteria of sarcoidosis, but found a few cases for which Group IV could not be ruled out.

Our failure to prove a single case of sarcoidosis has not discouraged our search for the disease in Korea. However, it may be a reflection of the fact that, although the prevalence of tuberculosis has been declining in Korea, the current rate of 4.2% is considerably higher than the rate of 3.0% in Japan 10 years ago when sarcoidosis began to appear in that country. It may still take a long time for tuberculosis to be substantially reduced and for sarcoidosis to emerge as a tangible clinical entity in Korea.

Sarcoidosis in Taiwan

Sze-Piao Yang and Min-Chien Wu

Department of Internal Medicine, National Taiwan University Hospital, Taiwan

Taiwan is an island located in the East China Sea between the Philippines and the Ryukyu Islands. It has a total area of nearly 14,000 square miles and population of 15 million, 99% of which are Chinese.

Sarcoidosis is a rare disease in Taiwan. Notification from major hospitals throughout the island revealed that only 6 cases have been found during the past 15 years. The clinical data of these cases are summarized as follows:

TABLE 1.

Case No. and name	Case 1 CYN	Case 2 WW	Case 3 TKF	Case 4 SSS	Case 5 TYS	Case 6 TCH
Age, & sex	36 M	29 F	56 F	27 M	28 M	27 M
Occupation	Teacher	Nurse	Housewife	Medical student	Dentist	Teacher
Source	NTUH	VGH	NTUH	TGH	NTUH	NTUH
Year diagnosed	1956	1962	1967	1968	1970	1971
Symptoms	Fatigue	Visual Dist.	Fatigue	Mild cough	None	None
Chest X-ray findings	Miliary	Miliary	BHL	BHL	BHL and parenchymatous patchy infilt.	BHL
Extrapulmonary manifestations	Heart, neck LN Liver Kidney	Eye, skin	None	None	None	None
Histological proof from	Neck LN	Skin	Med. LN	Med. LN	Med. LN	Not done
Tuberculin test	(−)	(−)	(−)	(+)	(±)	(−)
Kveim Test	Not done	Not done	Not done	(+)	Not done	Not done
Abnormal laboratory findings	Abnormal EKG; RBBB, VPC, RVH. A/G= 3.7/4.0 TTT 12.0 Slightly impaired KFT	Serum Ca 12.5– 17.0 mg% Urine Ca 44 mEq in 24 hour urine	α_2-Globulin 13.7%	ESR increased. No abnormal blood chemistry	Serum Ca 12.5 mg% Eosinophilia	None
Response to steroid	Fair	Good, Relapse after withdrawal	Good	Not given	Good	No effect
Outcome	Died of sudden heart attack on Sept. 10, 1959	Live and well in USA	Live and well	Live and well	Live and well in USA	Live and well

TABLE 1. Description of Thai sarcoidosis cases.

	Clinical	X-ray	Lab.	Skin tests	Biopsy	Rx
1952	No symptom, no signs	Thin infiltration bilat.	—	—	Thoracotomy +ve	—
1958	Female, 17 yrs fever, cough liver 3 fb.	RHL and reticulo-nodular mottlings bilat.	Serum prot. 9.3 g hypergammaglob. bld. Ca 15.3 mg Sulkowitch 4+	Tuberculin 1000 TU Histoplasmin neg.	Thoracotomy and liver +ve	Prednisone
1958	Female, 30 yrs cerv. lymph nodes bilat. liver and spleen 3 fb.	BHL c calc. primary complex	Serum prot. 8.5 g hypergammaglob. bld. Ca 15.3 mg Sulkowitch 2+	Tuberculin 100 TU Histoplasmin neg.	Lt. supraclav. lymph node +ve liver neg.	Prednisone
1964	Male, 37 yrs intractable flu liver 3 fb. spleen just palpable	BHL c calc.	Serum prot. 8.0 g hypergammaglob. bld. Ca 15.5 mg Sulkowitch 1+	Tuberculin 100 TU neg.	Liver, supraclav. lymph node and bronchus +ve	Triamcinolone
1967	Male, 53 yrs cough	Infiltration both upper and calc. primary complex	Serum prot. 7.3 g eugammaglob. bld. Ca 8.2 mg urine Ca 0.272 g/24 hrs	Tuberculin 100 TU neg. histoplasmin 10 mm Kveim neg.	Thoracotomy +ve	—
1968	Female, 32 yrs chest oppression and cough	BHL and infiltration rt. perihilar	Serum prot. 8.0 g eugammaglob. bld. Ca 10.2 mg urine Ca 0.026 g/24 hrs	Tuberculin 10 TU 14 mm Kveim neg.	Thoracotomy +ve liver, bronchus, and cerv. lymph node neg.	INH+PAS
1968	Male, 35 yrs cough	BHL	Eugammaglob.	Tuberculin 10 TU 17 mm Kveim +ve	—	INH+PAS

TABLE 2. Mass chest radiographical surveys and positive rates.

Mobile units (1963–71)			Chest clinics		
Provinces	No. exam.	No. +ve	Years	No. exam.	No. +ve
Northern	314,259	21,057	1969	140,072	27,255 (19.46%)
Northeastern	243,985	13,531	1970	137,889	32,759 (23.76%)
Central	1,036,181	46,795	1971	148,960	30,689 (20.60%)
Southern	189,794	9,669			
Overall	1,784,219	91,052 (5.1%)		426,921	90,703 (21.24%)

TABLE 3. Discordance of results of Kveim tests made with and without acid-fast staining.

		Without acid-fast stain			
		+	±	−	
With acid-fast stain	+	1	3	1	5 (12.5%)
	±			2	2
	−	8	1	24	33
		9 (22.5%)	4	27	40

TABLE 4a. Incidence of Kveim reactivity in clinical types of leprosy.

		Without acid-fast stain			
		+	±	−	
Leprosy	T	2 (12.5%)	2	12	16
	L	6 (27.27%)	1	15	22
	D	1 (50%)	1		2
		9 (22.5%)	4	27	40

TABLE 4b. Incidence of Kveim reactivity in clinical types of leprosy.

		Without acid-fast stain			
		+	±	−	
Leprosy	T	2 (12.5%)	1	13	16
	L	2 (9.09%)	1	19	22
	D	1 (50%)		1	2
		5 (12.5%)	2	33	40

CONCLUSIONS

(1)   Sarcoidosis is an extremely rare disease in Thailand, as in neighbouring countries, such as Cambodia, Laos, Vietnam, Malaysia, Singapore, Indonesia, Burma, India, Pakistan, Ceylon, the Philippines, Hong Kong, Taiwan, and Korea. So far there have been only 7 reported cases in Thailand. Mass radiography surveys did not seem to be particularly useful with this condition.

(2)   The Kveim test may be a good diagnostic aid in sarcoidosis, but positive reactions also occur in nonsarcoid conditions, such as leprosy.

REFERENCES

1.   Siltzbach, L. E. 1971. Sarcoidosis. Cecil-Loeb Textbook of Medicine (ed. Beeson, P. B., and McDermott, W.) (13th ed.) Philadelphia: W. B. Saunders. p. 827.

2.   Sirisampan, S. 1952. The Diagnosis of Pulmonary Diseases. *J. Med. Ass. Thailand.* Special number. p. 83.

3.   Bovornkitti, S., and Kangsadal, P. 1959. Sarcoidosis. A Report of Two Cases. *Siriraj Hosp. Gaz.* **11**: 69.

4.   Bovornkitti, S., Chatikavanich, K., Stitnimankarn, T., Purnabhavanga, S., Parnsingha, T., and Indaniyom, C. 1964. Sarcoidosis (Hutchinson-Boeck-Schaumann's Disease). *J. Med. Ass. Thailand* **47**: 689.

5.   Prijyanonda, B., Bovornkitti, S., Mettiyawongse, S., Suwanakul, L., Pushpakom, R., Thasnakorn, P., Keranpongse, Ch., and Viseskul, Ch. 1967. Epidemiological Study of Histoplasmosis in Thailand. VII. Clinical Investigation in Reactors with Intrathoracic Lesions. *J. Dept. Med. Serv.* **16**: 105.

6.   Bovornkitti, S., Prijyanonda, B., Pacharee, P., Chantarakul, N., and Limsila, Th. 1968. Clinical Diagnosis of Sarcoidosis Versus Kveim Test. Report of Three Cases. *J. Med. Ass. Thailand* **51**: 554.

7.   Sunakorn, B. 1972. (Tuberculosis Control Division, Dept. of Health, Bangkok). Personal Communication.

8.   Hurley, T. H., and Bartholomeusz, C. L. 1969. International Sarcoidosis Survey Australian (CSL) Siltzbach-Kveim Test Material. Presented at the *Fifth Int. Conf. on Sarcoidosis.* Prague.

9.   Bovornkitti, S., Ramasutra, Th., Chantarakul, N., Pacharee, P., and Hurley, T. H. 1972. The Kveim Reactivity in Thai Leprosy Patients. *J. Med. Ass. Thailand* **55**: 707.

Further Epidemiologic Investigation of Sarcoidosis in Yugoslavia

STEVAN GOLDMAN AND BRANISLAV DJURIĆ

Institute of Tuberculosis and Chest Diseases, Novi Sad, Yugoslavia

AND

HORST BEHREND

Medizinishe Hochschule Hannover, Hannover, Federal Republic of Germany

When we first presented our data on sarcoidosis in Yugoslavia at the congress in Paris in 1966, we thought it would be too pretentious to discuss the epidemiologic situation of the disease in our country. The only excuse for such an attempt was the view, which we wanted to investigate that sarcoidosis occurs in regions where tuberculosis is in retreat, i.e., the situation is due not to a more frequent occurrence of sarcoidosis, but rather is the result of more intensive diagnostics.

We have conducted a new survey covering the period 1967–1971 including practically the same regions of Yugoslavia as were included in the survey of 1966.

Before analyzing the results of our survey we want to present the epidemiologic situation of tuberculosis in Yugoslavia in brief. The incidence of tuberculosis in Yugoslavia was 267.2 per 100,000 in 1960, 167.6 per 100,000 in 1966, and 129.8 per 100,000 in 1970.

We may speak of intensive studies on sarcoidosis only in 2 regions where tuberculosis is least frequent. These are: Slovenia with a tuberculosis incidence of 208 per 100,000 in 1960, 121 per 100,000 in 1966 and 94.3 per 100,000 in 1970, and Vojvodina with 450 per

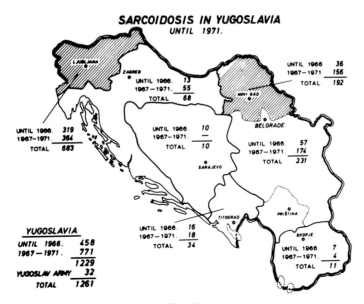

FIG. 1.

100,000 in 1960, 200 per 100,000 in 1966 and 135 per 100,000 in 1971.

Consider the following data on sarcoidosis in Yugoslavia for the year 1966:

A total of 458 cases of sarcoidosis was diagnosed in 1966, of which 190 were discovered radiophotographically. In the period 1967–1971, a total of 771 cases was discovered, almost twice as many as were discovered in 1966. However, we only have complete data for Slovenia and Vojvodina, which are very similar in population level. The remaining regions of Yugoslavia have not been included in the intensive investigation of sarcoidosis, with the exception of greater Belgrade, with a population about 2 million; Vojvodina and Slovenia have similar populations; the total population of Yugoslavia is about 20 million.

These patients were discovered by radiophotography in about the same number as by other methods. According to sex and age the pattern is as follows: women are in the majority; sarcoidosis was found in all age groups, being predominant in the 20–59 group, both in men and women.

The most frequent localization was in mediastinal lymph nodes, followed by the lungs. However, sarcoidosis was found in other organs in a considerable number of patients.

Of 771 cases, 550 (71.3%) were verified histologically. Two hundred Kveim tests were performed, of which 79.5% were found to be positive.

The morbidity in sarcoidosis for the past 5 years was 3.8 per 100,000 for Yugoslavia, 8 per 100,000 for Vojvodina and 21 per 100,000 for Slovenia. Incidence of sarcoidosis was about 5 per 100,000 in Slovenia for 1970 and 1971, whereas it was 3 per 100,000 in Vojvodina for the same period. (Slovenia has the best epidemiologic situation as regards tuberculosis.)

In the following table we can see a strikingly large number of radiophotographically discovered sarcoidosis cases, divided according to sex and age.

TABLE 1. Radiophotographically discovered sarcoidosis by sex and age.

	Age groups								Total
	0–14	15–19	20–29	30–39	40–49	50–59	60–69	over 70	
M	—	11	38	68	70	35	19	2	243
F	—	18	74	101	94	57	30	5	379
Total	—	29	112	169	164	92	49	7	622

Epidemiologic analysis does not provide facts relevant to the etiology, but it is statistically significant in showing that where tuberculosis is in retreat, a greater number of discovered cases of sarcoidosis exist, although we are unable to state whather they are torpid forms of tuberculosis or whether sarcoidosis is more frequent. We would suggest that the clinical picture of sarcoidosis was previously obscured by severe epidemic tuberculosis, and that now this disease has been revealed by modern diagnostic methods.

REFERENCES

1. Goldman S. 1966. Sarcoidosis in Yugoslavia. Paris.
2. Fortič B. 1972. Epidemiology of Sarcoidosis in Slovenia. Golnik.
3. Zengović J. et al. 1972. Sarcoidosis in the Yugoslav Army. Golnik.

On the Incidence of Sarcoidosis in Italy

A. Blasi, A. Giobbi, D. Olivieri, F. Calamari, G. D'Ambrosio, A. De Luca,
S. Marchese, A. Mariotti, G. Nai Fovino and A. Scozia

Clinic of Tuberculosis and Respiratory Diseases, Naples University, Naples, Italy

Our epidemiological data on the incidence of sarcoidosis in Italy are drawn from a limited sample study, performed in some districts of the continental part of Italy, the north, and parts of the peninsular region, the south.

Following the suggestions of Professor Hosoda, our investigations were carried out utilizing the cases discovered by mass X-ray and by clinical registration.

We think that our observations, although covering a fairly small area, may represent the real situation in our country and also explain some epidemiological differences between the north and the south of Italy.

Our study includes the centers of Milan, Alessandria, Venice, Udine and Genoa in the north, and those of Naples, Salerno, Ancona and Cosenza in the south.

In order to unify the data, the study was limited to the 5-year period 1967–1971. The format suggested by Dr Horwitz (Copenhagen) was used to collect information.

From an analysis of the results obtained, which are summarized in the tables, one can draw certain conclusions:

Table 1 shows a noticeable difference in the incidence of the disease between the continental and the peninsular regions of Italy. There are many more cases of sarcoidosis discovered either by mass X-ray or clinically in the north than in the south. Considering only those cases revealed by mass X-ray, in the north the incidence is 14.9 per 100,000, while in the south it is 1.31 per 100,000.

Table 2 shows all the cases detected over 5 years at mass X-ray examinations with

TABLE 1. Sarcoidosis cases detected in some italian cities between 1967 and 1971.

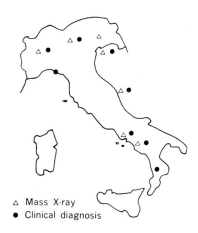

△ Mass X-ray
● Clinical diagnosis

	Detected at mass X-ray		Clinical diagnosis
	No. examined	No. cases	No. cases
Milan	1,396,253	251	180
Alexandria	79,459	6	26
Venice	668,914	25	29
Udine	440,000	104	—
Genoa	—	—	60
	2,584,626	386	295
Naples	77,205	—	4
Salerno	30,100	—	2
Ancona	252,000	5	9
Cosenza	—	—	2
	359,305	5	17

TABLE 2.   Detected at mass X-ray.

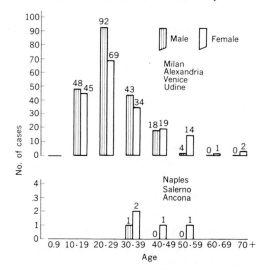

TABLE 3.   Clinical diagnosis.

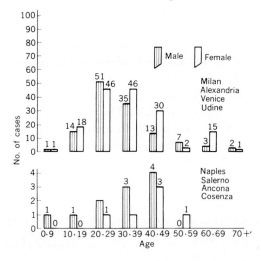

their distribution according to sex and age. Males are predominant in the first 4 decades, while from the fifth decade a higher incidence among females is noted. As regards age, the highest incidence is found in the third decade, with considerable elevations also in the second and fourth decades.

Table 3 collects all the cases clinically discovered over the 5 years. In the north of Italy there is a predominance of females (159 females and 136 males). In the south of Italy there is a predominance of males (11 males and 7 females). The highest incidences of the disease are found in the third, fourth and fifth decades; later than in the group revealed by mass X-ray. This fact is particularly important becouse it shows that mass X-ray can reveal cases which otherwise would not be discovered by clinical diagnosis until later.

The Frequency of Sarcoidosis in Finland

Olof Selroos

Fourth Department of Medicine, Helsinki University Central Hospital, Helsinki, Finland

During the past decade, considerable interest has been devoted to the frequency of sarcoidosis in Finland. In the neighbouring country, Sweden, the incidence of sarcoidosis is high, about 10 times as great as that in Finland.[1] Attempts to explain the difference have included divergent aspects of the diagnostic criteria applied, together with variations in tuberculosis, socioeconomic and enviromental situations. The BCG vaccination procedures are the same in the 2 countries.

For estimation of the true frequency of sarcoidosis in Finland, several prevalence and incidence studies have been carried out.

PREVALENCE OF SARCOIDOSIS IN FINLAND

In 1962–1967, a large prevalence study was carried out in 12 districts with divergences in the tuberculosis situation.[2] In all, 1,530,000 radiographs were taken and examined by 2 physicians; the final diagnosis was established in hospital. The prevalence of clinically verified sarcoidosis ranged from 2.3 to 16.7 per 100,000 examined, with a mean prevalence of 7.5 per 100,000. No correlation was observable with the situation in regard to tuberculosis. The highest prevalence was noted in the tuberculosis district of Raseborg, where the clinical staff had for many years been particularly interested in sarcoidosis.

INCIDENCE OF SARCOIDOSIS IN FINLAND

During the same period, 1961–1967, an incidence study was made in the same 12 districts as those selected for the prevalence study. All sarcoidosis patients were registered, irrespective of the mode of detection.[2] The average annual incidence of new cases ranged from 3.0 to 12.0 per 100,000 of population, with a mean value of 5.3 per 100,000 (6.8 per 100,000 of population above the age of 15). The differences between the districts were less than those noted in the prevalence study, and no correlation was apparent with the actual tuberculosis situation. It is noteworthy that no patient was detected below the age of 15.

The annual incidence of sarcoidosis has also been estimated by notification of all new cases diagnosed in hospitals throughout the entire country. The first registration was made in 1960; only 55 new cases were detected. Annual registration has been practicable since 1967. In 1967, 220 new cases were registered, and in 1968–1970 more than 300 annually (Table 1). For the period 1968–1970, the mean annual incidence of new cases was 7.5 per 100,000 of population, and 10.2 per 100,000 above the age of 15.

Of the 1,265 new sarcoidosis patients detected in 1967–1970, 789 (62.4%) were female. The highest incidence, irrespective of sex, was recorded in the age group 30–39

TABLE 1. Annual incidence of confirmed sarcoidosis in Finland in 1967–1970.

Year	No. of new cases			Incidence per 100,000 of population above the age of 15
	Women	Men	Total	
1967	146	74	220	6.4
1968	221	158	379	11.0
1969	199	123	322	9.4
1970	223	121	344	10.0

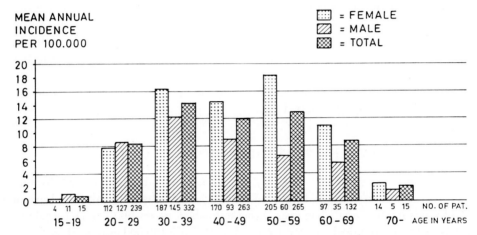

FIG. 1. Mean annual incidence of new sarcoidosis cases in Finland in 1967–1970 according to age and sex.

years. For females, the highest incidence was apparent in the age group 50–59 years (Fig. 1). Only 14.7% of the female patients were below the age of 30. This atypical age distribution of Finnish female sarcoidosis patients has been noted earlier.[2]

Of the new cases diagnosed in 1967–1970, 30% were detected at mass radiographic surveys, while 70% were diagnosed following the appearance of symptoms or signs of sarcoidosis. The diagnosis was established by a typical clinical picture in all cases, and in 73% of cases by a positive biopsy specimen and/or positive Kveim test.

DISCUSSION

It is probable that the frequency figures for the years in the early 1960's are too small, as a result of inadequate diagnostic methods and insufficient knowledge of the clinical features of the disease. The figures for recent years, which indicate an annual incidence of about 10 new cases per 100,000 of population above the age of 15, seem to be the closest approach to the truth, although a small proportion of cases always escapes recognition.

Divergences in the occurrence of tuberculosis in different areas of Finland do not explain regional differences in the frequency of sarcoidosis. It is thus improbable that a different incidence rate for tuberculosis accounts for the divergences in the incidence of sarcoidosis between Sweden and Finland. This investigation also excludes the possibility of unsatisfactory diagnostic procedures in the Finnish series. The real cause of the difference still remains obscure.

Since the 1950's, considerable emigration has been in progress from Finland to Sweden. To date, about 350,000 Finns, for the most part young people, are living in Sweden. Study of the frequency of sarcoidosis in this particular population might provide valuable information on the morbidity of sarcoidosis in the 2 countries.

REFERENCES

1. Bauer, H. J., and Löfgren, S. 1964. International study of pulmonary sarcoidosis in mass chest radiography. *Acta Med. Scand.* Suppl. **425**: 103–105.
2. Selroos, O. 1969. The frequency, clinical picture and prognosis of pulmonary sarcoidosis in Finland. *Acta Med. Scand.* Suppl. **503**: 1–73.

DISCUSSION

1

Chairmen: A. BLASI AND Å. HANNGREN

DR HIRAGA: Hokkaido has the highest incidence rate of sarcoidosis in Japan. In a village in Hokkaido, many cases of BHL were found by mass X-ray examination. As detailed examinations have not yet been completed, I shall report just the outline of the results. In Kamifuiano, in the center of Hokkaido, more than 20 cases of sarcoidosis out of 3,000 inhabitants were detected by mass X-ray. In Asahino, at the eastern end of the town, 6 BHL cases and 10 suspected BHL cases were found, out of the 889 examined. The age of the examined people ranged from 20 to 60, and the age of the BHL cases, between 20 and 30.

DR ISRAEL: The admirably thorough studies that have been carried out in Japan, Korea, Taiwan and Thailand seem to settle the question that has concerned us for some time:— whether sarcoidosis in the Orient is infrequent or merely unrecognized. I think it now clear that the frequency is indeed low. However the difference between Japan and European countries is not so very great.

Two countries from which data are available regarding annual attack rates are Denmark and England and there the annual attack rates are 5 per 100,000. I believe Dr Hosoda's figure for all of Japan is 1.5 per 100,000, which although lower is of the same order of magnitude. I think the most striking difference between the Japanese observations and those everywhere else, is in the age distribution. Apparently in Japan the disease is recognized or occurs at a younger age than it does elsewhere. This might be regarded as an argument for an infectious agent. The other remarkable feature of the Japanese study is that it shows a striking difference between northern and southern Japan, a similar pattern to that between northern and southern Europe. Yet English studies show no differences of significance between northern and southern counties, and studies of American war veterans now appear to show no real difference between the northern and southern states.

DR BYRNE: It is perhaps already being done, but if it's not, I would like to suggest that with this wonderful captive population you have, Dr Hosoda, which you are able to get in for periodic chest X-rays, that it would be an easy matter to collect a few ml of serum each time. Seroepidemiological studies similar to the one I reported yesterday then could be done in an attempt to relate different patterns of susceptibility or experience with various agents to the geographical distribution of the disease.

DR HOSODA: We have collected the sera from all over the country, and shall of course continue our collecting work in the Future.

DR HANNGREN: May Dr Hosoda's finding of higher prevalence in high school students fits with Dr Wu's presentation of the professions of his patients? The professions of those were connected with children or youths. Are those people more likely to have frequent X-rays examinations than other occupations, and hence increased likelihood of detections or is it an expression of a contagious disease in youth?

DR WU: Although correlation analyses were not performed, it is difficult to find any definite relationship between occupation and sarcoidosis from our limited number of cases.

DR HANNGREN: I should like to put another question to Dr James concerning epi-

322

demiology. Looking in the old book from the third Conference in Stockholm in 1963, I put the prevalence figures together and found Ireland among the group of countries which have a high prevalence, and Great Britain, with London, in the middle group, but also Northern Ireland. It therefore occured to me that it might be a "political" disease.

DR JAMES: Routine mass chest radiography in London reveals pulmonary sarcoidosis in about 20 per 100,000. If you restrict the sample to the Irish this figure becomes 100, and if the sample comprises only Irish women then the figure is 200 per 100,000. This situation is similar to the increased incidence noted by Dr Siltzbach amongst Puerto Ricans in New York City. It may be due to the migration of simple country folk to a sophisticated urban setting.

It would be interesting to note whether agricultural peasants of Asia are prone to develop it after they have lived in Tokyo for about 3 years. The other factor in the Irish women is hormonal, for they are all in the child-bearing years of life and are multiparous. The oral contraceptive pill is another hormonal factor which may provoke the appearance of erythema nodosum or uveitis.

I wish to congratulate those who are working hard, searching for sarcoidosis in different countries. I would advise them to establish a weekly Sarcoidosis Clinic in which a chest physician, ophthalmologist and dermatologist meet regularly. There is no doubt that the incidence of ocular sarcoidosis rises when slit lamp examination is undertaken routinely, or bone crysts are seen more often when X-rays are carried out selectively in those with chronic skin lesions.

2

Chairmen: Y. HOSODA AND B. DJURIĆ

DR ISRAEL: I would like to point out the great progress that has been made since earlier conferences in the presentation of epidemiologic data. At the 1960 conference, the reports were a meaningless mixture of incidence and prevalence data. A plea was made at that time to try to distinguish between studies which measured the prevalence of the disease in random surveys and hospital studies, and data reflecting the annual attack rate, the true incidence of the disease. In each subsequent conference, there has been a little progress. The present conference marks a real milestone since we now have precise data on the incidence in many countries. For the first time, we are able to compare the frequency or incidence of sarcoidosis in many parts of the world.

DR DJURIĆ: There is an age distribution between the northern and southern parts of Sweden as represented in the Uneå Hospital and the Karolinska Hospital in Stockholm. In females, there is a clear difference

between the 2 regions in age distribution. The same thing is seen for males. Annual distribution shows a different configuration, in the case of Uneå than in the Stockholm material. In the former, patients are found in inland areas where there are both familiar and enviromental connections with tuberculosis. In the Stockholm material, no such connection is found.

DR HOSODA: Before this conference, with the kind assistance of Dr Hororitz in Copenhagen, we had a project for the global epidemiological survey of sarcoidosis by participants from various countries, emphasising comparative age specific frequencies. We sent questionnaires to several participants in their countries. I shall show some of the results.

DR BLASI: I would like to say something about the comparative prevalence in Italy of sarcoidosis and tuberculosis. The respective trends in prevalence of sarcoidosis and

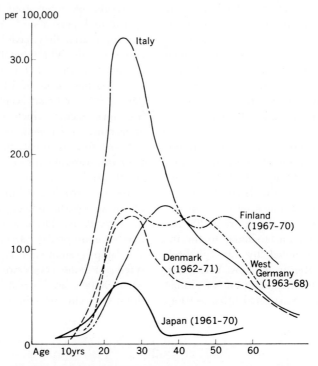

Incidence of Sarcoidosis by Age.
(Denmark reported by Horwitz, Finland by O. Selroos,
West Germany by H. Behrend, Italy by A. Blasi and
Japan by Y. Hosoda et al.)

tuberculosis have reversed themselves in Italy. At the present time, the highest number of sarcoidosis cases occur in young men, and youths, in their second decade, while the prevalence of tuberculosis is higher in older men. This has been the recent pattern of behaviour of tuberculosis in relation to sarcoidosis.

DR HOSODA: In the Second and Third Conferences in Washington and Stockholm, as Dr Israel mentioned, epidemiological studies were very active, but not complete. With the development of cellular immunity studies, the main interest in this disease has shifted to immunology. However, I am not convinced that the role of the epidemiology of sarcoidosis has seen an end. Epidemiology as a final goal will detect the cause of the disease. Shall we now start epidemiological studies aiming at its cause?

VII EXTRAPULMONARY INVOLVEMENT

A Case Report of Heerfordt's Syndrome

Ippei Fujimori, Katsuji Honda, Nobuyuki Gonda,
Hiroshi Koizumi and Masataka Katsu

Department of Internal Medicine, Kawasaki City Hospital, Kawasaki, Japan

Heerfordt's syndrome is a rare disorder characterised by a swelling of the parotid glands and uveitis, and is frequently associated with central nerve palsy. Recently we encounted 1 case, shedding light on previous reports of this illness in Japan.

The patient was a 34-year-old housewife with a chief complaint of swelling of the bilateral parotid glands. Her family history and past history were not contributory. In early July, in 1971, she noticed the onset of an intermittent low-grade fever, a general weakness and a feeling of pressure in the anterior chest. In the middle of July she noticed a swelling of the bilateral parotid glands. About the same time she also had photophobia. She was seen by an ophthalmologist who diagnosed uveitis. She was treated with an oral steroid hormone and eyedrops. In early August the swelling of the parotid glands was aggravated and she developed a continuous high fever. She was admitted to the department of medicine in this hospital. Physical examination on admission revealed a well-developed and well-nourished female. Her temperature was 37.5°C. There was same diffuse swelling and tenderness of the bilateral parotid glands and several hard, palpable, pea-sized lymph nodes were to be found on both sides of the neck. No dullness was noted on percussion of the lung and no rattle on auscultation. The abdomen was distended.

There were several erythematous nodules in the bilateral mid to lower abdominal walls. The liver, spleen and kidney were not palpable. There was no mass nor ascites. There was no edema in her extremities and no deformity in the joints. A neurological examination revealed no motor or sensory defect nor any pathologic reflex.

Laboratory data are shown in Tables 1 and 2. Urinalysis was normal.

Occult blood in her stool was positive. There was mild anemia of RBC 3.78 million; hemoglobin 11.2 g/dl; hematocrit 38%; WBC was slightly decreased to 4,100. The blood sedimentation rate was normal. Serum electrolyte was normal. The serum calcium level had a normal value of 4.5 mEq/L. Serum protein was normal. There was no elevation of gammaglobulin. CRP and LFT were negative. TA, TRC, ANF and anti-DNA antibody were all negative. An immunoglobulin study was within normal limits. Pulmonary function tests were normal. An electrocardiogram was normal. Schirmer's test gave normal results of 15 mm bilateral. Chest X-rays revealed an increase in pulmonary markings throughout tne lungs and showed a swelling of the bilateral hilar lymph nodes compatible with sarcoidosis. Hospital course is shown in Fig. 1. On admission, the patient was treated with prednisolone 20 mg daily.

In spite of this she continued to have fever. On the sixth hospital day she developed numbness in the left side of her face, a drooping of the left corner of the mouth and disappearance of the left nasolabial fold, suggesting left peripheral facial nerve palsy. On the eighth hospital day, INH 0.6 g daily and sulfisomezole 1.0 g were started. Fever

TABLE 1. Laboratory findings (1).

Urinalysis		ESR	11 mm/lh
protein	(−)	Blood chemistry	
glucose	(−)	Na	128 mEq/L
urobilinogen	(±)	Cl	107 mEq/L
Stool examination		K	3.3 mEq/L
occult blood	(+)	Ca	4.5 mEq/L
parasite eggs	(−)	BUN	13.3 mg/dl
Blood		Creati.	1.0 mg/dl
RBC	378×10^4	Uric acid	4.7 mg/dl
Hb	11.2 g/dl	Chol.	126 mg/dl
Ht	38%	TG	105 mg/dl
WBC	4100	Liver function tests	
Bands	9%	Icterus index	8
Neutrophils	40	ZTT	5.5 μ
Lymphocytes	45	AP	2.0 μ (Bessey)
Monocytes	3	SGOT	30 μ
Eosinophils	3	SGPT	33 μ
Platelet	11.5×10^4	LDH	290 μ

TABLE 2. Laboratory findings (2).

Serum protein fraction		Immunoglobulin	
TP	6.0 g/dl	IgA	128 mg/dl
A/G	1.71	IgG	880 mg/dl
albumin	63.1%	IgM	89 mg/dl
α-gl	6.6	Pulmonary function test	
β-	7.9	VC	3050 cc
γ-	22.4	%VC	140%
CRP	(−)	FEV 1.0	2600 cc
LFT	(−)	FEV 1.0%	85%
ASO	12 Todd unit	Index of	
Wa-R	(−)	air trapping	+1.6%
TA test	(−)	ECG within normal limits	
TRC	(−)	Schirmer's test	
ANF	(−)	l	15 mm
anti-DNA		r	15 mm
antibody	(−)		

decreased gradually in 10 days. The swelling of the parotid glands and the cervical lymph nodes disappeared between the twentieth and the thirtieth hospital day. However uveitis and facial nerve palsy existed even on the fiftieth hospital day and continued after discharge.

The blood sedimentation rate slightly increased after 30 hospital days. The serum calcium level remained within the normal range. Mantoux reaction was performed on the eighth hospital day and was negative. A scalene lymph node biopsy was performed on the sixteenth hospital day. No histological abnormality was found in the specimen. After discontinuation of the steroid hormone, a Kveim reaction was performed on the

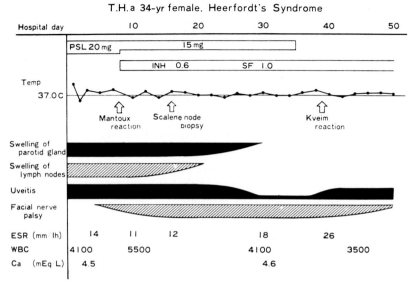

T.H. a 34-yr female. Heerfordt's Syndrome

FIG. 1. Clinical course.

TABLE 3. Nine patients with Heerfordt's syndrome in Japan (1956–1972).

Case	Age and sex	Uveitis	Parotid swelling	Facial palsy	Bilateral hilar lymph- adenopathy	Scalene node biopsy	Kveim reaction
1	58 W	+	+	+	+	−	Not
2	15 M	+	+	+	+	+	Not
3	15 M	+	+	+	Not	Not	Not
4	20 W	+	+	+	Not	Not	Not
5	36 W	+	+	−	+	+	+
6	34 W	+	+	+	+	+	+
7	43 W	+	+	+	+	+	Not
8	20 W	+	+	−	−	Not	Not
9	34 W	+	+	+	+	−	−

+ : Positive findings, − : Negative finding, Not : Not performed.

thirty-eighth hospital day and the result was negative. As for the uveitis, sediments in both sides of the rear cornea and warm stream were noted, but hypopyon was not evident and there was no visual disturbance.

With a negative Kveim reaction, a negative scalene node biopsy, and a typical bilateral hilar lymphnode adenopathy, this case should be classified as Group IV sarcoidosis according to the international classification. We diagnosed this case as Heerfordt's syndrome because of the association of the swelling of the parotid glands, uveitis and left facial nerve palsy. This syndrome was reported by Heerfordt for the first time in 1909. He reported 3 cases with swelling of the bilateral parotid glands, uveitis and facial palsy. Prior to this he reported an atypical form with ocular and salivary gland mani- festations which was called uveo-parotid fever in his article. However Heerfordt's syndrome with its 3 typical manifestations has been rare in the literature. Only 130 cases have been reported in Europe and America in 30 years since 1909. In Japan, as

Table 3 shows, only 9 cases have been reported in 16 years since Dr Kitamura's first report in 1956.

Age at the onset of cases ranged between 19 and 58 years old. However half of the cases were in the second and third decade. Seven cases were female, and 2 cases were male. Regarding the clinical manifestations, uveitis, bilateral parotid gland swellings and facial nerve palsy were noted in 6 cases, and 3 cases had only bilateral parotid gland swellings and uveitis. Chest X-rays were taken in 7 cases and in 6 out of these 7 there was bilateral hilar lymphadenopathy.

A scalene node biopsy was performed in 6 cases: 4 of them showed epithelioid cell granulomas and 2 cases, only epithelioid cell formation. In case 9 which I presented as uveitis, bilateral parotid gland swellings, and left facial nerve palsy were noted. There was bilateral lymphadenopathy. However epithelioid cell formation was not found by either scalene node biopsy or a Kveim reaction.

REFERENCES

1. Heerfordt, C. F. 1909. über eine "Febris uveo-parotidea subchronica" an der Glandula parotis und der Uvea des Auges lokalisiert und häufig mit paresen cerebrospinaler Nerven kompliziert, Albrecht v. Graefes Arch. Ophthal. **70**: 254–273.
2. Theobard, G. D., and Wilder, H. L. 1953. Heerfordt's Syndrome. *Trans. Amer. Acad. Ophthal. Otolarying.* **57**: 332–333.
3. Ebihara, I., Takayasu, S., and Ikeda, H. 1959. A Rare Case Of Heerfordt's Disease Complicated With Bilateral Perceptive Deafness. *J. Japan Otolaryng.* **62**: 1568–1572.
4. Greenberg, G., Anderson, R., Sharpstone, P., and James, D. G. 1964. Enlargement Of Parotid Gland Due To Sarcoidosis, *Brit. Med. J.* 861–862.
5. Jackson, H. 1970. Ocular Sarcoidosis. *Postgrad. Med. J.* **46**: 501–504.

Uveo-Parotid Fever (Heerfordt's Syndrome) or Sarcoid Affection of the Eyes and Parotid Glands

NILS STJERNBERG AND LARS-GÖSTA WIMAN

Departments of Lung Diseases and Diseases of Ear, Nose and Throat, University Hospital, Umeå, Sweden

SYNOPSIS

Since Heerfordt first described febris uveo-parotidea subchronica in 1909, only sporadic cases have been reported in the literature, with a few exceptions from Sweden and Great Britain. In 299 sarcoidosis patients from Northern Sweden during 1951–1971 we found 15 cases, most of which showed the complete syndrome with uveitis and parotid gland enlargement and a histopathological verification of sarcoidosis. Fever and cranial nerve pareses were observed in about 50%. Pulmonary lesions appeared in all but 1 patient. Differences in sex, age and geographic distribution are discussed with regard to the general sarcoidosis epidemiology. As in the total sarcoidosis material from this part of Sweden, the majority of patients with the diagnosis of uveo-parotid fever were middle-aged men. Sialometry was performed in 4 cases with inconclusive results. The method, however, is recommended as a diagnostic aid.

INTRODUCTION

In 1909 the Danish ophthalmologist Heerfordt described 3 patients showing pathological changes of the eyes and parotid glands. Two of them also displayed a unilateral facial palsy. All 3, as well as 2 more cases with similar symptoms which he found described in the literature by Daireaux,[1] Pechin[2] and Collomb,[3] ran a chronic and usually febrile course. As Heerfordt[4] considered an inflammatory cause to be the most probable, he suggested the name febris uveo-parotidea subchronica.

The clinical picture in uveo-parotid fever is distinctive and clearly separated from other conditions affecting the eyes and the parotid glands. The most constant finding is uveitis combined with enlargement, unilateral or bilateral, of the parotid gland. Complicating fever and pareses of cranial nerves, mostly the facial, are not always observed. A protracted course over months or years is characteristic of the disease. It is often part of a generalized sarcoidosis with lesions in various organs, such as lymph nodes, lungs, liver, spleen, kidneys, skin, etc.

The histopathological findings in sarcoidosis, however, are still difficult to distinguish from those of tuberculosis, the presence of central necrosis of the epithelioid granulomas being the important basis for differentiation. The diagnosis, therefore, is primarily a clinical one, which may be supported by characteristic histopathological findings in biopsies.

MATERIAL

During a 20-year period, 1951–1971, in the departments of lung diseases and diseases of the ear, nose and throat of the University Hospital in Umeå, 15 cases of uveo-parotid fever were diagnosed. The patients were 10 men and 5 women between 24 and 68 years of age. The mean age was close to 50 years (Table 1).

An increased body temperature of varying duration was found in 7 patients. In the remaining cases there was no fever, or a complete history was impossible to obtain in this respect.

Ocular discomfort of various kinds was present in all patients. A clear uveitis was diagnosed in 8 patients, and by the rose bengal staining test a kerato-conjunctivitis sicca was detected in 3. Conjunctivitis alone was found in 2 patients. Three more patients complained of a protracted course of ocular symptoms including photophobia, blurring of vision, watering, redness and aching or irritation of the eyes. At the first examination several months later these symptoms had disappeared, and an exact diagnosis was no longer possible.

Enlargement of the parotid gland on both sides was noticed in 11 patients. In 3 there was only a right-side swelling. A distinct affection of the parotid gland was missing in 1 patient only. This 53-year-old woman, however, displayed recidivant uveitis and recurrent facial palsies on both the left and right side. Generally the affected parotid gland was enlarged, firm and nontender, the condition lasting from weeks to several months. Six patients developed cranial nerve paralysis, involving the facial nerve in 5 and the oculomotor nerve in 1 case. In the first group they were all of the peripheral type, 3 bilateral and 2 unilateral. The duration varied from 1 month to 1 year.

Other organs were affected in all patients, except a 52-year-old man. Thus, in 13 patients enlarged hilar lymphomas were always found together with lesions of the lung parenchyma. Upon radiological examination of the chest a widespread, diffuse, mottled shadowing was found uniformly distributed in both lungs. Together with bilateral hilar lymphomas, this condition represented an early phase of the disease. Two patients showed a more cloudy shadowing, unequally distributed in the lungs, indicating a later stage of sarcoidosis. The fibrotic stage with irregular, dense shadows alternating with abnormal transradiency all over the lung fields and irreversible in type was disclosed in 3 patients showing disease of long standing. Further sarcoid changes were found in lymph nodes, liver, spleen, kidneys, striated muscle and bones. Hypercalcemia and/or hypercalciuria were demonstrated in many patients and urolithiasis was diagnosed in 2 cases.

In tuberculin testing according to Mantoux, old tuberculin was used at the beginning of the 20-year period. PPD-tuberculin was introduced during the last 5 years. A negative test result was obtained with 1 mg of the old tuberculin or 10 TU PPD-tuberculin in 11 patients, and a slightly positive reaction in 1 patient using 1 mg old tuberculin. In 2 cases the reaction was clearly positive using a low concentration of tuberculin. One patient was never tested.

Biopsy was performed in all patients but 2. The diagnosis of sarcoidosis was histopathologically verified in 12 of these 13 patients. Prescalene node biopsy according to Daniels was positive for sarcoidosis in 7 cases. Biopsy from the parotid gland in 5 patients and from a cervical lymph node in 1 showed sarcoidosis. Mediastinoscopy in 1 patient yielded material insufficient for histopathological diagnosis.

TABLE 1. Uveo-parotid fever, 1951–1971, University Hospital, Umeå, Sweden.

Pat. nr	Age and sex	Fever	Eyes	Parotid glands	Cranial nerves	Other organs affected	Calcium Serum mEq/l	Calcium Urine mg/24 h.	Tuberculin test	Histopathological verification
1.	24 M	No	Conjunctivitis Photophobia	Enlarged unilat.	—	Hilar lgll, lungs	5.1	392	Neg. 10 TU	Parotid gland
2.	36 M	Yes	Uveitis	Enlarged bilat.	—	Hilar lgll, lungs	—	—	Pos. 1 mg	Biopsy not performed
3.	43 F	Yes	Uveitis	Enlarged bilat.	—	Hilar lgll, lungs	—	—	Pos. 0.1 mg	Scalene node
4.	44 M	Yes	Iritis kerato-conjunctivitis	Enlarged bilat.	—	Hilar lgll, lungs	5.3	102	Neg. 10 TU	Scalene node
5.	45 F	No	Impairment of vision	Enlarged bilat.	—	Hilar lgll, lungs	5.4	330	Neg. 10 TU	Scalene node
6.	48 M	No	Kerato-conjunctivitis	Enlarged unilat.	—	Hilar lgll, lungs	4.8	340	Neg. 10 TU	Parotid gland
7.	49 F	Yes	Uveitis	Enlarged unilat.	Facial	Hilar lgll, lungs	—	—	Neg. 1 mg	Negative skin biopsy
8.	52 M	No	Blurring of vision Photophobia	Enlarged bilat.	Facial	Lungs normal	—	—	—	Parotid gland
9.	53 F	No	Iridocyclitis	Normal	Facial	Hilar lgll, lungs Cervical lgll	6.6	763	Neg. 1 mg	Cervical node
10.	53 M	Yes	Conjunctivitis	Enlarged bilat.	Facial	Hilar lgll	5.0 Urolithiasis	228	Pos. 2 TU	Negative mediastinoscopy
11.	54 M	Yes	Uveitis	Enlarged bilat.	—	Hilar lgll, lungs, bones	5.3	—	Neg. 1 mg	Scalene node Parotid gland
12.	55 F	No	Kerato-conjunctivitis	Enlarged bilat.	Facial	Hilar lgll	—	—	Neg. 1 mg	Parotid gland
13.	56 M	No	Uveitis	Enlarged bilat.	—	Hilar lgll, lungs spleen	6.5 Urolithiasis	448	Neg. 1 mg	Scalene node
14.	58 M	Yes	Conjunctivitis	Enlarged bilat.	Oculo-motor	Hilar lgll, lungs	—	—	Neg. 1/100	Scalene node
15.	68 M	No	Uveitis	Enlarged bilat.	—	Hilar lgll, lungs muscle	4.8	408	Neg. 10 TU	Scalene node Muscle

DISCUSSION

The prevalence of uveo-parotid fever largely depends on the prevalence of sarcoidosis in the area in question. During the 20-year period, 1951–1971, in the Västerbotten county in Northern Sweden, we found 299 cases of sarcoidosis among 235,000 inhabitants (1971) (Fig. 1). They were diagnosed clinically, with histopathological verification in about 65%, in hospital departments of lung diseases, internal medicine, diseases of ear, nose and throat and in dispensaries for tuberculosis. The number of true cases of uveo-parotid fever could not be exactly determined. Fifteen patients complied with the strict definition given above (Table 1). In a wider sense using the criteria of uveitis, parotid gland enlargement or cranial nerve pareses in various combinations with bilateral hilar lymphomas, pulmonary lesions or other sarcoid organs, 10 more patients with an incomplete form of Heerfordt's syndrome could be added. The prevalence of this disease is high in Sweden compared with Great Britain (Table 2). In a country-wide investiga-

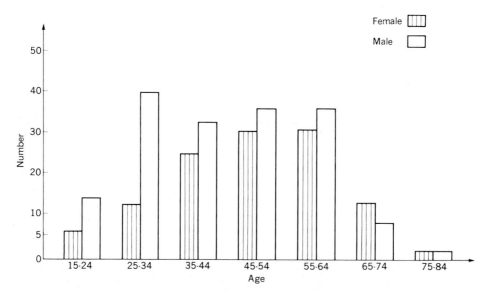

FIG. 1. Sarcoidosis, 1951–71, University Hospital, Umeå, Sweden, Distribution according to sex and age in 299 patients.

TABLE 2. The composition of some sarcoidosis materials with regard to uveo-parotid fever.

Investigator	Year	Sarcoidosis patients No.	Uveo-parotid fever patients	
			No.	%
Heerfordt[4]	1909	—	3	—
Löfgren[7]	1953	212	8	3.8
James[18]	1959	200	3	1.5
Rudberg-Roos[19]	1962	296	3	1.0
Greenberg et al.[16]	1964	388	8	2.1
Scadding[8]	1967	275	6	2.2
Selroos[9]	1969	140	0	—
Stjernberg and Wiman	1972	299	15	5.0

TABLE 3. Prevalence of sarcoidosis in mass chest radiography.

Country	Persons investigated millions	Sarcoidosis patients	
		Total No.	per 100,000
Finland I	1.4	111	8.1
Finland II	1.5	118	7.5
Norway	1.4	387	26.7
Sweden I	1.9	1,023	55
Sweden II	1.4	867	64
Sweden III	0.2	227	120
London	0.9	160	19
France	0.2	20	10
The Netherlands	4.6	994	21.6
Czechoslovakia	3.4	118	3.4
New Zealand	1.1	171	16
Japan	0.2	111	5.6

tion of sarcoidosis in Finland, Selroos (1969) was not able to find a single case of uveo-parotid fever. Compared with other parts of Sweden or other countries, there was a high prevalence of sarcoidosis in the investigated area of Northern Sweden (Table 3).

The sex and age distribution in our investigation differs from that in other materials. Usually females predominate among patients with uveo-parotid fever, as was shown by Garland and Thompson[5] in an analysis of 47 published cases. Berg[6] observed an equal distribution between the sexes among 40 cases selected from the literature. There is usually a predominance of females in all sarcoidosis investigations, e.g. Löfgren,[7] Scadding,[8] Selroos.[9] We found a male: female ratio of 2: 1. This, however, reflects the sex distribution of the total sarcoidosis material investigated in our district comprising 174 male and 125 female patients. The difference is most apparent in the younger age groups (Fig. 1).

Berg[6] found the majority of patients suffering from uveo-parotid fever to be between 11 and 35 years of age, and Garland and Thompson[5] found 62% to be under the age of 30. Two of Heerfordt's[4] cases were children, boys aged 11 and 14, and the third a 27-year-old man. The mean age of our 15 patients was close to 50, much higher than in other reports, but no correlation was made to life expectancy at different periods. Corresponding figures were found in our total sarcoidosis material, in which most of the patients belonged to age groups 45–54 and 55–64. Concerning the pathogenesis, a tuberculous etiology was anticipated in most publications appearing during the 2 and 3 decades following Heerfordt's report.[4] This opinion predominated among Scandinavian and German authors, e.g. Lehmann,[10] Bering[11] and Berg.[6] In Great Britain and America, however, the connection with tuberculosis was more widely questioned, e.g. by Merrill and Oaks.[12] In Sweden, Schaumann[13] collected various clinical conditions showing a similar histopathological picture and applied the name lymphogranulomatosis benigna, and Waldenström[14] demonstrated by clinical, histologic and postmortem examination that uveo-parotid fever must be regarded as a special manifestation of Schaumann's disease. This opinion was also presented by Bruins Slot et al.[15] and others.

In our material the diagnosis of uveo-parotid fever was based on clinical and histopathological features. Tuberculosis could be excluded epidemiologically and clinically, and tubercle bacilli could not be demonstrated in sputum or stomach washings. The negative or weakly positive results of the tuberculin tests were not consistent with tuberculosis in 12 patients, and in 2 positive reactors the biopsy or clinical picture including chest radiography were not conclusive for tuberculosis. A 52-year-old man was not tuberculin-tested, but he had a biopsy positive for sarcoidosis. The histopathological findings could always be regarded as supporting the diagnosis of sarcoidosis. Treatment with adrenocorticotropic hormone (ACTH) or corticosteroids was instituted in all patients and led to regression or full restitution. Today there seems to be no doubt regarding the sarcoid etiology of uveo-parotid fever.

With the introduction of sialometry as a diagnostic aid in diseases of the salivary glands, more exact information became available in parotid affections. The method was used in 4 of our patients. In patient 6 a completely normal secretion was found. No pareses of the cranial nerves were diagnosed in this case, although considerable swelling of the parotid glands on both sides was noticed. The salivary gland secretion was tested by sialometry several times in patient 12 during various phases of the disease. It was quite clear that the secretion varied concomitantly with the bilateral paresis and swelling of the parotid glands. In patient 1 no facial paralysis could be seen, but the test nevertheless showed a decreased secretion. Patient 8 had a very low secretion from all salivary glands, but only a slight paralysis of the left facial nerve.

Thus, the results of sialometry were rather difficult to evaluate and understand in these 4 cases. Sialometry should, however, be used in all cases of uveo-parotid affections, as a decreased secretion in combination with other clinical findings might support the diagnosis of sarcoidosis.

Clinical reports of dryness of the mouth and some degree of aptyalism in combination with facial palsy in uveo-parotid fever were published by Löfgren,[7] Greenberg et al.[16] and Scadding.[8] Hyposecretion of the lacrimal glands is usually found in kerato-conjunctivitis sicca or Sjögren's syndrome.[17] Three of our 15 patients showed signs of kerato-conjunctivitis sicca confirmed by the rose bengal test, but only 1 had a facial palsy (patient 12). In the last patient sialometry also disclosed decreased secretion. The same condition was also diagnosed in patient 6, who had normal secretion and no pareses. In patient 4, with the same diagnosis, sialometry was not performed.

In these few patients the results of clinical and laboratory investigations were inconclusive for an unequivocal diagnosis. Most evidence, however, favoured the diagnosis of sarcoidosis excluding Sjögren's syndrome.

REFERENCES

1. Daireaux. 1899. Paralysie faciale et iritis d'origine ourlienne. Des neurites ourliennes. *Le Bulletin Médical.* p. 227.
2. Pechin, A. 1901. Complications oculaires des oreillons. *Rev. Gén. d'Ophth.* **20**: 445.
3. Collomb, A. 1903. Un cas d'iritis ourlienne. *Revue médicale de la Suisse romande.* **23**: 43.
4. Heerfordt, C. F. 1909. über eine "Febris uveo-parotidea subchronica", an der Glandula parotis und der Uvea des Auges lokalisiert und häufig mit Paresen cerebrospinaler Nerven kompliziert. *v. Graefe's Archiv für Ophthalmologie* **70**: 254–273.
5. Garland, H. G., and Thompson, J. G. 1933. Uveo-parotid tuberculosis (febris uveo-parotidea of Heerfordt). *Quart. J. Med.* **26**: 157–177.
6. Berg, F. 1923. om "Febris uveo-parotidea" (Heerfordt). *Hygiea* **85**: 401–420.

7. Löfgren, S. 1953. Primary Pulmonary Sarcoidosis. *Acata Med. Scand.* **145**: 424–431, 465–474.

8. Scadding, J. G. 1967. Sarcoidosis. London: Eyre and Spottiswoode.

9. Selroos, O. 1969. The Frequency, Clinical Picture and Prognosis of Pulmonary Sarcoidosis in Finland. *Acta Med. Scand.* Suppl. 503.

10. Lehmann, K. 1916. Om Febris uveo-parotidea. *Hospitalstid.*, **9**: 117, 137.

11. Bering, F. 1910. Zur Kenntnis der Boeckschen Sarkoids. *Derm. Z.* **17**: 404.

12. Merril, H. G. and Oaks, L. W. 1931. Uveo-parotitis (Heerfordt): with case report. *Amer. J. Ophthalm.* **14**: 15.

13. Schaumann, J. 1936. Lymphogranulomatosis benigna in the light of prolonged clinical observations and autopsy findings. *Brit. J. Derm.* **48**: 399.

14. Waldenström, J. 1936–1937. Über gutartige, universelle, tuberkuloide Granulome mit Berücksichtigung der Uveoparotitis. Zentralbl. f. d. Ges. *Tuberk.-forschung* **45**: 249.

15. Bruins Slot, W. J., Goedbloed, J., and Goslings, J. 1938. Die Besnier-Boeck-(Schaumann-) sche Krankheit und die Uveo-Parotitis (Heerfordt). *Acta Med. Scand.* **94**: 74.

16. Greenberg, G., Anderson, R., Sharpstone, P., and James, D. G. 1964. Enlargement of Parotid Gland Due to Sarcoidosis. *Brit. Med. J.* **2**: 861–862.

17. Sjögren, H. 1933. Zur Kenntnis der Keratoconjunctivitis sicca. *Acta Ophthalm.* Suppl. 2.

18. James, D. G. 1959. Ocular Sarcoidosis. *Amer. J. Med.* **26**: 331.

19. Rudberg-Roos, I. 1962. The Course and Prognosis of Sarcoidosis as Observed in 296 Cases. *Acta Tuberc. Pneum. Scand.*, Suppl. 52.

Some Outstanding Problems in Sarcoidosis of the Central Nervous System

H. Urich

The London Hospital, London, Great Britain

While there is no doubt that cerebral sarcoidosis forms part of the generalised multisystemic disease, the problem turns up occasionally whether the condition can be limited to the central nervous system without involvement of other organs. Clinically this situation is not uncommon and leads to considerable diagnostic difficulties. However, at autopsy lesions are invariably found in other systems. Rabinowicz[1] in reviewing the literature reached the conclusion that there is no adequately examined case in which the lesions were confined to the CNS. My personal observations tend to confirm these views, although in 1 of my cases the lesions were scanty and could have been missed on cursory examination.

Another probable source of confusion may be giant-celled granulomatous angiitis of the cerebral vessels. In all probability this is a separate entity, unrelated to sarcoidosis, although the similarities are considerable. Some cases in the literature, such as that of Zollinger[2] are interpreted by some writers as examples of sarcoidosis, by others as granulomatous angiitis. The subject has recently been reviewed by Nurick, Blackwood and Mair[3] and I am indebted to Professor Blackwood for access to his material.

Comparison of the lesions in the 2 conditions reveals some subtle, yet important differences. In granulomatous angiitis the affected vessels are surrounded by a cuff of epithelioid cells, containing some giant cells which are generally smaller and less conspicuous than those seen in sarcoidosis. The vessel wall may be either normal with a well-preserved elastica, or may undergo necrosis with infiltration by fibrin which may extend into surrounding tissue. In sarcoidosis on the other hand most granulomas arise in the adventitia and lie to 1 side of the vessel wall. In some instances they erode the vessel wall, leading to localised destruction of the elastica and to encroachment of the granuloma upon the lumen, which may become completely obliterated. In some vessels only remnants of the elastica indicate the nature of the original structure. Apart from obliterative lesions due to involvement of vessels in epithelioid cell granulomas, rare acute necrotising lesions are encountered in some cases.[4, 5] In our case the acute lesions showed massive fibrinoid necrosis of the vessel wall with a surrounding acute inflammatory infiltrate. The lesions were indistinguishable from those of polyarteritis nodosa and were presumably due to precipitation of antigen-antibody complexes, though their exclusive localisation to the brain is difficult to explain.

A further difference between meningovascular sarcoidosis and granulomatous angiitis lies in the calibre of the vessels involved. In both conditions the pial and intracerebral branches are affected, but in granulomatous angiitis the larger arteries, such as the internal carotids and the vertebrals, may contain small intramural granulomas, a finding never observed in sarcoidosis.

Disturbances in calcium metabolism are not uncommon in sarcoidosis, yet their correlation with the rare intracerebral calcifications remains obscure. These calcifications are primarily pericapillary droplet calcifications which may become confluent. I have seen them in the hypothalamus in 2 cases, in 1 of which the cerebellar cortex was similarly affected. The distribution of these minimal deposits is totally different from the well-known localisation in Fahr's disease associated with hypoparathyroidism or pseudo-hypoparathyroidism.[6]

The final problem which I should like to discuss briefly is that of healed or burnt-out lesions of cerebral sarcoidosis. Fibrotic lesions in the form of nodules or plaques are encountered occasionally side by side with active granulomas. Yet the impression remains that sarcoidosis of the central, as opposed to the peripheral, nervous system is a progressive condition, with exacerbations and remissions, but ultimately leading to a fatal outcome. The search for an unequivocal example of a completely healed meningo-vascular sarcoidosis still goes on. A strongly suggestive case was presented by Rabinowicz at the European Symposium on Sarcoidosis; unfortunately the case was complicated by a terminal tuberculous meningitis which left the interpretation of some lesions open to doubt. The solution of the problem of healing, either spontaneous or therapeutic, would be of considerable importance, both in the study of the natural history of the disease and in the assessment of the value of therapeutic measures.

REFERENCES

1. Rabinowicz, T. 1971. *Communication to European Symposium on Sarcoidosis*. Geneva.
2. Zollinger, H. U. 1941. Grosszellig-granulomatöse Lymphagitis cerebri (Morbus Boeck) unter dem Bilde einer multiplen Sklerose verlaufend. *Virchows Arch. Path. Anat.* **307**: 597–615.
3. Nurick, S., Blackwood, W., and Mair, W. C. P. 1972. Giant cell granulomatous angiitis of the central nervous system. *Brain* **95**: 133–142.
4. Meyer, J. S., Foley, J. M., and Campagna-Pinto, D. 1953. Granulomatous angiitis of the meninges in sarcoidosis. *Arch. Neurol. Psychiat.* **69**: 587–600.
5. Herring, A. B., and Urich, H. 1969. Sarcoidosis of the central nervous system. *J. Neurol. Sci.* **9**: 405–422.
6. Norman, R. M., and Urich, H. 1960. The influence of a vascular factor on the distribution of symmetrical cerebral calcifications. *J. Neurol. Neurosurg. Psychiat.* **23**: 142–147.

Sarcoidosis of the Central Nervous System

ANDREW DOUGLAS

Department of Respiratory Diseases, University of Edinburgh,
Edinburgh, Great Britain

Involvement of the central nervous system in sarcoidosis is relatively rare and in the Edinburgh sarcoidosis register of more than 500 cases there are only 6 examples of this. They illustrate the infinite variety of the clinical expressions of CNS sarcoidosis, the difficulty in making the diagnosis in the absence of evidence of sarcoidosis in other systems, the chronicity of this form of the disease in most instances and its variable and usually poor prognosis even when corticosteroid therapy is employed (Table 1).

TABLE 1. Sarcoidosis of the central nervous system. Summary of findings in 6 patients.

Patient	Age and sex	Principal neurological features	Other sarcoid features	Diagnosis	Course
D. H.	44 F	Mental deterioration. Headache. Vomiting. Papilloedema. Diabetes insipidus.	Hilar and cervical adenopathy. ? Nasal granuloma.	Biopsy— Lymph gland.	Alive 11 yrs.+ Response to prednisolone.
F. McI.	38 M	Headache. Paraesthesiae. Right facial palsy. Epilepsy. Mental deterioration. Aphasia. Nerve deafness. Optic atrophy.	EN+Hilar adenopathy. Cervical adenopathy. Nasal granuloma. Skin sarcoid.	Biopsy— Lymph gland. Nasal granuloma. Brain	Progression despite prednisolone. Died 10 yrs.
E. F.	32 F	Amenorrhoea. Diabetes insipidus Headache. Epilepsy. Ataxia. Meningeal irritation. Coma.	Nil.	Autopsy—CNS	Died 2 yrs.+ Septicaemia.
T. C.	46 F	Right facial palsy. Palatal weakness Right hemiparesis Diplopia. Dysarthria. Headache.	Lupus pernio.	Presumptive.	Fluctuating course. No treatment. Permanent cerebral damage. Alive 13 yrs.+
J. O.	55 F	Rapid mental deterioration.	Nil.	Autopsy—CNS	Died 2/12. Pulmonary embolism.
J. S.	16 M	Somnolence. Papilloedema. Right hemiparesis Aphasia. Left facial palsy.	Nil.	Biopsy—Brain	Died 2 yrs. Deterioration despite prednisolone.

COMMENT

Any part of the central nervous system may be involved in sarcoidosis and any aspect of cerebrospinal function can be affected. Thus neurological presentations may vary from impairment of motor power in a limb to disturbance of the central control of respiration[2] or even mental deterioration or disorders of the personality. The possible combinations ol neurological manifestations are legion and there is no constant association of signs or symptoms which can be grouped together to describe a syndrome for sarcoidosis of the central nervous system.[7] It is, however, true that certain combinations may be suggestive (e.g. signs of chronic meningitis, diabetes insipidus, facial palsy) and when these occur examination of the CSF is mandatory and the usual investigations for sarcoidosis should be undertaken including a search for sarcoid lesions in other systems and a Kveim test if the tempo of the neurological picture permits. When there is evidence of coexisting sarcoid involvement of other organs, or a past history of this, the diagnosis of CNS sarcoidosis presents no great difficulties[4] and in this context the presumptive diagnosis usually proves to be correct. When, however, the neurological features are the only indication of the site of disease the diagnosis becomes a formidable problem. Random tissue biopsy (especially liver and scalene fat pad) may establish the diagnosis but will not if sarcoidosis is confined to the central nervous system (8; cases E.F. and J.O.). The value of the Kveim test in CNS sarcoidosis may be limited by the 4- to 6-week delay which is not always feasible before the need to initiate corticosteroid therapy. Moreover the positivity rate in sarcoidosis clinically or pathologically confined to the central nervous system is not known. A positive test would, however, be of inestimable value in cases of sarcoidosis manifesting with CNS symptoms and signs only.

Sometimes the diagnosis may be made after histological examination of tissue obtained at craniotomy undertaken for possible tumor or for the relief of CSF block. Rarely a tissue diagnosis is made after elective brain biopsy[9] as in case J.S. reported here. Even the ultimate procedure of brain biopsy may be unhelpful if needle biopsy is the technique used since the granulomata are frequently widely dispersed (Fig. 1) and a single biopsy may not include pathological tissue.

CSF examination may be of great importance in the diagnosis of CNS sarcoidosis (Table 2). The most consistent findings are a normal pressure and appearance, raised protein, normal sugar and a variable number of cells, mainly lymphocytes.[1,7] A low sugar has been occasionally reported.[1,3,7,10] Patient E.F. previously reported from this

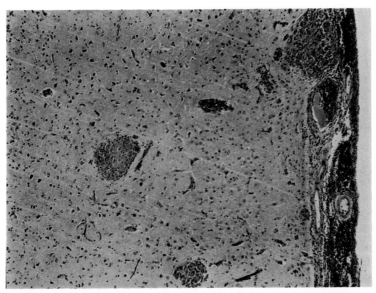

FIG. 1. Section of brain showing widely dispersed granulomata in cortex.

TABLE 2. Sarcoidosis of the central nervous system. CSF findings in 6 patients.

Patient	Protein (mg%)	Sugar (N=Normal)	Cells	
D. H.	200–300	N	0	
F. McI.	160	N	0	
	900	N	4	
E. F.	1800	N	0	
	1000	26 mg%	0	
	700	N	0	
	760	N	0	
T. C.	80	N	0	
J. O.	67	N	53	(L)
J. S.	64	N	31	(P)

unit[10] had a CSF protein of 1800 mg at one stage, the highest value for protein ever recorded in CNS sarcoidosis.

Absence of evidence of sarcoidosis in other systems in some cases is not surprising in view of the fact that CNS sarcoidosis tends to occur late in the timetable of the disease when coexisting multisystem involvement may be slight and not easily detectable. One would, however, expect that multisystem involvement would be proved at autopsy in such cases. In 2 patients reported here (E.F. and J.O.) full autopsy showed that the CNS was the only definable histological site of the disease and " isolated " CNS sarcoidosis has also been reported by others.[8] The alternative explanations would appear to be that " isolated " CNS sarcoidosis is an entity or, as seems much more likely, that preexisting asymptomatic lesions in other systems have resolved without demonstrable trace by the time the CNS lesions become predominant and symptomatic. Obviously there must be great caution about acceptance of a diagnosis of " isolated " CNS sarcoidosis and all alternative diagnoses must be thoroughly excluded before applying this label. In males under 20 it is important to include pineal teratoma in the differential diagnosis.

Sarcoid lesions have been found in almost every part of the central nervous system and vary from meningeal granulomas to actual tumor-like masses. The affinity of the sarcoid granuloma for cerebral vessels has been stressed by many authors[5, 6, 8, 9, 11] and was striking in the pathological material obtained from the cases reported here (Fig. 2). This probably offers 1 explanation for the variable response to corticosteroid therapy. Areas of cerebral ischaemia and infarction have been described in relation to granulomatous cerebral angiitis[6] and was found in case J.S. in this series. The development of meningeal fibrosis is another feature which may determine progression of neurological phenomena and limit response to corticosteroid drugs; it may sometimes compel surgical treatment for relief of hydrocephalus or of intractable epilepsy. (F.McI.)

The course of CNS sarcoidosis is unpredictable but it is generally agreed that involvement of the central nervous system indicates the use of corticosteroid therapy as the only hope of influencing the disease and modifying its effects on function. To be maximally effective treatment should be begun early but no matter how long the CNS features have been present it should always be tried. Unfortunately improvement does not always follow and deterioration may occur despite treatment (patients F.McI. and J.S.). If improvement does occur extreme caution must be observed in making reductions in dosage and treatment may require to be prolonged indefinitely.

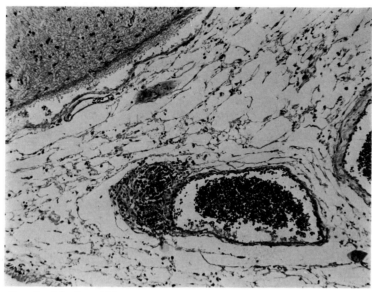

Fig. 2.   Meningeal blood vessel showing paravascular sarcoid granuloma.

By analogy with asymptomatic and symptomatic skeletal muscle sarcoidosis, it is reasonable to postulate that in the common forms of subacute, transient sarcoidosis there may be CNS involvement of a degree not disturbing function and that this resolves with no discernible residual damage. Why it is that the diffuse granulomatous process should become dominant in 1 organ or system remains one of the many inexplicable features of the disease.

REFERENCES

1. Colover, J. 1948. Sarcoidosis with involvement of nervous system. *Brain* **71**: 451.
2. Daum, J. J., Canter, H. G., and Katz, S. 1965. Central nervous system sarcoidosis with alveolar hypoventilation. *Amer. J. Med.* **38**: 893.
3. Ernsting, W., and Sillevis Smitt, W. G. 1944. Neurologische verschijnselen bij de ziekte van Beanier-Boeck-Schaumann. Geneesk. bl. Klin. *en Lab. Prakt.* **41**: 1.
4. Jefferson, M. 1957. Sarcoidosis of nervous system. *Brain* **80**: 540.
5. Longcope, W. T., and Freiman, D. G. 1952. A study of sarcoidosis. *Medicine* **31**: 1.
6. Meyer, J. S., Foley, J. M., and Compagna-Pinto, D. 1953. Granulomatous angiitis of the meninges in sarcoidosis. A.M.A. Arch. Neurol. *Psychiat.* **69**: 587.
7. Pennel, W. H. 1951. Boeck's sarcoid with involvement of the central nervous system. A.M.A. Arch. Neurol. *Psychiat.* **66**: 728.
8. Reske-Nielson, E., and Harmsen, A. 1962. Periangiitis and Panangiitis as manifestation of sarcoidosis of the brain: report of a case. *J. Nerv. Ment. Dis.* **135**: 399.
9. Robert, F. 1962. Sarcoidosis of the central nervous system. Report of a case and review of the literature. *Arch. Neurol.* (Chicago) **7**: 442.
10. Schonell, M. E., Gillespie, W. J., and Maloney, A. F. J. 1968. Cerebral sarcoidosis. *Brit. J. Dis. Chest* **62**: 195.
11. Urich, H. 1967. Pathological observations on six cases of cerebral sarcoidosis. In *La Sarcoidose: Reports Fourth Int. Conf. on Sarcoidosis* **1966**, Paris: Masson et cie.

Electroencephalography in Patients with Intrathoracic Sarcoidosis

Yasutaka Niitu, Masahiro Horikawa, Sumio Hasegawa, Hideo Kubota,
Shigeo Komatsu, Tomiko Suetake

*Department of Pediatrics, The Research Institute for Tuberculosis, Leprosy,
and Cancer, Tohoku University, Sendai, Japan*

AND

Takashi Mizuno

Mizuno Pediatric Dispensary, Sendai, Japan

Sarcoidosis is a systemic disease. It has been called an iceberg syndrome, in which the undiagnosed subclinical variants are far more common than is realized. Cases of sarcoidosis of the brain, in which sarcoid granulomas were demonstrated by autopsy or biopsy, have been reported.[1-3] Abnormalities of electroencephalography have been observed in cases of intrathoracic sarcoidosis with symptoms suggesting the involvement of the brain.[2,3] However, it seems that there has been no report dealing with electroencephalography in patients with intrathoracic sarcoidosis, who have no complaints and no clinical symptoms to suggest lesions of the central nervous system. We performed electroencephalography in patients with intrathoracic sarcoidosis without any clinical symptoms suggesting the presence of brain lesions for the purpose of detecting silent involvement of sarcoidosis of the brain.

MATERIALS AND METHODS

Twenty-eight patients with intrathoracic sarcoidosis, ranging from 8 to 38 years of age, were tested by electroencephalography. All cases except 1 had been found by chest X-ray surveys and had no complaints. None had symptoms suggesting the involvement of the brain. The chest X-ray findings revealed bilateral hilar lymphadenopathy in all cases except 1 and pulmonary involvements in 5 cases. Electroencephalography was analysed by Dr Mizuno, a specialist in electroencephalography and one of the present authors.

RESULTS AND DISCUSSION

Twenty-five cases were tested at the time of the presence of intrathoracic lesions and all except 1 within 3 months after the detection of the disease. Abnormalities of electroencephalography were observed in 8 cases, or 32%. Three cases were tested after the disappearance of abnormal chest X-ray findings and within 1 year after the detection of the disease. One of them revealed abnormalities in electroencephalography. Thus, 9 of the 28 cases tested, or 32%, showed abnormalities in electroencephalography (Table 1). The 9 cases with abnormalities in electroencephalography are shown in Table 2. Abnormal electroencephalograms of 4 cases are shown in Figs. 1 to 4.

TABLE 1. Electroencephalography in patients with intrathoracic sarcoidosis.

Chest X-ray shadow	No. of cases tested	Abnormal EEG	
		No.	%
Present	25	8	32
After disappeared	3	1	33
Total	28	9	32

TABLE 2. Abnormalities of electroencephalography in patients with inthrathoracic sarcoidosis.

Case	Age and sex	Date	Chest X-ray findings	Electroencephalography	Treatment with steroid
1. T. O.	14 M	1st exam.	BHL Lung	14 c/s positive spikes in right posterotemporal area and low voltage.	} Yes
		8 m later	Normal	Normal	
		2 y later	Normal	Normal	} Yes
2. M. E.	9 F	1st exam.	BHL Lung	Bursts of 4 c/s HVS (high voltage slow waves) in all areas in resting record.	} Yes
		2 m later	Normal	Normal	} No
		4 m later	Lung	Normal	
		7 m later	Normal	Normal	} Yes
3. T. K.	22 F	1st exam.	BHL	Irregular 1.5 c/s HVS occurring intermittently and paroxysmally in all areas.	} No
		2 y later	Normal	Normal	
4. Y. M.	13 M	1st exam.	Normal*	Bursts of 3 to 4 c/s HVS and 3 c/s spikes and waves in all areas and bursts of 6 c/s theta waves in bilateral frontal areas.	} Yes
		5 m later	Normal	3 to 4 c/s HVS and 6 c/s theta waves in bilateral frontal poles and mitten pattern in a part of record. Spikes and waves disappeared.	
		1 y and 4 m later	Normal	HVS and spikes and waves disappeared and only theta waves remained. The findings improved.	} No
5. F. F.	16 F	1st exam.	BHL Lung	5 to 6 c/s slow waves in basic pattern in occipital area and low voltage in activity in resting record.	} Yes
		8 m later	Normal	Low voltage was improved and slow waves remained.	
6. K. K.	17 M	1st exam.	BHL	Low voltage	} No
		4 m later	Normal	Low voltage	
		1 y later	Normal	Low voltage	} No
7. E. N.	14 F	1st exam.	BHL	Paroxysmal 4 to 5 c/s HVS and middle voltage slow waves in left parietal and vertex areas.	
8. Y. K.	9 F	1st exam.	BHL	Paroxysmal 3 to 4 c/s spikes and waves in all areas.	
9. K. M.	13 M	1st exam.	BHL	6 c/s positive spikes in right mid temporal area.	

[1] BHL: Bilateral hilar lymphadenopathy.

[2] *: BHL found 9 months before had disappeared after 2 months' treatment with steroid.

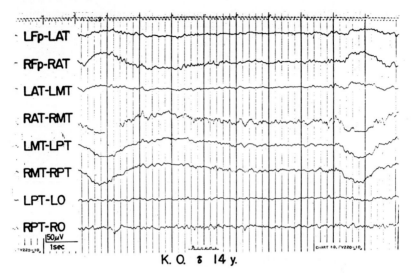

FIG. 1.   First electroencephalogram in case 1.

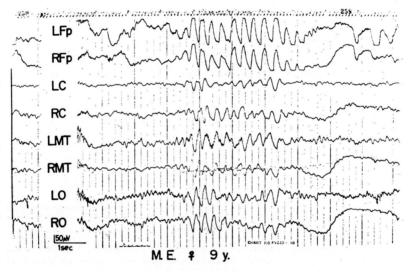

FIG. 2.   First electroencephalogram in case 2.

Of the 28 cases tested, 5 showed pulmonary shadows with or without bilateral hilar lymphadenopathy on the X-ray films. Three of the 5 cases or 60%, a high rate of incidence, showed abnormalities in electroencephalography.

Abnormal electroencephalography was followed up in 6 cases. The electroencephalographic findings had become normal in 3 of them and improved in 2 cases from 2 months to 2 years after the first examination. It thus appears that abnormalities of electroencephalography observed in patients with intrathoracic sarcoidosis disappear within rather short periods in most cases.

Considering the observations mentioned above that abnormalities of electroencephalography were observed in 32% of all cases tested and at a higher rate in cases with pulmonary involvement, which later became to normal or improved, it may be concluded

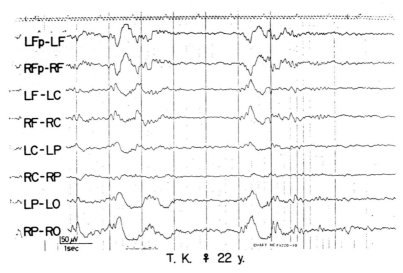

FIG. 3.   First electroencephalogram in case 3.

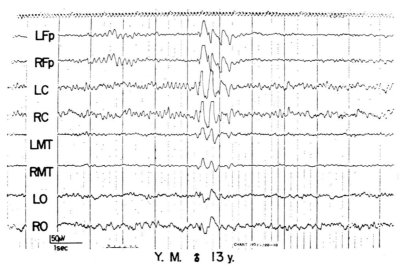

FIG. 4.   First electroencephalogram in case 4.

that silent sarcoidosis lesions might have existed in the brain in about one-third of symptomless patients with intrathoracic sarcoidosis.

SUMMARY

Electroencephalography performed in 28 patients with intrathoracic sarcoidosis and without any symptoms suggesting lesions of the brain, revealed abnormal findings in 9 patients. Of 5 patients with pulmonary involvement, 3 showed abnormal findings. Of 6 patients with abnormalities followed up, abnormal findings disappeared in 3 and improved in 2. Silent sarcoidosis lesions might have existed in the brain in about one-third of symptomless patients with intrathoracic sarcoidosis at the early stage.

REFERENCES

1. Yokoi, S. 1956. Sarcoidosis of central nervous system. *Seishinshinkeigaku Zassi* **58**: 431.
2. Silverstein, A., Feuer, M. M., and Siltzbach, L. E. 1965. Neurologic sarcoidosis. Study of 18 cases. *Arch. Neurol.* **12**: 1.
3. Wiederholt, W. C., and Siebert, R. G. 1965. Neurological manifestations of sarcoidosis. *Neurology* (Minneap.) **15**: 1147.

The Incidence and Course of Ocular Lesion in Sarcoidosis

FUMIKO KOBAYASHI

Department of Ophthalmology, Toranomon General Hospital, Tokyo, Japan

The present report is based on careful and repeated ophthalmological examinations in 61 cases with sarcoidosis during the period of July 1965 to the end of 1971 at Toranomon General Hospital (Fig. 1). In these examinations, special attention was paid to chorio-retinal lesions in the peripheral fundus, because their incidence and clinical course have not yet been sufficiently analysed in comparison with those of sarcoid uveitis.

Several examinations, at least 3 or 4 times at intervals of 2 or 3 weeks, were repeated in 61 cases, 36 male and 25 female aged from 15 to 60, until the diagnosis was confirmed. The follow-up study was continued at intervals of from 1 to 3 months for as long as the patient showed any clinical sign, and twice a year regularly after disappearance of these findings.

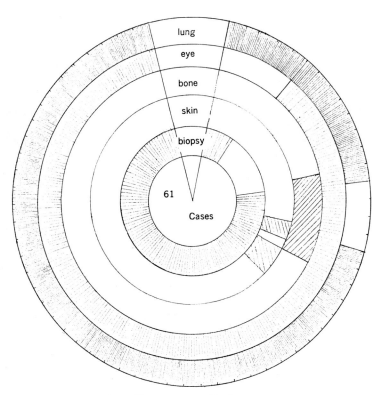

lung 57 cases skin 5 cases
eye 56 cases biopsy 52 cases
bone 7 cases

FIG. 1. Distribution of sarcoidosis.

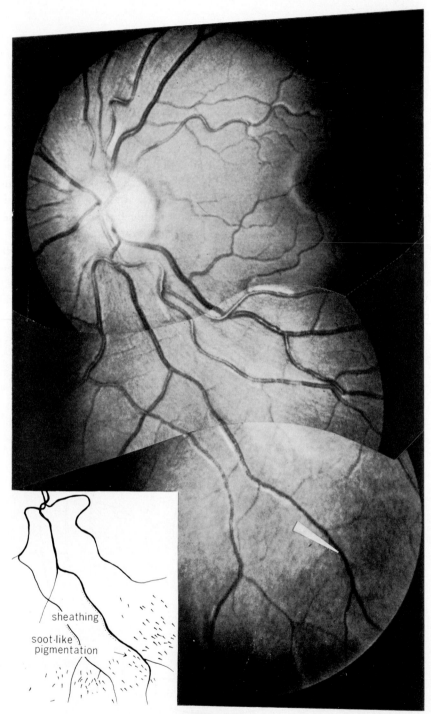

FIG. 2.

TABLE 1. Incidence of ocular sarcoidosis.

	No. of cases	Confirmed	Unconfirmed
Group I–III	52	48 (92%)	4 (8%)
Group IV	9	8 (92%)	1 (8%)
Tatal	61	56	5

TABLE 2. Ocular changes in 61 cases with sarcoidosis.

Serous uveitis	29
String of pearls	15
Periphlebitis	14
Peripheral—	
Sheathing of artery	55
Chorioretinitis	41
Chorioretinal atrophy	41
Black pigment patch	24

Distribution of sarcoid lesions among 61 cases is shown in Fig. 2. The ocular manifestations were found in 48 (92%) of 52 cases classified into Group 1 to 111 (histologically confirmed), and 8 (92%) of 9 in Group IV (clinically diagnosed), as shown in Table 1. Five cases were lost during the study. Types of ocular lesions observed and their incidence are listed in Table 2.

Thirty-eight (62%) of 56 with ocular changes showed active lesions including iritis, chorioretinitis, perivasculitis and other active forms, while the rest had inactive changes composed of deposits of iris pigment on the inner surface of the cornea or outer surface of the lense or of a characteristic soot-like pigmentation or large black pigment patches in the peripheral fundus.

Among 38 patients with initially active ocular changes, 27 (48%) showed clear improvement, 6 (11%) improved with no impairment of vision but were unstable. Two remained active and 1 had inactive lesions with moderate impairment of vision. Two cases were lost during the follow-up study. Eighteen cases with initially inactive lesions remained inactive except for 3 lost cases.

Recurrence was repeatedly observed in 16 cases judged initially as having an active form and in 2 cases of inactive form. The relapse of ocular lesion in these cases was more frequent and less predictive than had been expected. For instance, during a period of 6 and half years recurrence was noted every 3 or 6 months in one case, sometimes revealing an ocular fundus appearance without any changes in other lesions of sarcoidosis.

The effect of corticosteroids on the ocular lesions was usually transitory. Complete remission of the ocular lesions was observed in only 13 out of 48 cases, moderate improvement in 17 cases. In 14 cases out of the 17 cases, a temporary improvement was followed by worsening when the dose was reduced or soon after the cessation of the treatment. As far as the ocular lesions are concerned, the effect of corticosteroids is not predictable and the distinct indication for this treatment should only be limited only to those cases in which acute impairment of vision can be predicted.

The high incidence rate of ocular lesions in the present study is due to a careful checkup of the peripheral fundus in these patients. A typical example of a lesion in the fundus to which special attention was paid is shown in Fig. 3 where sheathing of the retinal

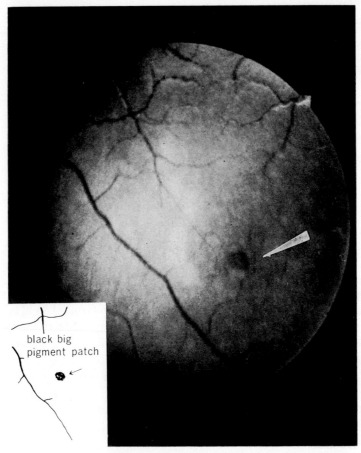

black big
pigment patch

FIG. 3.

artery accompanied by inflammatory patches simulated chorioretinitis in the periphery. Sheathing of the retinal artery might have resulted from inflammation affecting the wall of the artery. These inflammatory patches were later converted to focal atrophic lesions with fine soot-like pigmentation or large black pigment patches resembling pieces of black chips. These focal invasions of chorioretinitis and resulting scar formations were found more frequently in the periphery than in the central portion of the fundus. These scars were observable for many years after the active lesions had disappeared. The diagnostic value of these lesions was greater when their migratory nature was confirmed by follow-up observations.

CONCLUSION

1) The incidence rate of ocular lesion in sarcoidosis was 92% in the present study.

2) A careful check up of the peripheral fundus made it possible to obtain such a high incidence rate.

3) It might be useful to follow up the ocular changes in order to observe the clinical course of sarcoidosis as a whole, because the ocular changes were found easily at the on-set, recurrence or remission.

4)   A distinct indication for corticosteroid treatment should be limited to those cases in which acute inpairment of vision can be predicted.

REFERENCES

1.   Gould and Kaufman. 1961. Sarcoid of the Furndus *AMA. Arch. Ophthal.* **65**: 453–456.
2.   Chumbley and Kearns 1972. Retinopathy of Sarcoidosis *A. J. Ophthal.* **73**: 123–131.

Sarcoid Uveitis—Clinical course and treatment—

MASANOBU UYAMA

Department of Ophthalmology, Kyoto University, Kyoto, Japan

Sarcoidosis involving the eye is very common among Japanese sarcoidosis cases. In our clinic, ocular involvements were found in 60% of systemic sarcoidosis patients.

Among various types of ocular involvements of sarcoidosis, uveitis is the most frequent and important cause of visual disturbances. In our uveitis clinic, among 264 cases of endogenous uveitis during the past 4 years (1968–1971), sarcoidosis was ranked as the most common cause representing, 17% of all the cases, followed by Behçet's disease, toxoplasmosis, and Vogt-Koyanagi-Harada's disease.

The Tsuji-Izumi group at Kyoto University made the diagnosis of sarcoidosis in these patients, by chest roentgenogram, Kveim test, and histological confirmation by biopsy of the lymph nodes.

This report is derived from 52 cases, 100 eyes of sarcoid uveitis, treated and followed up by us.

The age at the apparent onset of sarcoid uveitis is shown in Fig. 1. The disease occurred most frequently at 20 years of age, and the prevalence was the same for both sexes in this generation. The disease also occurred in older age at the fourth, fifth and sixth decades. However, in the older age group, women were much more commonly affected than men. It is noteworthy that, there were late onsets in elderly patients.

Forty-eight cases were affected in both eyes, where clinical pictures were similar. The chronic, insidious course of uveitis was much more prevalent than the acute, transient type (Table 1). Serous, nodular, or fibrinous iritis and iridocyclitis, exudative retino-

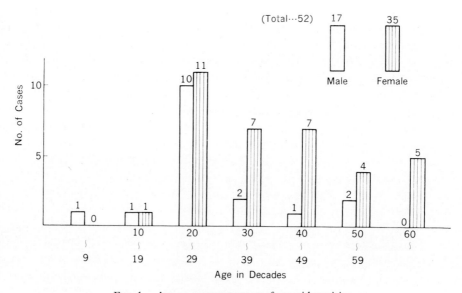

FIG. 1.   Age at apparent onset of sarcoid uveitis.

TABLE 1. Clinical pictures of sarcoid uveitis.

Course	Acute	11 cases
	Chronic	41 cases
	Total	52 cases
Anterior uveitis (Iritis, Iridocyclitis)		11 Eyes
Posterior uveitis (Retinochoroiditis)		5 Eyes
Panuveitis		84 Eyes
anterior, predominant		29
posterior, predominant		10
	Total	100 Eyes

TABLE 2. Complications of sarcoid uveitis.

(No. of eyes)

Glaucoma	acute		9	26
	chronic	Goniosynechia 12	17	
		Iris bombe 5		
Cataract				28

choroiditis, and retinal angiitis were seen in both acute and chronic courses. Iritis and iridocyclitis, that is anterior uveitis, were usually more predominant than posterior uveitis.

Intraocular inflammations of sarcoidosis lasted such a long time, that several complications appeared frequently during the course of the disease, severely impairing visual functions of the eyes (Table 2).

Secondary glaucomas were commonly seen; acute elevation of the intraocular pressure occurred sometimes in acute iritis. This type of glaucoma was one of the characteristics of acute iritis of sarcoidosis. Chronic glaucomas were also common in chronic iritis cases. Among them, 5 eyes had to undergo surgery.

Cataract formation was also a hazard and a frequent complication in long-term cases. Among the cases, 12 eyes were so severe that they had to have the lens removed.

Treatment, the use of topical and systemic corticosteroid, was effective in all cases. The response to the steroid was dramatic, especially in the case of acute iridocyclitis. Retinochoroiditis, however, showed a slow response to steroid.

Two cases will be shown here as examples.

The first is a case of a 20-year-old male, who had a slight ciliary injection, numerous mutton-fat keratic precipitates, marked turbidity of aqueous, nodular exudates on the iris, and opacities of the vitreous in both eyes. On the fundus, moderate retinal angiitis was seen in the periphery to equator. His acute panuveitis, predominantly in the anterior segment was due to sarcoidosis.

Eye drops of mydriatics (atropine) and subconjunctival and oral stereoid were given. Following the treatment, inflammations in the anterior segment of the eye disappeared rapidly within a few days, and all inflammatory findings cleared up within a month. However, retinal angiitis remained for several months. A relative high dose of oral steroid was given by the physician to cure intrathoracic involvements, but a slight degree of retinal angiitis remained and did not disappear during the succeeding 2 years of observation.

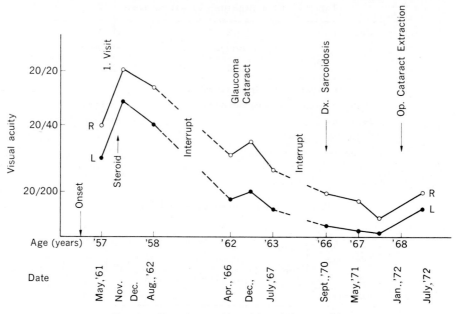

FIG. 2.   Chronic sarcoid uveitis.   (66 years, ♀)

Almost all cases of acute iridocyclitis showed a clinical course similar to this case.

The second example is one of the chronic iridocyclitis cases. A 66-year-old woman had been treated for 9 years at our clinic for chronic iridocyclitis of unknown etiology, before she was referred to the present author. The apparent onset of her eye symptoms dated back to 1961 when she was 57 years of age. When she first visited the clinic, both her eyes were affected to a moderate degree by subacute iridocyclitis. The use of oral steroid was effective and her vision improved to 20/20 in her right eye and 20/30 in her left eye (Fig. 2). Thereafter, during a period of 9 years without proper attention, her eyes suffered several relapses, followed by remissions with the use of steroid. Because of development of chronic glaucomas and cataracts resulting from the formation of posterior synechia and goniosynechia of the iris, her visual acuity had gradually been decreasing. In 1970, the etiology of uveitis was confirmed as sarcoidsis. The examination revealed the final stage of sarcoid uveitis, and her vision was nearly lost (20/400 in the right eye, 20/2,000 in the left eye). Recently, cataract extractions were performed and her vision recoverded to 20/200 in the right eye, and 20/300 in the left eye.

In this case, uveitis occurred at a relatively old age. At the beginning, topical and systemic steroid therapy cleared up the ocular imflammation. But, because of the insidious course of the disease without sustained adequate treatment, severe complications of uveitis developed in her eyes. Many instances of eye disease of this type have been observed at the clinic.

In addition to steroid therapy, immunosuppressive therapy was tried in 2 cases of chronic panuveitis.

One case was a 32-year-old woman, whose eyes showed clinical findings of chronic uveitis of sarcoidosis (Fig. 3). A high dose of oral steroid was effective for iridocyclitis. It was less effective, however, for exudative retinochoroiditis. Relapses of uveitis occurred so frequently, following the reduction or cessation of steroid, that her visual

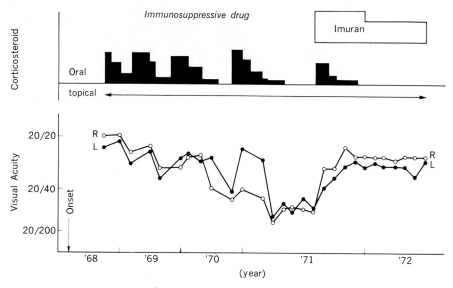

FIG. 3. Chronic sarcoid uveitis. (33 years, ♀)

TABLE 3. Prognosis of sarcoid uveitis.

	(No. of cases)
Healed, completely	5
Improved	20
Continued, not worse	16
Worse	9

acuity worsened (20/80 in both eyes). Azathioprine (Imuran: 3 tablets a day), with some amounts of steroid was given and the eyes were maintained in a silent condition. Two months later, the dose of Imuran was reduced to 2 tablets a day and oral steroid was discontinued. The patient has not shown any recurrence of uveitis, and has exhibited no side effects from the drug for 12 months, and her visual acuity has been maintained at 20/30 in both eyes.

We have another case, in which Imuran was effective in keeping the eye quiet after the withdrawal of oral steroid.

Prognosis of sarcoid uveitis was good in general (Table 3). However, there were only 5 cases which healed completely without any imflammation. In 20 cases, most of the imflammation subsided and visual acuity improved following treatment, but slight imflammatory findings remained on some parts of the eye for a long term. In 15 cases, a moderate degree of uveitis has sometimes recurred, but relatively good vision has been maintained. In 9 cases, relapse occurred frequently, complications developed, and visual acuity worsened.

The prognosis of sarcoid uveitis was chiefly dependent upon the timing and the method of treatment. An intensive therapy with topical and oral steroid initiated during the early stages of the disease brought about satisfactory clinical cures. Delay in initiation of treatment frequently resulted in a protracted course or recurrences.

In sarcoid uveitis, relatively good visual acuity was obtained in most cases. However,

TABLE 4. Visual acuity of sarcoid uveitis.

	Before treatment	After treatment
−20/20	55	64
20/25–20/60	21	17
20/100–20/2,000	19	13
Hand movement—	5	6
	100	100 eyes

one-quarter of the patients remained with poor vision (Table 4). Visual functions were impaired mainly due to massive vitreous opacity, and developments of glaucoma and cataract complications.

SUMMARY

1) Sarcoidosis is one of the common causes of uveitis among Japanese people.

2) In sarcoid uveitis, there are 2 types of uveitis, i.e., acute and chronic.

3) Acute uveitis occurs in young people in their twenties of both sexes, and affects both eyes abruptly. Iritis and iridocyclitis are more dominant than posterior uveitis.

4) Chronic uveitis occurs among older women, affecting both eyes, and follows a protracted course.

5) Corticosteroid is effective for ocular sarcoidosis. Prognosis of this disease is generally good. However, some degree of relapse may frequently occur. A complete cure may be difficult to obtain.

6) Patients should therefore be subjected to long-term observation.

7) In protracted cases, hazardous glaucoma and cataract complications impair visual acuity irreversibly.

8) Immunosuppressive therapy (Azathioprine) may be effective in protracted cases.

ACKNOWLEDGEMENTS

The author wishes to express his thanks to Dr Masao Kishimoto, Professor and Chairman of our department for his encouragment and advice during this study, and to Drs Fumie Okamoto, Masato Okuma, and Kunio Asayama for their association in the uveitis clinic.

The author is also grateful to Drs Syusuke Tsuji, Takahide Izumi, and Shigeharu Morioka of the Chest Disease Research Institute, Kyoto University for their diagnosis of sarcoidosis in the patients.

REFERENCES

1. Uyama, M. 1971. Ocular Sarcoidosis as a Clinical Uveitis Entity. *Japanese J. Clin. Ophthal.* **25**: 1513–1522.

2. Yamada, N., et al. 1971. Studies of Ocular Lesions in Sarcoidosis. *Japanese J. Clin. Ophthal.* **25**: 697–703.

3. Yamada, N., et al. 1971. Studies of Ocular Lesions in Sarcoidosis, found in Mass Screening by X-ray. *Japanese J. Clin. Ophthal.* **25**: 704–706.

4. Yamada, N., et al. 1971. Studies of Ocular Lesions in Sarcoidosis, Diagnosis. *Japanese J. Clin. Ophthal.* **25**: 707–711.

5. Yamada, N., et al. 1971. Follow-up Studies of Ocular Sarcoidosis. *Japanese J. Clin. Ophthal.* **25**: 719–723.

6. Yamada, N. 1972. Some Problems on Ocular Sarcoidosis. *Jap. Rev. Clin. Ophthal.* **66**: 103–110.

7. Nielsen, R. H. 1959. Ocular Sarcoidosis. *Arch. Ophthal.* **61**: 657–663.

8. Gould, H., and Kaufman, H. E. 1961. Sarcoid of the Fundus. *Arch. Ophthal.* **65**: 453–456.

9. Crick, R. P., Hoyle, C., and Smellie, H. 1961. The Eye in Sarcoidosis. *Brit. J. Ophthal.* **45**: 461–481.

10. Geeraets, W. J., et al. 1962. Retinopathy in Sarcoidosis. *Acta Ophthal.* **40**: 492–514.

11. James, D. G., Anderson, R., et al. 1964. Ocular Sarcoidosis. *Brit J. Ophthal.* **48**: 461–470.

12. Simpson, G. V. 1968. Diagnosis and Treatment of Uveitis in Association with Sarcoidosis. *Tr. Amer. Ophthal. Soc.* **66**: 117–140.

13. James, D. G. 1968. Uveitis—Immunopathy or Infection? *Trans. Ophthal. Soc. U.K.* **88**: 711–729.

Asymptomatic Electrocardiographic Alterations in Eighty Patients with Sarcoidosis

E. STEIN, I. JACKLER, B. STIMMEL, W. STEIN AND L. E. SILTZBACH

Division of Cardiology and Thoracic Diseases, Department of Medicine,
The Mount Sinai School of Medicine, New York, U.S.A.

Although sarcoidosis is not a rare disease, clinical recognition of intrinsic involvement of the heart is infrequent. This is irrespective of the finding that up to 20% of patients with sarcoidosis at postmortem can be demonstrated to have some degree of myocardial involvement.[1,2] As of 1971 however, only 70 cases of documented clinical involvement of the heart in sarcoidosis have been reported in the literature. The major manifestations of intrinsic cardiac involvement have been conduction disturbances, disorders of impulse formation and progressive myocardial failure.[3-7]

Recently, we observed an unusual aggregation of patients with suspected cardiac sarcoidosis at the sarcoidosis clinic of the Mount Sinai Hospital. These patients had potentially life-threatening episodes requiring hospitalization in a cardiac intensive care unit, where they were continuously monitored.

The appearance of these serious cardiac complications prompted us to survey systematically, over a 3-month period of time, the electrocardiographic findings of 80 patients attending our sarcoidosis clinic.

PATIENT MATERIAL

In addition to the usual clinical, radiologic and laboratory investigations for the presence of tissue-confirmed sarcoidosis, these patients were scrutinized with special attention to possible cardiac abnormalities. Patients were included in the study only if the following criteria were present: 1) under 40 years of age; 2) no past or present history of cardiac or hypertensive vascular disease; 3) absence of a murmur on physical examination; 4) no history of current or past cardiotonic or antihypertensive regimens; 5) absence of cardiomegaly on X-ray. We found 80 patients who satisfied these criteria and they comprise the present study population. All patients were classified as to the duration of sarcoidosis, i.e., subacute or chronic—and according to stage on the basis of chest X-ray findings.

There were 51 women and 29 men (Table 1); 61 were black, 14 were Puerto Rican-born and 5 were Caucasians. Subacute sarcoidosis (less than 2 years duration) existed in 33 patients and chronic sarcoidosis in 47 patients. Chest X-rays at the time the electrocardiograms were made showed hilar adenopathy alone (stage I) in 32 patients, hilar adenopathy with parenchymal mottling (stage II) in 31 patients and mottling only (stage III) in 17 patients.

This work was supported by a research grant from the National Heart and Lung Institute, Public Health Service (HE–13853–14).

TABLE 1. Electrocardiographic alterations in 80 patients with sarcoidosis.

	Patients with abnormal EKG No. of pts. (41)	Patients with normal EKG No. of pts. (39)	Total patients
Sex			
Male	15	14	29
Female	26	25	51
Ethnic Group			
Black	35	26	61
Puerto Rican-born	4	10	14
Caucasian	2	3	5
Estimated duration			
Subacute	17	16	33
Chronic	24	23	47
Chest X-ray			
Stage I	19	13	32
Stage II	13	18	31
Stage III	9	8	17

RESULTS

Some electrocardiographic abnormality was surprisingly detected in 41 of these 80 patients with no cardiac symptoms. They exhibited, in all, 57 separate deviations from the normal. Abnormalities in rhythm and conduction were seen in 18 instances occurring in 15 patients (Table 2). First-degree heart block was noted in 7 patients and a shortened PR interval in 5. Intra-atrial conduction defects were seen in 2 patients and premature atrial contraction in 1 patient. One patient presented with episodes of AV dissociation, ventricular premature contractions, and AV dissociation with junctional premature contractions.

There were also 39 repolarization abnormalities among 26 of the patients in this study (Table 3). T wave changes were noted in 21 instances and consisted of flat T waves in 5, inverted in 6, notched in 9 and peaked in 1. U waves in the absence of bradycardia were seen in 9 patients. ST segment elevation occurred in 4 patients and depression was noted in 4 others. One patient had a prolonged QT interval.

Factors including the sex of the patient, ethnic background, duration of sarcoidosis,

TABLE 2. Alterations in rhythm and conduction in 15 of 80 patients with sarcoidosis.

Alterations		No. of pts.
PR intervals	>0.20 sec	7
	<0.1 sec	5
Intra-atrial conduction defects		2
Premature atrial contractions		1
A-V dissociation		1
Ventricular premature contractions		1
A-V dissociation with junctional premature contractions		1

TABLE 3. 39 Repolarization abnormalities in 26 of 80 patients.

	No. of pts.
Flat T waves	5
Inverted T waves	6
Notched T waves	9
Peaked T waves	1
U wave (no bradycardia)	9
ST segment elevations	4
ST segment depressions	4
Prolonged QT interval	1

radiographic stage and corticosteroid therapy did not appear to influence the frequency and character of the electrocardiographic abnormalities which were found. None of the patients observed in this study exhibited clinical evidence of cardiac disease during a 6-month period of subsequent observation.

DISCUSSION

The essential question that this study poses is the nature of the underlying histopathological myocardial changes which account for the electrocardiographic alterations among these relatively young patients with sarcoidosis. The most plausible hypothesis would seem to be the fortuitous but critical placement of sarcoid granulomas within various locations of the cardiac conducting system as simply another representation of systemic involvement in this disorder. Such a hypothesis is supported by findings of granulomas in the cardiac conducting system of patients succumbing to fatal arrhythmias.[3, 4, 7, 8] Whether or not myocardial granulomas have a predilection for the conducting system cannot be determined from available autopsy data or from clinical studies. Numerous granulomas are almost invariably found at autopsy in the cardiac muscle as well as in the more usual locations, suggesting that involvement of the conduction system occurs haphazardly in a hit-or-miss fashion.[3, 5]

The most common electrocardiographic findings reported in cases of myocardial sarcoidosis are conduction disturbances and arrhythmias consisting of frequent premature ventricular contractions, paroxysmal atrial and ventricular tachycardias and disturbances in sinoatrial function.[13–16] However, on occasion, extensive involvement of the myocardium has been seen associated with only minor ST segment and T wave changes noted on the electrocardiogram.[17] In one instance, the electrocardiogram in a patient with extensive myocardial sarcoidosis revealed only the presence of a sinus tachycardia.[18]

In the literature, up to two-thirds of those patients whose deaths are considered to be directly related to intrinsic cardiac sarcoidosis died suddenly.[4, 19, 20] In 25% of these fatalities no previous cardiac symptoms have been experienced. The average age at the time of death varied from 35 to 44 years.[4, 21] Porter,[4] reported fatal cardiac sarcoidosis to be twice as frequent in males as in females. However, in a series published by Mayaji, the frequency in the 2 sexes was found to be reversed.[21] In the asymptomatic patients of our study abnormal ECG findings were equally common in both sexes.

The mechanisms leading to sudden cardiac death in sarcoidosis have not been conclusively demonstrated. However, it is not unlikely that the presence of fatal arrhythmias is the common mode of exitus. It is known that individuals with abnormalities of repolarization may be more prone to develop arrhythmias through reentry phenomena or by initiation and persistance of ectopic foci.[22,23] Twenty-six of our 80 patients demonstrated repolarization abnormalities a potentially dangerous manifestation. Fifteen patients or 18% had changes in rhythm and conduction which might also represent a threat of future difficulty. The ECG alterations here reported did not correlate with ethnic group, the duration of sarcoidosis or the severity of pulmonary sarcoidosis as determined by chest X-ray staging.

It is difficult to prove without histologic evidence that these electrocardiographic changes are a direct result of myocardial involvement. However, the age of the patients studied, the absence of a past or present history of treated or untreated hypertension or heart disease, and the presence of a normal-sized heart on chest film make other pathogenetic mechanisms less likely. In a large series of patients with proven myocardial sarcoidosis reported by Gozo,[24] Porter[4] and Bashor[3] the electrocardiographic disturbances in rhythm and conduction which they described are similar to those seen in our series of patients.

At the present time, prospective studies are under way in our clinic to determine which of the asymptomatic electrocardiographic abnormalities occurring in patients with sarcoidosis may represent precursors of more serious and potentially dangerous cardiac arrhythmias secondary to myocardial involvement by sarcoid granulomas or fibrosis.

SUMMARY

Among 80 patients with tissue-confirmed sarcoidosis attending the sarcoidosis clinic of the Mount Sinai Hospital, electrocardiographic abnormalities of varying import were noted in 41 patients despite the fact that these patients were entirely without cardiac complaints and exhibited no evidence of previous or current cardiac disease on thorough examination. All these patients were under 40 years of age.

The ECG alterations included repolarization abnormalities and alterations in rhythm and conduction. Because of the potential hazards of some of these ECG abnormalities prospective studies are being undertaken to determine which of them may represent precursors of dangerous intrinsic cardiac sarcoidosis.

REFERENCES

1. Longcope, W., and Freiman, D. 1952. A study of sarcoidosis based on combined investigations of 160 cases, including 30 autopsies from the Johns-Hopkins Hospital and Massachusetts General Hospital. *Medicine* **31**: 1.
2. Branson, J., and Park, J. 1954. Sarcoidosis—hepatic involvement: presentation of case with fatal liver involvement, including autopsy findings and review of evidence of sarcoid involvement of liver- as found in literature. *Ann. Int. Med.* **40**: 111.
3. Bashour, F. A., McConnell, T., Skinner, W., and Hanson, M. 1968. Myocardial Sarcoidosis, *Diseases Chest* **53**: 413.
4. Porter, G. H. 1960. Sarcoid Heart Disease. *N. Engl. J. Med.* **263**: 1350.
5. Duvernoy, W. F. D., and Garcia, R. 1971. Sarcoidosis of the Heart Presenting with Ventricular Tachycardia and Atrioventricular Block, *Amer. J. Cardiol.* **28**: 348.

6. Longcope, W. T., and Freiman, D. G. 1952. A study of sarcoidosis based on combined investigation of 160 cases including 30 autopsies from Johns Hopkins Hospital and Massachusetts General Hospital. *Medicine* (Balt.) **31**: 1–132.

7. Contreras, R., Sanchez, Torres, G., and Duran Rodriguez. P. 1967. Sarcoidosis cardiaea. *Arch. Inst. Cardiol. Mex.* **37**: 20–37.

8. Shimada, N., Ishihara, Y., Kojima, A., et al. 1967. Three cases of granulomatous myocarditis with giant cells. *Acta Path. Jap.* **17**: 503–515.

9. Scadding, J. G. 1967. Sarcoidosis. London: Eyre and Spottiswoode. p. 293.

10. Schaumann, J. 1936. Lymphogranulomatosis benigna in light of prolonged clinical observations and autopsy findings. *Brit. J. Dermat.* **48**: 399, 446.

11. Horton, R., Lincoln, N. S., and Pinner, M. 1939. Noncaseating tuberculosis: case reports. *Amer. Rev. Tuberc.* **39**: 186–203.

12. Hauser, H. 1946. Pulmonary sarcoidosis. *J. Oklahoma M. A.* **39**: 395–402.

13. Salvesen, H. A. 1935. Sarcoid of Boeck, disease of importance to internal medicine: report on 4 cases. *Acta Med. Scand.* **86**: 127–151.

14. Cotter, E. F. 1939. Boeck's sarcoid: autopsy in case with visceral lesions. *Arch. Internal Med.* **64**: 286–295.

15. Johnson, J. B., and Jason, R. S. 1944. Sarcoidosis of heart: report of case and review of literature. *Amer. Heart J.* **27**: 246–258.

16. First, S. R. 1949. Electrocardiographic evaluation of Boeck's sarcoid and advanced pulmonary tuberculosis: special reference to interpretation of multiple unipolar leads. *Amer. J. Med.* **7**: 760–764.

17. Johnson, J. B., and Jason, R. S. 1944. Sarcoidosis of heart: report of case and review of literature. *Amer. Heart J.* **27**: 246–258.

18. Laroche, C., de Gennes, J. L., Hazard, J., and Samarcq, P. 1955. Maladie de Besnier-Boeck- chaumann avec manifestations polyarticulaires et localisations endomyo-pericardiques mortelles. *Bull. Mem. Soc. Med. d. Hop de Paris* **71**: 908–913.

19. Longcope, W. T., and Freiman, D. G. 1952. A study of sarcoidosis based on a combined investigation of 160 cases including 30 autopsies from the Johns Hopkins Hospital and Massachusetts General Hospital. *Medicine* (Balt.) **31**: 1–132.

20. Nisses, A. W., and Berte, J. B. 1964. Cardiac arrhythmias in sarcoidosis. *Arch. Internal Med.* (Chicago) **113**: 275–282.

21. Miyaji, T., Ohara, M., Funaki, M., et al. 1967. A case of myocardial sarcoidosis with Adams-Stokes syndrome. *J. Jap. Soc. Internal Med.* **56**: 260–266.

22. Goldreyer, B. N. 1972. Intracardiac electrocardiography in the analysis and understanding of cardiac arrhythmias. *Ann. Internal Med.* **77**: 117–136.

23. Kisten, A. D., and Landowe, M. 1951. Retrograde conduction from premature ventricular contractions—a common occurrence in the human heart. *Circulation* **3**: 738–751.

24. Gozo, E. G., Cosnow, I., Cohen, H., and Okun, L. 1971. The Heart in Sarcoidosis. *Chest* **60**: 379.

Abnormal Electrocardiographic Findings in Sarcoidosis

J. R. MIKHAIL, D. N. MITCHELL AND K. P. BALL

*Central Middlesex Hospital and MRC Tuberculosis and Chest Diseases Research Unit,
Brompton Hospital, London, Great Britain*

INTRODUCTION

Involvement of the heart by sarcoidosis is uncommon and the majority of cases described in the literature have been found at postmortem examination. It therefore seemed possible that electrocardiographic abnormalities might in fact be more common among patients with sarcoidosis than has hitherto been recognised. Accordingly, a full electrocardiographic examination was included in the investigation of 147 consecutive cases of histologically confirmed sarcoidosis. These patients came predominantly from Britain, Ireland and the Caribbean[1] and were mainly in the 20- to 44-year-old age group with females predominating, approximately 2:1. The majority of the immigrants had been in Great Britain for 5 years or more.

RESULTS

The results of our routine ECG examinations are shown in Table 1 which analyses the 14 cases with abnormal findings. There were 3 patients who had abnormal ECG findings in whom the evidence that these were attributable to sarcoidosis is doubtful. The first case was an Indian lady of 72 years who had bilateral hilar lymphadenopathy with pulmonary mottling, a positive Kveim test and a mediastinal lymph node biopsy showing noncaseating epithelioid and giant cell granulomata. She had bilateral iridocyclitis; the ECG showed a right bundle branch block. There was no evidence to suggest that this was necessarily associated with her sarcoidosis. The second case was a 47-year-old lady from Guyana with bilateral hilar lymphadenopathy, a positive Kveim test and a mediastinal lymph node showing noncaseating granulomata. She had arthralgia and a left facial palsy and gave a long history of angina pectoris. Her ECG showed evidence of a transmural anterior infarction and a previous ECG 2 years earlier had shown ischaemic changes. The third case was an Indian lady of 47 years with a normal chest radiograph and noncaseating granulomata in her abdominal lymph nodes. She developed cardiomyopathy. It was never satisfactorily established whether her initial condition was attributable to sarcoidosis, tuberculosis or Crohn's disease.

TABLE 1. Abnormal ECG findings in 147 histologically
confirmed cases of sarcoidosis.

1.	Abnormal ECG findings of doubtful significance	3
2.	Abnormal ECG in acute active sarcoidosis:	
	a) Ventricular tachycardia	1
	b) T wave changes	10
	Total	14

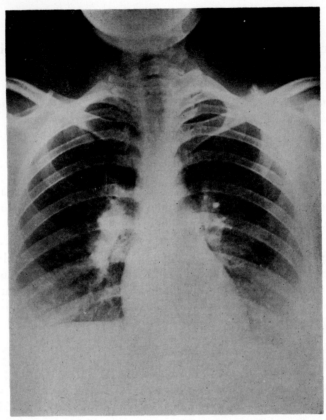

F<small>IG</small>. 1.   P. A. chest radiograph of case 1 on presentation, showing bilateral hilar lymphadenopathy.

The other 11 cases had abnormal ECG's in the presence of acute active sarcoidosis, and it is felt that the findings are strongly suggestive of an association. The following 5 case histories illustrate these findings.

The first is that of a 19-year-old Caucasian female who had a classical Löfgren's syndrome, namely erythema nodosum and arthralgia, bilateral hilar lymphadenopathy (Fig. 1), a negative tuberculin test and a positive Kveim test. Noncaseating granulomata were found on biopsy of her mediastinal lymph nodes. The ECG on diagnosis showed T wave inversion in leads II and III, AVF, V_5 and V_6; and, with regression of her acute disease the tracing returned to normal (Fig. 2).

The second is a 38-year-old coloured male with bilateral hilar lymphadenopathy and pulmonary mottling, a negative tuberculin test and a positive Kveim test. Mediastinal lymph node biopsy showed noncaseating granulomata. An ECG on diagnosis was normal. Ten months later he deteriorated clinically and radiologically and treatment with steroids was commenced. Ten days later he was admitted to hospital as an emergency with ventricular tachycardia. He was treated with practolol, with continuation of steroid therapy. He reverted to normal rhythm (Fig. 3) and has remained well for the last year.

The third case is a 23-year-old coloured female with bilateral hilar lymphadenopathy and pulmonary mottling. She had a negative tuberculin and a positive Kveim test; noncaseating granulomata were found on biopsy of her mediastinal lymph nodes. Her ECG

pt :   J.V.

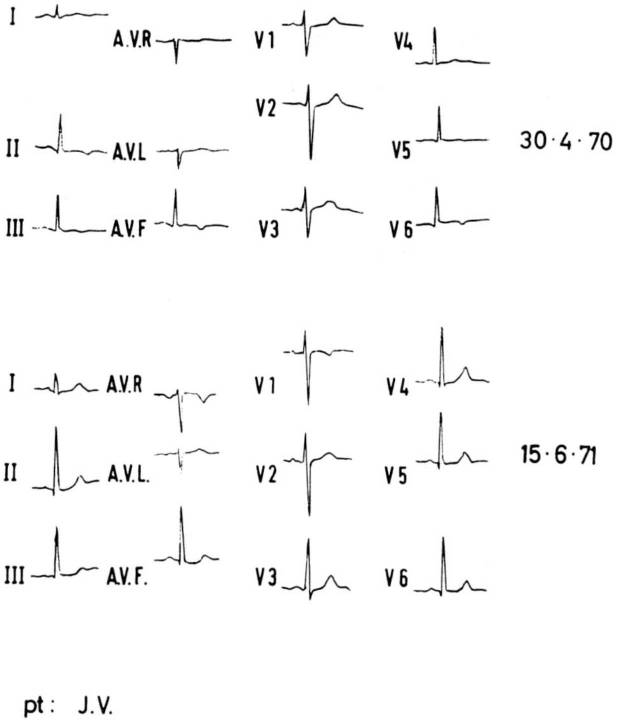

FIG. 2.   ECG showing T wave inversion in leads 2 and 3, AVF, V_5 and V_6; and, with regression of sarcoidosis the return of the tracing to normal.

on diagnosis (Fig. 4) showed T wave inversion in V_1 to V_3 and flat T waves in V_4. Because of increasing dyspnoea she required steroid therapy. Her ECG 2 months later showed some improvement and eventually returned to normal. She remains well with a normal ECG tracing 4 years later. Her sarcoidosis has regressed and her chest radiograph is within normal limits.

The fourth case[2] is that of a 41-year-old coloured male with bilateral hilar lymphadenopathy and pulmonary mottling (Fig. 5), a negative tuberculin test and a positive Kveim test. He showed evidence of extrathoracic sarcoidosis in many organs and noncaseating granulomata were found in biopsy from a subcutaneous skin nodule and from his mediastinal lymph nodes. He had a blocked nose and a hoarse voice, biopsy of the nasal mucosa and larynx both revealed noncaseating granulomata. Both epididymii were grossly swollen and biopsy of 1 epididymis showed noncaseating granulomata (Fig. 6). The ECG on diagnosis showed coronary sinus rhythm, T wave inversion in leads I and AVL, ST elevation V_5 and V_6 (Fig. 7). Because of his extensive multisystem sarcoidosis he was treated with steroid therapy with dramatic clinical improvement. Three months later the ECG showed a normal tracing.

The last case (case 5) is that of a 25-year-old Irish girl who had been in this country for 8 years. Negative tuberculin test. Chest X-ray shows bilateral hilar lymphadenopathy (Fig. 8). Mediastinal lymph node showed noncaseating granulomata. Kveim test was positive. Her lacrimal secretions were reduced to 40% in both eyes. ECG on diagnosis showed T waves to be flat in leads III, AVF, V_4, V_5 and V_6. A further ECG 1 month later

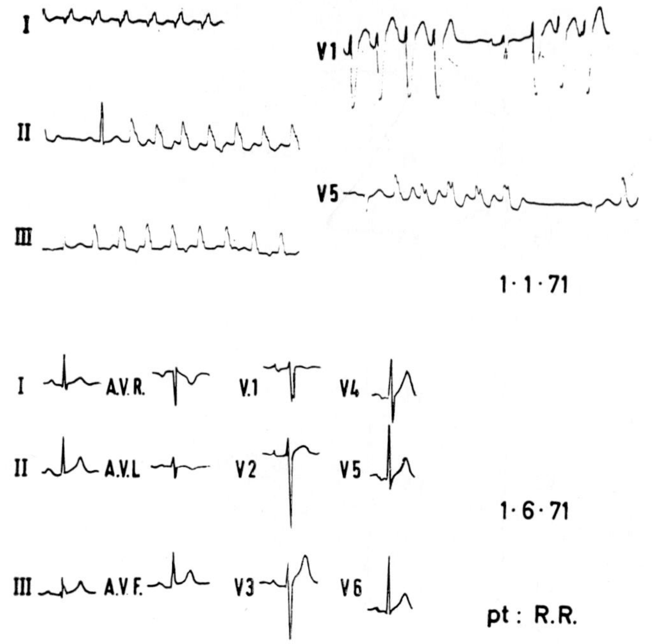

FIG. 3. ECG showing ventricular tachycardia associated with clinical and radiological deterioration of sarcoidosis and the return to a normal tracing after treatment with practolol and continuation of steroid therapy.

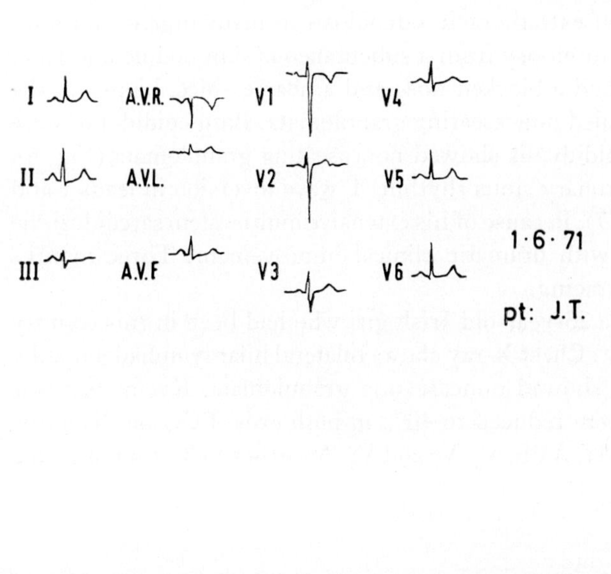

FIG. 4. ECG showing T wave inversion in V_1 to V_3 and flat T wave in V_4 with eventual return to a normal tracing following treatment with steroids and regression of her sarcoidosis.

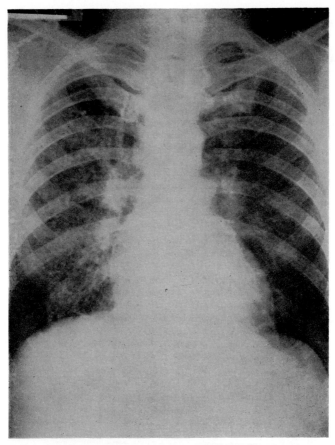

FIG. 5. P. A. chest radiograph of case 4 on presentation, showing bilateral hilar lymphadenopathy and pulmonary mottling.

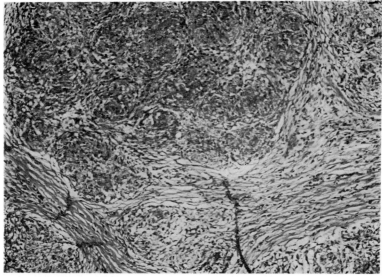

FIG. 6.   Histology of epididymis (case 4) showing noncaseating epithelioid and giant cell granulomata.   Haematoxylin and eosin, Mag. × 120.

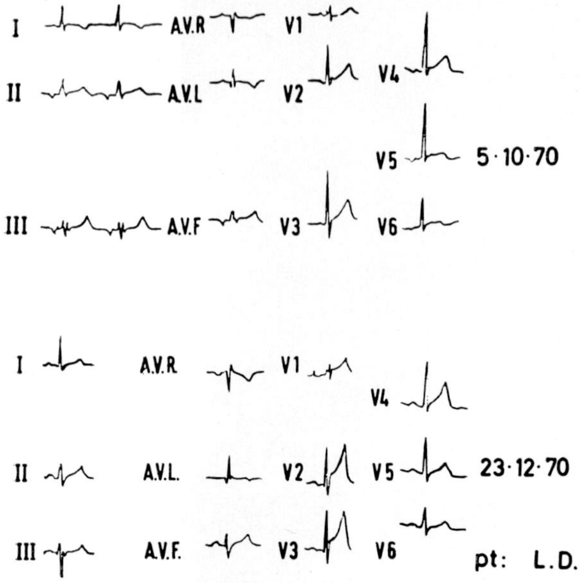

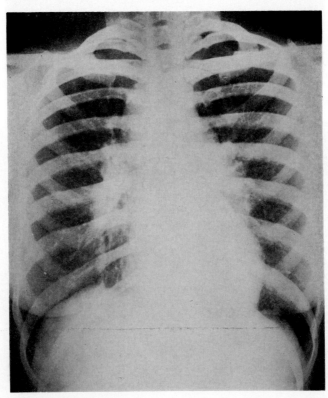

FIG. 7. ECG showing T wave inversion in leads I and AVL with ST elevation in V_5 and V_6 and the later return to a normal tracing following treatment with steroid therapy.

FIG. 8. P. A. Chest radiograph of case 5 on presentation, showing bilateral hilar lymphadenopathy.

showed frequent ventricular ectopics had appeared with post-ectopic T wave inversion. A subsequent ECG 1 month later showed no change. A further ECG 2 years later showed that the ventricular ectopics persisted, the T wave was inverted in leads V_5 and V_6 (Fig. 9).

SUMMARY

On hundred and forty-seven histologically confirmed cases of sarcoidosis were submitted to a series of routine investigations which included electrocardiography. Fourteen of these patients (13 being asymptomatic) were found to have abnormal ECG changes of which 3 were probably not attributable to sarcoidosis.

In 11 cases, the ECG showed a changing pattern coinciding with resolution of the sarcoidosis. These changes are highly suggestive of myocardial involvement by sarcoidosis.

ACKNOWLEDGEMENT

We thank Mr A. G. Booker and Miss J. O. Williams for the photographs.

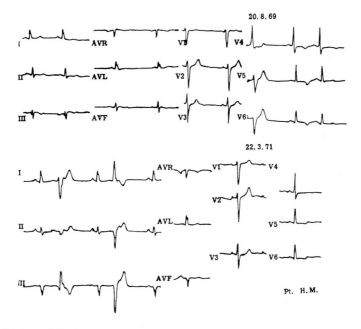

FIG. 9.   ECG on 20.8.69 showing flat T waves in leads III, AVF, V_4, V_5 and V_6. On 22.3.71 the change were still present with postectopic T wave inversion.

REFERENCES

1. Mikhail, J. R., Mitchell, D. N., and Ball, K. P. 1972. Electrocardiographic abnormalities found in patients with sarcoidosis. La Sarcoidose particulierement dans ses localisations endothoraciques. *Rapp. Symp. Europeen de la Sarcoidose.* Geneva: Edition Hallwag SA. p. 99.

2. Mikhail, J. R., Mitchell, D. N., Dyson, J. L., Williams, W. J., Ogunlesi, T. O. O., and Van Hein-Wallace, S. E. 1972. Sarcoidosis with genital involvement. *Amer. Rev. Res. Dis.* **106**: 465.

Sarcoidosis of the Pleura

E. Leslie Chusid, L. O. B. D. Vieira and Louis E. Siltzbach

The Mount Sinai School of Medicine, The Mount Sinai Hospital and the City Hospital Center (Elmhurst), New York, U.S.A.

Pleural sarcoidosis, like sarcoidosis of other serosal membranes, is uncommon. Pleural involvement in sarcoidosis requires corroboration by findings of a pleural effusion in association with visceral and parietal pleural granulomas, or by pleural granulomas without effusion.

Among 950 patients with sarcoidosis observed at the Sarcoidosis Clinic of the Mount

Age range	26–59
Sex	6 male, 1 female
Diagnostic features of sarcoidosis	chronic disease, 5/7 pulmonary mottling, 5/7 multi-organ
Tuberculin status	negative (7)
Pleural effusion	4/7
Diagnosis of pleural involvement	biopsy—3 open, 2 closed
Characteristics of effusion	exudate ; 99–100%
	lymphocytes ; small to massive

FIG. 1. Seven cases of sarcoidosis (The Mount Sinai Hospital, N.Y.C.).

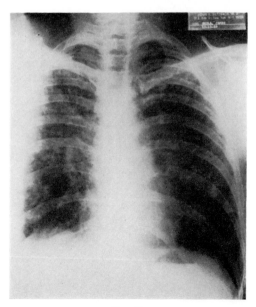

FIG. 2.

373

Sinai Hospital during the past quarter century, seven patients were encountered with pleural involvement (Fig. 1). A histologic confirmation was obtained in 5 of the 7 patients; in 3 by open pleural biopsy, and in 2 by Abrams needle biopsy. In the remaining 2 patients pleural effusions occurred in association with extensive pulmonary involvement and multiorgan extrathoracic sarcoidosis. In none of the 7 was there evidence of infection, cardiac failure, or pulmonary infarction.

The patients ranged in age from 26 to 59 years old and the tuberculin test (250 TU) was negative in all of them. A pleural effusion occurred in 4 patients and it was an exudate, containing mostly lymphocytes (99–100%), and at times was massive in quantity (up to 3500 cc).

Three examples of pleural sarcoidosis will be presented. The first is a 30-year-old man with a chief complaint of dyspnea on exertion. Five years before being seen at the Mount Sinai Hospital he was told of hilar node enlargement. Physicial examination now showed hepatosplenomegaly and a chest film (Fig. 2) showed diffuse bilateral nodular pulmonary disease. A tuberculin test and a Kveim test were negative. Thoracotomy and biopsy of lung, pleura, and mediastinal nodes revealed noncaseating epithelioid cell granulomas in all specimens (Fig. 3). He was treated with corticosteroids with moderate clearing of his chest film.

The second patient was a 38-year-old male with a chief complaint of increasing dyspnea, fatigue, and cough for one year. His chest film (Fig. 4) showed a diffuse haziness in the right lower lung field with bilateral interstitial densities and full hilar shadows. A

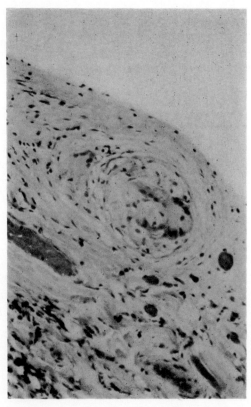

FIG. 3.

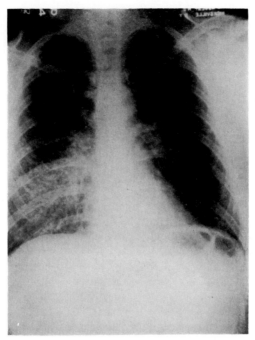

FIG. 4.

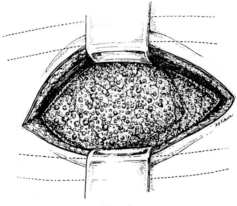

FIG. 5.

tuberculin test was negative and a Kveim test was positive. An open-lung biopsy was performed and Fig. 5 shows a sketch of the lung and pleural surface at the time of surgery. Grape-like lesions can be seen to project from visceral and parietal pleura. Microscopically (Fig. 6) specimens from both visceral and parietal pleura showed sarcoid granulomas.

The third patient was a 55-year-old male with abdominal pain, enlarged parotid glands, peripheral adenopathy, and hepatosplenomegaly. The initial chest film was normal, but a liver biopsy showed noncaseating granulomas. The tuberculin test was negative and the Kveim test was positive. He was treated with corticosteroids, but the patient stopped the medication on his own. Eighteen months later, he complained of dyspnea, and a new chest film (Fig. 7) showed a massive pleural effusion. A tuberculin

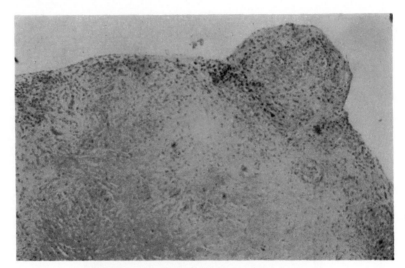

FIG. 6.

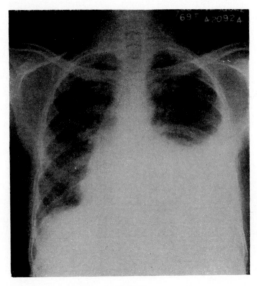

FIG. 7.

test (250 TU) was negative and a closed pleural biopsy (Fig. 8) showed noncaseating granulomas. The pleural fluid resorbed with the use of corticosteroids which were later discontinued, only to have the patient return with recurrent bilateral effusions. A biopsy of the right parietal pleura with an Abrams needle also showed noncaseating granulomas. The tuberculin tests were still negative. The effusions disappeared again with reinstitution of corticosteroids.

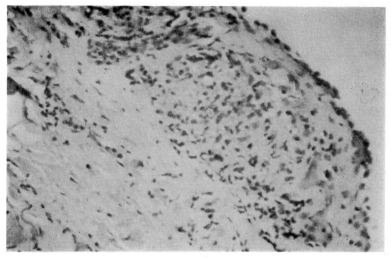

FIG. 8.

DISCUSSION

The 7 cases from the Mount Sinai Hospital were analyzed along with other reports of pleural sarcoidosis in the literature with respect to the time of pleural involvement, the frequency of its occurrence and the characteristics of pleural effusions when present. Figure 9 shows that from 1947 to 1971, 22 instances of pleural involvement were mentioned among 2,410 patients reported in 11 large reviews of sarcoidosis, an overall frequency of 0.9%.

Figure 10 indicates that 23 other cases of sarcoidosis with pleural envolvement, not included in the larger series, have been reported in the literature from 1933 to 1972. In patients with pleural effusions, none had a coexisting disease which might cause such an

	Investigator	Year	Total cases of sarcoidosis	Number with pleural involvement
1.	McCort	1947	28	2
2.	Longcope	1952	160	*
3.	Israel	1958	160	3
4.	Mayock	1963	145	2
5.	Kamfer	1964	245	2
6.	Lebacq	1964	100	3
7.	Scadding	1967	234	2
8.	Siltzbach	1967	311	3
9.	James	1968	537	*
10.	Selroos	1969	140	5
11.	Turiaf	1971	350	*
	Total		2410	22 (0.9%)

* Not mentioned.

FIG. 9. Reported pleural involvement in sarcoidosis.

Years in which reported	1933–1968
Number of cases	23
Age range	20–79
Sex	9 male, 10 female*
Tuberculin status	14 negative, 2 positive**
No. cases with effusion	17/23
Features of sarcoidosis	20/23 with multi-organ disease
Timing of pleural involvement	19/23 with chronic disease, up to 16 yrs. after onset of sarcoidosis

  * 4 cases not mentioned.
  ** 7 cases not mentioned.

Fig. 10. Sarcoidosis with pleural involvement reported in literature.

effusion. In each instance, the diagnosis of sarcoidosis was established by Kveim test, tissue biopsy specimen, or the typical clinical findings. In all instances pleural disease was associated with extensive pulmonary lesions and/or extrathoracic localization of sarcoidosis. Pleural involvement occurred at times up to 16 years after the initial diagnosis of sarcoidosis was made. Generally, in both the previously reported patients and the patients from Mount Sinai Hospital pleural sarcoidosis was virtually always associated with stage II or III pulmonary sarcoidosis.

SUMMARY

(Fig. 11), pleural involvement in sarcoidosis appears to occur with a minimum frequency of 0.9%. Pleural sarcoidosis occurs usually in association with extensive pulmonary disease and/or multiorgan extrathoracic granulomas. Sarcoid pleural effusions are usually exudates, contain 60%–100% lymphocytes, are not characterized by pain or fever, may be yellow, serosanguinous or bloody, and may be minimal or massive in quantity (up to 3500 cc).

Frequency	0.9%
Pleural fluid	
Amount	none / small / massive
Color	yellow / serosanguinous / bloody
Composition	exudate, high protein, normal sugar
Cells	60%–100% lymphocytes
Timing of pleural involvement	usually in chronic stage, up to 16 years after onset
Clinical manifestations	no pleuritic pain or fever, virtually always associated with pulmonary sarcoidosis or extrapulmonary involvement

Fig. 11. Pleural effusion and pleural disease in sarcoidosis.

Two Cases of Sarcoidosis with Radiographic Findings Indicative of an Enlarged Thymus

Masami Matusima

Department of Pediatrics, Gunma University, Maebashi, Gunma, Japan

AND

Toshisada Kimura

Tomo Hospital, Ota, Gunma, Japan

There is scarcely any organ or tissue which is free from involvement of sarcoidosis, with the exception of the adrenals. Although the thymus is related closely to lymphoid tissue, which is most susceptible to sarcoidosis, there has been no report of thymus sarcoidosis to date. In McGovern and Merrit's world review of 113 cases of sarcoidosis in children, and Jasper and Denney's review of 68 such cases no case of thymus involvement was reported. As the thymus usually becomes atrophic with age, the involvement of this organ may have been overlooked in the past. However, a recent wider use of the pneumo-mediastinum technique has revealed that enlargement of the thymus is not very rare even in older children, suggesting the possibility of involvement of the thymus in sarcoidosis for this age group. We have observed 2 cases of sarcoidosis aged 15 and 13 years with abnormal mediastinal shadows suggesting a thymic enlargement.

Case 1. A 15-year-old boy developed uveitis with granulomas in his left iris. He had generalized enlargements of superficial lymph nodes. A biopsy of the femoral lymph node revealed epithelioid cell tubercles with scanty necrosis and without caseation. A biopsy of nodules in the conjunctiva and nasal mucosa also demonstrated epithelioid cell granulomas. The tuberculin reaction was positive 6 months prior to admission but negative at the time of admission. Physical findings revealed dullness to percussion over

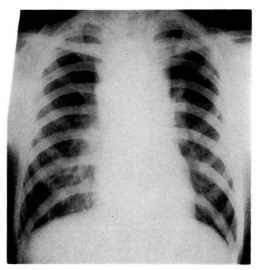

Fig. 1.   Case 1.   BHL and broad mediastinal shadow with bilateral straight borders.

379

the superior aspect of the sternum. A chest radiograph showed bilateral enlargement of the hilar lymphnodes, with faint mottling in both lungs. The mediastinal shadow was markedly enlarged with bilateral straight borders (Fig. 1). Lateral radiography showed a shadow occupying the upper portion of the anterior mediastinum. On a tomograph, this shadow was well-defined behind the sternum. After the administration of 850 mg of Prednisolone over a 52-day period, the broad mediastinal shadow and enlarged hilar lymph nodes regressed rapidly and 1 month later subsided almost completely.

Case 2. A 13-year-old girl was found to have bilateral hilar lymphnode enlargement on a routine radiograph. The right inguinal lymph nodes were enlarged. A biopsy revealed noncaseating epithelioid cell tubercles with giant cells. Tuberculin reaction was positive for 7 consecutive years prior to admission but was negative at the time

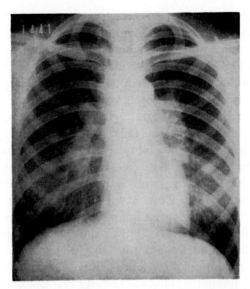

FIG. 2.   Case 2.   BHL and broad mediastinal shadow.

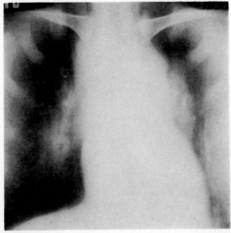

FIG. 3.   Pneumomediastinum.   Tomograph, 10 cm from back, just behind the sternum, showing the broad mediastinal shadow.

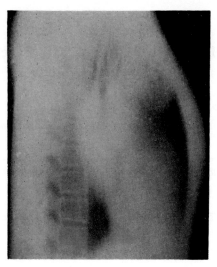

FIG. 4. Pneumomediastinum. Lateral tomograph, 13 cm from right. A tumorous shadow occupying the upper portion of the anterior mediastinum.

of admission. Chest radiographs showed enlargements of the bilateral hilar lymph nodes and mediastinal shadow (Fig. 2). The lateral radiographs showed a tumorous shadow occupying the upper portion of the anterior mediastinum. A pneumomediastinum was performed by injecting 2,700 ml of air into the mediastinum. On tomographs the broad mediastinal shadow was well-defined behind the sternum (Fig. 3). Lateral tomographs demonstrated a tumorous shadow in the upper portion of the anterior mediastinum just behind the sternum and anterior to the great vessels (Fig. 4). Prednisolone was administered for 75 days in a total dosage of 1,225 mg. The tumorous mediastinal shadow and the enlarged hilar lymphnodes regressed rapidly and subsided almost completely within 3 months. A pneumomediastinum was performed 3 months thereafter, and revealed no tumorous shadow in the mediastinum.

These tumorous shadows in the upper portion of the anterior mediastinum, just behind the sternum, suggest an enlargement of the thymus or anterior mediastinal lymph nodes. The differentiation between the two is difficult radiographically. Whether these shadows represent thymus sarcoidosis or not, must be proved by biopsy with a mediastinoscope in the future.

Clinical Course of Patients with Sarcoidosis with Hepatic Lesions

Teruo Tachibana and Kazuhiko Aratake

Osaka Prefectural Hospital, Osaka, Japan

Shizuo Okada

Japan Antituberculosis Association, Osaka Branch, Osaka, Japan

Minoru Matsuda

Center for Adult Diseases, Osaka, Japan

AND

Shiro Kato, Matao Naito and Yoko Akiyama

Research Institute for Microbial Diseases, Osaka University, Osaka, Japan

It must be emphasized that subclinical extrathoracic lesions may exist in sarcoidosis patients and may be disclosed by appropriate procedures. We have already reported that hepatic invasion could be revealed in a high percentage of cases by peritoneoscopy and a liver biopsy in sarcoidosis patients.[1] We have followed up the chest radiographic findings of sarcoidosis patients with or without hepatic lesions.

MATERIALS AND METHODS

Peritoneoscopy and liver biopsy were performed on 50 sarcoidosis patients with normal hepatic function. Chest radiographs were taken every month for follow-up. A

TABLE 1. 37 cases of sarcoidosis with hepatic lesion demonstrated by peritoneoscopy and liver biopsy.

1.	Sex		
	male	17	(23)
	female	20	(27)
2.	Age		
	−10	0	(1)
	10–19	17	(20)
	20–29	14	(21)
	30–39	4	(6)
	40–49	1	(1)
	50–59	1	(1)
3.	Intrathoracic lesion on chest film		
	BHL	21	(32)
	BHL with parenchymal lesion	15	(17)
	Parenchymal lesion	1	(1)

( ) indicates the number of total cases performed peritoneoscopy and liver biopsy.

382

second peritoneoscopy and liver biopsy were performed after improvement of the chest radiographs in 10 cases.

RESULTS

In 37 of the 50 cases hepatic lesions were demonstrated, as shown in Table 1. Those patients with or without hepatic lesion were divided into 4 groups; group A without hepatic lesions, group B with a slight hepatic lesions, group C with moderate hepatic lesions and group D with marked hepatic lesions. Slight hepatic lesions means only a few sarcoid nodules on the liver surface, where only 1 or 2 were found in the liver biopsy specimen. Moderate hepatic lesions means many sarcoid nodules on the liver surface, where several sarcoid nodules were found in the liver biopsy specimen. Marked hepatic lesions means numerous sarcoid nodules on the liver surface and about 10 to 20 sarcoid nodules in the liver biopsy specimen. Hepatic lesions of the last group included large sarcoid nodules up to 1 cm in diameter on the liver surface and conglomerated sarcoid nodules in the liver biopsy specimen.

CHEST-RADIOGRAPHIC COURSE OF SARCOIDOSIS PATIENTS WITH OR WITHOUT HEPATIC LESIONS

The radiographic course in all the patients in groups A and B was good. However, in 2 of 12 cases in group C and in 2 of 10 cases in group D, the radiographic improvement was slow. Furthermore, in 2 cases of group D relapse occurred (Fig. 1). These cases had eye and other extrathoracic lesions.

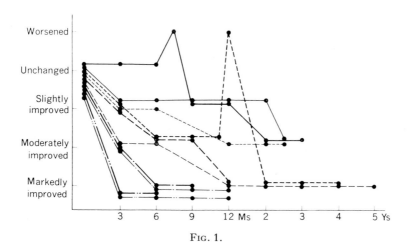

Fig. 1.

PERSISTENCE OF TYPICAL SARCOID GRANULOMAS IN THE LIVER

In 5 of 10 cases, sarcoid nodules were still demonstrated on the liver surface and epithelioid cell granulomas were still found in the liver biopsy specimen, after the improvement of chest X-ray results.

ANTIBODY TITERS TO EB VIRUS IN SARCOIDOSIS PATIENTS WITH AND WITHOUT HEPATIC LESION

Antibody titers to EB virus were determined by the indirect immunofluorescence method. Anti-EB virus titers in sarcoidosis patients were higher than in the healthy

TABLE 2. Distribution of anti-EBV (VCA) titers among normal subjects and selected diseases.

Group	Anti-EBV (VCA) titers					Total cases	$1:640 \leq$ positive %	Ridit analysis
	$<1:4$	$1:40$	$1:160$	$1:640$	$1:2560\leq$			
Sarcoidosis	0	11	46	47	39	143	60.1	0.733 ± 0.048
Control group	12	42	31	16	7	108	21.3	0.500 ± 0.056
Sarcoidosis								
Before treatment	0	6	17	22	19	64	64.1	0.831 ± 0.072
Under treatment	0	1	18	17	20	56	66.1	0.867 ± 0.077
After clearing of X-ray changes	0	4	11	8	0	23	34.8	0.722 ± 0.120
Tuberculosis	1	6	2	3	2	14	35.7	0.591 ± 0.154
Other diseases	3	15	10	9	3	40	30.0	0.593 ± 0.091
Normal subjects	8	21 (2)	19 (2)	4	2 (2)	54 (6)	11.1	0.500 ± 0.079

( ) Family of patients.

TABLE 3. Antibody titers to EBV in sera from sarcoidosis patient with and without hepatic lesions.

Patient No.	Age and sex	Lesions			Anti-VCA titers			Anti-EA	Sampling interval (months)
		Eyes	Skin	Liver	Before treatment	Under treatment	After clearing of X-ray changes		
10	18 F	−	−	‖	2560	640, 640, 2560		−	12, 14, 6
18	49 F	+	+	‖	2560	2560, 2560		+	3, 6
19	22 M	−	−	‖	640	2560		+	12
36	12 M	+	−	‖	160, 640	160, 160	40	−	21, 14, 13, 7
21	16 M	−	−	‖		640, 2560	640	−	2, 6
27	11 F	−	−	‖	640	640	640, 160	−	25, 27, 3
25	14 M	+	−	‖	160	160, 160, 2560		−	11, 7, 13
86	22 F	−	−	‖	2560	640, 160	640, 160	−	5, 13, 3, 14
38	23 F	−	−	‖	2560	2560		−	7
3	35 M	+	−	‖	640	160	160	−	7, 8
80	10 F	−	−	‖	640	160		N.T.	4
24	21 M	−	+	‖	160	640, 160, 160		−	5, 13, 4
41	16 M	−	−	‖	2560	2560, 640	160, 40	+	5, 17, 5, 1
33	22 F	−	−	‖	40	160		+	13
17	28 M	−	−	−	2560	160		−	10
84	9 F	−	−	−	640	2560	640, 40	+	6, 5, 8
82	27 M	−	−	−	160	640, 640	640	−	2, 10, 12
26	25 M	−	−	−	40	2560		−	7

controls and in patients with other diseases, as shown in Table 2. These higher titers showed a tendency to become lower after the clearing of chest X-rays. No such difference was observed in sarcoidosis patients with and without hepatic lesions (Table 3).

DISCUSSION

It has been widely considered that prognosis of sarcoidosis patients with extrathoracic lesions such as eye or skin lesions is worse.[2,3] We would regard marked hepatic lesions as an important factor in the prognosis of sarcoidosis.

SUMMARY

1)   Hepatic lesions were demonstrated in 37 of 50 patients with sarcoidosis.

2)   The chest radiographic course in sarcoidosis patients with a slight hepatic lesion was as good as in those without hepatic lesions. However, in some patients with marked hepatic lesions worsening occured or radiographic improvement was slow.

REFERENCES

1.   Tachibana, T., et al. 1969. *Fifth Int. Conf. on Sarcoidosis* p. 559.
2.   James, D. G. 1961. *Amer. Rev. Resp. Dis.* **84**: 66.
3.   Sones, M., and Israel, H. L. 1961. *Amer. Rev. Resp. Dis.* **84**: 60.

Symptomatic Sarcoidosis of Skeletal Muscle

ANDREW DOUGLAS

*Department of Respiratory Diseases, University of Edinburgh,
Edinburgh, Great Britain*

Symptomatic involvement of skeletal muscle is rare, and fewer than 50 cases have been recorded. In more than 500 patients with sarcoidosis seen in the Edinburgh area over the past 20 years there have been only 2 cases of symptomatic muscle sarcoidosis. Both were examples of chronic sarcoid polymyositis and both showed pseudohypertrophy. The principal features are summarised in Table 1.

TABLE 1. Skeletal muscle sarcoidosis (Chronic myopathy):
Summary of findings in 2 patients.

Age and sex	Presenting symptoms	Other sarcoid features	EMG	Method of diagnosis	Course
59 F	Painful swelling and weakness of thighs and calves Weakness of proximal muscles of upper limbs	Nil	Myopathy (Widespread)	Biopsy— Quadriceps	Initial improvement with prednisolone Later relapse Death from pulmonary embolism .... Autopsy showed multisystem sarcoid involvement
56 F	Weakness of thighs, calves and abdominal muscles	Subcutaneous swelling of fingers Bilateral hilar adenopathy Bilateral parotid swellings Retinal vasculitis CSF— Lymphocytes+ Protein 128 mg%	Neuro-myopathy	Biopsy— Gastrocnemius Quadriceps Rectus abdominis	Maintained improvement with prednisolone (1 year+)

COMMENT

Why granulomatous involvement of skeletal muscle should be symptomatic in some patients but asymptomatic in most is not understood nor is there any known reason why the disease process should become dominant in skeletal muscle. It has been suggested that previous nonsarcoid muscle disease may predispose but this is not borne out by most case histories. The predilection for menopausal women has led to speculation about an endocrine factor but there is no proof of this.

Although the muscle disorder in the 2 patients reported here was very similar clinically, the extent of granuloma formation was strikingly different. In 1 the volume of granuloma and its effect on muscle fibres (Fig. 1) was sufficient to explain the muscle weakness and EMG confirmed a pure myopathy. In the other the sarcoid lesions were scanty (Fig. 2) and an associated neuropathy, confirmed by EMG, contributed importantly

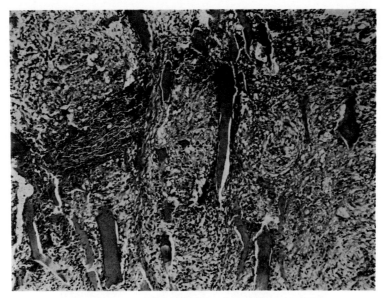

FIG. 1. Quadriceps biopsy showing exuberant granuloma formation widely separating muscle fibres.

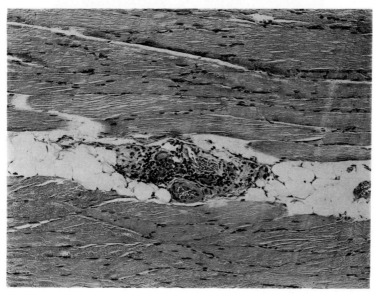

FIG. 2. Muscle biopsy showing sarcoid granuloma between bundles of apparently normal muscle fibres.

to the symptomatology. This patient also showed evidence of CNS involvement.

The patients contrast in other respects. Whereas 1 had extensive clinical evidence of sarcoidosis when the muscle symptoms developed the other did not, although in this patient multisystem involvement was demonstrated at autopsy, supporting the view that isolated muscle sarcoidosis probably never occurs. An unexpected autopsy finding was the presence of hyaline droplets in the convoluted tubules of the kidney (Fig. 3). These had the characteristics of protein in the process of transport and it is possible that

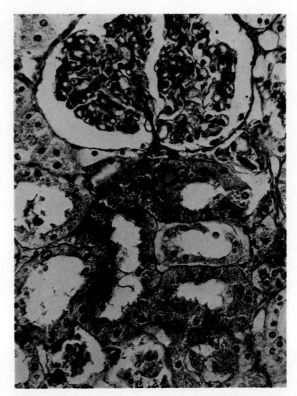

FIG. 3.   Section of kidney showing hyaline droplets in convoluted tubules.

myoglobin contributed to their formation since breakdown of muscle fibers was so marked.

Treatment with prednisolone was initially effective in both but there was later relapse in 1, occurring after an attempt at reduction in the maintenance dosage of prednisolone below 10 mg daily because of intractable peptic ulcer symptoms. Increased dosage of prednisolone failed to control the deterioration. In the other patient the muscle symptoms have been satisfactorily controlled for over a year by prednisolone in a dosage of 20 mg daily.

The principal features of sarcoid myopathy can be summarised as follows (see also Refs. 1–11):

1)   Onset in middle age or later as a rule.

2)   A chronic form of sarcoidosis.

3)   Usually diffuse, symmetrical polymyositis with muscle atrophy. Occasionally palpable nodules, pseudohypertrophy, fibrosis and induration, contractures.

4)   Proximal muscles most frequently involved clinically but often widespread muscle involvement histologically.

5)   May simulate progressive muscular atrophy or muscular dystrophy.

6)   Neuropathy may coexist. EMG useful.

7)   May (+) or may not (+) be evidence of sarcoidosis elsewhere.

8)   Muscle biopsy plays definitive role in diagnosis.

9)   Muscle fibres not invaded by granuloma. May be pressure atrophy or degeneration with fibrosis.

10) Effect of corticosteroids variable but should always be tried. Dosage must be adequate and treatment may require to be indefinitely prolonged.

REFERENCES

1. Ammitzböll, F. 1956. A case of Boeck's sarcoid with isolated localization in the musculature. *Acta Rheum. Scand.* **2**: 3.
2. Brun, A. 1961. Chronic polymyositis on the basis of sarcoidosis. *Acta Psychiat. Neurologic. Scand.* **36**: 515.
3. Crompton, M. R., and MacDermot, V. 1961. Sarcoidosis associated with progressive muscular wasting and weakness. *Brain* **84**: 62.
4. Devic, M., Masson, R., and Bonnefoy, R. 1955. A propos d'une observation de myosite a nodules de Besnier-Boeck. *Rev. Neurol.* **92**: 563.
5. Erbsloh, F., and Dietel, W. 1959. Ubor etogene Spatmyophthien: I Die Polymyositis Granulomatosa Boeck. *Arch. Psychiat. Nervenkr.* **199**: 215.
6. Harvey, J. C. 1959. A myopathy of Boeck's sarcoid. *Amer. J. Med.* **26**: 356.
7. Hinterbuchner, Catherine N., and Hinterbuchner, L. P. 1964. Myopathic syndrome in muscular sarcoidosis. *Brain* **87**: 355.
8. Hofstetter, J. C. 1967. Forme amyotrophique grave de sarcoidose: Traitement a la prednisone. *Proc. Fourth Int. Conf. on Sarcoidosis*. Paris: Masson et cie. p. 678.
9. Kryger, J., and Rnnov-Jessen, V. 1959. Myopathy in Boeck's sarcoid. *Acta Rheum. Scand.* **5**: 314.
10. McConkey, B. 1958. Muscular dystrophy in sarcoidosis. *Arch. Internal Med.* **102**: 443.
11. Talbot, P. S. 1967. Sarcoid myopathy. *Brit. Med. J.* **4**: 465.

The Role of the Otolaryngologist in the Diagnosis
of Sarcoidosis

Toshio Ohnishi, Kenichi Takino and Tadashi Hinohara

Department of Otolaryngology, St. Luke's International Hospital, Tokyo, Japan

Sarcoidosis manifests a variety of changes in the ear, nose and throat. Otolaryngologists, however, rarely make an initial diagnosis of this disease because the changes in the otolaryngology are very inconspicuous. A case of Heerfordt's syndrome which showed interesting otolaryngological manifestations is presented together with a review of 14 other sarcoidosis cases that have been treated at St. Luke's International Hospital, Tokyo, during the past 10 years, in order to show how otolaryngologists can contribute to the diagnosis of this disease.

The patient was a 17-year-old high school girl student who was referred to the Department of Otolaryngology in June, 1971. Her initial symptom was right facial palsy, which improved in about 4 weeks on conservative treatment. Swelling of both parotid glands followed, associated with facial palsy of the other side. She complained of a low-grade fever, dryness of the mouth and general fatigue. Lymph nodes were palpable in the right supraclavicular region, the left axilla and the inguinal region. Blood tests showed no abnormalities. Sialography of the left parotid gland revealed destruction of the fine structures of the gland.

Chest X-ray revealed bilateral hilar lymphadenopathy and scattered lesions in both lung fields compatible with sarcoidosis. Ophthalmological examinations revealed left uveitis, bilateral choked discs and perivasculitis of the retina. Her vision was 0.3 on the left and 0.4 on the right. A swollen left inguinal lymph node was biopsied and numerous epithelioid cell granulomas with Langhans-type foreign-body cells were found.

A tuberculin test was negative although the patient's history revealed a positive reaction in a previous test. A Kveim test was positive.

Careful intranasal examination revealed changes of the septal mucosa, characterized by formation of nodules on the mucosa, some of which had yellowish-white points.

A biopsy of one of the nodules revealed typical epithelioid cell granulomas but X-rays of the paranasal sinuses showed no abnormalities. No changes were seen in the pharynx, tonsils and larynx but biopsy of the left tonsil again showed epithelioid cell granulomas. Silver stain revealed absorption of the reticulin fiber. Both tympanic membranes were turbid. An audiogram revealed combined deafness, more severe in the low frequency range. Bronchoscopic findings were characterized by a mesh-like appearance of the engorged blood vessels in the bronchial mucosa. During the past 10 years from 1962 to 1971 a total of 15 confirmed cases of sarcoidosis were treated at St. Luke's International Hospital, Tokyo. Table 1 shows a list of the patients reviewed in this report. Of 15 patients, 8 were female and 7 were male. Nine of the patients were in the twenties. The main symptoms included ophthalmologic symptoms in 8 cases, general fatigue in 5 cases, facial paralysis in 3 cases, cough and fever in 2 cases and a skin node in 1 case.

Seven were without any subjective symptoms and the abnormality was suspected

Table 1. List of cases.

Case No.	Age and sex	Chief compl.	ENT sympt.	Bronchoscopy.	Swollen lymph node	BHL	Posit. biopsy	Kveim	Mant. test	Ocular sympt.	Nerve invol.	Prog.
1.	23 M	X-ray*			cervical	+	lung	+	–	periphlebitis		good
2.	39 M	cough X-ray		white nodules	cervical	+	prescal.		+			good
3.	24 M	visual dist. lassitude		nodules		+	prescal.		–	uveitis		good
4.	50 F	skin nodes	deafness, loss of taste	white spots				+	+	iritis, turbid lens	facial	trans
5.	21 M	X-ray			cervical	+	prescal.		±	uveitis		good
6.	25 M	pain in chest			cervical	+	prescal.		–			good
7.	63 F	X-ray		uneven mucosa	cervical	+	prescal.					good
8.	29 M	lassitude		uneven mucosa	cervical inguinal axillary	+	prescal. inguinal axillary		–			good
9.	27 F	visual distur.	deafness vestib. sym. loss of taste			+				choked disc	facial	good
10.	14 M	cough		uneven mucosa	inguinal, cervical	+	inguinal		–			good
11.	20 F	X-ray		uneven mucosa	cervical	+	cervical		+			good
12.	25 F	X-ray		white spots	cervical	+						good
13.	31 F	X-ray		engorged blood v.	mediast.	+	mediast.	+	–	iritis		good
14.	21 F	rash		engorged b. v. network		+			+	visual distur.		good
15.	17 F	swollen parotis	nose' tonsil deafness parotis	injected	inguinal	+	inguinal nose tonsil	+	–	uveitis	facial	good

* Found in periodical X-ray examination of the chest.

initially by routine, periodic X-ray examination of the chest. All of the cases but 1 showed bilateral hilar lymphadenopathy, which was the most frequent symptom in this series. Uveitis was encountered in 5 cases. Changes in the fundus oculi included choked edema, and periphlebitis in 4 cases. Lymph nodes were palpable in 10 cases in either the neck, supraclavicular region or inguinal region.

A biopsy was done in 14 cases, including Daniels' biopsy, open-chest lung biopsy, and biopsies of the mediastinum, bronchial mucosa and the upper respiratory mucosa.

The specimens were positive for pathological evidence of sarcoidosis in 11 cases. A Kveim test was positive in 4 cases, and the Mantoux test showed 7 negative, 4 positive and 1 doubtful positive. Bronchoscopic examinations in 11 cases revealed nodules in 2 cases, coarse mucosal surface in 4 cases, engorged blood vessels in 6 cases. Biopsies of the bronchial wall, however, failed to show any conclusive histopathological evidence which was pathognomonic of sarcoidosis. As for otolaryngological findings, deafness was found in 3 cases, cases 4, 9 and 15.

All 3 cases had facial paralysis and taste disturbances. Case 15 showed Heerfordt's syndrome characterized by a marked swelling of both parotid glands.

An audiogram of case 4 revealed a moderate hearing loss in the low and middle frequency ranges with a marked decline in the high frequency range. Hearing loss in case 9 was also sensorineural in type with a marked depression in the high frequency range. This patient showed vestibular dysfunction besides cochlear and facial involvement.

Deafness in case 15 was a conductive type caused by sarcoidosis pathology probably involving the Eustachian tubes. Her hearing loss returned to normal level within 2 months after initiation of predonine therapy.

Rhinological and laryngological examinations revealed typical sarcoidosis nodules on the nasal septal mucosa in case 15. Biopsy from the nasal septum, lower turbinates and the tonsils revealed positive sarcoidosis in case 15 although there were no discernible changes in the lower turbinate and the tonsil.

DISCUSSION

A variety of changes can be manifested by sarcoidosis in the field of otolaryngology. Most of the changes, however, are not specific and pathognomonic for sarcoidosis.

Otolaryngologists who encounter an early case of sarcoidosis may overlook the disease because the changes are so inconspicuous. Important changes in the ear, nose and throat caused by sarcoidosis may be classified into cranial nerve disturbances and changes of the mucosa in the upper respiratory tract. Major nerve symptoms include facial paralysis, sensorineural deafness, loss of taste, dysphagia and hoarseness. Changes of the mucosa can occur in any part of the upper respiratory tract such as the nasal mucosa, turbinates, paranasal sinuses pharynx, middle ear, larynx and trachea or bronchial mucosa. The nasal mucosa and tonsils are frequently invoved among other parts of the upper respiratory system.

Lindsay and Perlman reported an incidence of nasal involvement of 100% and Boeck 67%. Schaumann found involvement of the tonsils in 100% of his series of 21 cases. Although cranial nerve disturbances are not specific to sarcoidosis, production of nodules in the upper respiratory tract seems to be the most important change, because the biopsy in many instances presents sufficient evidence on which to base a diagnosis of sarcoidosis. A biopsy of the upper respiratory tract can be readily obtained at the office without causing discomfort to the patient. A biopsy is taken from the site of mucosal changes. Even in cases where mucosal change is not prominent, blind biopsy should be done at several places, including the septal mucosa, the lower turbinate and tonsils. By doing so, the otolaryngologist can make a most significant contribution to the diagnosis of sarcoidosis because the incidence of involvement of the upper respiratory tract in sarcoidosis is considered to be very high.

DISCUSSION

1

Chairmen: A. S. Teirstein and Y. Hiraga

Dr Stork: The calcification in the central nervous system mentioned by Professor Urich is very interesting to me because we have seen so much, particularly in older patients with sarcoidosis, of arteriosclerotic calcification of the vessels in our skull series. One of our sarcoid cases showed eggshell-type calcification of the lungs, not associated with silicosis, and had a peculiar nontubular calcification of the skull. Would Professor Urich comment on this—whether or not the nontubular calcification I have indicated as seen in our skull series is similar to that he describes as sarcoidosis of the central nervous system?

Dr Urich: To answer this question first, the calcifications which I have seen in my material are in my opinion too fine to be seen in an X-ray. As for the eggshell calcifications in the lung, I have seen them in hypercalcemic states though not in sarcoidosis. I should also like to make two comments on Dr Douglas' paper. In two of his cases he has been unable to show, at postmortem, any lesions outside the central nervous system. I had one case in which that very nearly happened, and it was only owing to a wide sampling of apparently normal lymph nodes and of all major salivary glands, that I have been able to prove that there were extraneural lesions. The second point is about the value of cerebral biopsies. I have been very disappointed in cerebral biopsies in sarcoidosis. The reason is the distribution of sarcoid lesions: they predominate in the hypothalamus, basal cisterns and brain stem, and can be few and far between over the cortical surface. A random cortical biopsy will as often as not be negative. A biopsy is not devoid of risk of infection and therefore

I would strongly advise against it as a diagnostic procedure, unless there is another clinical indication for surgery. As for Dr Niitu's paper, I was very interested to hear about the EEG changes in acute sarcoidosis. I am not convinced that they indicate sarcoid lesions in the brain. Diffuse changes in the EEG can happen in a variety of conditions. I would like to hear something about other parameters such as pulmonary function, or the level of blood calcium, as all these can affect the EEG. Obviously only autopsy will reveal whether there are specific lesions in the brain in acute sarcoidosis.

Dr Young: Dr Douglas' case 1, the 44-year-old female, disturbed me because it was very suggestive of the possibility of another diagnosis—of Wegener's granulomatosis. There have been many incomplete forms. Dr Carrington and Dr Liebow have suggested the incomplete forms, and they respond to steroid therapy, and also to immunosuppressive drugs. To Dr Kobayashi, I suggest that her incidence of ocular sarcoidosis of 92% is overwhemingly high, and I suspect that this may have been due to a biased population which she may have been working with. The world incidence is somewhere about 38%, and this is our incidence, too.

Dr Douglas: With regard to Dr Young's query about my first case, he will recall that this was a patient who had bilateral hilar adenopathy and who had a positive cervical gland biopsy. It seems entirely appropriate to label the associated neurological features as central nervous system sarcoidosis and certainly I think I can fit atrophic rhinitis and perforated nasal septum much more properly into a diagnosis of CNS sarcoidosis than he could into Wegener's granulomatosis.

May I ask a question of DR Urich? Does he ever find thrombosis of vessels in his material? What impressed me about our own material was that, although there was a great deal of paravascular granuloma, we very rarely, if ever, were convinced that there was thrombosis of cerebral vessels.

Finally, seeing that the problems which Dr Urich has outlined are unlikely to be solved except by pooling all resources, would not something be said for any of us who came across possible cases in the future referring pathological case material to a centre? Perhaps Dr Urich wouldn't mind taking this on, himself.

DR URICH: I am of course more than willing to cooperate. With regard to the question about thrombosis of the vessels, I suppose Dr Douglas meant occlusive lesions of the vessels, irrespective of whether they are thrombotic or granulomatous. Thrombosis of the vessels is rare; occlusive lesions of small vessels are quite common, and if you look at the brain in some detail you will almost invariably find at least minor areas of ischaemic necrosis.

DR SULAVIK: I would like to reemphasise the association of cryptococcosis with sarcoidosis. Over 50% of cases where the association is present will have meningitis or meningoencephalitis, or a presentation of a brain-occupying lesion. Now, if one starts with a series of cryptococal meningitis, approximately 3% (being a report from England) will be associated with sarcoidosis. The feeling is, that for a patient who has stage II sarcoid and also has menigitis, that the first diagnosis to consider is cryptococcus. This diagnosis is to be ruled out since there is almost a 100% mortality in untreated cryptococcal menigitis. The treatment for cryptococcal meningitis is relatively good. Latex agglutination test, testing for polysaccharide antigen of the cryptococcus are performed on the spinal fluid is a very fine test. In most cases of sarcoid CNS lesions, as pointed out today, the diagnosis is tremendously difficult to make, short of biopsy and autopsy material. I don't think

we know a great deal about CNS sarcoid. It may well be that many cases who die indeed have had cryptococcal meningitis. Calcification of the eggshell type is not seen in very many diseases and is by far most common in silicosis. In hyperparathyroid states, we have not seen eggshell calcifications. The interesting point is that the eggshell calcification occurs in the anterior mediastinum, a place where we rarely see adenopathy in sarcoid; a peculiar distribution. Regarding Dr Young's comment about Liebow and Carrington' work, the hallmark for diagnosis of Wegeners' is not only the granuloma, but also vasculitis of arteriale and venules.

DR TEIRSTEIN: Are we now prepared to make a diagnosis of sarcoidosis in patients who have nonspecific granulomas localized in one organ or organ system without any evidence of sarcoidosis elsewhere?

DR JOHNS: It seems to me that there is enough that is confusing about this disease, without extending it to include those that involve only one system. I find myself most reluctant to put that label upon a patient who has evidence limited to the nervous system. We are likely to learn more if we admit our lack of understanding in these puzzling problems.

DR ISRAEL: I should like to comment on the criteria for a diagnosis of sarcoidosis. One extreme is exemplified by American resident physicians who are likely to take a quite obvious case of sarcoidosis with hilar adenopathy and consider it necessary to get, not just a single biopsy, but 2 or 3 to establish that the patient has systemic granulomatosis. That is really excessive zeal. On the other hand, when one is dealing with atypical cases, efforts should be made to secure evidence of granulomatosis in more than 1 organ or tissue. The problem is not confined to the central nervous system. It is a very general one which comes up when seemingly isolated granulomas are found in the kidney, bones, liver or upper respiratory tract. The best way of establishing the presence of systemic disease is by mediastinoscopy. The diagnosis of sarcoidosis must be questioned when an autopsy reveals granulomas in only a single organ or tissue.

DR NIITU: Thank you for your comments on my electroencephalography presentation. We performed electroencephalography successfully in all patients with pulmonary sarcoidosis over the last 2 years. In Japan it has been reported that abnormalities are found in 10%, at the most, of children and teen-agers. The rate of abnormalities was very high, 30%, in patients with pulmonary sarcoidosis. These abnormalities disappeared or improved within a relatively short period. The results suggest the frequent presence of sarcoid lesions in the brain in patients with pulmonary sarcoidosis.

DR TACHIBANA: I am presenting here a case of a 14-year-old boy with typical BHL. Since the time of detection, epileptic attacks have occurred. This boy presented abnormal EEG findings, and Dr. Silverstein includes such cases as neurological manifestation of sarcoidosis in the "Archives of Neurology".

DR TEIRSTEIN: This would seem to be another case of a patient with bilateral hilar lymphadenopathy and abnormal electroencephalography similar to the patient presented before. I am always reluctant, as a chest doctor, to denigrate what the electroencephalographists tell me, or what the ophthalmologists tell me. I find that when I send my patients to the ophthalmologist, they see a great deal more than I ever see, looking in their eyes. I would not be a bit surprised if, in this disease, which I think of as systemic, the true incidence of ocular involvement is a great deal more than the 30% that most of us recognise. I am not terribly surprised that the electroencephalograms seemed to indicate, although they did not prove, that there may be disseminated brain disease as well, in most cases with sarcoidosis. I am particularly impressed, and would like to have seen in the cases just shown, a subsequent follow-up encephalogram, which shows improvement through clearing, concomitant with the clearing of the lymph nodes. I should also like to second the last remark that Dr Israel made. In the first case of Heerfordt's syndrome, who had a clinical picture compatible with sarcoidosis, we did not have a positive biopsy; both the Kveim and the scalene biopsy were negative. If the patient had undergone mediastinoscopy, a positive diagnosis probably could have been made. In fact, I suspect, today, that there must be a very rare patient who has sarcoidosis, in whom one cannot establish a diagnosis by some sort of biopsy.

2

Chairmen: E. CARLENS AND O. HONGO

DR KOSUDA: I wish to make an additional presentation of a case of pleural sarcoidosis where confirmation was made by open-lung biopsy. The patient was a 64-year-old woman outpatient, suffering from hypertension. Her lung roentgenogram showed BHL with a dense shadow, suggesting plueral affection in the right phrenicocostal sinus. There was no complaint of fever, chest pains or other signs of inflammation. A tuberculin test was negative; a Kveim test was not done. An open-biopsy was performed to exclude the possibility of malignancy, although the scalene node biopsy showed typical sarcoid granulomas. The histological findings on the biopsy specimen showed many small but rather typical sarcoid granulomas, just under the pleura or in the pluera itself. Tuberculous lesions were not detected microscopically, and mycobacteria or fungi were not cultured from the specimens. Nine months later, she was well, and BHL became smaller, though the pleural shadow remained unchanged.

DR TACHIBANA: I would like to show evidence of muscular involvement in sarcoidosis. I collected at least 12 cases in Japan. The tumor-forming cases comprising 6 males and 4 females, from the second to sixth decade in age. Involved muscles were mainly those of the extremities. Intrathoracic lesions were found, and some of these cases had other extrathoracic lesions such as eye and skin lesions. Tuberculin reaction was negative in 6 cases, and doubtful positive in 1 case.

DR CARLENS: Both Drs. Teirstein and Mitchell presented electrocardiographic changes in a large precentage of their patients, but they were of a rather mild character. In Stockholm, we have found routine electrocardiographic changes in about 400 of our mediastinoscoped patients among whom were 3 young patients with complete heartblock. In two of the patients we suspected sarcoidosis from clinical symptoms and chest findings. They were immediately put on pace makers, first on a fixed-rate pace maker with the stimulating electrode intravenously introduced into the right ventricle. As both of them were very young, with a normally beating atrium, atrial-triggered pacing was considered. We performed mediastinoscopy to reach a diagnosis. Removed paratracheal lymph nodes were typical of sarcoidosis and then we introduced the atrial electrode. The third patient had sarcoidosis, which we hadn't suspected at all. He was also a young man with sudden heartblock. When we introduced the atrial electrode mediastinoscopically, I was astonished to find a large bundle of typical sarcoid lymph nodes, and these were proved microscopically. I think therefore there are cases with severe heart lesions of sarcoid origin. It would appear that the acute stages had passed.

DR MITCHELL: May I briefly show slides, which exemplify 1 further patient with a persistent, changing ECG abnormality. She is a 25-year-old Irish girl who has been in Great Britain for 8 years. Her tuberculin test was negative, her Kveim, positive. She had bilateral hilar nodes which histologically showed noncaseating granulomas. ECG on diagnosis showed T waves to be flat in leads

III AVF, V4, V5 and V6. A further ECG later showed that frequent ventricular ectopics had appeared with post-ectopic T wave inversion. A subsequent ECG, 1 month later, showed no change. A further ECG, 2 years later, showed that ventricular ectopies persisted and that the T wave was inverted in V5 and V6.

DR TEIRSTEIN: We are all seeing more sarcoidosis with heartblock, and arrhythmias. The almost epidemic number of patients we had seen in a period of about 6 months, some requiring acute intensive therapy because of arrhythmias and near death, impelled us to establish a routine for evaluating all patients electrocardiographically in the hope of finding abnomalities in the asymptomatic patients. This might give us a hint concerning the patients that should be followed closely, since apparently some of these people will suddenly experience life-threatening arrhythmias.

DR VILLAR: I was particularly interested in the series of cases of pleural involvement in sarcoidosis from Mount Sinai and the 1 from Japan. The outlook of physicians working in countries where tuberculosis is still quite prevalent and sarcoidosis scarce, as against that of those working in areas where there is very little tuberculosis and a lot of sarcoidosis, has necessarily to be different.

Due to this fact I was quite disturbed over case 2 of the Mount Sinai series. Pleural biopsy, by itself, cannot give the diagnosis of sarcoidosis. In Lisbon we do systematic needle biopsies in all pleural effusions to try and get an etiological diagnosis because of following up treatment. In some cases it has been possible to follow the course of a pleurisy by taking a biopsy every time fluid is removed. In this way we have seen cases of active pleural tuberculosis with sclerosing, and even calcifying, tuberculoid granulomas at the first or second biopsies. Healing may set in even spontaneously, as early as 2 weeks after the effusion appears. So you can get this type of picture in tuberculosis. In Mount Sinai case 2, I did not see any other proof of sarcoidosis such as there was in the other Mount

Sinai cases and in the Japanese case. I would like to know if the picture showed parietal or visceral pleura. Quite frequently we see nothing on X-ray, but a tuberculous pleural effusion exists. Pleuroscopy or open thoracotomy will show nodules right under the pleura that can even be felt by the surgeon. The characteristics of the fluid were also those we usually find in tuberculosis. Some of the cases had negative tuberculin tests but we have also seen this happen for a time in tuberculous pleurisy.

DR MILLER: Those 3 cases from Mount. Sinai all had negative tuberculin. All had microscopic examinations and culture tests for mycobacteria which were negative. None of the cases, including the second, was treated with antituberculosis medication, but with steroids, to which they responded. The third case, for example, went through this several times, responding to steroids. The second patient, specifically, had a negative tuberculin and a positive Kveim test. He showed noncaseating granulomas in his lung and in his visceral pleura, at the same time.

DR YAMAMOTO: I should like to report another case of pleural sarcoidosis—that of a female of 35 years, with BHL, negative tuberculin reaction, and positive Kveim reaction, diagnosed by scalene node biopsy. Worsening with pleural involvement was observed 4 years after diagnosis. Pleural needle biopsy was performed, revealing noncaseating epithelioid cell granulomas.

DR JAMES: We are dealing with a multisystem disorder and comparative incidence of various tissues is similar in all countries. Some of the conditions we have discussed this morning, the comparative incidence in Japan, are very much like ours in London.

DR MITCHELL: A short while ago I heard of the development in Japan of a tiny implement which could be used with minimal risk, and with which nice tiny cores of endocardium were obtained. In the postmortem reports, many of the granulomata found in cardiac muscle have been bizarre, and one wonders whether anyone has any experience of this implement in a broader context.

DR CARLENS: I will raise the question of whether you think it is possible to have sarcoidosis in the thymus. As far as I know it has never been shown earlier. Dr Matsushima has presented 2 young patients with enlarged thymuses. Unfortunately he has not been able to prove defenitely that it was sarcoidosis in the thymus. In 40 patients with sarcoidosis in whom diagnostic mediastinoscopy has been performed I have also removed a small piece of the thymus. In none of them was the pathologist able to find the slightest sign of sarcoidosis in the thymus although all of them showed a typical picture in all the lymphnodes. I would also like to ask those who know more about immunology if they think it is possible to have sarcoidosis in the thymus. We also know from patients with myasthenia gravis that when they are put on steroid treatment there is a rapid involution of the thymus. In the 2 presented cases it must therefore be difficult to draw a definite conclusion as to whether the diagnosis was sarcoidosis or not.

DR MATUSIMA: I am looking forward to the next patient with the same radiographic finding to decide this question by mediastinoscopy.

DR CARLENS: It is also very interesting that both these patients were very young. We very seldom see such young sarcoidosis patents in Sweden as our Japanese colleagues have presented here today.

DR MATUSIMA: I think it may be possible to have sarcoidosis in the thymus in children.

DR KOSUDA: Dr. James presented a valuable paper at the last conference in Prague on the corticosteroid therapy of sarcoidosis. Do you think that pleural sarcoidosis without symptoms is one of the indications for corticosteroid therapy or not?

DR JAMES: Let's put pleural sarcoidosis into a proper perspective. It is rare, for it is only recognised in less than 1% of patients with sarcoidosis.

Dr Miller: Again to put pleural sarcoidosis in perspective, most, if not all, of these patients had multisystem and severe pulmonary involvement with symptoms which themselves would require steroid therapy, so I think that the question could be decided by the other organ involvement and the symptomatic pulmonary involvement.

Dr Turiaf: Je m'excuse de revenir sur le problème des localisations pleurales qui a été fort bien exposé dans la communication de mon ami le Professeur Siltzbach. En effect les localisations pleurales chiffrent environ 1%. Pour ma part, sur 400 cas de sarcoïdose que j'ai réunis en 20 ans dans mon service de l'Hôpital Bichat à Paris, j'en ai vu qui se sont manifestées cliniquement dans 4 cas seulement. Ces 4 cas étaient une pleurésie, une pachy-pleurite qui a subi la résolution sous corticostéroïdes, et 2 cas de pleuro-péricardite récidivante. En aucun de ces 4 cas je n'ai pu faire de ponction biopsie pleurale, mais, à deux autres reprises, à propos d'une thoracotomie chirurgicale pour biopsie pulmonaire, le chirurgien a pu prélever une fraction de plèvre dans laquelle nous avons identifié des granulomes sarcoïdiens pleuraux alors que, sur la radiographie, il n'y avait pas d'épaississement pleural. Si bien qu'il se peut, mais c'est une hypothèse, que l'atteinte pleurale soit plus fréquemment présente anatomiquement qu'elle ne s'inscrit sur les radiographies.

VIII VARIOUS TOPICS

Clinical and Histopathological Features in the Course of Spontaneously Healed Cases of Sarcoidosis

Ichiro Ohira, Masao Ogihara and Akira Yamaguchi

Department of Internal Medicine, Tokyo Jikeikai University School of Medicine, Tokyo, Japan

In the study of sarcoidosis, it is very important to observe in detail the histological and clinical features in the process of spontaneous healing in cases of sarcoidosis. In this connection, 2 cases will be given here, where some characteristic clinicopathological features were observed, without treatment by drugs, for 6 or 8 months after the onset.

Case 1

A 24-year-old Japanese man complaining of general tiredness and many swollen lymph nodes was admitted to our hospital. Thirty lymph nodes were distinctly palpable in the cervical, axillar, inguinal and the upper arm area on both sides and histological features of the lymph nodes, biopsied at monthly intervals, were compared with clinical findings.

On admission, a tuberculin skin test was negative, Kveim test was negative, sputum was negative for acid-fast bacilli and the serum calcium value was elevated slightly.

The first chest X-ray picture showed enlargement of the hilar lymph nodes and diffuses miliary infiltration in both lung fields. The histological finding on the first lymph node biopsy, which helped us diagnose sarcoidosis, revealed clusters of noncaseating tubercles composed of epithelioid cells with scattered Langhans-type giant cells including so-called asteroid bodies; the individual tubercles were of the same size, form and structure, being well demarcated from the surrounding tissue (Fig. 1).

Two months later, the lymph nodes revealed features of advanced fibrosis around the tubercles (Fig. 2). Chest X-ray findings at this time showed that the hilar lymph nodes and the miliary densities in both lungs were less than those 1 month earlier.

Three months later, resected lymph nodes showed decreased fibrosis around tubercles and the reappearance of the fundamental structure of lymph node tissue taking the place of fibrosis in places. The chest X-ray picture at the same stage showed a minimal enlargment of the hilar lymph nodes.

Five months later, only scattered giant cells and no remarkable granulomas of fibrosis were observed on the histological section in lymph node tissue. It is very interesting to know that the finding of *giant cells* which in lymph node tissue was in the latest state of spontaneous healing in sarcoidosis (Fig. 3).

At this stage, the chest X-ray picture did not show any abnormalities, and only 4 small lymph nodes were palpable, 2 of which were identified by biopsy.

Six months later, no indications for lymph node biopsy exist, because no symptoms or signs of the disease were observed at this stage.

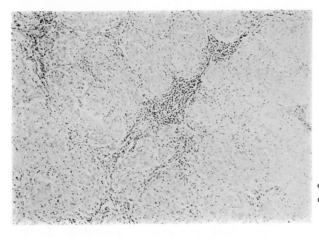

FIG. 1. On admission. Granuloma composed of giant cell and epithelioid cell.

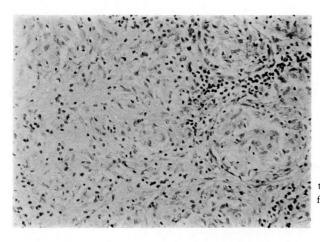

FIG. 2. Two months later. No caseation in the granuloma and advanced fibrosis around the granuloma.

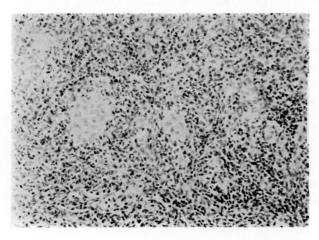

FIG. 3. Five months later. Giant cells in the tissue of lymph node.

Case 2

A 31-year-old man. He complained of general tiredness and anorexia and had been placed under our care for 8 months without treatment with drugs.

On admission, a Kveim test revealed a typically positive reaction, a tuberculin skin test was negative, acid-fast bacilli in sputum was negative and hypergammaglobulinemia was noted. The findings in the eye showed typical features of sarcoidosis. The chest X-ray picture showed distinctly enlarged bilateral hilar lymph nodes. The histological findings of liver biopsy specimen showed suspected sarcoidosis.

The patient was followed in detail clinically and pathologically for 8 months, but no improvement was observed except conversion of tuberculin reaction from negative to positive.

It is suspected that in a great many spontaneously healed cases of sarcoidosis cured in a short period of time the lymph glands would be chiefly involved and in protracted cases organs other than the lymph glands would be involved to a great extent.

REFERENCES

1. Riker, W., and Clark, M. 1949. Sarcoidosis. *Amer. J. Clin. Path.* **19**: 725.
2. Rubin, E., and Pinner, M. 1949. *Amer. Rev. Tuberc.* **49**: 146.
3. Uehlinger, E. A. 1961. *Amer. Rev. Resp. Dis.* **84**: 6.

Clinical Observation of Sarcoidosis
at Kitano Hospital, Osaka

H. Muromoto, J. Majima, T. Shigematsu, J. Akita and M. Kurata

Tazuke Kofukai Medical Research Institute, Kitano Hospital, Osaka, Japan

Our report covers about 30 cases of " probable sarcoidosis " experienced at the Kitano hospital during the last 4 years.

Organ biopsies, immunological studies, and steroid therapy in each case are also discussed in the light of their clinical significance.

As is generally accepted, sarcoidosis occurs more frequently in males than in females by a ratio of 3 to 2.

1) It has been our experience that an awareness of symptoms by the individual patient himself leads to discovery of the disease much more often than does mass examination.

2) More than half of the patients had sarcoidosis in both sides of the lungs.

3) Half of the 18 cases which had tissue biopsies of such organs as the mediastinal or scalene lymph nodes, liver and/or skin proved to be positive, while Kveim tests more frequently gave negative results using different antigens.

There has been much discussion on the specificity of the Kveim test for sarcoidosis recently. We also have found typical sarcoidosis to have negative results in the Kveim test using various antigens. This fact seems to reflect an immunological disorder, rather than a relationship between the antigen and the activity in sarcoidosis.

During the past 4 years from 1969 to 1972, 56 cases of probable sarcoidosis were examined at the Kitano hospital, Osaka. Thirty-eight of them were demonstrated by our clinical observations and other results.

EPIDEMIOLOGICAL STUDIES

Age distribution, sex difference and the onset of the disease.

This disease was more frequently found in males, 23 cases (60.5%), than in females, 15 cases (39.5%). In males, 87.5% were between the ages of 20 and 49, while in females 60% were between 10 and 29 years of age. The age distribution, as a whole, resembled that given in the national statistics.

Clues to the discovery of the disease and the organ involved.

By mass examination, a total of 11 cases were discovered, about equal numbers of both sexes. Seven were discovered by intrathoracic changes such as BHL.

Twenty-seven were discovered because of the patients' own complaints. Of these, 17 had sarcoidosis of the lung combined with other organs, and 14 had BHL. In both groups, BHL and other involvement appeared in more than 50% of the total number of cases.

CLINICAL EXAMINATIONS AND THEIR RESULTS

Organ biopsy and Kveim test

Results of biopsy and Kveim test performed on 15 patients were obtained. Of the cases which underwent biopsy of the scalene nodes, mediastinal node or liver, 50% were positive and 50% were negative. Both biopsies and Kveim tests were positive in 5 cases, and both were negative in 7 cases. The Kveim-positive rates were influenced by the kind of antigens employed.

Tuberculin test

The tuberculin test was negative in 29% of the cases. A similar insensitivity to tuberculin and other delayed-type hypersensitivity antigens has been noted in many other sarcoidosis reports.

Pulmonary function test

More than 33 cases were normal or nearly normal in pulmonary function tests, such as vital capacity and FEV.

Lymphocyte, protein fraction and others

The lymphocyte count was also in a normal range, but 7 cases (18%) were below 1.000. Hyperglobulinemia with an elevation of the gammaglobulin fraction was encountered in 10% of cases. Serum Ca level, RAT, and LDH were also almost within normal limits.

CASE REPORT

Case 5 (C.M.)

A 22-year-old woman with a history of aphthous stomatitis at the age of 18 was seen at the Kitano hospital in June, 1969, for evaluation of a slight fever and subsequently, from July, 1969, for blurred vision. She had had cutaneous lesions over the lower legs since April, 1969. Physical examinations revealed symmetrical erythema with papules in both lower legs and uveitis bilaterally. Roentgenogram of the chest disclosed UHL. A Kveim test was negative. A tuberculin test (0.05 r) gave an area of induration 3.0×5.0 mm in diameter in 48 hours. A diagnosis of sarcoidosis was established from the findings of cutaneous biopsy. Steroid treatment was started with prednisolone, 30 mg a day. Skin lesions disappeared completely and uveitis improved. The slight fever, however, had persisted, and subsided with methotrexate and an increased dosage of steroid (40 mg a day). She continued to make favorable progress and was discharged on December, 1969.

Case 9 (Y.O.)

A 24-year-old woman in her, fourth month of pregnancy, gravida II, para I, had been noticing, since February 1970, a mild chest pain in the right side without any other symptoms. A routine roentogenogram of the chest at that time showed a " suspicious " BHL, which had not been discovered 1 year before. The Kveim test was positive. A tuberculin skin test (0.05 r) gave an area of induration of 4.0×4.0 mm in diameter in 48 hours. A clinical diagnosis of sarcoidosis was made. Sarcoidosis had also been diagnosed previously at another hospital in her brother 3 years ago. This case suggested an instance of familial occurrence of sarcoidosis.

Case 25 (S.T.)

A 38-year-old man who had been suffering from subcutaneous nodules and exertional dyspnea over the previous 4 months was referred to Kitano hospital on 23rd December 1970. His past history included 2 episodes of gastric ulcer at the age of 30 and 37. A biopsy of the nodules revealed a pathological picture of sarcoidosis. He was admitted to the hospital on 28th, February, 1971. Chest X-ray films showed minimal BHL and an increase in reticular shadow throughout both lung fields. A Kveim reaction was positive. He had no visual disturbance but granulomas were demonstrated in the vitreous body. Subcutaneous nodules and abnormal chest X-ray findings rapidly disappeared with steroid therapy. He was discharged in June, 1971 and was doing well until April, 1972, when he noticed some nodules on his face. These nodules also disappeared with increased doses of the steroid.

TREATMENT

Indications for treatment are progressive impairment of the lung, visual acuity and cutaneous lesions.

The majority of patients with a mild form of the disease will have spontaneous remission and need no therapy. A first choice of drugs would be adrenocorticosteroids. The duration and types of treatment are variable. If a contraindication to corticoid therapy is given, other drugs, such as immunosuppressive agents may be used.

The Concomittance of Feverish Onset of Sarcoidosis and Necrosis Formation in the Lymph Nodes

Eric Carlens, Åke Hanngren and Biörn Ivemark

Karolinska Hospital, Stockholm, Sweden

Although clinical manifestations of sarcoidosis are variable, most cases of sarcoidosis have an insidious onset and many patients pass through the whole course of the disease without any constitutional symptoms. In a small proportion, however, sarcoidosis presents clinically as an acute febrile illness, nearly always accompanied by erythema nodosum or arthralgia or a combination of both. Scadding found out of 275 cases of sarcoidosis 12 patients with constitutional symptoms such as lassitude, malaise and fever. Among the latter BHL was always found.[1]

Pathologically it is characterised by the presence in almost any organ of the body of epitheloid cell tubercles with inconspicuous or no necrosis. If necrosis exists it is described as eosinophilic granular necrosis, distinguishable from caseation by the persistence of an intact reticulum, demonstrable by silver staining methods. This distinction is, however, not absolute. True caseous necrosis has been described and the granular

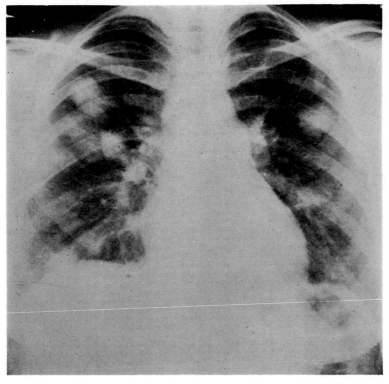

Fig. 1. Chest radiograph of a 22-year-old woman with acute febrile illness and pronounced mottled shadowing in both lungs.

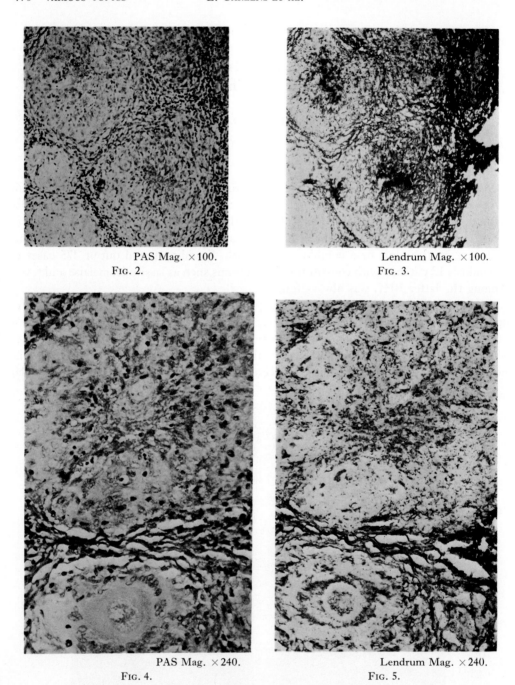

PAS Mag. ×100.
FIG. 2.

Lendrum Mag. ×100.
FIG. 3.

PAS Mag. ×240.
FIG. 4.

Lendrum Mag. ×240.
FIG. 5.

FIGS. 2–5.   Sarcoidosis. Sections from mediastinal lymph nodes from a case with acute, febrile onset.   Granulomas with central granular necrosis and large giant cells.   Figs. 2 and 4 are PAS-stained, and Figs. 3 and 5 are silver-impregnated (Lendrum).   Note prominent reticulin network in the center of granulomas.   Figures 2 and 3, Mag. ×100; Figs. 4 and 5, Mag. ×240.

necrosis can be so pronounced that it gives the pathologist the impression of being of the caseous type. This was the case in 15 out of 250 patients with sarcoidosis in whom mediastinoscopy with lymph node biopsy was performed. All these 15 patients also presented an acute febrile illness, nearly always accompanied by erythema nodosum or arthralgia. None of them, however, were accompanied by BHL. In 6 out of 15 the tuberculin skin test was also positive, and tuberculosis was difficult to exclude. However, in 2 patients the positive tuberculin test converted to negative during the short observation time. The following case report illustrates these points:

A woman aged 22, whose mother had tuberculosis when the patient was a child, first complained of rather ill-defined aching round the costal margin with fever and lassitude for 2 weeks. There was no skin rash. A chest radiograph (Fig. 1) showed pronounced mottled shadowing in both lungs but no definite enlargement of the hilar lymph nodes. The tuberculin skin test was positive to 1 mg tuberculin. A slight enlargement of the thyroid gland was also found. Tuberculosis or metastases from a cancer of the thyroid gland was suspected. Transthoracic needle biopsy was performed. Microscopic examination showed tubercle-like groups of epitheloid cells and signs of necrosis. Although tubercle bacilli were not demonstrated, the clinical picture spoke in favour of tuberculosis and antituberculous therapy was instituted. At this time mediastinoscopy was performed and to the right of the trachea a large bundle of yellow, firm and well-defined lymph nodes of typical sarcoid appearence was found. Microscopic examination (Figs. 2–5) showed epitheloid cell tubercles some of which were confluent and occasionally large giant cells of the Langhans type. In many places necroses were found which gave the impression of being caseous. Silver staining, however, demonstrated the persistance of an intact reticulum. Culture both with lymph node material and gastric lavage fluid grew no tubercle bacilli. Although the antituberculous therapy was discontinued and no other therapy was introduced the recovery was uneventful and after 1 year the patient showed an almost normal chest radiograph.

Several authors have attempted to correlate the histological picture of sarcoidosis with the clinical findings but no definite conclusions concerning the severity or prognosis have been drawn. As to the central necrosis of the granuloma, however, Beckert and coworkers state, without any further description, that it occurs only in cases of progression; Zettergren[2] stresses that necrobiotic lesion of the granulomata, which is certainly often mistaken for caseous necrosis, seems more prevalent in those cases in which lesions are relative recent. For example, in 1 case a lymph node was removed early in the disease and another later. There were marked necrobiotic lesions in the former and only very slight ones in the latter.

Our findings agree with the opinion that necrobiotic lesion of the granuloma is connected with the acute and active phase of the disease. If we accept that necrosis of epitheloid cell granuloma is caused by transformed thymus-derived lymphocytes, so called T cells, we may explain the lack of necrosis in sarcoid material by a defective T cell function. The incomplete or false necrosis found in our material suggests that this T cell defect may be partial or that some other mechanism causes this kind of necrosis. As it is found in acute stages, we may speculate that the T cell-depressing mechanism is not yet fully developed. Our finding of conversion of positive tuberculin skin reactivity to negative during the short observation period in some patients supports the assumption of a successive T cell depression. Those patients may represent good material in the search for the T cell-depressing agent.

REFERENCES

1. Scadding, J. G.: 1967. Sarcoidosis. London: Eyre & Spottiswoode.
2. Zettergren, L.: 1954. Lymphogranulomatosis benigna. A clinical and histo-pathological study of its relation to tuberculosis. *Acta Soc. Med.* Upsaliensis, Suppl. 5.

Hypercalciuria and Sarcoidosis

Robert A. Goldstein, Harold L. Israel, Kenneth L. Becker
and John J. Ryan

*VA-George Washington University Medical Center, Washington, D. C. and
The Jefferson Medical College, Thomas Jefferson University, Philadelphia, U.S.A.*

INTRODUCTION

In a recent study of serum calcium in patients with sarcoidosis, we found that hyper-calcemia occurred infrequently and was almost always associated with disseminated disease.[1] This contrasted with the view that sarcoidosis was a common cause of disordered calcium metabolism even in persons with minimal disease. However, many of the metabolic studies in support of the latter view had been performed in selected patients who already had manifest calcium disturbances. Furthermore, many studies of urinary calcium excretion had been performed in outpatients without strict dietary regulations. We therefore initiated a study in unselected patients with sarcoidosis who were not hypercalcemic in order to determine whether or not hypercalciuria is in fact a subclinical feature in many patients with sarcoidosis.

MATERIALS AND METHODS

Eighteen patients with biopsy-proven subacute or chronic active sarcoidosis and normal serum calcium were admitted to a research metabolic unit for 10 days. Patients were ambulatory, none were receiving therapy and all were carefully supervised to insure adequacy of 24-hour urinary collections and adherence to dietary restrictions. Calcium intake was as follows: 1120 mg for 3 days, 120 mg for the next 3 days, 0 intake for 1 day and 5120 mg for the final 3 days. Twelve healthy control subjects were studied in a similar fashion.

RESULTS

To allow for an adequate period of equilibration for each successive dietary change only values from the final day of each collection period were utilized. The mean 24-hour calcium excretion in sarcoidosis patients on a " normal " (1120 mg) calcium intake was 156 mg; on a " low " (120 mg) intake, mean excretion was reduced to 75 mg; during the fast day, mean excretion was 80 mg; and following a " high " (5120 mg) intake mean excretion rose to 207 mg. These values were not significantly different from those found in 12 healthy persons. Mean 24-hour urinary calcium excretion in the latter group was 145 mg, 100 mg, 68 mg, and 282 mg respectively. Phosphate excretion was slightly but not significantly lower in sarcoidosis when compared with control subjects.

Eight of the patients were studied in the Thomas Jefferson University Clinical Research Center (Funded by PHS Grant RR 72–08).

DISCUSSION

The reported frequency of hypercalciuria in sarcoidosis varies widely. Although it has been stated that most patients with sarcoidosis are hypercalciuric, few studies have been reported in which both the diet and urinary collection was closely supervised. Nordin and co-workers[2] have called attention to the problem of dietary control in the definition of hypercalciuria and have pointed out the wide variation in values encountered in normal subjects. It is of interest that Putkonen et al.,[3] who also studied unselected patients under strict supervision found hypercalciuria (24-hour excretion greater than 300 mg) in 15% of 39 patients with sarcoidosis compared to 6% in controls. Mean values of calcium excretion were identical in both groups. On a " normal " calcium intake, the accepted range of 24-hour urinary calcium excretion in normal men is 300 mg or less and in women 250 mg or less. Some authors however, think that these limits should be raised.[4] Using these criteria no persons in the present study were hypercalciuric.

By first restricting and then by supplementing dietary calcium, we had hoped to " provoke " abnormalities of calcium excretion not evident in persons on a " normal " intake. We found, however, that calcium excretion was closely related to dietary intake in both sarcoidosis patients and healthy control subjects.

Although we have studied relatively few patients, all had active sarcoidosis. Based on previous estimates, we would have expected several persons to manifest hypercalciuria. It is concluded that when dietary intake of calcium is strictly controlled and urinary excretion closely monitored, hypercalciuria is an uncommon feature of sarcoidosis. Furthermore, recognizing that few patients are available for prolonged and tedious studies such as these, it would appear that measurements of serum calcium alone would uncover those few persons with sarcoidosis who have clinically significant disorders of calcium metabolism. Of course, detailed metabolic studies in the latter group are still of great interest since the pathophysiologic explanation of hypercalciuria and/or hypercalcemia is still not known with certainty.[5]

REFERENCES

1. Goldstein, R. A., Israel, H. L., Becker, K. L., and Moore, C. F. 1971. The infrequency of hypercalcemia in sarcoidosis. *Amer. J. Med.* **51**: 21.
2. Nordin, B. E. L., Hodgkinson, A., and Peacock, M. 1967. The measurement and the meaning of urinary calcium. *Clin. Ortho.* **52**: 293.
3. Putkonen, R., Hannuksela, M., and Holme, H. 1965. Calcium and phosphorus metabolism in sarcoidosis. *Acta Med. Scand.* **177**: 327.
4. Davis, R. H., Morgan, D. B., and Rivlin, R. S. 1970. The excretion of calcium in the urine and its relation to calcium intake, sex and age. *Clin. Sci.* **39**: 1.
5. Miller, B., Schaumloffel, E., Baltzer, G., Behrend, H., and Kessler, G. F. 1971. Investigation of calcium metabolism in sarcoidosis by isotope methods. *Proc. Fifth Int. Conf. on Sarcoidosis.* Prague: Univ. Karlova. p. 319.

The Calcium Infusion Test in Sarcoidosis

H. MORII, T. OKAMOTO AND N. HAMADA

Second Department of Internal Medicine, Osaka City University, Osaka, Japan

H. TANIMOTO, M. TAMURA, H. MOCHIZUKI, M. WASHIZAKI AND H. OKANO

Toranomon Hospital, Tokyo, Japan

R. MIKAMI

Third Department of Internal Medicine, University of Tokyo, Tokyo, Japan

H. IBAYASHI

Third Department of Internal Medicine, Kyushu University, Fukuoka, Japan

AND

H. HOMMA

Juntendo School of Medicine, Tokyo, Japan

Abnormalities of calcium metabolism are common in sarcoidosis. Hypercalcemia and excessive absorption of calcium[1] have been reported. The cause of hypercalcemia is considered to be increased sensitivity of the intestinal tract to vitamin D[2] and enhanced absorption of calcium. Bell et al. demonstrated that the calcium excretion and resorption rates in the bone were elevated in patients with sarcoidosis and they postulated that such derangements were caused by abnormal sensitivity of the bone to vitamin D.[3] Although information as to parathyroid function in sarcoidosis has been conflicting, Cushard et al. recently reported that the parathyroid hormone (PTH) level was extremely low in sarcoidosis by the direct measurement of serum PTH using radioimmunoassay.[4]

The calcium infusion test has been utilized in order to assess the parathyroid function, by measuring phosphate clearance before and after calcium infusion. However, it was also demonstrated that the recovery of serum calcium level after calcium infusion is dependent on the secretory activity of calcitonin.[5] While the secretion of calcitonin is considered to be deranged in some of the thyroid diseases and hypoparathyroidism, the response to calcium infusion was abnormal in these diseases.[6, 7] The present study was undertaken to determine the response to calcium loading in sarcoidosis.

PATIENTS AND METHODS

Healthy subjects and patients with minimal pulmonary tuberculosis were chosen as controls. The diagnosis of sarcoidosis was made according to the criteria which were established at the Second International Conference on Sarcoidosis in 1960. Sixty-seven cases, 27 female and 40 male patients, were studied. The age of the patients ranged from 15 to 59. Calcium loading tests were performed in 31 nontreated cases and 5 cases treated with corticosteroids. Three patients with idiopathic hypoparathyroidism were also investigated. In the early stage of this study, the serum calcium concentration was measured, for the purpose of screening, in 49 patients. The serum calcium was determined by the method of Clark and Collip[8] or by the O-cresolphthalein complexone method.[9]

Calcium loading test

A dose of 4 mg of calcium per kg of body weight, in the form of calcium gluconate containing 0.86% calcium, was injected intravenously during a period of 10 minutes. Venous blood was drawn before and 5, 60, 120 and 180 minutes after injection for analysis of serum calcium by Webster's method.[10] Any increase above the preinjection level of serum calcium was investigated in every specimen. Phosphate clearance and urinary excretion of calcium were also determined before and after calcium infusion. Phosphate was determined by the method of Fiske and Subbarow[11] and serum alkaline phosphatase by the method of King and Armstrong.

RESULTS

In the early stage of the study, in which calcium determination was carried out by the method of Clark and Collip method or by the O-cresolphthalein complexone method, serum calcium was 9.60 ± 0.07 mg/dl (mean $\pm$ SE) and exceeded the normal range (8.6–10.0 mg/dl) in 7 cases out of 49. In subjects in whom the calcium infusion test was performed, serum calcium was 9.20 ± 0.17 mg/dl (mean $\pm$ SE) in 22 control subjects and 9.25 ± 0.16 mg/dl in 31 nontreated patients with sarcoidosis. There was no significant difference between these 2 values. Two nontreated patients showed serum calcium of 11.0 mg/dl, but other patients showed serum calcium of less than 10.6 mg/dl. Although 24-hour urinary excretion did not exceed 300 mg in 8 patients, 3 others recorded 340, 958 and 1419 mg respectively.

Although the increase at 5 minutes after injection of calcium gluconate in patients with sarcoidosis was not significantly different from that in normal subjects, significant increases were observed at 60, 120 and 180 minutes after calcium injection between values obtained in control subjects and those obtained in nontreated patients with sarcoidosis (Fig. 1a). There were no significant differences in mean values in the increase of serum calcium at 60, 120 and 180 minutes after injection of calcium gluconate among the 4 types of diagnostic criteria in sarcoidosis (Table 1). In 5 treated patients with sarcoidosis, significantly lower values were found in the increase above preinjection level of serum calcium at 60 and 180 minutes after injection of calcium gluconate, compared with in-

TABLE 1. Comparison of increases of serum calcium above preinjection levels among 4 types of sarcoidosis.

Type	Increase of serum Ca (mg/dl) above preinjection level		
	60 min	120 min	180 min
I.	1.20 ± 0.11* (10)	0.99 ± 0.11 (10)	0.92 ± 0.14 (9)
II.	1.20 ± 0.12 (4)	1.03 ± 0.08 (4)	0.60 ± 0.10 (3)
III.	1.21 ± 0.09 (9)	0.97 ± 0.09 (9)	0.70 ± 0.10 (6)
IV.	1.27 ± 0.18 (3)	0.70 ± 0.30 (3)	0.50 ± 0.20 (3)

* Mean $\pm$ SE

There were no significant differences in means of increase of serum calcium above preinjection level at each time among 4 types of nontreated sarcoidosis.

Numbers in parentheses are numbers of patients.

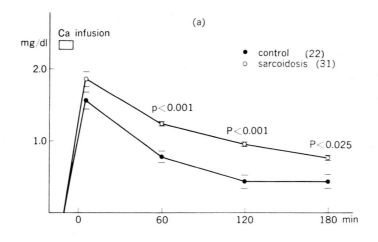

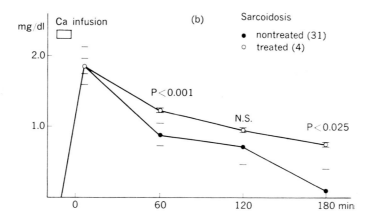

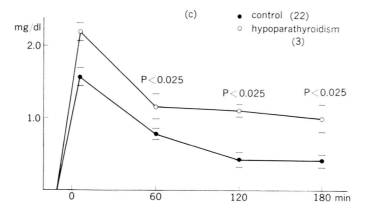

FIG. 1. Increases of serum calcium after calcium injection above preinjection level in a) control subjects versus nontreated patients with sarcoidosis, b) nontreated patients with sarcoidosis versus treated patients with sarcoidosis and c) control subjects versus patients with idiopathic hypoparathyroidism.

Each point indicates mean±SE. of increases of serum calcium above preinjection levels.

crease values in a nontreated group of sarcoidosis cases (Fig. 1b).

Similar patterns of response in serum calcium were observed in patients with idiopathic hypoparathyroidism (Fig. 1c).

Serum alkaline phosphatase was normal in most of the patients with sarcoidosis. Renal function was also normal in patients studied. Mean urinary excretion of calcium in sarcoidosis cases before and after calcium injection showed higher values than for normal subjects, but the difference was not significant.

Concerning phosphate metabolism, the serum phosphate level was 3.54 ± 0.06 mg/dl (mean $\pm$ SE) (normal range: 2.5–4.3 mg/dl) in 43 sarcoidosis patients studied. Mean serum phosphate levels showed a gradual rise after calcium infusion both in control subjects and patients with sarcoidosis. However, there was no significant difference in serum phosphate at each sampling after calcium infusion.

Phosphate clearance was suppressed after calcium infusion in normal subjects (Table 2). While the ratios of mean phosphate clearance after calcium infusion to that before calcium infusion were 43, 66, 77 and 88% in 4 normal subjects, those of 4 patients with sarcoidosis were 78, 95, 133 and 232%. In 2 cases in the latter group whose values of phosphate clearance were not suppressed after calcium infusion, mean values of phosphate clearance before calcium injection were 3.76 and 2.54 ml/min (patients M. O. and K. T.) respectively, while 2 cases in the former group, whose values of phosphate clearance were suppressed showed mean values of phosphate clearance of 5.44 and 16.02 ml/min (patients Y. K. and F. F.) before calcium injection (Table 2).

TABLE 2. Phosphate clearance (ml/min) before and after calcium infusion.

			Period before Ca infusion		Period after Ca infusion		
			1*	2*	3*	4*	5*
a) Controls							
Y. H.	22	M	6.90	1.90	1.06	2.27	2.36
H. M.	39	M	11.01	11.30	12.44	9.00	7.83
T. O.	30	M	12.10	8.64	7.58	5.57	7.40
N. H.	25	M	11.24	8.33	10.78	4.25	—
b) Patients with sarcoidosis							
Y. K.	34	F	3.73	7.14	6.13	3.37	3.23
K. T.	20	F	2.77	2.30	9.09	4.44	4.12
M. O.	51	M	3.76	—	5.92	3.55	5.51
F. F.	32	M	14.24	17.80	18.18	14.22	13.18

Periods 1 and 2 cover 60 minutes periods immediately before and periods 3, 4 and 5 cover those after Ca infusion.

DISCUSSION

Although the frequency of hypercalcemia in sarcoidosis varied widely from 1.3[12] to 63%[13] and a large survey reported a frequency of 16.5%[14], the survey of the Japan Sarcoidosis Committee in 1964 indicated a frequency of 20 to 35%. While 7 patients (14%) out of 49 showed higher values than normal in our earlier study, the present study showed that 2 out of 31 patients had serum calcium of 11.0 mg/dl and others that of less than 10.6 mg/dl.

Exaggerated response in serum calcium was observed in patients with sarcoidosis in the present study. An explanation for such an unusual phenomenon is possible from one standpoint. The equilibrium of calcium in the bone and extracellular fluids, and renal and fecal excretion of calcium are factors contributing to the response of serum calcium to calcium administration. Parathyroid hormone, calcitonin and vitamin D would also influence the response. By utilizing the calcium infusion method, Roos proposed that parathyroid activity is increased in sarcoidosis,[15] because the changes in serum phosphate and urinary phosphate resembled those seen in hyperparathyroidism.[15] However, the present study indicated that patients whose values of phosphate clearance were low showed an abnormal response in phosphate clearance after calcium infusion. Moreover, a similar pattern of response in serum calcium after calcium infusion was observed in patients with idiopathic hypoparathyroidism. These facts strongly suggest that some of the patients with sarcoidosis were in a state of hypoparathyroidism. Rhodes reported an enhanced calcemic response to the intravenous administration of parathyroid hormone. This pattern of response is more typical of hypoparathyroidism.[16] Cushard proposed that the parathyroid hormone level was extremely low in the active form of sarcoidosis.[4]

However, we still cannot explain why the serum calcium level was higher in sarcoidosis than in controls after calcium infusion. Dent suggested that hypercalcemia and hypercalciuria result from active bone destruction due to generalized sarcoidosis.[17] Serum alkaline phosphatase levels were normal in our patients. As far as the international classification of sarcoidosis is concerned, the values of serum calcium above preinjection levels at 60, 120 and 180 minutes after calcium gluconate administration did not seem to correlate with clinical manifestations, histological findings or the Kveim reaction. According to Nagle[18] hypercalcemia was more likely to occur in association with renal complications, but most of our patients showed normal renal function.

It is known that calcitonin secretion may be impaired in hypoparathyroidism.[7] Therefore, if excessive absorption of calcium is a stimulus for the secretion of calcitonin, the secretion of parathyroid hormone would be inhibited and additional secretion of calcitonin after calcium infusion impaired, in sarcoidosis. Another possibility is the inhibition of calcitonin secretion due to the pathological changes in thyroid tissues. It was reported that thyroid tissues were involved in sarcoidosis with a frequency of 4.2% in one of the large surveys.[19]

Corticosteroids are useful in differentiating hypercalcemia in sarcoidosis from that of other causes.[17] While hypercalcemia in sarcoidosis could be corrected by corticosteroid therapy, normalization of the response to calcium infusion was also observed in our patients. There was a significant decrease in the response 60 and 180 minutes after calcium infusion.

REFERENCES

1. Bell, N. H., Gill, J. R. Jr., and Bartter, F. C. 1961. *Amer. J. Resp. Dis.* **84**: 27.
2. Anderson, J., Dent, C. E., Harper, C., and Philopot. G. R. 1954. *Lancet* 2: 720.
3. Bell, N. H., and Bartter, F. C. 1967. *Acta Endocrinol.* **54**: 173.
4. Cushard, W. G., Simon, A. B., Canterbury, J. M., and Reiss, E. 1972. *New Engl. J. Med.* **286**: 395.
5. Talmage, R. V., Neuenschwander, J., and Kraintz, L. 1965. *Endocrinology* **76**: 103.
6. Williams, G. A., Hargis, G. K., Galloway, W. B., and Henderson, W. J. 1963. *Proc. Soc.*

Exp. Biol. Med. **122**: 1273.

7. Mazzuoli, G. F., Coen, G., and Antonozzi, I., 1967. Israel J. *Med. Sci.* **3**: 627.
8. Clark, E. P., and Collip, J. B. 1925. *J. Biol. Chem.* **63**: 461.
9. Kessler, G., and Walfman, M. 1964. *Clin. Chem.* **10**: 686.
10. Webster, W. W. Jr. 1962. *Amer. J. Clin. Pathol.* **37**: 330.
11. Fiske, C. H., and Subbarow Y. 1925. *J. Biol. Chem.* **66**: 375.
12. Israel, H. L., and Sones, M. 1958. *Arch. Internal Med.* **102**: 766.
13. McCort, J. J., Wood, R. H., Hamilton, J. B., and Ehrlich, D. E. 1947. *Arch. Internal Med.* **80**: 293.
14. Taylor, R. L., Lynch, H. J. Jr., and Wysor, W. G. Jr. 1963. *Amer. J. Med.* **34**: 221.
15. Roos, B. E. 1958–1959. *Acta Tuberc. Scand.* **36**: 152.
16. Rhodes, J., Reynolds, E. H., Fitzgerald, J. D., and Fourman, P. 1963. *Lancet* **2**: 598.
17. Dent C. E., Flynn, F. V., and Nabarro, J. D. N. 1953. *Brit. Med. J.* **2**: 808.
18. Nagle, R., 1961. *J. Mt. Sinai Hosp.* **28**: 268.
19. Branson, J. H., and Park, J. H. 1954. *Ann. Internal Med.* **40**: 111.

Evidence of Airway Involvement in Late Pulmonary Sarcoidosis Using Flow-Volume Curves and N_2 Washout

ALBERT MILLER, ALVIN S. TEIRSTEIN, IRA JACKLER AND LOUIS E. SILTZBACH

The Pulmonary Laboratory and Division of Thoracic Diseases, The Mount Sinai Hospital and The Mount Sinai School of Medicine, City University of New York, New York, U.S.A.

We studied 16 patients with pulmonary fibrosis caused by sarcoidosis for evidence of airway involvement, using single-breath nitrogen washout and maximum expiratory flow-volume curves, as well as conventional lung volumes and indices of airflow (VC, FRC by He dilution, MMF, $FEV_1\%$ and MVV). Unlike results of previously reported studies, 75% of our patients exhibited airway obstruction and virtually all showed impaired distribution of inspired air.

CRITERIA

The X-ray criteria for fibrosis were:
1)   Unchanging coarse streaking.
2)   Confluence.
3)   Retraction of trachea and/or hila or distortion of diaphragm.
4)   All patients also had large upper lobe bullae or hair lines, numerous 1–2 cm cysts or microcysts.

The diagnosis of sarcoidosis was established by biopsy, Kveim test or both in all patients.

RESULTS

From the flow-volume curve, flow at the middle and end of the forced vital capacity can be related to volume as flow at 50% VC over FVC ($\dot{V}50/FVC$), flow at 25% VC (remaining in the lungs) over FVC ($\dot{V}25/FVC$) and change in flow over change in volume over the corresponding range of the FVC ($\Delta\dot{V}/\Delta V$ 50–25). Loss of flow relative to volume (reduced ratios) would indicate airway obstruction; proportional loss of flow and volume

TABLE 1.   Normal values for flow-volume ratios.

	Mt. Sinai, 1972	Lapp and Hyatt, 1967[1]
$\dot{V}50*/FVC$	1.1	0.98
$\dot{V}25**/FVC$	0.48	0.45
$\Delta\dot{V}/\Delta V***$	2.45	2.36

* Flow at 50% of FVC.
** Flow at 25% of FVC remaining in the lungs.
*** Change in flow over change in volume for 50–25% of the FVC.

TABLE 2. Lung volumes, air flow, flow-volume ratios and single-breath N_2 gradients in late (fibrotic) pulmonary sarcoidosis.

	Patient (yrs*)	VC % pred.	FRC % pred.	FEV$_1$ % FVC	MMF % pred.	MVV % pred.	V̇50 L/sec.	V̇50/FVC	V̇25 L/sec.	V̇22/FVC	ΔV/V	N$_2$ Δ%
1)	P.L. 37 NF (13)	63	60	58	19	70	0.64	0.27	0.22	0.09	0.92	3.5
2)	A.T. 39 NM (5)	49	93	65	20	41	0.98	0.41	0.60	0.25	0.64	5.3
3)	B.L. 51 NM (20)	66	—	99	97	59	7.8	2.80	3.9	1.40	6.16	—
4)	C.W. 53 NF (17)	51	84	80	63	54	0.76	0.47	0.34	0.21	1.00	1.5
5)	J.P. 29 NF (5)	41	38	85	56	60	1.5	0.97	0.70	0.46	2.10	6.0
6)	C.R. 56 WF (27)	59	75	71	26	33	0.36	0.34	0.26	0.25	0.39	8.0
7)	J.K. 36 NF (10)	55	47	71	50	71	1.2	0.68	0.60	0.34	1.33	6.6
8)	J.L. 47 NF (14)	51	44	70	29	62	0.78	0.49	0.38	0.24	1.00	7.4
9)	D.M. 34 WF (4)	43	56	88	42	38	0.98	0.74	0.36	0.27	1.82	5.4
10)	R.M. 42 WM (7)	61	53	74	25	64	0.8	0.28	0.24	0.09	0.76	3.9
11)	L.C. 44 WM (18)	73	66	40	19	59	0.45	0.11	0.19	0.05	0.40	4.1
12)	P.P. 52 WM (11)	82	95	57	25	80	0.7	0.22	0.30	0.09	0.52	3.6
13)	M.H. 38 NF (12)	43	55	51	10	39	0.2	0.15	0.06	0.05	0.43	9.5
14)	J.R. 44 WM (6)	85	83	66	59	69	2.1	0.47	0.82	0.19	1.12	1.1
15)	B.M. 43 NF (13)	49	58	72	19	53	0.58	0.45	0.19	0.15	0.89	5.2
16)	S.W. 57 WF (11)	79	64	80	78	118	2.12	0.90	0.60	0.25	2.58	2.7
	Mean for all patients:	59.4	64.8	70.4	39.8	64.7	1.37	0.65	0.61	0.27	1.38	4.9
	Mean for the 12 patients with obstruction:	60.1	67.8	64.6	30.3	57.9		0.36		0.17	0.78	4.9

* Duration of disease shown in parenthesis.

would mean that a diminished flow rate is secondary to diminished volume. Normal values for these ratios are shown in Table 1.[1] Reduction in all three flow-volume ratios was used as the criterion for airway obstruction.

Results of pulmonary function tests in our 16 patients are shown in Table 2. Note that VC was reduced in 14 of the 16 cases (mean 59.4% of pred.) and FRC was reduced in 12 (mean 64.8% of pred.). In no case was the FRC increased.

MMF was diminished in 15 cases (mean 39.8% of pred.), $FEV_1\%$ (below 75) in 11 and MVV in 14.

$\dot{V}25/FVC$ was reduced in 14 patients (mean for all patients 0.27, mean for the 12 with an obstructive pattern 0.17), $\dot{V}50/FVC$ in 12 (mean for all patients 0.65, for the 12 with obstruction 0.36) and the slope of the flow-volume curve ($\Delta\dot{V}/\Delta V$) in 12 (mean for all patients 1.38, for the 12 with obstruction 0.78).

The single-breath nitrogen washout was impaired in 13 of 15 patients tested (mean gradient 4.9%).

CONCLUSIONS

1) A pattern of airway obstruction was present in 12 of our 16 patients with pulmonary fibrosis due to sarcoidosis. Values for flow-volume ratios were similar to those reported in airway obstruction[1] (Table 3). This pattern has not received adequate recognition in sarcoidosis, which is generally believed to show restricted lung volumes with normal airflow.[2, 3] Where airway obstruction has been noted in fibrotic pulmonary sarcoidosis, it was not as severe or as uniform a finding as in our series.[4, 5] The airway obstruction in our patients was not attributable to smoking.

TABLE 3.   Values for flow-volume ratios in airway obstruction.

	Mt. Sinai, 1972	Lapp and Hyatt, 1967[1]
	12 of 16 patients with fibrotic pulmonary sarcoidosis	COPD
$\dot{V}50/FVC$	0.36	0.32
$\dot{V}25/FVC$	0.17	0.18
$\Delta\dot{V}/\Delta V$	0.78	0.78

2) Four patients (cases 3, 5, 9 and 16) had flow-volume ratios indicative of restriction; the decrease in MMF in 3 of these is attributable to reduced volume. Note that FEV_1 exceeds 80% of FVC. All but one of the 4 had decreased MVV.

3) MMF, which is readily obtained, is a good index of diminished airflow while analysis of flow-volume relationships indicates whether diminished flow is independent of diminished volume.

4) Distribution of inspired air was significantly impaired in the patients with both obstructive and restrictive patterns. Impaired distribution of ventilation has not generally been recognized in sarcoidosis.[2, 3]

REFERENCES

1. Lapp, N. L., and Hyatt, R. E. 1967. Some Factors Affecting the Relationship of Maximal

Expiratory Flow to Lung Volume in Health and Disease. *Diseases Chest* **51**: 475–481.

2. Marshall, R., and Karlish, A. J. 1971. Lung Function in Sarcoidosis: An Investigation of the Disease as Seen at a Clinic in England and a Comparison of the Value of Various Lung Function Tests. *Thorax* **26**: 402–405.

3. Scadding, J. G. 1970. The Late Stages of Pulmonary Sarcoidosis. *Postgrad. Med. J.* **46**: 530–536.

4. Svanborg, N. 1961. Studies of the Cardiopulmonary Function in Sarcoidosis III. Cases with Fibrosis of the Lungs. *Acta Med. Scand.* Suppl. **366**: 75–117.

5. Emirgil, C., Sobol, B. J., Herbert, W. H., and Trout, K. 1971. The Lesser Circulation in Pulmonary Fibrosis Secondary to Sarcoidosis and Its Relationship to Respiratory Function. *Chest* **60**: 371–378.

Simultaneous Biopsy of Mediastinal Lymph Nodes, Lungs and Pleura in Sarcoidosis

Ivan Fajgelj and Branislav Djurić

Institute of Tuberculosis and Chest Diseases, Novi Sad, Yugoslavia

At present combined biopsies are more frequently used during single anaesthesia. That way a higher percentage of positive findings is obtained, and if sarcoid granulomas are discovered in 2 different organs, the diagnosis is proven with accuracy.

Bronchobiopsy and mediastinoscopy are most frequently performed during single anaesthesia. Addrizzo and his collaborators[1] recommended triple biopsy: prescalene lymph nodes, mediastinal and lung. Otte[2] obtained positive findings in 85% of diseased cases by bronchobiopsy and transbronchial puncture of lymph nodes. Otte[2] suggested the best diagnostic combination to be the following: first, bronchoscopy and bronchobiopsy followed by transbronchial puncture of lymph nodes, and if insufficient tissue was obtained, to proceed immediately with mediastinoscopy.

In addition, it is of interest for the pathogenesis of sarcoidosis to find whether lung changes already exist in the glandular stage of the disease and whether pleura was involved in the process. Stavenow reported sarcoid granulomas in the lung in 2 out of 3 cases with bilateral hilar lymphadenopathies after biopsy. Eule[3] found sarcoid granulomas histologically even in the lungs using lung biopsy in 36 (95%) out of 38 patients with bilateral hilar lymphadenopathies.

We employed different techniques of approach which proved to be more or less satisfactory in solving the above problem. Special techniques enabling approach to the lungs and mediastinal lymph nodes were the only choice. First, we tried isolated mediastinoscopies after Carlens and easily showed the desired diagnosis in the lymph nodes themselves, but our investigations were limited to the paratracheal glands. Thus, the entire mediastinum, where sometimes lymph nodes may be affected even very early, remained completely unknown. Since this large part of the mediastinum is inaccessible by Carlens exploration of the mediastinum, not to mention the inaccessibility of the lung parenchyma, we have employed pure lung biopsy after Klassen. This very popular approach always yields excellent results concerning lung changes, but it does not offer any chance of discovering changes in the lymph apparatus of the mediastinum.

Therefore, we decided to modify our former paramediastinal approach to the mediastinum, first employed in 1966, and aimed to determine the operability of lung malignoma. The modification consists of simultaneous thorough exploration of the entire anterior mediastinum, midmediastinum of the corresponding side up to the spine, as well as a specially detailed lung biopsy.

In addition to technical advantages, parasternal approach offers good visualization of all desired structures, the possibility of reliable palpable exploration, and of taking rather large pieces of tissue for analysis. Besides wide lung sections, this approach yields whole conglomerates of lymph nodes weighing several tenths of gram and occasionally whole lymph tumefaction.

Encouraged by our first attempts, we decided to apply our method on a large scale. The method may be performed both with local and general anaesthesia; this being its advantage. The usual recumbent position on the back, if necessary, can be changed for semisedentary and lateral positions.

Skin and subcutaneous tissue were cut longitudinally to a length of 6 cm at about 2 cm laterally from the margin of the sternum on the chosen side (although the right side is more frequent and, regarding lymph drainage, more suitable) and the pectoral muscles up to the ribs. An attack was made against the second rib, less frequently the second and the third, thus providing a better approach. Costal cartilage was resected subperiosteally for 4 cm up to the sternum. By gradual preparation the posterior side of the sternum was delivered at once and a step-by-step approach was made into the anterior mediastinum without opening the pleura. In time, a definite palpable sensation was acquired which is almost specific for sarcoid lymph nodes. By this approach environmental areas, particularly the lungs, may be explored and biopsy materials can be taken under control of the eye.

TABLE 1. Simultaneous parasternal biopsy of mediastinal lymph nodes, lungs and pleura performed in 17 cases of I stage intrathoracic sarcoidosis.

Sarcoid granulomas found in lungs and lymph nodes	14
In lungs only	2
In lymph nodes only	1
In pleura	Ø
Total	17

Parasternal mediastinal biopsy was performed in 42 patients with intrathoracic sarcoidosis; in 17 out of the above 42 cases biopsy of mediastinal lymph nodes, lungs and pleura was conducted simultaneously. Biopsy material was sent for histopathological examination, BK and biogram. Sarcoid granulomas were found both in mediastinal lymph nodes and lungs in 14 cases; in lungs in 2 cases and in mediastinal lymph nodes in 1 case. In 12 out of 17 cases, no changes in the lungs were visualized radiologically. Thus, only in 1 case out of 17 no sarcoid granulomas were found in the lungs. Sarcoid granulomas were not found in the pleura in any of the examined cases.

All culture media, seeded both for BK and the other bacteria, remained sterile.

In 2 cases granulomas were found in the lungs whereas they were absent in the mediastinal lymph nodes, which suggests that sampling of the material was not technically accurate as the nodes were coalesced with the blood vessels and bronchi, and the lymph nodes could not be removed completely. Since we have found pulmonary changes to occur almost regularly in the glandular stage of the disease, this means that sarcoidosis is not localized only in the mediastinal lymph nodes. However, it is very likely that the disease is not localized intrathoracically only, but from the beginning a disseminated process exists, being difficult to discover.

SUMMARY

Parasternal mediastinal biopsy was performed in 42 patients with intrathoracic sarcoidosis, whereas simultaneous biopsy of the mediastinal lymph nodes of the lungs and pleura was conducted in 17 out of 42. Sarcoid granulomas were discovered both in mediastinal lymph nodes and lung in 14 cases and sarcoid granulomas in the lungs in 2 cases, whereas they were found in mediastinal lymph nodes in 1 case. Thus, sarcoid granulomas in the lung were absent in 1 case only. In 12 out of 17 cases no changes were obtained radiologically. In the pleura, granulomas were not discovered histologically in any of the examined cases. Modified parasternal biopsy was used for the intrathoracic approach.

REFERENCES

1. Addrizzo, et al. 1969. Triple Biopsy in the Diagnosis of Sarcoidosis. Sarcoidosis. Prague: Univ. Karlova. p. 476.
2. Otte. 1968. Bronchologie der Sarkoidose. Sarkoidose Tagung in Höchenschwand. p. 52.
3. Eule. 1969. Findings by Lung Biopsy in Patients with Löfgren's Syndome Sarcoidosis. Prague: Univ. Karlova. p. 469.

Lymphographic Studies in Sarcoidosis

O. ISHIDA, H. UCHIDA, S. SONE, Y. TAJI AND T. TACHIBANA

Osaka University School of Medicine and Osaka Prefectural Hospital, Osaka, Japan

Sarcoidosis has gradually come to be recognized as a systemic disease of undetermined etiology. The mechanism of the disease and changes in the extrathoracic lymph nodes have not been fully ascertained as yet. The authors of the present paper have therefore made a study of lymphographic patterns, and relationships between extrathoracic lymphadenopathy and hilar lymphadenopathy involving pulmonary lesions, and other lesions.

MATERIALS AND METHOD

Lymphographies were performed by injection of oily contrast medium into the dorsum of each foot, in 23 cases of sarcoidosis, verified by the Kveim reaction or biopsy. Six of them, however, had been treated with varying doses of steroid before lymphography.

The patients were 16 males and 7 females whose ages ranged from 12 to 48 years. Modes of detection, examination results and classification are listed in Table 1.

The swelling of the hilar and the paratracheal lymph nodes in chest radiograms was divided into the 3 categories, fixed by the Japanese Sarcoidosis Committee, which are slight, moderate and remarkable, according to the size of the nodes. The slight degree of swelling (+) is below 1.4 cm diameter of the nodes, the moderate degree (++) is 1.5 to 2.4 cm, and the remarkable degree (+++) is above 2.5 cm. Pulmonary lesions were classified radiographically as nodular (N), linear (L) and confluent (C) shadows. These chest X-ray findings are summarized in Table 2.

RESULTS

Lymphographic patterns (Table 3)

Abnormal structures of the lymph nodes were divided roughly into granulated and foamy patterns, and further subdivided according to the nature of the pattern into coarsely granulated (G-1), irregularly distributed and more coarsely granulated (G-2), a few small round filling defects of about 1 mm diameter (F-1), more filling defects with partial confluence (F-2), and many foamy defects occupying almost all parts of the nodes (F-3) (Figs. 1–4).

The granulated pattern was observed in 18 cases (78%), the foamy pattern, typical or atypical, in all cases, and both patterns in 78% of cases. The F-2 nodes were in 83% of the cases and F-3 nodes were observed in 1 case (case 10).

The foamy filling defects were mostly situated in the central portion of the nodes and the contour of the nodes was usually smooth, but nodes with irregularity of outline and marginal defects (M) were found in 7 cases.

These abnormal patterns were sometimes confined to a few nodes, and sometimes

TABLE 1. Examinations and classification.

Case	Age and sex		Reaction Mantoux	Reaction Kveim	Lymph node	Biopsy Liver	Biopsy Others	Eye	Other symptoms	International classification
1. R. A.	17 M	Mass examination	−		C	+				III
2. H. K.	28 M	Mass examination	−		C	−				III
3. M. S.	12 M	Cough, conjunctivitis	±		C	++		Uveitis		III
4. S. M.	23 M	Malaise	±		C	+				III
5. M. N.	23 F	Mass examination	±		C	+				III
6. K. N.	21 M	Swollen parotic glands	−		C	+	Parotis, skin			III
7. H. S.	48 F	Malaise	+		C			Uveitis		III
8. S. K.	15 M	Mass examination	−		C I	++	Tonsils	Uveitis	Epilepsy	III
9. S. Y.	22 M	Mass examination	−	−	C			Uveitis	Palpable nodes	III
10. M. H.	18 F	Subfever, malaise	−		C	++			Palpable nodes	III
11. A. H.	22 F	Subfever, visual disturbance	−	+				Periphlebitis retinae		II
12. A. M.	16 M	Common cold	−		C	+			Nephritis Extrasystole	III
13. N. S.	28 M	Common cold	−	+						II
14. I. N.	36 M	Visual disturbance	−		C	+		Uveitis		III
15. S. M.	23 M	Mass examination	−		C	+		Uveitis		III
16. Y. I.	28 M	Mass examination	−		C	+				III
17. Y. Y.	12 M	Mass examination	−	+	I				Palpable nodes	I
18. C. I.	26 M	Visual disturbance	−	−	C			Periphlebitis retinae		III
19. K. N.	22 F	Common cold	−	−	C	+				III
20. H. S.	25 F	Mass examination	−	−	C					III
21. E. H.	30 F	Mass examination	±	−	C	+				III
22. Y. T.	23 M	Visual disturbance	−	−	C			Uveitis	Shenkel block	III
23. S. I.	25 M	Visual disturbance	−		C	+		Uveitis		III

TABLE 2. X-ray findings in the chest.

Case	Duration of prelymphographic therapy	Lymph nodes		Pulmonary lesions
		Bronchopulmonary	Paratracheal	
1	—	⧺	+	—
2	—	⧺	+	L, N
3	—	⧺	⧺	N
4	—	⧺	—	—
5	—	⧺	—	—
6	—	+	+	—
7	—	+	—	—
8	—	⧺	⧺	—
9	—	⧺	⧺	—
10	—	⧺	⧺	—
11	—	⧺	⧺	—
12	—	⧺	⧺	N
13	—	⧺	+	N
14	—	⧺	+	N
15	—	⧺	+	N, C
16	—	⧺	+	—
17	—	⧺	⧺	N
18	2 ws	(⧻) +	+	N, C
19	1 m	(⧻) ⧺	—	L, N
20	3 ms	(⧻) ⧺	⧺	N
21	6 ms	(⧻) +	—	N, C
22	3 ms	(⧻) ⧺	+	—
23	7 ws	(⧻) +	—	—

( ) before therapy.

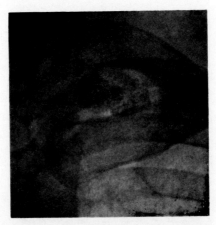

FIG. 1. (Case 18), Coarse granulated pattern with a small filling defects are seen in the supraclavicular nodes (G-1, F-1).

TABLE 3. Lymphographic findings.

Case	Lymph nodes				Increase		Femoral retention	Thoracic duct	Mediastinum	Cervical reflux
	Inguinal	Iliac	Lumbar	Supraclav.	Number	Size				
1	G_1F_2M	F_2M	G_2	F_1	$+$	$\pm$	L, R			
2	G_1F_2	F_2	G_1F_1		$-$	$-$	L, R			
3	G_1	F_1	G_1		$-$	$-$	$-$			
4	G_2F_2M	G_2F_2	F_1		$\pm$	Small	$-$			$+$
5	F_1	F_2M	F_2		$-$	Small	L			
6	G_1F_2	G_1F_1	F_2		$+$	$-$	$-$			
7	F_1	F_1	F_1		$-$	$-$	$-$			
8	G_1F_2	G_1F_2	G_1F_2	G_1F_1	$-$	$-$	$-$	Displace.		$+$
9	F_1	F_1	F_1	F_1	$-$	Small	L		Lymph vessel	$+$
10	G_2F_3	G_2F_3M	G_2F_3M	F_1	$\pm$	$\pm$	L, R			
11	G_1F_1	F_2	G_1F_2	F_1	$+$	$\pm$	$-$			
12	F_1	F_2	F_1	F_2M	$-$	$-$	L			
13	G_1F_2	G_1F_1	F_1	F_2M	$\pm$	$\pm$	L			
14	G_1F_1	G_1F_1			$-$	$-$	$-$			
15	G_1F_2	G_1F_2	G_1F_2	G_1F_2	$-$	$-$	$-$			
16	G_1F_2	G_1F_2			$+$	Small	$-$			
17	G_1F_1	G_1F_2M	G_1F_2		$\pm$	$+$	$-$			
18	F_2	F_2	F_1	F_2	$\pm$	$-$	L, R		Lymph node	
19	F_2	F_2	F_1		$-$	$-$	L			
20	G_1	F_2	G_1F_1		$+$	$-$	$-$			
21	G_1F_1M	G_2F_2M	G_1F_1	G_1F_2	$\pm$	$-$	L	Displace.	Lymph node	
22	G_1F_1	F_2	F_1	G_1F_1	$+$	$-$	L		Lymph node	
23	G_1F_1				$-$	Small	$-$			

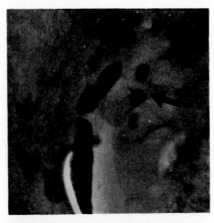

FIG. 2. (Case 3), A small filling defect is observed in a few small iliac nodes (F-1).

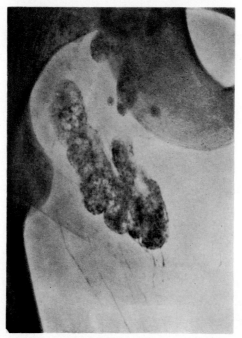

FIG. 3. (Case 1), Multiple foamy defects and a more coarsely granulated pattern with slight retention are to be seen in the femoral lymphatics (G-2, F-2).

occupied almost all nodes in 1 region or all regions. As for the involved region, the iliac lymph nodes were most frequently invaded in 70% of cases, the inguinal in 56%, the lumbar in 35%, and the supraclavicular nodes in 10 out of 14 stained cases.

There was a slight tendency for increase in size and number of the lymph nodes. The abnormal patterns were marked in larger lymph nodes but were apparently detected even in small lymph nodes.

The abnormal patterns were observed in all cases before and after therapy. Very slight changes such as G-1 or F-1, however, were occasionally observed even in normal persons. Therefore if the cases with such slight changes were excluded abnormal patterns would have been detected in 18 (78%) cases.

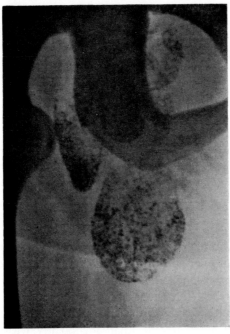

FIG. 4. (Case 10), Nearly all parts of the swollen nodes are occupied by foamy filling defects with marginal defects and coarse granulated pattern (G-2, F-3, M).

Decrease in size of the hilar lymph nodes with or without steroid therapy was usually accompanied by a decrease in size of the extrathoracic lymph nodes, but some cases showed no simultaneous decrease in size. When the lymph nodes decreased in size, their filling defects also decreased in both size and number, and they were filled with granulated patterns.

Retention of the contrast medium in the femoral lymph vessels was observed (1 day after the injection) in 10 cases, where a moderate degree of abnormal inguinal or iliac lymph nodes was usually confirmed X-rays revealed that the thoracic duct was displaced slightly in 2 cases at the level of the pulmonary hilum. The cervical reflux and staining of the mediastinal lymphatics were observed in 3 cases, but no congestive signs were perceived.

Relationship between the lymphadenopathy and the other lesions (Table 4)

In 7 out of 8 cases (cases 1, 4, 8, 10, 15, 17, 21) where an extrathoracic lymphadenopathy occurred in marked degree, such as G-2, F-2, F-3, and M, a remarkable hilar adenopathy and also hepatic lesions were confirmed except for 1 nonbiopsied case, but ocular lesions were detected in only 2 cases.

In the other 15 cases with a slight extrathoracic lymphadenopathy, a remarkable hilar adenopathy and hepatic lesions were apparent in 8 cases, and ocular lesions were found in 6 cases.

In 15 cases with a remarkable hilar adenopathy, marked extrathoracic lymphadenopathy, ocular lesions, and hepatic lesions, were present in 7, 6, and 9 cases, respectively.

Of the other 8 cases with a slight hilar adenopathy, both a marked extrathoracic lymphadenopathy and ocular lesions were found in 1 case, and hepatic lesions in 5.

TABLE 4. Relationship between the extrathoracic and the hilar lymphadenopathy, and the other lesions

Lymphadenopathy	Extrathoracic (卌)	Hilar (卌)	Lesion		
			Eye	Liver	No liver biopsy
Extrathoracic					
(卌)	8	7	2	6	2
(+)	15	8	6	8	4
Total	23	15	8	14	6
Hilar					
(卌)	15	7	6	9	3
(+)	8	1	3	5	3
Total	23	8	9	14	6

All of 11 cases with pulmonary lesions also showed a remarkable hilar adenopathy, and 15 cases with a slight hilar adenopathy had no pulmonary lesions at all.

Of 9 cases with ocular lesions, 3 had a remarkable hilar adenopathy, and of 14 cases with hepatic lesions, 9 revealed a remarkable hilar adenopathy.

These results suggest that cases with a marked extrathoracic lymphadenopathy are usually accompanied by a remarkable hilar adenopathy with pulmonary lesions and hepatic lesions, but seldom by any ocular lesion.

On the other hand, the cases with pulmonary lesions and a remarkable hilar adenopathy were not always accompanied by a marked extrathoracic lymphadenopathy and ocular lesions, but frequently by hepatic lesions.

Therefore it may be concluded that extrathoracic lymphadenopathy and hepatic lesions have a tendency to maintain a relatively parallel relationship with the hilar adenopathy and pulmonary lesions, but seem to show scarcely any relationship to the ocular lesions.

SUMMARY

Lymphographic studies were made on 23 cases of sarcoidosis, which had been verified by the Kveim test or visceral biopsy.

Lymphographically, the small round filling defects or foamy pattern and coarsely granulated pattern were observed in varying degrees in the extrathoracic lymph nodes of almost all the cases.

The iliac lymph nodes were most frequently invaded, and the inguinal, the lumbar and the supraclavicular lymph nodes, in that order, were also severely affected.

An increase in size and number of lymph nodes was observed to a slight degree.

The outline of the lymph nodes was usually smooth, but marginal filling defects and irregular outline were also detected in some cases.

A small degree of passage disturbance in the femoral lymphatics was observed in about 50% of cases, and cervical reflux and staining of the mediastinal lymphatics were occasionally observed.

When the extrathoracic lymph nodes were severely affected, the hilar lymphadenopathy and the hepatic lesions were also remarkable, but ocular lesions were apparent in only a few cases. On the other hand, when the hilar lymphadenopathy was remarkable, the extrathoracic lymph nodes were not always seriously affected, but hepatic lesions were greatly in evidence.

The decrease in size of the hilar lymph nodes brought about by steroid therapy was usually accompanied by a decrease in size of the extrathoracic lymph nodes, but there was no parallel relationship between them in some cases.

REFERENCES

1. Akisada, M., Tasaka, A., and Mikami, R. 1970. Roentgenographic studies of fifteen cases of sarcoidosis. *Nipp. Acta Radiol.* **29**: 1415.
2. Albrecht, A., Taenzer, V., and Nickling, H. 1967. Lymphographische Befunde bei Sarkoidose und Lymphknotentuberkulose. *Fortschr. Röntgenstr.* **106**: 178.
3. Bacsa, S., and Mandi, L. 1966. Abdominal lymphography in thoracic sarcoidosis. *Scand. J. Resp. Dis.* **47**: 244.
4. Becker, W. F., and Coleman, W. O. 1961. Surgical significance of abdominal sarcoidosis. *Ann. Surg.* **153**: 987.
5. Ishida, O., Sone, S., Uchida, H., Taji, Y., Kuroda, C., Kinjyo, T., and Tachibana, T. 1972. Lymphographic patterns in sarcoidosis. *Saishin-igaku* **27**: 1372.
6. Strickstrock, K. H., und Weißleder, H. 1969. Lymphographische Diagnose und Differentialdiagnose bei der Sarkoidose. Fortschr. *Röntgenstr.* **108**: 577.
7. Tachibana, T., Donomae, I., Aratake, M., Murata, Y., Kiyonaga, G., Takase, K., Seki, K., and Shinji, K. 1971. Peritoneoscopy and liver biopsy in intrathoracic sarcoidosis. *Fifth Int. Conf. on Sarcoidosis.* Prague: Univ. Karlova.
8. Viamonte, M., Attman, D., Parkers, R., Blum, E., Benilacqua, M., and Recher, L. 1963. Radiographic pathologic correlation in the interpretation of lymphangiograms. *Radiology* **80**: 903.
9. Walther, H. H. 1962. Kasuistischer Beitrag zum Frühstadium des Lungen-Boeck. *Fortschr. Röntgenstr.* **96**: 986.
10. Wiljasalo, M. 1968. Thoracic sarcoidosis and lymphography. *Scand. J. Resp. Dis.* Suppl. **65**: 251.

α_1-Antitrypsin Levels in Sarcoidosis
—Relationship to disease activity—

ROSCOE C. YOUNG, JR, VERLE E. HEADINGS, SIKTA BOSE, K. ALBERT HARDEN,
EDWARD D. CROCKETT, JR AND ROBERT L. HACKNEY, JR

Pulmonary Function Laboratory, Pulmonary Disease Division, Department of
Medicine and Medical Genetics Unit, Department of Pediatrics,
Howard University College of Medicine and Freedmen's Hospital,
Washington, D.C., U.S.A.

In the course of an ethnic group study of black persons for α_1-antitrypsin deficiency associated with pulmonary disease, it became apparent that some patients with sarcoidosis had higher levels of α_1-antitrypsin (α_1-AT) than healthy subjects or persons with a variety of other pulmonary diseases.

Since a deficiency of α_1-AT, a glycoprotein of molecular weight over 45,000, has been genetically associated with some cases of emphysema[1] and also a juvenile form of liver cirrhosis,[2] an attempt was made to correlate increases in α_1-AT with disease activity, airways obstruction and environmental factors of cigarette smoking and occupation in sarcoidosis patients.

MATERIALS AND METHODS

Forty black patients with organ biopsy and/or Kveim-Siltzbach test positive sarcoidosis were studied. They were divided into 2 groups, active and inactive, depending upon the presence or absence of constitutional symptoms such as fever, hypercalcemia, hyperglobulinema with reversal of the A/G ratio, Kveim reactivity and elevation of the erythrocyte sedmentation rate. An equal group of healthy black subjects, matched for age and sex, served as controls.

Clinical characteristics of the sarcoidosis patients were similar to those described earlier.[3] Additional information was obtained from a modification of the Medical Research Council questionnaire, history, physical examination and radiographs of each subject. Radiologic stage of disease, smoking habits and occupational environments of sarcoidosis patients are shown in Tables 1, 2 and 3, respectively.

None of the subjects studied were on adrenocorticoid therapy, had had recent surgery, were pregnant, had evidence of infection or were taking oral contraceptives at the time of study, situations known to increase α_1-AT levels in all but homozygotes.[4–6]

Procedures used were those standardized for National Heart and Lung Institute Epidemiologic studies.[7] Spirography was performed on all subjects with a water-seal respirometer. Predicted normal values were those of Goldman and Becklake.[8] Arterial oxygen saturation was measured with an ear oximeter.[9] Calculations and interpretations were made using a time-sharing computer technique.[10]

Work supported by National Heart and Lung Institute Contract 71–14 and Research Grant HE–13854–07, NIH.

TABLE 1. Radiologic stage of sarcoidosis.*

Stage	Active	Inactive	Totals
0	1	6	7
1	9	9	18
2	7	2	9
3	4	0	4
4	2	0	2
Totals	23	17	40

* Stage 0, normal chest X-ray; 1, bilateral hilar adenopathy (BHL); 2, BHL and parenchymal infiltration; 3, parenchymal infiltration only; 4, pulmonary fibrosis, mediastinal distortion, honeycomb lung, sarcoidosis for over 2 years.

TABLE 2. Smoking habits of sarcoidosis patients.

	Active	Inactive	Totals
Non-smokers	12	10	22
0–4 pack/years	3	1	4
0–9	3	2	5
10–20	5	4	9
>20	0	0	0
Totals	23	17	40

TABLE 3. Occupational environment of sarcoidosis patients.*

	Active	Inactive	Totals
Civil servant	4	1	5
Clerical	7	4	11
Education	5	4	9
Food service	1	0	1
Health care	1	4	5
Homemaking	3	2	5
Utilities	2	2	4
Totals	23	17	40

* Entertainment, farming, industrial, mining, transportation occupations were not represented.

Eight patients with active sarcoidosis underwent more extensive tests. Diffusing capacity for carbon monoxide was measured by the breath-holding technique[11] modified for gas chromatography.[12] Thoracic gas volume was measured at functional residual capacity and airway resistance measured in a variable pressure body plethysmograph, using accepted methods.[13, 14] Airway resistance was expressed as specific conductance.

Assessment of obstruction in small airways less than 2 to 3 mm in diameter was done by measurement of static lung compliance followed by dynamic lung compliance at several respiratory frequencies up to 92 breaths per minute, using the esophageal balloon technique of Woolcock et al.[15] Dynamic compliance at different respiratory frequencies was expressed as percentage of its static value.

Three methods were used to evaluate a_1-AT: trypsin inhibitory capacity (TIC), cellulose acetate electrophoresis and radial immunodiffusion. The quantitative estimation of serum antitrypsin activity was obtained on 40 patients and their age and sex matched controls by a modification (used by Dr Richard Talamo) of the method of Erlanger et al.[16] Quality control of the method used in the writers' laboratory was assured by analysis of unknown sera from a standard reference laboratory (laboratory of Dr John A. Pierce, Washington University, St. Louis, Missouri, U.S.A.). The quantitative determination of serum a_1-AT on 12 patients and 2 controls was performed by radial immunodiffusion using the Partigen plate (distributed by Behring Diagnostics, Inc.).

This single radial immunodiffusion is a modified method of Mancini et al.[17] The principle of this method depends upon the diffusion of protein from a small cylindrical well into a thin antibody-containing agar gel layer. As the antigen diffuses into the agar gel, a precipitin ring is formed around the well, the diameter of which is proportional to antigen concentration. Lastly, also on 12 patients and 2 control subjects, electrophoresis of human serum proteins (stored at $-20°C$ until tested) was performed on cellulose acetate membranes using high resolution buffer and stained with Ponceau-S stain. The cleared strips were then examined in a densitometer for scanning[18,19] (Densicord Integraph, Integrater Model 49, Photovolt, 1115 Broadway, New York, New York 10010, U.S.A.).

RESULTS

A comparison was made between TIC levels of 23 patients with active sarcoidosis against values in age and sex matched healthy control subjects (Fig. 1a). The mean TIC for active sarcoidosis patients was 1.88 mg/ml, SD$\pm$0.40, SE$\pm$0.08. The maximum was 2.72 and the minimum was 1.30. Their age and sex matched controls had a mean TIC of 1.42 mg/ml, SD$\pm$0.24, SE$\pm$0.05. The maximum was 1.94 and minimum was 0.99. Student's T Test was applied and the difference of the means of these 2 groups was highly significant $P<0.001$.

On the other hand, 17 patients with inactive sarcoidosis and an equal number of control subjects were similar. For the inactive sarcoidosis patients, mean TIC was 1.39 mg/ml, SD$\pm$0.20, SE$\pm$0.05, maximum 1.82, minimum was 1.04, while for their matched controls TIC was 1.52, SD$\pm$0.30, SE$\pm$0.07, maximum was 2.38 and minimum was 1.08. The difference between means of these two groups was not significant.

The entire control population analyzed as a group had a mean TIC of 1.46 mg/ml, SD$\pm$0.27, SE$\pm$0.04, maximum of 2.38 and minimum of 0.99.

Interrelationships between different methods of measuring a_1-AT were examined. The relationship of TIC with a_1-globulin measured by cellulose acetate electrophoresis and expressed as percent of total protein in 14 subjects is shown in Fig. 2a. Patients with active sarcoidosis cluster at the upper right, while those with inactive disease and 2 healthy controls are below and to the left. The correlation was r=0.7, SEE= $\pm$0.34. The significance of the regression was tested by analysis of variance, F=11.5, P<0.01.

The relationship of immunodiffusion with TIC is shown in Fig. 2b. The pattern is similar to Fig. 2a. The correlation for 2b was r=0.77, SEE= $\pm$0.37. Analysis of variance for the regression F=17.7, P<0.01.

Not shown is the correlation between a_1-globulin and immunodiffusion. Results were below the level of significance.

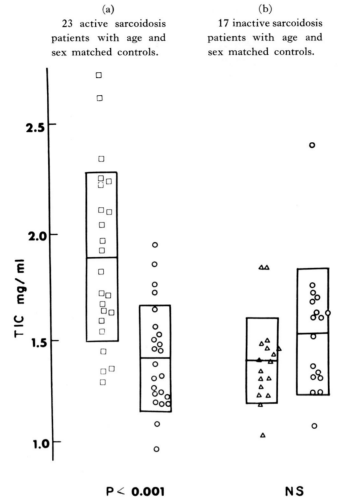

FIG. 1. (a) Difference in TIC in 23 patients with active sarcoidosis (squares) against an equal number of age- and sex-matched control subjects (circles).

(b) Similarity between TIC of patients with inactive sarcoidosis (triangles) and an equal number of age- and sex-matched controls (circles). Total of 80 subjects.

Spirographic patterns of 40 sarcoidosis patients are shown in Table 4. Three patients in the active group and 2 in the inactive group had obstructive airways disease in their larger airways as judged by prolonged FVC, $FEV_{1.0}\%$ less than 70 and air velocity index less than unity. Five patients in the active group had a combined ventilatory defect. No relationship existed between either cigarette smoking, occupational environment or TIC and airways abstraction.

Arterial oxygen saturation at rest, breathing room air, in the patients is shown in Table 5. Ninety-two% is taken as the lower limit of normal. In about half the patients with active disease and a quarter with inactive disease, saturation was decreased suggesting inhomogeneity of distribution of ventilation and perfusion as cause of hypoxemia. Again, no significant relationships could be demonstrated between resting oxygen saturation and cigarette smoking, occupational environment and TIC.

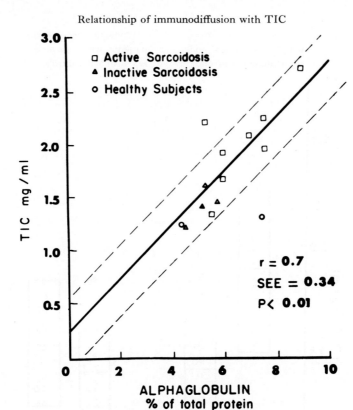

FIG. 2a.   TIC vs α_1-globulin by cellulose acetate electrophoresis in 14 subjects.   The regression line is solid.   Confidence limits are shown by the dashed lines.

TABLE 4.   Spirographic patterns in sarcoidosis.

	Active	Inactive	Totals
Normal	9	12	21
Obstructive	3	2	5
Combined	5	0	5
Restrictive	6	3	9
Totals	23	17	40

TABLE 5.   Arterial oxygen saturation at rest in sarcoidosis.*

	Active	Inactive	Totals
Normal	11	13	24
Low	12	4	16
Totals	23	17	40

* Saturations below 92% were regarded as low.

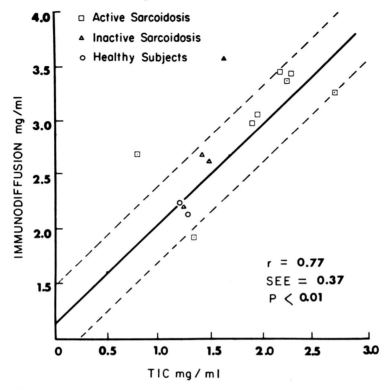

Relationship of immunodiffusion with TIC

FIG. 2b. Immunodiffusion vs TIC in the same subjects. In both Figs. 2a and 2b, patients with active sarcoidosis (squares) are shown in upper right while those with inactive disease (triangles) and healthy controls (circles) are shown in lower left.

TABLE 6. Additional pulmonary function tests in patients with peripheral airways obstruction.*

	Mean	SD	Maximum	Minimum
R_A (CmH$_2$0/L/Sec)	1.8	1.04	3.5	0.49
V_{TG} (L)	2.57	0.68	3.36	1.69
SG_{aw} (Sec^{-1}cmH$_2$0^{-1})	0.35	0.19	0.67	0.09
$C_{L\ STAT}$ (L/cmH$_2$0)	0.08	0.03	0.14	0.05
$D_{L_{CO}}$ (ml/min/mmHg)	15 (60%)	5.6	25	9

* R_A, airway resistance; V_{TG}, thoracic gas volume measured at FRC; SG_{aw}, specific airway conductance; $C_{L\ Stat}$, static lung compliance; $D_{L_{CO}}$, breath-holding diffusing capacity for carbon monoxide.

Table 6 shows statistical values of additional pulmonary function tests performed on 8 patients with active sarcoidosis, 5 of whom are cigarette smokers. Two of the 8 had pure airways obstruction, 1 had a combined ventilatory defect and the remainder had restrictive lung disease as assessed by conventional pulmonary function tests.

Dynamic lung compliance of these 8 patients, plotted as percentage of their static compliance at multiple respiratory frequencies, is shown in Fig. 3. All patients had frequency dependent compliances (greater than a 20% decrease from static compliance)

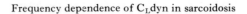

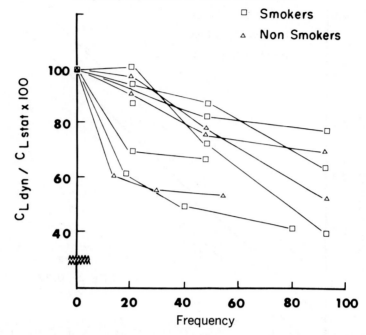

FIG. 3.   Dynamic lung compliance in 8 patients with active sarcoidosis measured at
multiple respiratory frequencies and plotted as percentage of static value.   Smokers are
represented by squares, nonsmokers by triangles.

Although only 3 patients had evidence of airways obstruction by conventional tests, all
patients had frequency dependent compliances, indicating disease in peripheral airways.

denoting small airways disease. Obstruction in peripheral airways was, therefore, present in all sarcoidosis patients tested regardless of their spirographic pattern or smoking
habits.

DISCUSSION

The present study indicates that sarcoidosis is a disease in which protease inhibitor
activity is increased during the active phase. Jacobsson's discovery that 90% of protease
inhibitor lies in the α_1-globulin and 10% in the α_1-globulin[20] may explain the mechanism
of increased protease inhibitors in sarcoidosis.

Although Salvensen[21] first called attention to hyperglobulinemia in sarcoidosis, much
investigation in the current literature is concerned with immunoglobins. Relatively
little attention has been given to increases in α_1- and α_2-globulins in this disease. Sunderman and Sunderman's "step-like" pattern in this disease suggested elevations of globu-
lin fractions gamma, beta, α_2 and α_1 in that order of magnitude.[22] Shelton et al.[23] found a
34% increase in α_2-globulin and a 19% increase in α_1 but found no difference in black
patients with active sarcoidosis when compared with a "quiescent" group. In a comparison of chronic idopathic dysproteinemia with sarcoidosis, Petera and Sach[24] found
α_1- and α_2-globulins to be increased in 54% of 104 sarcoidosis patients. On the other
hand, Scadding[25] found slight increases in the α_2- and lesser increases in α_1-globulin in

sarcoidosis, while greater increases were in the gamma and beta fractions. Finally, Bottiger and Norberg[26] noted that serum-bound carbohydrate, seromucoids and α_2-globulin seemed to correlate well with disease activity in sarcoidosis.

All globulin fractions are produced in reticuloendothelial cells, 80% of which is in the liver. Gammaglobulins, however, are mainly produced by the lymphocyte-plasma cell axis.[27] Since sarcoidosis commonly involves the liver[28] and collars of lymphocytes surround granulomata, it is not surprising to find all globulin fractions increased in active sarcoidosis. Increase in protease activity, especially α_1-AT follows. It is tempting to speculate that an increase in α_1-AT in sarcoidosis may help protect structurally damaged lungs from infectious complications since protease inhibitors possess antibiotic action.[29]

It might be well to point out that the increase in α_1-AT in active sarcoidosis is by no means specific. Increased levels of protease activity have been described in pancreatitis, malignancy, acute bacterial infections, tuberculosis, rheumatic fever, nephritis, hyperthyroidism and postoperatively.[20,30] It has been previously suggested that ethnic group variations exist in α_1-AT levels in normal subjects.[31,32] Persons of nordic ancestry have more frequent deficiencies than persons of dark-skinned ancestry. The possibility also exists that a normal quantity for one ethnic group may be abnormal for another. The mean level of TIC of 1.49 mg/ml in healthy blacks of the present study is greater than a mean of 1.09 in ethnic mixtures of normal subjects taken from the literature.[33-35] Data is still scanty and its significance has yet to be tested.

The popular concept that restrictive lung disease is the most common spirographic abnormality associated with sarcoidosis must not go unchallenged. Airways obstruction is common in sarcoidosis.[36,37] Further, airway resistance rather than tissue viscous resistance constitutes the greater portion of mechanical resistance in sarcoidosis.[38] Macklem and Mead's demonstration that 20 to 30% of resistance to airflow is in small airways less than 2 to 3 mm in diameter[39] suggests that considerable occlusion of small airways by epithelioid granuloma could occur in sarcoidosis and yet obstruction could go undetected by conventional forced expirograms as well as by the more sensitive plethysmographic method for measuring airways resistance. Dynamic lung compliance, a test for small airways disease,[15] was found to be frequency dependent in all 8 randomly selected sarcoidosis patients in the present study, 5 of whom were nonsmokers. Because of its invasiveness, however, this test failed to gain wide patient acceptance. Perhaps the other test for small airways disease, " closing lung volume "[40] would have been better tolerated. Other causes for frequency dependence of compliance could be regional differences in lung compliance. The measurement of dynamic lung compliance is an extremely difficult and meticulous test requiring great attention to detail both in terms of the maneuvers the patient makes and the frequency response of the equipment. Macklem (personal communication; Dr Peter T. Macklem, Royal Victoria Hospital, Montreal, Quebec, Canada) suggests the latter may account for such variable results in the literature.

Lack of a relationship between airways obstruction and α_1-AT levels in sarcoidosis may be explained by the occurrence of obstruction in the early active stages when protease inhibitor is apt to be increased, and obstruction in the late inactive fibrotic stage when it tends towards normal levels. Unlike airways obstruction in emphysema, that in sarcoidosis is not due to loss of elastic lung recoil. Mean static compliance was decreased in patients in whom it was measured denoting " stiff " lungs (Table 6).

Methods used to measure α_1-AT in the present study shed no light on the genetic susceptibility for development of sarcoidosis. In other studies, genetic phenotyping was not helpful. Fagerhol and Hauge[41] studied serum-inherited variants of a_1-AT (the Pi system) in pulmonary disease and found the phenotype of sarcoidosis patients to be that most commonly found in normal individuals, Pi MM.

SUMMARY

a_1-Antitrypsin levels were increased in active sarcoidosis patients not under treatment when compared with inactive patients or matched healthy control subjects. This increase follows the same trend as it does in other types of inflammation and may be related to an increase in globulins in active sarcoidosis.

Airways obstruction in sarcoidosis was common particularly disease of the smaller peripheral airways. No relationship existed between a_1-antitrypsin level, airways obstruction and environmental factors of occupation and smoking habits.

Methods used to measure a_1-antitrypsin shed no light on the genetic susceptibility for developing sarcoidosis.

ACKNOWLEDGEMENT

The authors wish to acknowledge the technical assistance of Mrs Adora Ogunye, Mr William G. Pennix, Mrs Maria J. Ewell and Mr James Miller.

REFERENCES

1. Laurell, C. B., and Eriksson, K. 1963. Studies in a_1-Antitrypsin Deficiency. *Scand. J. Clin. Lab. Invest.* **15**: 132.
2. Sharp, H. L. 1971. a_1-Antitrypsin Deficiency. *Hosp. Pract.* **6**: 83.
3. Young, R. C. Jr, Titus-Dillon, P. Y., Schneider, M. L., Shelton, T. G., Hackney, R. L. Jr, and Harden, K. A. 1971. Sarcoidosis in Washington, D. C., Clinical Observations in 105 Black Patients. Levinsky, L., and Macholda, F. *Fifth Int. Conf. on Sarcoidosis.* Prague: Univ. Karlova. p. 513.
4. Faarvang, H. J., and Lauristen, O. S. 1963. Increase of Trypsin Inhibitor in Serum During Pregnancy. *Nature* **199**: 290.
5. Faarvang, H. J., and Lauristen, O. S. 1963. Relationship Between Serum Concentration and Urinary Output of Trypsin Inhibitor after Cortisone Administrator. *Scand. J. Clin. Lab. Invest.* **15**: 483.
6. Talamo, R. C., Blennarhassett, J. B., and Austin, K. F. 1966. Familial Emphysema and a_1-Antitrypsin Deficiency. *New Engl. J. Med.* **275**: 1301.
7. National Heart and Lung Institute Workshop on Epidemiology of Respiratory Disease. 1972. *Amer. Rev. Resp. Dis.* **105**: 484.
8. Goldman, H. I., and Becklake, M. R. 1959. Respiratory Function Tests: Normal Values at Median Altitudes and the Prediction of Normal Results. *Amer. Rev. Tuberc.* **79**: 457.
9. Wood, E. H., and Geraci, J. E. 1949. Photoelectric Determination of Arterial Saturation in Man. *J. Lab. Clin. Med.* **34**: 387.
10. Young, R. C. Jr, Pennix, W. C., Ewell, M. J., and Sampson, C. C. 1971. Pulmonary Function Compatibility of the Time-Sharing Computer System. *JNMA* **63**: 346.
11. Ogilvie, C. M., Forster, R. E., Blakemore, W. S., and Morton, J. W. 1957. Standardized Breath-holding Technique for the Clinical Measurement of Diffusing Capacity of the Lung for Carbon Monoxide. *J. Clin. Invest.* **36**: 1.

12. Smith, J. R., and Hamilton, L. H. 1962. DLCO Measurements with Gas Chromatography. *J. Appl. Physiol.* **17**: 856.

13. DuBois, A. B., Betelho, S. Y., Bedell, G. N., Marshall, R., and Comroe, J. H. Jr. 1956. A Rapid Plethysmographic Method for Measuring Thoracic Gas Volume: A Comparison with a Nitrogen Washout Method for Measuring Functional Residual Capacity in Normal Subjects. *J. Clin. Invest.* **35**: 322.

14. DuBois, A. B., Betelho, S. Y., and Comroe, J. H. Jr. 1956. A New Method for Measuring Airway Resistance in Man Using a Body Plethysmograph: Values in Normal Subjects and in Patients with Respiratory Disease. *J. Clin. Invest.* **35**: 327.

15. Woolcock, A. J., Vincent, N. J., and Macklem, P. T. 1969. Frequency Dependence of Compliance as a Test for Obstruction in the Small Airways. *J. Clin. Invest.* **48**: 1097.

16. Erlanger, B. F., Kokowsky, N., and Cohen, W. 1961. The Preparation and Properties of Two New Chromogenic Substrates of Trypsin. *Arch. Biochem.* **95**: 271.

17. Mancini, G., Carbonara, A. O., and Heremans, J. F. 1965. Immunochemical Quantitation of Antigens by Single Radial Immunodiffusion. *Immunochem.* **2**: 235.

18. Lieberman, J., Mittman, C., and Schneider, A. S. 1969. Screening for Homozygous and Heterozygous α_1-Antitrypsin Deficiency. *JAMA* **210**: 2055.

19. Lieberman, J., and Mittman, C. 1970. Screening for Heterozygous α_1-Antitrypsin Deficiency. *Ann. Internal Med.* **73**: 9.

20. Jacobsson, K. 1955. Studies on the Trypsin and Plasmin Inhibitors in Human Blood Serum. *Scand. J. Clin. Lab. Invest.* Suppl. **14–22**: 7.

21. Salvensen, H. A. 1935. The Sarcoid of Boeck. A Disease of Importance to Internal Medicine: Report of Four Cases. *Acta Med. Scand.* **86**: 127.

22. Sunderman, F. W. Jr, and Sunderman, F. W. 1957. Clinical Applications of the Fractionation of Serum Proteins by Paper Electrophoresis, *Amer. J. Clin. Path.* **27**: 125.

23. Shelton, T. G., Cherrie, A. L., and Harden, K. A. 1966. Blood and Sarcoidosis I, Paper Electrophoresis of the Serum Proteins. *JNMA* **58**: 99.

24. Petera, J., and Sach, J. 1970. Syndrome of Idiopathic Chronic Dysproteinemia and Sarcoidosis. Levinsky, L. and Macholda, F. *Proc. Fifth Int. Conf. on Sarcoidosis*. Prague: Univ. Karlova. p. 209.

25. Scadding, J. G. 1967. Sarcoidosis. London: Erye and Spottiswoode. p. 378.

26. Bottiger, L. E., and Norberg, R. 1964. Studies in Sarcoidosis II, Serum Bound Carbohydrates. *Acta. Med. Scand.* **175**: 373.

27. Best, C. H., and Taylor, N. B. 1966. The Physiologic Basis of Medical Practice (8th ed.). Baltimore: Williams and Wilkins. p. 476.

28. Maddrey, W. C., Johns, C. J., Boitnott, J. K., and Iber, F. L. 1970. Sarcoidosis and Chronic Hepatic Disease: A Clinical and Pathologic Study of 20 Patients. *Medicine* **49**: 375.

29. Mirsky, I. A., and Foley, G. 1945. Antibiotic Action of Trypsin Inhibitors, *Proc. Exper. Biol. Med.* **59**: 34.

30. Homer, G. M., Zipf, R. E., Hieber, T. E., and Katchman, B. J. 1960. The Trypsin Inhibitor Capacity of Serums in Normal and Disease States, *Amer. J. Clin. Path.* **34**: 99.

31. Mittman, C., and Lieberman, J. 1970. Ethnic Group Variation in the Incidence of α_1-Antitrypsin Deficiency. *Clin. Res.* **18**: 488. (Abstract.)

32. Lieberman, J. 1972. New Test Makes Screening for Emphysema Prone. *Int. Med. News.* p. 3 (February 1).

33. Eriksson, S. 1965. Studies in α_1-Antitrypsin Deficiency. *Acta. Med. Scand.* Suppl. **432**: 177, 1.

34. Lieberman, J. 1969. Heterozygous and Homozygous α_1-Antitrypsin Deficiency in Patients with Pulmonary Emphysema. *New Engl. J. Med.* **281**: 279.

35. Welch, M. H., Reineke, M. E., Hammarsten, J. F., and Guenter, C. A. 1969. Antitrypsin Deficiency in Pulmonary Disease: The Significance of Intermediate Levels. *Ann. Internal Med.* **71**: 533.
36. Harden, K. A., Barthakur, A., and Carr, C. 1959. Sarcoidosis: A Functional Classification. *Med. Ann. D.C.* **28**: 129.
37. Young, R. C. Jr, Carr, C., Shelton, T. G., Mann, M., Ferrin, A., Laurey, J. R., and Harden, K. A. 1967. Sarcoidosis: Relationship Between Changes in Lung Structure and Function. Turiaf, J., and Chabot, J. La Sarcoidose. *Rapp. IV Conf. Int.* Paris: Masson et cie. p. 455.
38. Young, R. C. Jr, Johnson, M., Pennix, W. G., Barnes, B. B., and Harden, K. A. 1970. Further Studies of Respiratory Bellows Dynamics in Sarcoidosis. *JNMA* **62**: 441.
39. Macklem, P. T., and Mead, J. 1967. Resistance of Central and Peripheral Airways Measured by a Retrograde Catheter. *J. Appl. Physiol.* **22**: 395.
40. Anthonisen, N. R., Danson, J., Robertson, P. C., and Ross, W. R. D. 1969–1970. Airway Closure as a Function of Age. *Resp. Physiol.* **8**: 58.
41. Fagerhol, M. K., and Hauge, H. E. 1969. Serum Pi Types in Patients with Pulmonary Diseases. *Acta. Allerg.* **24**: 107.

DISCUSSION

Chairmen: K. VISKUM AND T. KOSUDA

DR VISKUM: The problem of the frequency of hypercalcemia would present a good topic for this part of the discussion. From Copenhangen we have 250 cases of proven sarcoidosis and among these we only had between 2 and 3% of patients with significant hypercalcemia. Here I have to disagree with Dr Israel. The cause of this low percentage is hardly an increase in the use of steroids, which were given to only 10–15% of the patients. Probably there is a variation from country to country in this frequency.

DR ISRAEL: What we are suggesting is that in the United States, the two-thirds of patients who don't need steroids, don't get steroids; they also never have hypercalcuria or hypercalcemia. It is the smaller group who require steroids for eye, skin, pulmonary lesions that represent the more serious forms of sarcoidosis, who probably have more osseous involvement even though it isn't demonstrated by ordinary roentgenograms. Also there is evidence that it is the patients with renal granulomas that have disturbed calcium metabolism. I think it is among the ill patients, that all of the calcium problems are concentrated: They are also the ones who get steroids.

DR MORII: Could I ask Dr Israel one thing? I have been thinking that it is generally accepted that the primary event as to calcium derangement in sarcoidosis is enhanced absorption of calcium from the intestine. What is the destination of calcium ingested in your cases?

DR ISRAEL: This is an inference and not an established fact, I admit it's the one that was held by most authorities, but I think it's inconsistent with the data we have collected. The balanced studies carried out by Hendrixs of Rockfeller University of New York, also failed to show increased absorption.

DR JAMES: Before stating dogmatically that abnormal calcium metabolism is frequent or infrequent it is first necessary to define the clinical material the investigator is studying. It is frequent at the onset of acute sarcoidosis but since it is transient and self-limiting it may disappear undiscovered. It tends to persist in a small group of patients with chronic fibrotic sarcoidosis. Its presence poses 2 queries. What is there about these patients and their type of disease which allows a continuation of abnormal calcium metabolism? Secondly, what is the mechanism of the disorder? At the stage of acute sarcoidosis, sarcoid granulomas are actively involving many tissues of the body. Could they be invading the thyroid and interfering in some way with calcitonin?

DR MITCHELL: I would just like to congratulate Dr Carlens on his magnificent presentation and to say that in a series of over 200 mediastinoscopies amongst patients with sarcoidosis, Dr Mikhail, Dr Drury and I have noted just the same histological features in several patients with a symptomatic onset of their sarcoidosis. In these, as Dr Carlens has stressed, eosinophilic necrosis of collagen can be quite extensive and is often difficult to differentiate from caseation. One further point: Sven Löfgren in his clinical essays mentions the occasional occurrence and persistence of 'nodal fever' among patients presenting with hilar lymphadenopathy, apart of course from the fever associated with Löfgren's syndrome itself.

DR REFVEM: I'm examining routinely the serum calcium of every sarcoid patient under my care, and it's my experience that if you don't find hypercalcemia on the first occasion, you will not find it later.

447

DR HANNGREN: If I had understand Dr Israel and Dr James right, we should stop examining the calcium in urine and in blood? When regarding the tremendous increase of costs in medical care today this will save at least some money.

DR ISRAEL: That is what we intend to convey. The ordinary asymptomatic patient with sarcoidosis or even the patient with chronic sarcoidosis who is not severely ill has neither hypercalciuria or hypercalcemia and does not require routine investigation of calcium metabolism. The patient who is ill with severe sarcoidosis is the subject who should be studied. I should like to emphasize that each of the 12 patients in our metabolic study had active sarcoidosis. These were not people with asymptomatic hilar adenopathy, but were moderately ill with various manifestations of sarcoidosis.

DR TEIRSTEIN: We have experienced 26 deaths due to sarcoidosis in our first 311 patients. Two of these deaths were due to hypercalcemia and associated renal failure. These two patients were symptomatic only when in the terminal stages of renal failure as a consequence of years of chronic hypercalcemia. Neither of these 2 patients had hilar lymph node enlargement or significant pulmonary insufficiency. They had no other symptoms of chronic sarcoidosis. In fact, there was nothing in their presenting clinical status that lead us to suspect hypercalcemia and it was detected only after a routine serum calcium determination. It is difficult to predict from the clinical presentation which patient will suffer from hypercalcemia. One patient was particularly sensitive to prednisone therapy. A decrease of only 5 mgm in the steroid dosage would result in a rise in her serum calcium and blood urea nitrogen. So I think that we are on somewhat dangerous ground if we stop performing routine serum calcium studies. With our present automated chemistry laboratories, it costs only a few pennies to add calcium to the other 18 or so routine tests done on a single blood specimen. Economies can be better made elsewhere.

DR JAMES: If you are discussing the economics and the cost of investigating patients with sarcoidosis, then it is more important to carry out serum calcium rather than serum globulin determinations. The former will provide guidelines for management whereas knowing the serum globulin levels is of no practical benefit to the patient.

DR KIRA: I have a question for Dr Miller. You presented results of lung function studies especially in patients who are in late stage and have diffuse fibrotic change within the lung, i.e., not in the granulomatous stage. I think the same type of functional disturbance may be expected also in pulmonary fibrosis due to any other, know or unknown, causes. How about pulmonary blood gas exchange?

DR MILLER: Our study did not concern itself with blood gas changes. These patients presented were ambulatory and not terribly sick at the time of study. They do not have CO_2 retention.

We certainly see cor pulmonale at a late stage of fibrotic pulmonary sarcoidosis, and this is a main cause of death. As is the doctor from Tokyo University, we are also asking the question whether the changes in airway function in late pulmonary sarcoidosis are the result of fibrosis or whether they are more specifically a result of granulomatous disease. We are studying other patients with other kinds of diffuse fibrotic disease, as well as patients in other stages of sarcoidosis.

DR KIRA: How about the incidence of cor pulmonale in those patients?

DR MILLER: Dr Teirstein from our institution could comment on his data on mortality.

DR TEIRSTEIN: We recorded 24 deaths in our first 311 patients with sarcoidosis. Sarcoidosis, or its complications, was the cause of death in 19 of the 26 patients. Of the 19 deaths due to sarcoidosis, 13 were due to cardiorespiratory failure. There was clinical, pathologic, and/or electrocardiographic evidence of "cor pulmonale" in the majority of these patients whose lungs were scarred by chronic sarcoidosis. Thus, "cor pulmonale" was the most important clinical cardiac abnormality. However, Dr Miller's data indicate that many patients with sarcoidosis have subclinical cardiac involvement with granulomatous disease as manifested by abnormalities seen on the routine electrocardiogram. This cardiac involvement is, of course, not "cor pulmonale".

Dr Kira: One more question to Dr Young. You divided the patients into 2 groups, active and inactive. In the active group, they showed disseminated parenchymal changes throughout the lung and increase of antitrypsin level. The bilateral lymphoadenopathy and minimal pulmonary lesions are also active. Do such patients also show any disturbance in antitrypsin?

Dr Young: Inactivity in sarcoidosis does not mean that no physiologic changes exist in the organ system involved. In fact, physiologic changes of a mechanical nature often occur as a result of morphological damage. We feel that activity is better related to the constitutional symptoms, headache, weight loss, anorexia, dizzyness and fever. We have found these constitutional symptoms very common amongst active sarcoidosis patients, perhaps more common than among the population as a whole. Activity is also indicated by some of the chemical changes in the blood such as hypercalcemia, hyperglobulinemia, elevated alkaline phosphatase, elevated erythrocyte sedimentation rate, and hypercalciuria and elevated hydroxyproline excretion. Elevation in α_1-antitrypsin in the active phase most likely is related to the slight increases in α_1-globulin.

Dr Israel: I would like to ask Dr Teirstein when the deaths occurred from renal damage from hypercalcemia, because our autopsy experience has been, that renal damage is less frequent and important in the last 10 or 15 years.

Dr Viskum: Our last death occurred about 18 months ago. This was a relatively young girl of about 32 who had had hypercalcemia and azotemia for at least 10 years. The participating cause of death was an acute gastroenteritis with fever and her renal function just could not take all of this fluid

loss, but I think it is fair to say that she died from sarcoidosis of her kidneys associated with hypercalcemia throughout the course of the disease.

Dr Refvem: One late evening, I had a telephone call from the State Hospital in Oslo, where they were just operating on a case of hypercalcemia thought to be primary hyperparathyroidism. The Cortisone administered beforehand for 10 days made the calcium values fall slightly from about 16 mg% to about 14. There had been no manifestations of sarcoidosis. But during the operation they had just removed a lymph node which showed sarcoidosis on freeze-section. Were they ought to consider this case of hypercalcemia as being caused only by sarcoidosis, or ought they to go on trying to find hyperplastic parathyroid? I instructed them to just go on searching for hyperplastic parathyroid.

Dr Kosuda: Dr Carlens, you have pointed out the possibility of the presence of rather predominant necrosis in the sarcoid granuloma. You have also said such a necrosis is sometimes difficult to differentiate from tuberculous necrosis.

Now, I wish to ask the opinion, of Dr Iwai. He is a pathologist of the Japan Sarcoidosis Committee. Have you any comment about the difference between the necrosis of sarcoidosis and that of tuberculosis?

Dr Iwai: I am impressed with Dr Carlens' slide, showing the silver stain of the sarcoid granuloma which reveals necrosis. The reticulin fiber remaining in the necrotic area seems to show a swelling, to be somewhat fragmented and of an ill-defined nature, so it looks to me as if this silver stain shows an early stage of swelling or melting of the reticulin fiber, and I think that sarcoidosis is distinguishable from tuberculosis, when the reticulin fiber remains intact. Such differentiation of necrosis of sarcoid granulomas from tuberculous ones is important but not 100% dependable.

Dr Carlens: I agree with what you have said. I would only like to stress that without the silver staining method, at least in these 15 cases, it may be very difficult to distinguish between sarcoidosis and tuberculosis. I have heard that sometimes even with silver staining there may be some difficulty. These 15 cases were the only ones who presented some difficulties. In all the other ones, almost 400, there were no difficulties at all, even without the silver staining method.

DR JONES WHILLIAMS: Our fine structure studies of the small areas of 'necrosis' in sarcoid granulomas have shown a mixture of fine fibrils—reticulin—and thicker fibers with and without 650 Å banding, considered to be collagen. The difficulty arises that in healing, fibrosing tuberculous caseation you also get similar appearances. I think that silver staining is helpful but not diagnostic. It is worth noting that tuberculous but not sarcoid necrosis is often finely granular.

IX PROGNOSIS

Sarcoidosis with Accurately Dated Onset
—A study of 100 patients with initial erythema nodosum—

A. S. Teirstein and L. E. Siltzbach

Division of Thoracic Diseases, Department of Medicine, The Mount Sinai School of Medicine, New York, U.S.A.

You are all familiar with chest radiographs demonstrating the most typical intra-thoracic roentgen pattern seen in sarcoidosis, bilateral hilar and right paratracheal lymph node enlargement—radiologic stage I sarcoidosis. If one would predict the duration of the disease after viewing this radiograph, acute sarcoidosis would be favored. And in 4 out of 5 instances this forecast would be correct.[1]

However, radiographs of the some patients in the chronic phase of sarcoidosis, demonstrate the same stage I radiographic pattern. Thus, the finding of hilar adenopathy does not, in a minority of patients, support the supposition that the disease had a recent onset.

One of the major problems in assessing the duration of sarcoidosis is the difficulty of accurately dating its inception. In the main, the clinical presentation of sarcoidosis is marked by its insidious onset. Indeed, it is probable that most patients endure the entire course of sarcoidosis without ever experiencing symptoms severe enough to spur them to seek medical care. When the disease does come to the attention of the patient and his physician, in 40% the first evidence is the finding of an abnormal chest radiograph in an individual totally without symptoms.

An accurate marker of the onset of sarcoidosis is required by the physician who finds himself presented with a bewildering array of varying patterns of distribution and activity of lesions, so that he may properly estimate the true duration and prognosis of the disease. Such a marker is available in studies of patients who had normal chest radiographs within 1 year of the clinical presentation of the disease. Similarly, erythema nodosum is universally regarded as a reliable indicator of the beginning of sarcoidosis and most observers believe that the subsequent course in this unique group of patients differs little from that of patients without erythema nodosum in whom the onset can be accurately dated radiologically.[2, 3]

In the present study we have observed the clinical course of 101 patients, at the sarcoidosis clinic, Mount Sinai Hospital, New York, with biopsy-proven sarcoidosis initiated by an attack of erythema nodosum.

Table 1 shows the ethnic and sex distribution of the 101 patients. You will note that almost half of our patients are Puerto Rican-born and that all but 5 of this ethnic group are females. This preponderance of Puerto Rican-born females closely resembles the high incidence of sarcoidosis with erythema nodosum previously reported among young Swedish and Irish women.[4, 5] Approximately one-third of our patients are Caucasians and less than one-fifth are Negroes. However, quite contrary to reports from other centers where erythema nodosum is rarely encountered among Negroes, in this study 18%

This work was supported by USPHS grant, HL–1383, and by Louis & Sadie Elow Foundation.

TABLE 1.   101 Patients with sorcoidosis and erythema nodosum
Mount Sinai Hospital, New York.

	Female	Male	Total
Puerto Rican-born	42	5	47
Caucasian	21	13	34
Negro	15	3	18
Oriental	1	1	2
Total	79	22	101

TABLE 2.   Radiographic presentation: 101 patients
with erythema nodosum.

Stage I. (hilar nodes)	79
Stage II. (hilar nodes plus mottling)	12
Stage III. (mottling alone)	4
Normal	6

began their sarcoidosis in this fashion. Parenthetically, the rarity of erythema nodosum among Japanese patients with sarcoidosis is striking and unexplained.[6]

In Table 2, we show the radiographic stage of the presenting chest X-ray. As you see, four-fifths of all patients with sarcoidosis and erythema nodosum presented with bilateral hilar and right paratracheal lymph node enlargement, stage I. Only 5 of these 79 patients were noted later to progress to radiologically demonstrable lung granulomas, stage II. Twelve of the 101 patients with a history of erythema nodosum-exhibited radiographic stage II sarcoidosis when first seen by us. Of these 12, 7 either had overt erythema nodosum at the time that this chest X-ray already showed lung involvement, or the erythema nodosum had been present within 3 months of the radiograph demonstrating stage II disease. In the other 5 of the 12 patients with stage II X-rays, the eruption had subsided from 6 months to 7 years prior to the performance of the chest radiograph. Were we now to add all the patients who demonstrated stage II radiographs together, we find that 17 of the 101 patients who had erythema nodosum progressed to radiographic stage II patterns at some time in the course of their disease.

Four other patients had diffuse pulmonary disease, *without* evident hilar adenopathy, radiograph stage III, at the time of presentation to our clinic. But in 3 of these, the history of erythema nodosum went back 3, 4 and 19 years, respectively. In a single patient, erythema nodosum had been present only 1 month prior to the chest radiograph demonstrating stage III disease.

We have come to recognize that radiologic stage III sarcoidosis, i.e., pulmonary densities without hilar adenopathy, may be present in at least 2 patterns. The first, and by far the most common, is the presence of diffuse scarring with microcystic and bullous transformation, while a second, considerably rarer, pattern consists of diffuse small and larger areas of mottling occasionally mimicking bronchopneumonia or metastatic infiltrations in the patient's X-ray.

Six patients had normal chest radiographs at presentation. Four of the 6 had their erythema nodosum within 7 weeks of the normal X-ray. Two had a history of erythema nodosum 3 and 15 years prior to the normal radiograph. None of these 6 ever developed radiologic abnormalities during the follow-up period.

We can now return to the use of erythema nodosum as a marker of the onset of sarcoidosis. Sixty-six of the 76 patients who had subacute disease (less than 2 years duration), presented with bilateral hilar adenopathy or normal chest X-rays, emphasizing the generally accepted correlation between subacute sarcoidosis and radiographic stage I disease. However, 15 of the 25 patients with chronic sarcoidosis (more than 2 years duration) had persistent hilar node enlargement.

More than half of the 101 patients complained of arthralgias or arthritis. With 1 exception, these joint symptoms involved the ankles and accompanied the erythema nodosum, usually subsiding when the eruption abated, occasionally lingering for several months. In the 1 exceptional patient, chronic arthritis evolved later in his course, did not accompany the erythema nodosum, involved the ankles, knees and wrists and smoldered for more than 3 years. We will not at this time consider insidiously occurring sarcoid arthritis, which is a subject unto itself.

Twenty-one patients at some time in their course exhibited ocular, salivary gland, lymph node and cutaneous sarcoids. As expected, these extrathoracic manifestations occurred almost twice as often in the chronic than they did in the subacute phase. Noteworthy is the fact that cutaneous sarcoids occurred only in chronic sarcoidosis. It is an interesting paradox, that just as the nonspecific cutaneous manifestation of erythema nodosum is a reliable indicator of acute sarcoidosis, granulomatous sarcoids of the skin are invariably an indicator of chronic sarcoidosis.

CONCLUSIONS

Erythema nodosum is an accurate marker of the onset of sarcoidosis, especially in certain population groups. It can be utilized as a reliable indicator to predict the course and prognosis of sarcoidosis in general.

Our data confirm that most patients with sarcoidosis manifest hilar lymphadenopathy without pulmonary densities (radiographic stage I) at the onset of their disease. However, almost one-fifth of these patients will show persistence of the enlarged hilar lymph nodes even into the chronic phase. Thus a stage I radiographic pattern is not always a certain indicator of subacute sarcoidosis. Almost all patients with pulmonary infiltrations of some duration, without demonstrable hilar adenopathy (radiographic stage III) are in the chronic phase of their illness. However, a rare patient may show a pattern of diffuse mottling caused by fresh granulomatous deposits in the lungs which is compatible with sarcoidosis of short duration.

REFERENCES

1. Siltzbach, L. E. 1955. *Amer. J. Surgery* **89**: 556.
2. Stavenow, S. 1964. *Acta Med. Scand.* Suppl. **425**: 176, 289.
3. Mandi, L. 1964. *Acta Med. Scand.* Suppl. **425**: 176, 287.
4. Lofgren, S. 1953. *Acta Med. Scand.* **145**: 465.
5. James, D. G. 1961. *Brit. Med. J.* **1**: 853.
6. Nobechi, K. 1964. *Acta Med. Scand.* Suppl. **425**: 176, 165.

General Prognosis on Mediastino-Pulmonary Sarcoidosis at Stage II

J. Turiaf, J. P. Battesti, R. Georges and G. Saumon

Bichat Hospital, University of Paris, Paris, France

At stage II, pulmonary sarcoidosis is anatomically represented by diffuse interstitial granulomatous infiltration without parenchymal fibrosis. At this stage, recovery from pulmonary involvement may be recognized by 2 means:
1) Complete and definitive fading of chest X-ray pathological pictures.
2) Disappearance of functional respiratory disorders

Treatment, when applied, starts 1 to 3 months after illness recognition. It consists in all cases in giving cortisone uninterruptedly for about 2 years, the initial daily dose equivalent to 40 mg of Prednisone. It is later progressively and slowly reduced, and suppressed consecutively with the fading of X-ray pathological pictures, surveyed every 3 months, and with progressive restoration of respiratory function parameters, surveyed every 6 months (Table 1).

All cases shown in this paper were X-rayed every 3 months and subjected to respiratory function investigation for about 5 years, i.e., for some patients, during at least 3 years after the end of the treatment, when recovery took place, and for others, during 5 years or more, sometimes because of relapses or because of resistance of pulmonary lesions to therapy.

Radiological prognosis (Table 2)

We gathered 72 cases in order to isolate data for the first part of this paper.

Results recorded in this series of 72 cases of stage II sarcoidosis confirm those shown in previous publications.[1]

TABLE 1. Protocol of corticosteroid treatment.

Prednisone		
	40 mg	3 months
	30 mg	3 months
	20 mg	3 to 6 months
	15 mg	3 to 6 months
	10 mg	3 to 6 months
	5 mg	6 months

Average duration: 2 years

TABLE 2. Mediastino-Pulmonary sarcoidosis stage II—72 cases.

Evolution according to X-ray pictures

Spontaneous recovery	13 cases	18%	67%
Recovery after corticosteroids	35 cases	49%	
Partial resistance to treatment	8 cases	11%	33%
Relapse after 2 years treatment	16 cases	22%	

SPONTANEOUS RECOVERY

Recovery occurred spontaneously in 13 cases, that is 18%. This happened in cases characterized by micronodular or reticulonodular pictures, without associated mediastinal adenopathies. Delay was always less than 6 months. Pictures of large infiltrated areas never underwent spontaneous resolution.

RECOVERY WITH CORTICOSTEROIDS

Definitive fading of pathological X-ray pictures was obtained by corticosteroids in 35 cases (49%). All radiological evidence (nodular and reticulonodular pictures, large infiltrated areas of various size and opacity, with or without mediastinal adenopathies) very rapidly shows, simultaneously with lymphomediastinal intumescence, the resolving influence of cortisone.

Pictures recalling miliary and reticulomicronodular aspect, as well as a cloudy and slightly dense infiltration, show a greater rendency to fade under corticosteroid action. In about half the cases, the thoracic picture becomes normal after 6 or 9 months treatment. In the other half, complete eradication of pathological pictures is reached at the end of the first year of treatment, or between the twelfth and fifteenth month. Experience taught us that in sarcoidosis, premature interruption of treatment in the first month following disappearance of X-ray pictures leads to very rapid and frequent relapses. This is why we have established the treatment, proposed nearly 15 years ago, which is shown at the beginning of this paper.

This treatment, lasting 2 years, proposes that for safety while the thoracic picture clears, the patient will receive for another 9 to 12 months a daily dose equivalent to 15 mg of Prednisone, which will be reduced as the months go by, and finally suppressed.

PULMONARY SARCOIDOSIS RESISTANT TO CORTICOSTEROIDS

Corticosteroids are never totally inefficient on pulmonary alterations of stage II. But in a small number of cases there is a phenomenon representing a kind of relative resistance to cortisonic drugs. It acts in the following manner: treatment applied according to above rules starts by being very effective. Complete eradication of radiological pictures occurs, in the usual lapse of time, but toward the eighteenth to twentieth month of treatment, when the daily dose is about 7.5 to 5 mg of Prednisone, the thoracic picture becomes abnormal again. Pulmonary parenchyma takes a diffuse and generalized reticulonodular aspect, discrete at first, but which reveals renewed activity of sarcoidosis, while treatment has not yet stopped. Then it becomes impossible to reduce the dose of corticosteroids, or even to maintain it, without risking reappearance of previous images. It must be substantially but temporarily increased, to induce fading of the newly appeared pictures, which regularly happens in 4 to 6 weeks. The daily dose is then progressively decreased, under frequent X-ray controls, and a daily maintainance dose is fixed, preventing the reappearance of pathological pictures. In spite of the low corticosteroid dose which controls pulmonary lesions, this kind of sarcoidosis is more severe than the previous ones, because it needs a treatment that cannot be interrupted. It should be installed for life, because of the long-term threat of an eventual transformation of granulomatous lesions into pulmonary fibrosis. We proposed to call this clinical form " partly corticoresistant pulmonary sarcoidosis ". Eight of our cases, or 11%, belong to this category of pulmonary sarcoidosis. Nevertheless, in 1 case, we succeeded in suppressing treatment definitively, after 15 years, 11 of which were at a dose of 4 mg of Triamcinolone. This fact indicates the curability of this clinical form, even after a long time. Among the 8 cases composing this small group, 5 were patients lately treated or subjected to a prematurely interrupted corticosteroid cure, and having had 1 or more severe relapses. The 3 others were half-breeds from the French West Indies, who in spite of an early and correctly applied treatment, progressed towards this type of pulmonary sarcoidosis. The influence of a racial factor in this group of patients perhaps intervenes in their resistance to corticosteroids, as it frequently increases the severeness of the general prognosis.[3]

RELAPSES OF PULMONARY SARCOIDOSIS AFTER CORTICOSTEROID TREATMENT

Mediastino-pulmonary sarcoidosis, healing spontaneously, an eventuality noted in our statistics in 70% of cases at stage I and 18% of cases at stage II, recurs exceptionally. When the disease shows new activity, after a variable time of apparent healing, pulmonary involvement having receded without therapeutic intervention, sarcoidosis manifests itself usually elsewhere than in the mediastino-pulmonary regions. This does not occur when pulmonary lesions, with radiological evidence, fade under the effect of corticosteroids. One knows that at stage II, radiologically indicated relapses happen for less than 6 months.[4] We have recorded among our 47 treated cases, 16 cases of relapse (22%). In 14 cases relapse started as soon the third month after interruption of treatment. In another case, it happened a year later, and in another, at the beginning of the third year after suppression of corticosteroids. Evidence of relapse is usually shown by a bilateral and diffuse, reticular or reticulonodular image. Sometimes, but less frequently (3 cases), there is also reappearance of nodular mediastinal intumescence. Relapses must be submitted to the same treatment as previously untreated sarcoidosis. But if the picture is identified early, while it is still at its initial reticular phase, without nodules, one can start treatment by a daily dose of 30 or even 25 mg of Prednisone, instead of 40 mg. Reduction or suppression of the dose must obey the same rules as a first treatment. The majority of our cases, did not relapse at the end of the second treatment, but in 1 case there were 2 relapses and in 3 others there were 3 relapses.

To sum up, pulmonary or mediastino-pulmonary stage II sarcoidosis heals in 67% of cases without relapse or radiological sequelae, but in 33% of our patients, pulmonary disease treatment and consequently its prognosis set problems hard to solve. The difficulties come from either a partial corticoresistance of pulmonary changes requiring a lifetime prescription of corticosteroids in 11% of our cases, or they come from a tendency to relapse which occurs in 22% of our cases in spite of a lengthy corticotherapy.

FUNCTIONAL PROGNOSIS

Functional respiratory investigation is an indispensable part in the whole range of examinations to judge evolution, and to fix a prognosis on the pulmonary localization of sarcoidosis. Functional data cannot be guessed from radiological readings: about 50% of cases of stage II pulmonary sarcoidosis are free from respiratory disorders, while in cases showing mild X-ray evidence, various functional parameters appear sometimes substantially altered.[5] Respiratory function tests in cases of sarcoidosis must be done as exhaustively as possible so that the principal components might be measured: particularly pulmonary volumes, respiratory mechanics, CO transfer, which at stage II are more frequently affected. We selected 42 suitable patients.

Cases having a normal respiratory function

Among these 42 cases, 17 had an absolutely normal functional respiratory investigation all along evolution. In all those patients, chest X-ray showed variable pulmonary changes (Table 3).

TABLE 3. Pulmonary sarcoidosis—Stage II.

Normal functional respiratory investigation 17 cases	
Spontaneous fading of pathological pictures	4 cases
Fading of pathological pictures with corticosteroids	8 cases
Corticosteroid treatment maintained for a life time to ensure fading of pathological pictures	5 cases

In 4 cases pathological pictures disappeared spontaneously and in 8 cases they progressed towards definitive resolution under corticotherapy; finally in 5 cases they belong to a kind of sarcoidosis that we label partly corticoresistant sarcoidosis. These clinical forms need a permanent and uninterrupted low dose of cortisone to control their activity and to prevent reappearance of radiological signs.

Cases with functional alterations

In 25 other patients, significant perturbation of various parameters of functional respiratory investigation (FRI) were clearly expressed, but diversely associated: the most frequent were volume restriction, decreased compliance, reduction of CO transfer, and more rarely inhomogeneity of air and blood distribution.

TABLE 4. Pulmonary sarcoidosis—Stage II.

Functional respiratory investigation, initially pathological		
Restoration of FRI and spontaneous disappearance of pulmonary opacities	1 case	
Restoration of FRI and disappearance of pulmonary opacities with corticosteroids	12 cases	13 cases
Persistence of FRI disorders in spite of spontaneous disappearance of pulmonary opacities	1 case	
Persistence of FRI disorders in spite of disappearance of pulmonary opacities with corticosteroids	11 cases	12 cases

Among these 25 cases, restoration of FRI happened in 13 cases, together with disappearance of chest X-ray abnormalities, spontaneously in 1 case and with corticosteroids in 12 cases. In 12 other cases functional disorders remained, in spite of the disappearance of pulmonary X-ray changes, spontaneously in 1 case, despite corticosteroids for many years in 11 cases.

J. TURIAF ET AL.

TABLE 5. Pulmonary sarcoidosis—Stage II.

Persistence of disorders in respiratory function 12 cases	
Restrictive syndrome	7 cases
Respiratory mechanics alteration	5 cases
Reduction of Co transfer	4 cases
Obstructive syndrome	2 cases
Distribution disturbance	1 case

There was a restrictive syndrome in 7 cases (Table 5), respiratory mechanics alteration in 5 cases, reduction of CO transfer in 4 cases, an obstructive syndrome in 2 cases and distribution disturbances in 1 case.

This short analysis of a homogenous series of cases of pulmonary sarcoidosis carefully recorded many times during at least 5 years, shows that disorders identified by FRI, if less frequent than radiological evidence of granulomatosis without fibrosis at stage II (25 cases out of 42) have a lesser tendency towards spontaneous resolution, but a similar sensitivity to corticosteroids. Actually, we have noted in this series of 42 patients that total and definitive disappearance of pulmonary opacities took place spontaneously in 6 cases, and in 20 cases through corticosteroid treatment, i.e., in 26 cases out of 42 (62%). We noted as well that reestablishment of respiratory function in the 25 cases with functional abnormalities, happened once spontaneously, and 12 times with corticosteroid treatment, i.e., 13 times out of 25 (52%). It should be emphasized that the disappearance of X-ray abnormalities, either spontaneous or maintained under corticotherapy, is compatible with the presence of significant functional disorders. This was so in 12 cases out of 25, i.e., 48%, which at the first examination showed alteration of 1 or more parameters of respiratory function. In these cases prognosis for respiratory function is severe on a more-or-less long-term basis. Patients must be frequently controlled to obtain, by a well-adapted corticosteroid treatment, the restoration of respiratory function, or to prevent its progressive degradation.

Extrathoracic lesions of sarcoidosis progress in most cases completely independently of pulmonary localizations. They do not interfere in their prognosis.

SUMMARY

At stage II, radiological records are insufficient for pulmonary sarcoidosis prognosis. Chest X-ray abnormalities disappear sometimes spontaneously or after corticotherapy in 67% of cases. To keep the chest X-ray integrity, 33% of cases require uninterrupted treatment with small doses of corticosteroids.

On the other hand, spontaneous or therapeutic improvement of respiratory function happened only in 52% of cases (13/25). Persistence in 48% of cases (12/25) contrasts with the absence of pathological chest X-ray pictures. Functional abnormalities remained in cases of partly corticoresistant sarcoidosis. Late application of corticotherapy and its premature interruption, bringing relapses, and probably also a racial factor (West Indian half-breed), contribute to the severeness of the prognosis in pulmonary alterations in stage II sarcoidosis.

REFERENCES

1. Basset, G., Georges, R., and Turiaf, J. 1967. Intéret de l'étude de la fonction respiratoire dans la sarcoidose pulmonaire. *Poumon et Coeur* **23**: 569.
2. Scadding, J. G. 1967. Sarcoidosis. London: Eyre and Spottiswoode. Vol. 1.
3. James, D. G., Siltzbach, L. E., Sharma, O. P., and Carstairs, L. S. 1969. A tale of two cities. A comparison of sarcoidosis in London and New York. *Arch. Internal Med.* **123**: p. 187.
4. Turiaf, J., Battesti, J. P., Basset, G., and Georges, R. 1971. La sarcoidose médiastino-pulmonaire imparfaitement résolutive par la cortisonothérapie. *Rapp. Ve Conf. Int. sur la Sarcoïdose.* Prague: Univ. Karlova. Vol. 1. p. 629.
5. Turiaf, J., and Battesti, J. P. 1971. La sarcoïdose d'apres l'étude de 350 cas inventoriés depuis 15 ans dans un service de Pneumologie. *Rev. Tuberc.* (Paris) **35**: 569.

Fatal Sarcoidosis

Walter J. Stork, S. Donald Greenberg and Carlos W. M. Bedrossian

*Departments of Radiology and Pathology, Baylor College of Medicine,
Jefferson Davis Hospital, Houston, Texas, U.S.A.*

INTRODUCTION

Sarcoidosis still puzzles the clinician, radiologist and pathologist. Although posing no major immediate hazard to the patient's health, this disease can mimic malignancy, tuberculosis, and mycosis. Many clinical reviews of sarcoidosis are available,[1-3] but studies correlating the radiological and pathological findings in fatal cases are relatively few.[4]

Over a period of 10 years we had the opportunity of seeing 186 cases of sarcoidosis. Of these patients, 14 died, and 6 came to autopsy. The purpose of this report is to review our experience in dealing with these patients. Emphasis will be placed on the radiologic and pathologic data of the fatal cases.

MATERIALS AND METHODS

Of the total of 186 cases of sarcoidosis seen at Jefferson Davis Hospital since 1960, 82 had a tissue diagnosis of sarcoidosis, and 104 were diagnosed on a clinical and radiologic basis. Fourteen of these cases, with an average age of 45.5 years, were fatal, and 6 of these had autopsies. Young blacks between 19 and 40 years of age were most severely affected by the disease. The female to male ratio was 134: 52 (approximately 5: 2). The youngest patient was 11 years of age; the oldest was 76, with a mean age of 36.4 years. There were only 3 Caucasians in the total series.

Chest roentgenograms on the 14 fatal cases were reviewed. Six of these cases had autopsy material for evaluation. Also, biopsies of the remaining fatal cases which did not come to autopsy were reviewed in order to assess the body involvement by sarcoid granulomata. Clinical data were extensive, but only selected aspects will be included in this report. Two case histories are given, showing a fairly typical course of the disease through fatal termination following cardiac involvement.

Case B.L. (Fig. 1)

A 29-year-old black female, first seen at the age of 19, with uveo-parotid fever. Biopsies of the parotid gland, bronchial mucosa and skin, all showed noncaseating granulomata. Pulmonary function studies revealed a ventilatory defect with mild obstructive airway component. Incision, drainage, and curettage of a lytic lesion in the right calcaneous was performed. Liver and bone biopsies were done, and a diagnosis of disseminated cryptococcus was established from cultures of urine, gastric contents, and bone fragments.

This patient was admitted 8 times in 10 years. A clinical diagnosis of cor pulmonale was made. Therapy was instituted, but the patient continued to complain of dyspnea on

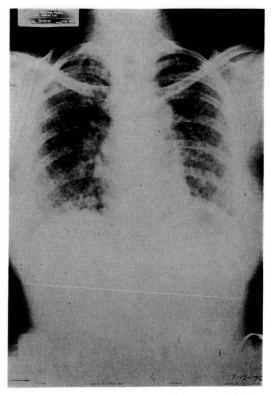

FIG. 1.   Case B. L. Combined diffuse pulmonary disease and lymph node involvement.
There has been some regression of the hilar adenitis while the parenchymal fibrosis progressed, in this fatal case.

exertion and right upper quadrant pain. Eighteen days after her last admission she
developed fever up to 103°F, and expired of a cardiac arrest.

Postmortem examination revealed sarcoidosis involving lungs, heart, liver, spleen,
kidneys, and mediastinal and periportal lymph nodes; diffuse fibrosis and apical fibrotic
adhesions of the lungs; hypertrophy and dilatation of the right heart ventricle (history
of cor pulmonale); atrophy of the adrenals, slight; bronchopneumonia, confluent, left
lower lobe; and thrombosis of the common carotid arteries.

Case J.M. (Fig. 2)

A 27-year-old black male admitted in March, 1969, with incapacitating dyspnea on
exertion. He had intermittent asthma and episodic production of white to yellow sputum.
No palpable adenopathy or hepatosplenomegaly was noted. Roentgenographic examination showed diffuse fibrotic changes with soft nodular densities throughout the lung
fields. Two sputum cultures were positive for *Mycobacterium tuberculosis*, and the patient
was started on antituberculosis therapy. His obstructive disease was treated with intermittent positive-pressure breathing and bronchodilators, with some response.

In February, and December, 1971, and in February, 1972, sputa cultures were negative for tuberculosis but became positive for Aspergillus. Aspergillus skin tests were
negative, and a precipitin Aspergillus test was nonreactive. The patient refused mediastinoscopy and open-lung biopsy. He developed an acute respiratory infection and was

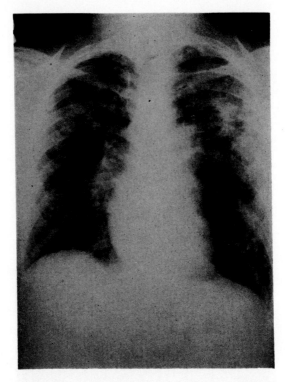

FIG. 2. Case J. M. Lymph node enlargement with some clearing and eventual extensive pulmonary fibrosis in this fatal case.

noted to have ventricular tachycardia. He developed severe respiratory failure. He initially responded to treatment, with some improvement, but expired of cardiac arrest 8 days after his final admission.

Postmortem examination (limited to heart and lungs) showed extensive noncaseous granulomatous disease, consistent with sarcoidosis, involving the lungs, hilar lymph nodes and heart (myocardium of left ventricle).

RESULTS

All 186 cases presented with thoracic involvement as seen by chest roentgenograms. Fifty cases had hilar lymphadenopathy; 115 had pulmonary changes plus hilar lymphadenopathy; and 21 cases showed lung involvement without hilar lymph node enlargement. Of these, 82 had proven diagnosis by tissue biopsy. Thirty had tissue biopsy from the thorax, and 52 from extrathoracic sites.

Table 1 summarizes important concurrent diseases and complications in 60 cases. In the remaining 126 cases, sarcoidosis was uncomplicated. Of the total, 14 cases were fatal. The average duration of the illness was 5.41 years in the fatal cases. The shortest duration was 6 months in a 44-year-old black female; the longest duration was 24 years in a 50-year-old black female who had therapeutic pneumoperitoneum. Pertinent clinical, radiologic, and anatomical findings are summarized in Tables 1, 2, 3 and 4.

TABLE 1. Important concurrent diseases and
complications in 60 cases.

Disease	No. cases
Tuberculosis	14
Congestive heart failure	10
Cor pulmonale	6
Acute and chronic bronchitis	4
Osteomyelitis	3
Epididymitis	2
Silicosis	2
Histoplasmosis	2
Severe dermatitis	2
Diabetes	2
Spontaneous pneumothorax	2
Parotid gland involvement	2
Pneumoperitoneum	1
Bronchiectasis	1
Cryptococcus	1
Coccidioides	1
Optic neuritis	1
Atrial defect in offspring	1
Colon lesion	1
Adenocarcinoma	1
Severe uveitis and blepharitis	1

Roentgenographic Findings in 14 Fatal Cases

On roentgenographic examination, 12 of the fatal cases initially showed a predominantly reticulofibronodular pattern in the lung parenchyma bilaterally, which progressed.
Two cases initially had bilateral massive hilar and paratracheal adenitis which later
changed to a reticulofibronodular terminal pattern in the lungs. As the fibrosis in the
lung parenchyma progressed, the adenitis receded. This was typical in all of our cases.
Kerley lines were noted in the cardiac cases, but were frequently vaguely defined, because of predominant fibrosis of the lungs. In 1 case a pneumonic-type infiltrate which
faded was seen initially in the left upper lobe of the lungs.

Pathologic Findings in 14 Fatal Cases

Histological examination was available in 14 cases of fatal sarcoidosis. In 3 of these,
the diagnosis was made at autopsy, and in the remaining 11, biopsies were performed of
the following sites: skin—1 case; parotid—1 case; mediastinal lymph nodes—1 case;
lungs—2 cases; scalene lymph nodes—4 cases. The typical lesion consisted of multiple
discrete noncaseating granulomata composed of epithelioid cells, and a scattering of
lymphocytes. There was no central necrosis and no specific etiologic agents were identified, either by acid-fast or fungal stains. When affecting the lungs, sarcoid granulomata
were found not only in the submucosa of the large bronchi, but peripherally around
bronchioles or within alveolar septae (Fig. 3). Diffuse pulmonary fibrosis was invariably
present in the late stage of lung involvement. Myocardial involvement was evidenced by

TABLE 2.

Case	Clinical findings
LB/29/F	Dyspnea; skin rash; uveo-parotid fever; aspergillus-positive sputa culture; AFB sputa negative
PG/52/F	Dyspnea; pedal edema; cough; clubbing of fingers; AFB sputa negative
GS/73/M	Dyspnea; dysuria; cough; AFB sputa negative
KR/43/F	Dyspnea; skin lesions; fever; AFB sputa negative
KB/44/F	Dyspnea; cough; acute hemoptysis; AFB sputa negative
DS/60/F	Dyspnea; cough; weight loss; AFB sputa positive
CJ/32/F	Dyspnes; cough; weight loss; AFB negative
GP/28/F	Dyspnea; cough; weight loss; AFB sputa negative
AM/68/F	Cough; hemoptysis; dyspnea; weight loss; irregular pulse; deafness; TB in past; AFB sputa positive
GA/56/F	Dyspnea; skin rash; cough; AFB sputa negative
BC/49/M	Dyspnea; cough; skin rash; AFB sputa negative
SM/52/F	Dyspnea; cough; hemoptysis; AFB sputa positive
MJ/30/M	Dyspnea; cough; tachycardia; pedal edema; AFB negative
HE/40/F	Dyspnea; hemoptysis; parotid swelling; hepatomegaly; AFB sputa negative
LB/29/F	Predominantly pulmonary fibrosis; cardiomegaly; cor pulmonale
PG/52/F	Progressive pulmonary and fibrocystic pattern; cor pulmonale
GS/73/M	Pulmonary fibronodular infiltrate; progressive LUL infiltrate; primary adenocarcinoma
KR/43/F	Initially hilar adenitis; later predominantly pulmonary fibrosis
KB/44/F	Progressive pulmonary fibrosis; hilar adenitis, acute
DS/60/F	Predominantly pulmonary fibrosis, bilateral; cardiomegaly
CJ/32/F	Cor pulmonale; cardiomegaly; pulmonary fibrosis; confluent bilateral infiltrate never resolved
GP/28/F	Extensive pulmonary fibrosis simulating Hamman-Rich syndrome; cor pulmonale
AM/68/F	Large apical bullae; LUL infiltrate simulating cavitary tuberculosis; extensive pulmonary fibrosis; spontaneous pneumothorax
GA/56/F	Cor pulmonale; predominantly bilateral fibrocystic infiltrate of lungs; large bilateral bullae
BC/49/M	Extensive pulmonary fibrosis, bilateral; hilar adenitis
SM/52/F	Initially pulmonary fibrois, progressive; high left diaphragm
MJ/30/M	Progressive pulmonary reticulofibronodular pattern; cor pulmonale
HE/40/F	Initially hilar adenitis only; later predominantly pulmonary fibrosis

the findings of noncaseating granulomata interspersed amidst cardiac muscle fibers (Fig. 4).

DISCUSSION

The causative agent of sarcoidosis remains unknown (5). On the basis of the distribution of sarcoid granulomata in the body, it is tempting to assume that a causative agent enters through the lungs, whence it may disseminate to virtually any organ or tissue (Fig. 5). We agree with the hypothesis that both an infectious agent and altered immunity must be present to explain the pathogenesis of sarcoidosis. Clay eating, chewing tobacco, and the cultivation of peanuts have been proposed as possibly related to development of sarcoidosis in the past.[6] Also, the pollen of pine trees has been implicated in the etiology

TABLE 3.

Case	Anatomical findings
*LB/29/F	Sarcoidosis proven by biopsy involving parotids, eyes, lymph nodes, lungs, heart, liver, spleen, kidneys; cryptococcus, right heel; cor pulmonale
*PG/52/F	Noncaseating granulomata consistent with sarcoidosis of lungs, spleen, liver, lymph nodes; previous hysterectomy; hemothorax, right (350 cc), left (300 cc); therapeutic pneumoperitoneum
GS/73/M	Sarcoidosis by scalene biopsy; heart failure; fibrotic lungs; triangular infiltrate LUL never resolved; lymphadenopathy; bronchogenic carcinoma
KR/43/F	Sarcoidosis by scalene biopsy; lymph node hyperplasia; squamous metaplasia of bronchial mucosa; fibrosis of lungs; hepatomegaly; thoracotomy; skin rash; heart failure
*KB/44/F	Sarcoidosis involving mediastinal lymph nodes, heart, skin; fibrocystic lungs with bullae; hypocalcemia
DS/60/F	Sarcoidosis by scalene biopsy, involving heart, lungs, lymph nodes, bronchial mucosa; bronchogenic carcinoma; heart failure; hepatomegaly; fibrotic lungs
CJ/32/F	Sarcoidosis by lung biopsy, involving mediastinal lymph nodes; fibrotic lungs; confluent bilateral infiltrate, never resolved
*GP/28/F	Pulmonary fibrosis simulating Hamman-Rich syndrome; cor pulmonale; lymphadenitis
AM/68/F	Sarcoidosis involving skin, heart, lymph nodes; fibrocystic lungs; large apical bullae simulating tuberculosis; perforated nasal septum
GA/56/F	Sarcoidosis; skin rash; heart failure; fibrotic lungs; heart failure; lymph node hypertrophy; scalene biopsy
BC/49/M	Biopsy proven sarcoidosis; skin rash, severe, incapacitating; fibrotic lungs; heart failure; lymph node hypertrophy
*SM/52/F	Sarcoidosis by scalene biopsy; liver atrophy (880 g); hydrothorax, right (150 cc); bronchiectasis; fibrocystic lungs; terminal tuberculosis
*MJ/30/M	Noncaseating granulomata, left ventricle, lungs, spleen, liver, kidneys, lymph nodes; heart failure
HE/40/F	Sarcoidosis by liver biopsy; heart failure; noncaseating granulomata, lymph nodes; hilar and paratracheal adenitis, progressing to fibrotic lungs

* Autopsy.

TABLE 4.

Case	Cause of death
LB/29/F	Cardiorespiratory failure (lived 9 years)
PG/52/F	Cardiorespiratory failure (lived 24 years)
GS/73/M	Heart failure (lived 2 years)
KR/43/F	Cardiorespiratory failure (lived 11 years)
KB/44/F	Respiratory failure (lived 6 months)
DS/60/F	Heart failure (lived 2.5 years)
CJ/32/F	Cardiac arrest (lived 4 years)
GP/28/F	Cardiorespiratory failure (lived 6 months)
AM/68/F	Cardiorespiratory failure (lived 8 years)
GA/56/F	Cardiorespiratory failure (lived 9 years)
BC/49/M	Cardiorespiratory failure (lived 5.5 months)
SM/52/F	Cardiorespiratory failure (lived 8 years)
MJ/30/M	Cardiorespiratory failure (lived 3 years)
HE/40/F	Cardiorespiratory failure (lived 2 years)

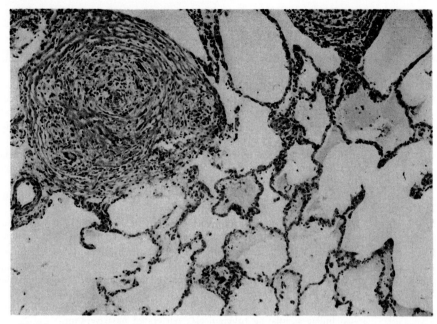

FIG. 3. Photomicrograph showing the noncaseating granulomata in the pulmonary alveolar septum (H & E ; ×).

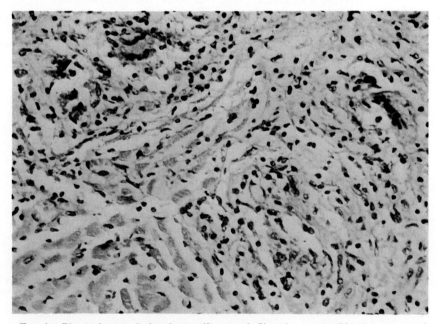

FIG. 4. Photomicrograph showing cardiac muscle fibers interspersed by the noncaseating sarcoid granulomas (H & E ; ×).

Involvement of regional lymphatics and organs

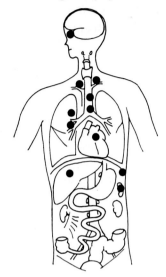

FIG. 5.   Artist's sketch of the distribution of sarcoid granulomas in the body.   On the basis of the distribution it is tempting to assume that the causative organism enters through the lungs.

of sarcoidosis, and all of our patients admitted having many pine trees in their neighborhoods. However, concrete proof of any relationship is lacking.[7]

The clinical findings in our series were similar to other studies reported in the literature.[1-3] Eye and skin lesions were common among sarcoid patients; erythema nodosa was infrequent, or perhaps not always recorded because this malady produced few symptoms. Polyarthralgia was not uncommon; pleural effusion was extremely rare. No proven cases of sarcoidosis of the pleura were recorded in our series, nor was calcification noted within the pleura.

In our series, 1 familial case—mother and daughter—was observed. Similar observations have been reported by Sharma et al.[8] Sarcoidosis rarely produced complications in pregnancy. One of our patients had 10 children, the last 4 after she was known to have sarcoidosis. Eight patients produced at least 1 normal healthy infant. Some childhood cases of sarcoidosis may have been overlooked because children with bilateral hilar adenitis and negative tuberculin tests made spontaneous recovery without ever coming to biopsy. Such a clinical course may account for the rarity of reported cases of childhood sarcoidosis.[9]

The majority of our patients were treated on an outpatient basis, indicating that most of them were asymptomatic or only mildly affected. Few required more than routine medical care. Six of our arrested cases are employees of our hospitals with good working records. However, relapses of sarcoidosis do occur and were documented in approximately 13% of our cases.

The tissue diagnosis of sarcoidosis was made by biopsy in 82 cases. The remaining 104 cases had only presumptive clinical and radiologic diagnoses. In reviewing the literature regarding pathologic findings in sarcoidosis, it becomes apparent that the tissue diagnosis is made by exclusion with the findings of noncaseating granulomata in the absence of specific etiologic agents.[10]

In the majority of our cases hilar and paratracheal adenitis was noted,[11] and this often was the extent of the disease. Lesions of the lungs were mostly reticulofibronodular and increased as the disease progressed. Roentgenographic changes of the lungs, with or without hilar and perihilar adenitis, may simulate widespread bronchopneumonia or consist of a fine stippling which resembles miliary tuberculosis, or even silicosis. Frazer and Pare's textbook points out that it is not uncommon to find localized noncaseating granulomata in association with carcinoma, Hodgkin's disease, ulcerative colitis, or secondary to trauma.[12]

Large and variable size bullae are often seen in the extensive pulmonary fibrotic stages of sarcoidosis. Aspergillomas have been recorded,[13] but not among our patients. Unexplained hemoptysis did occur, however, and in these cases fungus balls were excluded. " Eggshell " calcifications in the anterior mediastinum were noted in 2 cases. As pointed out by Israel et al., mediastinal " eggshell " calcifications are not pathognomonic for silicosis.[14]

In the differential diagnosis of sarcoidosis, berylliosis, histoplasmosis, alveolar cell carcinoma, Wegener's granulomatosis, metastatic carcinoma, septic emboli, hydatid cyst, histocytosis X, and others must be excluded.[15] Diagnosis by chest roentgenogram alone is almost axiomatic in our geographic area if the patient is a young black with the findings of massive bilateral hilar and paratracheal adenitis, showing a normal air bronchogram in the right lower lobe bronchus (Fig. 6).

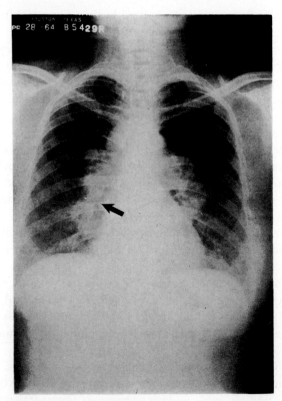

FIG. 6.   Case E. J. H. This 40-year-old black female, asymptomatic, shows massive hilar and paratracheal adenitis, contrasted against the air in the right lower lobe bronchus (arrow). Diagnosis of sarcoidosis is axiomatic.

Lesions of the bones occurred in 7 cases, always in the last stages, and never early. These appeared as small destructive cystic areas in the distal ends of the phalanges, metacarpals, and metatarsals. A typical foamy rarefication on the margins of the phalanges with swelling of the soft tissues was characteristic of young patients with sarcoidosis. Two of our patients, in addition to involvement of the phalanges of the feet and hands, had lesions of the knees, lower legs and nasal bones.

A high incidence of renal calculus in sarcoidosis has been reported, but this was not borne out in our study.[16] Toomey and Bautista reported sarcoidosis in the kidneys of a 4.5-year-old Caucasian proven by biopsy.[17] Incapacitating dermatitis occurred in only 1 of our cases, although some authors suggest skin lesions as an accesible means of diagnosis.[18]

Dyspnea was the chief clinical symptom in all 14 of our fatal cases. Thirteen died of cardiorespiratory failure, and 1 of lung hemorrhage. In the fatal cases, clinical findings of conduction defects and cardiac failure were frequent (10 in our series). Clinical cor pulmonale resulting from end-stage interstitial fibrosis and scarring of the lungs was present in 6 of our cases. This, coupled with primary myocardial involvement with sarcoid granulomata would explain cardiac deaths among patients with sarcoidosis.[19]

At autopsy, in our cases, sarcoidosis was found in the lungs, heart, liver, spleen, and mediastinal and periportal lymph nodes. The review of autopsy findings in 6 of our fatal cases showed the cause of death to be respiratory failure in 4, and cardiac failure in 2. These last 2 cases had definite myocardial involvement by sarcoid granulomata. In 1 of the sarcoidosis cases, proven by biopsy 8 years earlier, advanced tuberculosis was found at autopsy. No history of exposure to tuberculosis was obtained. This points to the tubercle bacillus as another possible etiologic agent in sarcoidosis. Indeed, even cases of proven tuberculosis have apparently undergone complete healing after chemotherapy and later presented with a clinicopathological picture indistinguishable from sarcoidosis.[20]

SUMMARY

From a total of 186 cases of sarcoidosis seen in a chest disease hospital during a 10-year interval, 82 had tissue diagnosis and had close clinical observation. Fourteen cases proved to be fatal in a period ranging from 6 months to 24 years after initial diagnosis.

Distribution of the lesions was consistent with the assumption of a pulmonary portal of entry of the causative agent, followed by lymphatic spread to other organs, including the lymph nodes of the mediastinum and neck, and to the heart, liver, parotid glands and skin. Of the 14 fatal cases, 10 had a clinical history of cardiac involvement. Autopsy findings in 6 cases revealed extensive pulmonary granulomata and interstitial fibrosis. In 2 cases myocardial involvement was documented.

It is interesting to note that 1 of our fatal cases of sarcoidosis had pulmonary tuberculosis in the past, whereas another case of biopsy-proven sarcoidosis revealed extensive tuberculosis at autopsy.

ACKNOWLEDGEMENT

We wish to thank Dr Jorge Gonzales, Connie Buentello, Maydel Massey, and the entire staff of the Radiology Department, Jefferson Davis Hospital, for their valuable assistance in the preparation of this paper.

REFERENCES

1. Reisner, D. 1944. Boeck's sarcoid and systemic sarcoidosis. *Amer. Rev. Tuberc.* **49**: 289.
2. Cummings, M. M., Dunner, E., and Williams, J. H., Jr. 1950. Epidemiologic and clinical. observations in sarcoidosis. *Ann. Internal Med.* **50**: 879.
3. Mayock, R. L., Bertrand, P., Morrison, C. E., and Scott, J. H. 1963. Manifestations of sarcoidosis. *Amer. J. Med.* **25**: 67.
4. Iwai, K. and Oka H. 1964. Sarcoidosis: Report of 10 autopsy cases in Japan. *Amer. Rev. Resp. Dis.* **89**: 612.
5. Hardy, H. L. 1961. Definition of sarcoidosis. Int. Conf. on Sarcoidosis. *Amer. Rev. Resp. Dis.* Suppl. **84**: 2.
6. Scadding, J. G. 1967. Sarcoidosis. London: Eyre and Spottiswood. p. 97.
7. Cummings, M. M. 1964. An evaluation of the possible relationship of pine pollen to sarcoidosis (A critical summary). Proc. Third Int. Conf. on Sarcoidosis. *Acta. Med. Scand.* Suppl. **425**: 48.
8. Sharma, P. O., Johnson, C. S., and Balchum, O. J. 1971. Familial sarcoidosis. *Amer. Rev. Resp. Dis.* **104**: 255.
9. Kending, E. 1961. Sarcoidosis in Children, Int. Conf. on Sarcoidosis. *Amer. Rev. Resp Dis.* Suppl. **84**: 49.
10. Uehlinger, E. A. 1961. The morbid anatomy of sarcoidosis, Int. Conf. on Sarcoidosis. *Amer. Rev. Resp. Dis.* Suppl. **84**: 6.
11. Ellis, K, Renthal, G. 1962. Pulmonary sarcoidosis: Roentgenologic observations in course of disease. *Amer. J. Radium Ther. Nucl. Med.* **88**: 1070.
12. Fraser, R. G., and Pare, J. A. P. 1970. Diagnosis of Diseases of the Chest. Philadelphia: W. B. Saunders Co. p. 1087.
13. Israel, H. Personal communication.
14. Israel, H., Sones, M., Roy, R. L., and Stein, G. N. 1961. The occurrence of intrathoracic calcification in sarcoidosis. *Amer. Rev. Resp. Dis.* **64**: 541.
15. Hahn, R. 1971. Unusual forms of sarcoidosis. *South. Med. J.* **64**: 541.
16. Scholz, D. A. 1956. Renal insufficiency, renal calculi, and nephrocalcinosis in sarcoidosis. *Amer. J. Med.* **21**: 75.
17. Toomey, F., and Bautista, A. 1970. Rare manifestations of sarcoidosis in children. *Radiology* **94**: 569
18. Crofton, J. and Douglas, A. 1969. Respiratory diseases. Oxford: Blackwell Scientific Publications. p. 386.
19. Gozo, E. G., Cosnow, I., Cowen, H. C., and Okun, L. 1971. The heart in sarcoidosis. *Chest* **60**: 379.
20. Scadding, J. G. 1967. Sarcoidosis. London: Eyre and Spottiswood. p. 418.

Course and Prognosis in Pulmonary Sarcoidosis
—A ten-year clinical and cardiopulmonary follow-up study—

P. CARLENS, A. HOLMGREN, N. SVANBORG AND O. WIDSTRÖM

Karolinska Hospital, Stockholm, Sweden

Although the prognosis in sarcoidosis has been studied in many previous investigations, there is still some uncertainty concerning the functional prognosis in different kinds of pulmonary sarcoidosis. In 1958–1960 a clinical and physiological investigation was made by Svanborg and Holmgren in patients grouped according to the clinical and roentgenological picture. These patients are now being reinvestigated 10–14 years after the first study.

MATERIAL

Thirty-seven consecutive cases of patients with sarcoidosis of the lungs in Stockholm 1958–1960 were studied. The diagnosis was supported histologically after biopsy of scalene or mediastinal lymph glands.

The patients were classified into 3 groups clinically and according to the X-ray picture. Group I; patients with hilar lymphomas but without radiographical signs of parenchymal involvement. Group II; patients with parenchymal changes but without signs of fibrosis and group III; patients with signs of fibrosis of varying degree.

The number of patients and the composition of the groups can be seen in Fig. 1.

	1958–60	1969–72	Dead	Cortisone treatment
Group I	11	10	0	2
Group II	11	8	(1)	5
Group III	15	6	4	8

FIG. 1. Ten-year follow-up of patients with pulmonary sarcoidosis.

Among the patients in group I, 7/11 never had parenchymal infiltrations on X-ray, 2/11 patients had minor infiltrations in 1960–1961 which later disappeared and 2/11 had a more severe course ending in fibrosis and respiratory disability.

In groups II and III there are, as could be expected, cases with both regressive and progressive course, and many have become stationary at all levels from total healing to fibrosis with manifest respiratory insufficiency.

In group II, 1 patient died of hypernephroma, in group III 4 patients died in complications to sarcoidosis 8–24 years after the known debut of the disease.

The patients have been treated with corticosteroids with comparatively restrictive indications and in small doses. Usually prednisolone ≤ 15 mg has been given to patients with long-lasting progression, cases with complications as hypercalcemia, uveitis etc., or with respiratory distress. The number of patients given corticosteroid treatment for a shorter or longer time is shown in Fig. 1.

473

METHODS

The methods employed have been reported in detail earlier (Svanborg, 1961).

RESULTS

The dimensions of the cardiovascular system have been studied in terms of total hemoglobin, blood volume and heart volume in supine in order to see whether these important determinants of the working capacity had changed. The results are presented below.

Total hemoglobin had decreased systematically in all groups. To eliminate the influence of an increase in body weight the total hemoglobin was expressed as g/kg in Fig. 2.

Blood volume was however unchanged in most patients (Fig. 3) but decreases of 25% were noted in patients from groups II and III.

Heart volume (ml) measured in supine did not show any systematic changes. In 11 patients it remained unchanged, in 3 it decreased markedly and in 8 patients there was a marked increase (Fig. 4).

Working capacity (kpm/min, W_{max}) determined as the highest work load the subject could perform, and calculated as suggested by Strandell (1964) varied markedly (Fig. 5). Increases of more than 25% were found in women belonging to all groups. Marked decreases were found in 2 respiratory cripples, both women belonging to group III.

Static lung volumes are represented here briefly by vital capacity, VC, only. There is no systematic variation in either group (Fig. 6). Marked decreases were observed in re-

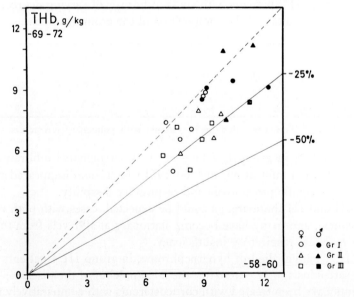

FIG. 2. Total hemoglobin, THb (g), at the first investigation 1958–60 in 21 patients with sarcoidosis of the lung in relation to THb in 1969–72. Thin broken line indicates identity. Thin full lines indicate a decrease of 25 and 50% of the 1958–60 values. Open symbols represent women, filled symbols men, circles represent group I, triangles group II and squares group III.

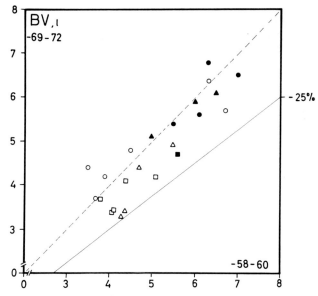

FIG. 3. Blood volume, BV (l), in 1958–60 in relation to that 1969–72. Material and symbols as in Fig. 2.

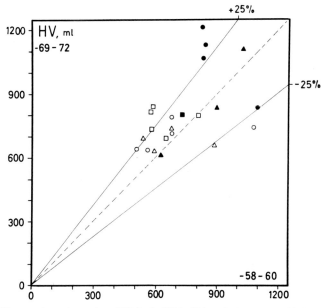

FIG. 4. Heart volume in supine, HV (ml), 1958–60 in relation to that 1969–72. Material and symbols as in Fig. 2.

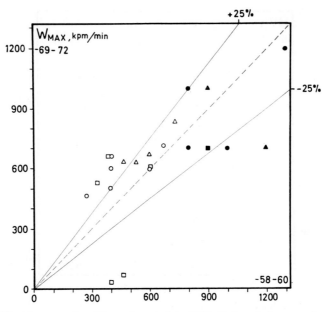

FIG. 5. Working capacity, W_{max} (kpm/min), 1958–60 in relation to that 1969–72. Material and symbols as in Fig. 2.

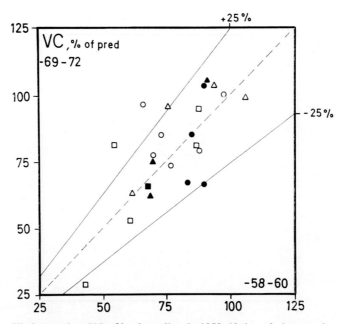

FIG. 6. Vital capacity, VC, % of predicted, 1958–60 in relation to that 1969–72. Material and symbols as in Fig. 2.

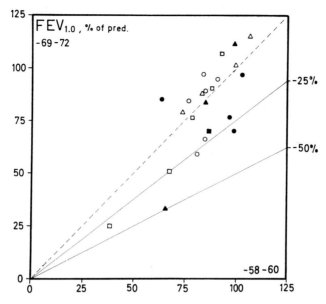

Fig. 7. Forced expiratory volume in 1 second FEV$_{1.0}$, % of predicted 1958–60 in relation to that in 1969–72. Material and symbols as in Fig. 2.

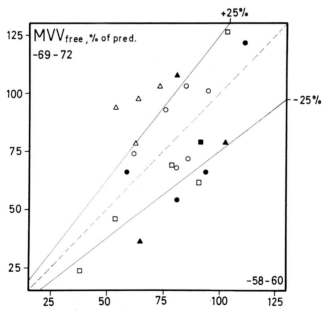

Fig. 8. Maximum voluntary ventilation, at free rate, MVV$_{free}$ in % of predicted 1958–60 in relation to that 1969–72. Material and symbols as in Fig. 2.

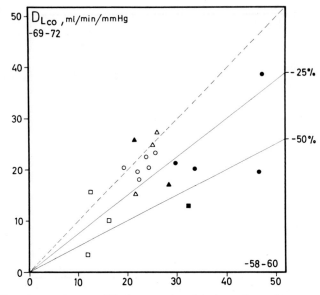

FIG. 9. Exercise steady-state diffusing capacity of the lungs for carbon monoxide, $D_{L_{CO}}$ (ml/min/mm Hg) in 1958–60 in relation to that at the same work load in 1969–72. Material and symbols as in Fig. 2.

spiratory cripples in group III and those 2 patients of group I that showed a progressive course.

Dynamic lung volumes. The dynamic lung volumes are here represented only by $FEV_{1.0}$ and MVV_{free}.

In most patients the $FEV_{1.0}$ remained unchanged but in 4/group I, 1/group II and 3/group III there were marked decreases seemingly related to the progress of the disease. These patients also had a lower MVV while in the rest of the material MVV had increased (Figs. 7 and 8).

Exercise, steady-state $D_{L_{CO}}$ remained unchanged in half the material but decreased markedly in 4/group I, 1/group II and 3/group III (Fig. 8).

DISCUSSION

A material consisting of patients of different age and investigated with intervals of many years is problematic to evaluate. Intercurrent disease, changes in activity and phenomena of aging may interfere. This report is preliminary because all patients have not yet been reinvestigated.

The dimensional parameters of the cardiovascular system, blood volume and heart volume, shows no systematic trend in the 10-year reinvestigation. Total hemoglobin anyhow seems to be distinctly lower in the reinvestigation, which could not be explained by type or activity of disease, weight variations, or ageing. Maximal working capacity is unchanged or tends to increase except in 4 cases with clinical progression and in 2 patients from group I, 1 healed and 1 still after 10 years with bilateral hilar lymphomas but no signs of lung infiltrations. These patients, as do those with clinical progression, show decreased static and dynamic lung volumes and diffusion capacity. In common lung volumes, mechanics of breathing, gas mixing, diffusion capacity etc., tend to be fairly unchanged during the years except in cases with clinical progression. In some patients with a benign clinical course and even normalized radiographical picture, the functional parameters show marked deterioration. The discrepancy between clinical and functional findings in cases treated with steroids and with radiological healing but without functional improvement is well-known, but this occurs also in patients from group I with supposed healing but marked functional impairment years afterwards. In our material there is possibly a better functional trend in females than in males.

Generally the relationship between the clinical severity of the disease and functional findings is good in the advanced cases, but in moderate cases the functional changes are sometimes surprisingly pronounced and clinically marked. A tendency to progressive course is most pronounced in the fibrotic patients but a functional progression can occur also in patients with minor or no parenchymal changes in X-ray and little clinical distress.

REFERENCES

1. Bousky, S. F., Kurtzman, R. S. Mashin, N. D., and Lewis, B. M. 1965. *Amer. Internal Med.* **6215**: 939–955.
2. Coates, E. O., and Comroe, J. H. Jr. 1951. *J. Clin. Invest.* **30**: 848.
3. Hamer, N. A. J. 1963. *Thorax.* **18**: 275.
4. Löfgren, S. 1953. *Acta Med. Scand.* **145**.
5. Marshall, R., Smellie, H., Baylis, J. H., Hoyle, C., and Bates, D. V. 1958. *Thorax.* **13**: 48–58.
6. Sharma, O. P., Colp, C., and Williams, M. H. J. 1966. *Amer. J. Med.* **41**: 541–551.
7. Stone, D. J., Scwartz, A., Feltman, J. A., and Lovelock. 1953. *Amer. J. Med.* **15**: 468–76.
8. Strandell, T. 1964. *Acta Med. Scand.* Suppl. **414**.
9. Svanborg, N. 1961. *Acta Med. Scand.* **170**: Suppl. 366.
10. Svanborg, N. 1971. *Proc. Fifth Int. Conf. on Sarcoidosis.* Prague.
11. Turiaf, J., Basset, Y., and Georges, R. 1969. *Poumon Coer.* **25**: 1–15.

Prognosis of Intrathoracic Sarcoidosis

K. Viskum and K. Thygesen

Department of Pulmonary Medicine, Bispebjerg Hospital, Copenhagen, Denmark

In this study, 254 patients have been included in whom the diagnosis of sarcoidosis was established during admission to the Department of Pulmonary Medicine, Bispebjerg Hospital, in Copenhagen in the period January 1954 to April 1970. All patients had a convincing clinical picture and/or chest X-ray findings compatible with sarcoidosis. A histological verification was obtained in 192 patients (76%). The 62 patients with a negative biopsy have been included in the study, as the exclusion of these patients who, on clinical criteria have sarcoidosis, would have biased the material.

The distribution according to age and sex follows closely the pattern reported by other Danish investigators (Fig. 1). The equal number of men and women is unusual, as women most often dominate.

During the year 1971 the patients were followed up. The average observation time is 7.4 years.

The chest X-ray findings at the follow-up were correlated with the findings at the initial admission (Table 1). As in other studies a normal chest X-ray was most often found at the follow-up in patients who initially had hilar adenopathy as a solitary finding. If parenchymal lesions were initially present, the chest X-ray at the follow-up was more likely to be normal if the parenchymal lesion was combined with hilar adenopathy, than if it was not. The percentage of patients who at the follow-up had a normal chest X-ray in this study is lower in all groups than in most other studies.

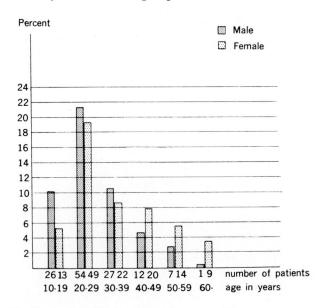

Fig. 1. Distribution according to age and sex of 254 patients with intrathoracic sarcoidosis.

TABLE 1. Correlation of the initial chest X-ray and the chest X-ray at the follow-up.

	Hilar adenopathy	Hilar adenopathy and parenchymal lung lesion	Paren-chymal lung lesion	Total	Mean duration of observation
Cleared	26	37	13	76 (30%)	7.9 years
Improved	8	23	17	48 (19%)	6.0 years
Unchanged	11	39	25	75 (30%)	7.6 years
Worse	1	5	4	10 (4%)	6.3 years
Died	3	19	7	29 (11%)	6.1 years
Chest X-ray unknown	4	10	2	16 (6%)	5.9 years
Total	53 (21%)	133 (52%)	68 (27%)	254	7.4 years

TABLE 2. The initial chest X-ray finding related to clinical status at the follow-up.

	Hilar adenopathy	Hilar adenopathy and parenchymal lung lesion	Parenchymal lung lesion	Total
Working or obtaining old-age pension	45	102	48	195
On the sick list or obtaining disablement pension	2	10	12	24
Dead	3	19	7	29
Unknown	3	2	1	6
Total	53	133	68	254

At the follow-up the working ability was evaluated (Table 2). The prognosis, as related to work, was best for patients with hilar adenopathy, followed by patients with hilar adenopathy and parenchymal lung lesions and worst for patients with parenchymal lung lesions.

In the estimation of the vital prognosis of sarcoidosis it was possible to obtain information concerning 250 or 98.4% of the 254 patients. The observed number of deaths among the 250 patients has been compared to the expected number of deaths in a similar portion of the general population of Copenhagen.

Table 3 shows that there is approximately 4 times the expected number of deaths: 29 against 7.35. There is virtually no difference between men and women or between cases verified by biopsy and those not so verified. Therefore no distinction has been made between these groups in the figures and tables.

Due to the varying observation times, the survival of the patients in the study as compared to that expected, has been illustrated using the decrement method (Fig. 2). As can be seen, 159 of the patients have been observed for 5 or more years, 35 for at least 15 years. The broken line indicates the expected survival rate, the unbroken the observed. As indicated at 5- and 10-year observation periods, the difference is in excess of 2 standard deviations. As seen, the observed survival rate steadily decreases following a nearly straight line. This must indicate that sarcoidosis does not become appreciably more lethal, the longer the disease has existed.

TABLE 3. The expected and observed deaths among 250 patients with pulmonary sarcoidosis. The patients have been divided according to sex and result of biopsy.

Men

	Number	Expected deaths	Total number of observed deaths	Observed deaths / Expected deaths
Biopsy positive	93	2,69	11	4,1
Biopsy negative	32	0,94	4	4,3
Total	125	3,63	15	4,1

Women

	Number	Expected deaths	Total number of observed deaths	Observed deaths / Expected deaths
Biopsy positive	95	3,14	11	3,5
Biopsy negative	30	0,58	3	5,2
Total	125	3,72	14	3,8

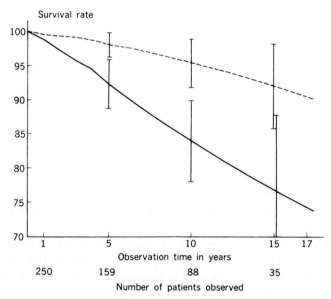

FIG. 2. The survival rate of 250 patients with intrathoracic sarcoidosis. (Expected survival rate : broken line, observed : unbroken.)

TABLE 4. The expected and observed deaths among 250 patients with sarcoidosis divided according to the cause of admission to hospital.

	Number	Expected deaths	Observed deaths all causes	Observed deaths / Expected deaths
No symptoms	133	3,55	12	3,4
Erythema nodosum	22	0,56	1	1,8
Pulmonary symptoms	95	3,24	16	4,9

TABLE 5. The observed and expected deaths among 250 patients with sarcoidosis divided according to the chest X-ray at the admission.

Chest X-ray	Number	Expected deaths	Observed deaths all causes	Observed deaths / Expected deaths
Hilar adenopathy	50	0,86	3	3,5
Parenchymal lung lesions	200	6,49	26	4,0

TABLE 6. The observed and expected deaths among patients with sarcoidosis divided to the outcome of the initial spirometry.

Spirometry	Number	Expected deaths	Observed deaths all causes	Observed deaths / Expected deaths
Normal	175	4,31	12	2,8
Abnormal	46	2,41	14	5,8
Not performed	29	0,63	3	4,8

The influence of the initial symptoms on the prognosis is seen in Table 4. The patients listed as having " no symptoms " have been detected by mass chest X-ray screening of the population. The common complaints in the group of patients with " pulmonary symptoms " were cough and/or shortness of breath. This group has the poorest prognosis. Those patients under the category " no symptoms " have a better chance of survival but nevertheless not so good as those with " erythema nodosum ". The differences however are not statistically significant. The more favourable prognosis of patients with erythema nodosum is well-known, but nevertheless the death rate was twice the expected value in this study.

Hilar adenopathy as an isolated finding is often considered to give a better prognosis than parenchymal lung lesions. This could not be confirmed in the present study, where there was virtually no difference between the 2 groups (Table 5).

A spirometry was performed during the first admission in 221 patients. In 46 there was a modest decrease in lung function (Table 6). The patients with an initially normal spirometry had a lower excess death than those with decreased lung function, but surprisingly the difference did not reach levels of significance.

During the period of observation, 29 patients had died as opposed to 7.35 expected, an excess death of approximately 4 times. Fifteen of these deaths were due to cor pulmonale or respiratory insufficiency and 1 patient died during a diagnostic mediastinoscopy. Thus 16 deaths were directly related to sarcoidosis. Among the remaining 13 patients who died due to causes unrelated to sarcoidosis, there was no uniform pattern of disease. The death rate in this group was almost twice the expected number. This suggests an increased susceptibility of an as yet unknown nature towards other diseases in patients in whom sarcoidosis has been diagnosed.

SUMMARY

In a follow-up study of 254 patients with intrathoracic sarcoidosis with an average observation time of 7.4 years, it was found that patients with hilar adenopathy as a solitary initial finding had the best chance of a complete normalisation of the chest X-ray and the best chance of retaining normal working ability.

The survival rate for patients with sarcoidosis was significantly lower than that for a similar portion of the population at large. The observed number of deaths was 4 times as high as the expected value. The excess death was correlated to the initial chest X-ray finding, to various symptoms and to the outcome of the initial spirometry, but no statistically significant differences were found.

Prognosis of Sarcoidosis

K. Wurm

University of Freiburg, Freiburg, Federal Republic of Germany

The prognosis of sarcoidosis is matter of primary interest firstly for the doctor of whom the patients expects such a prognosis and secondly for the social physician, who from the point of view of preventive medicine needs information about the importance of sarcoidosis with regard to epidemology, morbidity, planning for social welfare and insurance provisions. Also the results of recovery, disability, invalidity or death are of importance to him. Thirdly for the research-worker, who is able to draw nosological conclusions from the disease's course and its consequences.

Statistics from former periods regarding mortality and lethality are too unfavourable and are no longer valid today, as in former times the acute and latent forms of sarcoidosis were not included comprehensively in a high percentage in statistics, and moreover, with the help of modern steroid therapy the prognosis has become better. Further improvements are to be expected if sarcoidosis is diagnosed at an early stage and from a general mastering the therapeutic technique.

Three years ago, at the Fifth International Sarcoidosis Congress in Prague, I[5] reported the first results of our study to which the present notes are a supplement. The number of patients whose course of disease has been followed up, amounts to 3,000 in this report and the period of observation extends from 1950 to 1972. The total number of patients suffering from sarcoidosis and who were treated between 1950 and 1972 has increased to 7,500 up to this date. The patients with the longest observation have been statistically evaluated. They came for treatment in the years from 1950 to 1966 in our clinic. This new statistics also includes patients, regarding whom we reported in Prague in 1969. However, the continuance of observation of the course of their disease was extended by 3 years. The method of examination is the same. As to the *individual prognosis* the doctor has principally to differentiate between sarcoidosis with an acute, resp. subacute syndrome (Loefgren's syndrome, acute form of sarcoidosis) and the form of sarcoidosis starting latently and becoming chronic. The prognosis of the *acute course* is extremely favourable. We confirm Loefgren's[3] quotation of 80% spontaneous recovery within 1 year.

With regard to its duration and consequences the prognosis of the *latent-chronic course* of sarcoidosis in its totality is very different and uncertain. In spite of this the *individual case* permits a prognostic statement. The results of general statistics give an orientation even for the particular case; its prospective course can be predicted, if one takes into consideration the sarcoid-specific course of stages.[2]

In particular, the results of extended statistics are of importance for social medicine and research work. The results of our studies are demonstrated in Table 1.

I shall omit a detailed discussion of all registered dates. I only should like to point out the following important observations: Beyond the 3,000 examined patients are 337 patients with an observation time of more than 15 years. Only these allow a reliable conclusion: 72% healed, and the other 28% still are active after this long time. Fifteen

TABLE 1. Prognosis of sarcoidosis (Analysis of 3,000 Patients).

Age	Duration of observation	Number	Cured		Still active		Died						No information	
							Sarcoidosis		No sarcoidosis		Cause unknown			
			abs.	%	abs.	%	abs.	%	abs.	%	abs.	%	abs.	%
>25 years	more than 15 years	128	101	79	23	17.9	1	0.78	0	—	1	0.78	2	1.54
	4–9 years	288	150	52.1	136	47.2	2	0.7	0	—	0	—	0	—
	1–4 years	458	161	35.2	295	64.5	2	0.3	0	—	0	—	0	—
		874	412	47.2	454	51.9	5	0.57	0	—	1	0.11	2	0.22
26–40 years	more than 15 years	109	84	77	18	16.6	3	2.75	0	—	0	—	4	3.65
	4–9 years	473	215	45.4	244	51.5	11	2.3	2	0.4	1	0.2	1	0.2
	1–4 years	840	270	32	566	66.6	3	1.4	0	—	0	—	0	—
		1422	569	40	828	58.2	17	1.2	2	0.14	1	0.07	5	0.39
<40 years	more than 15 years	100	57	57	27	27	11	11	2	2	0	—	3	3
	4–9 years	224	63	28	143	63.8	13	5.8	4	2.4	0	—	0	—
	1–4 years	380	81	21.3	295	77.6	4	0.95	1	0.15	0	—	0	—
		704	201	28.6	465	66.1	28	3.98	7	0.99	0	—	3	0.33
		3000												

of these 337 patients died of sarcoidosis, whilst the outcome of 75 still uncured cases is unknown at present. The known lethality amounts to 3% up to now but will be increased by the outcome of the 75 cases which are still active. The rate of death is dependent on age. Within the 3 age groups in the cases with an observation of more than 15 years it shows an increase from 0.78% to 11%, i.e., 14-fold. Altogether the results of this extensive study are in accordance with our report in Prague, 1969.

The analyses of our data are far from being closed and are being further investigated from other points of view. Definitive and more differentiated results obtained with the aid of a computer will be reported in the future.

Evaluation of the outcome of the disease

Autopsy findings show that the anatomical lesions which are characteristic for sarcoidosis may still be present in cases which the clinician has considered to be cured long time ago. A *general agreement* would be very desirable under what conditions in sarcoidosis cases a complete recovery or recovery with defect or a latent outcome should be assumed. Such clarification would not only be of value to the clinician as a means of orientation for further treatment, but it is above all a scientific requirement to compare the statistics of authors.

May I bring up the following suggestions for discussion by all sarcoidosis experts.

Healing in the sense of a restitutio ad integrum is present, if within 3 years (or 5?) after discontinuing the medication no relapse has occured and, with completely intact organic functions, no more clinicopathological findings are present. In untreated cases a final recovery can be assumed if for 3 (or 5?) years there have been no more pathological findings.

Recovery with defect is present if within 3 (or 5?) years after discontinuation of the medication no relapse has occured, but however, anatomical or functional lesions persist (limited function of the lungs, hilar calcifications, diminished strength of vision, disturbing skin scars, myocardial scars etc.). In these cases a further gradual distinction between clinically insignificant, clinically significant and life-shortening is necessary.

Outcome into clinical latency is to be assumed if 3 (or 5?) years after the discontinuation of the medication neither a relapse has occured nor any functional disturbances of an organ can be proven. However, anatomical organic lesions (e.g. mediastinal lymphomas, splenectasis) may persist. The evaluation of untreated cases after disappearance of a clinical symptomatology is analogous.

Finally it has to be noted that the acute and the chronic form of sarcoidosis a priori have a very different prognosis, so that a separate statistical work-up of the acute form (Loefgren's syndrome) and of the sarcoidosis which primarily starts latently and becomes chronic, is indicated.

REFERENCES

1. Wurm, K. 1961. Arch. Klin. *Exp. Dermat.* **213**: 522.
2. Wurm, K. 1971. *Fifth. Int. Conf. on Sarcoidosis* Prague. p. 483.
3. Loefgren, S. 1955. *Beitr. Klin. Tuberk.* **114**: 75.
4. Wurm, K., Ewert, E. G., Romacker, E. M. 1969. Beitr. Klin. *Erfschg. Tuberk. Lungenkr.* **140**: 279.
5. Wurm, K. 1971. *Fifth Int. Conf. on Sarcoidosis*. Prague: Univ. Karlova. p. 529.

Factors Relating to the Course of Sarcoidosis

Masahiko Yamamoto

Second Department of Internal Medicine, Nagoya City University Medical School, Nagoya, Japan

AND

Daishiro Kawazoe, Kaoru Shimokata and Koo Fujii

First Department of Internal Medicine, Nagoya University School of Medicine, Nagoya, Japan

INTRODUCTION

The manifestations of sarcoidosis in most cases can be resolved, leaving no residue; however, in some cases, the sarcoid manifestations remain for a long time with repeated relapses.

In this paper, the factors relating to the course of sarcoidosis were studied by multiple factor analysis, in order to quantify the significance of the factors affecting the prognosis of sarcoidosis.

MATERIALS AND METHODS

The background factors of 118 cases of sarcoidosis studied in this series were as follows: male in 40% of the cases and female in 60%; younger than 25 years in 27%, between 25 and 35 years in 19%, and older than 35 years in 19%; histologically diagnosed in 57% and clinically diagnosed in 43%; negative tuberculin reaction in 59% and positive or equivocal in 41%; with hilar lymphadenopathy in 100%; with mediastinal lymphadenopathy in 70% and without in 30%; with pulmonary involvement in 50% and without in 50%; with extrapulmonary lesions in 38% and without in 62%. The sites of extrapulmonary lesions were eye in 35 cases, peripheral lymph node in 6, skin in 5, liver in 5, parotis in 2 and skeletal muscle in 1 case.

The period of observation of the cases was less than 1 year in 8%, between 1 and 2 years in 39%, between 2 and 3 years in 18%, and more than 3 years in 36%. The mean period of observations was 2.7 years.

In order to find an index to separate the cases with excellent prognosis from the cases with poor prognosis, the percentage disappearance of sarcoid manifestations and frequency of relapse during every 6 months were observed.

Multiple factor analysis was performed according to Hayashi's model[1] in order to quantify the factors affecting prognosis of sarcoidosis. All cases of sarcoidosis were separated into 2 groups: in group I, all sarcoid manifestations disappeared within 18 months after diagnosis, and in group II, the sarcoid manifestations had not disappeared within 18 months of diagnosis. The items and categories adopted here are as follows: age (younger than 25 years, between 25 and 35 years, or older than 35 years); tuberculin reaction (positive or negative); previous history of tuberculosis (presence or absence); hilar lymphadenopathy (less than 25 mm or 25 mm and more); pulmonary involvement (none, nodular, or reticular); extrapulmonary involvement (present or absent); and gammaglobulin (less than 18.5% or 18.5% and more). A category score (x_{jk}) was given to each category (k) of each item (j), so as to minimize the dispersion of the sample score ($a_i = \sum_j \sum_k \delta i(jk)x_{jk}$), which was obtainable from the sum of the category scores of cases in the same group, and to maximize the dispersion in all cases. Partial correlation coefficient of the items to the prognosis of sarcoidosis was calculated using the category score of each case in the 2 groups.

RESULTS

The status of sarcoid manifestations at the final observation in this series was as follows: disappeared in 53% of cases, improved in 28%, unchanged in 5% and deteriorated in 14%.

Percentage disappearance of manifestations of sarcoidosis during the 6-month observation periods after diagnosis was 16.1% in the first 6 months, 32.0% in the second 6 months and 18.9% in the third 6 months, but it became low after the fourth 6 months (Table 1). The percentage of relapse during the 6 months after and before the disappearance of the sarcoid manifestations is shown in Table 2. The relapse rate became very low after all the manifestations of sarcoidosis disappeared, while the relapse rate before the disappearance remained high, even 24 months after the diagnosis.

Multiple factor analysis was performed to quantify the significance of the factors affecting the prognosis of sarcoidosis both in cases whose sarcoid manifestations disappeared within 18 months and cases whose sarcoid manifestations did not disappear within the same period.

TABLE 1. Percentage of disappearance of sarcoid manifestations at 6-month intervals after diagnosis.

Months after diagnosis	Cases observed	Cases where sarcoid manifestations disappeared	Percentage (%)
0–6	118	19	16.1
7–12	97	31	32.0
13–18	53	10	18.9
19–24	32	1	3.1
25–30	25	0	0
31–36	20	1	5.0
37–42	15	1	6.7
43–48	13	1	7.7

TABLE 2. Percentage of relapse.

Period of observation (months)	After disappearance of sarcoid manifestations		Before disappearance of sarcoid manifestations	
0–6	0/63	0%	22/94	23.4%
7–12	0/53	0%	7/40	17.5%
13–18	0/35	0%	5/25	20.0%
19–24	1/28	3.6%	3/16	18.8%
25–30	0/20	0%	3/11	27.3%
31–36	0/16	0%	1/4	25.0%

TABLE 3. Partial correlation coefficient of items and category scores.

Item	Partial corr. coeff.	Category score		$\times 10^2$
Age	0.45	~24y 0	25~34y −1.43	35y −2.12
Tuberculin reaction	0.10	+ 0	− −0.35	
Previous history of TBC	0.06	no 0	yes −0.34	
Hilar lymphadenopathy	0.06	less than 2.5 cm 0	2.5 cm or more −0.19	
Pulmonary involvement	0.25	no 0	nodular −0.47	reticular −1.18
Extrapulmonary involvement	0.03	no 0	yes 0.13	
Gammaglobulin	0.12	less than 18.5% 0	18.5% or more −0.4	

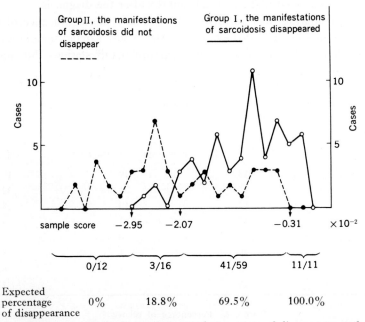

FIG. 1. Frequency distribution and expected percentage of disappearance of sarcoid-manifestations according to the sample score.

Example of calculation of sample score
    Age: −24 y, Tuberculin reaction: negative,
          0   −0.35
    Hilar L. Ad.: 3.0 mm, Pul. invol. nodular,
        −0.19   −0.47
    Extra pul. inv.: no, gamma globulin: normal
          0   0
    Sample score $= (−0.35) + (−0.19) + (−0.47) = −1.01$

Table 3 shows the results of the calculation. The most important item affecting prognosis was age, with a partial correlation coefficient of 0.45, and the second was pulmonary involvement, with 0.25. The most disadvantageous category was the older-than-35 age group. The next was the 25-to-35 age group, and the presence of reticular-type pulmonary lesions. Less important items were negative tuberculin reaction, presence of a previous history of tuberculosis, presence of nodular-type pulmonary lesions, and hypergammaglobulinaemia.

Figure 1 shows the frequency distribution of the 2 groups and expected percentage of disappearance of sarcoid manifestations according to the sample score. The expected percentage of disappearance would be 100% if the sample score of the cases is more than -0.31×10^{-2}, 69.5% between -0.3×10^{-2} and -2.07×10^{-2}, 18.8% between -2.07×10^{-2} and -2.96×10^{-2}, and 0% less than -2.96×10^{-2}.

The reliability of this program was calculated from the cumulative curve of the cases of both groups, and 72% of the cases could be separated by this program from the results of the calculation.

DISCUSSION

The course of sarcoidosis in this study was similar to that of 369 cases followed by the Japan Sarcoidosis Committee,[2] and showed better prognosis than that reported by Sones,[4] Reisner,[5] and James.[1] In Japan, mild cases of sarcoidosis have been discovered by the nationwide antituberculosis chest survey.

The Japan Sarcoidosis Committee pointed out that a disadvantageous factor of sarcoidosis was the presence of eye lesion,[2] and Sones[3] considered race and the extension of sarcoid lesions as important factors affecting the prognosis of sarcoidosis. In this study, however, age seemed the most important factor. Since the onset of sarcoidosis in this study was not always clear, there is a possibility that more chronic cases were included in the older group than in the younger group, and further analysis may be necessary for cases where the date of onset can be established.

SUMMARY

1) The disappearance of manifestations of sarcoidosis was observed to occur mostly within 18 months after diagnosis.

2) The relapse rate of sarcoidosis became very low after all manifestations disappeared.

3) The most disadvantageous factor of sarcoidosis was the above-35 age group, the next being the 25-to-35 age group and the presence of reticular-type pulmonary lesions.

REFERENCES

1. Hayashi, C., and Murayama, T. 1964. Planning of Market Research (in Japanese). Nittkan Kogyo Shinbun Sha. Tokyo.
2. Japan Sarcoidosis Committee. 1968. *Japanese J. Thoracic Dis.* (in Japanese). **6**: 105.
3. Sones, M., and Israel, H. L. 1961. *Amer. Rev. Resp. Dis.* **84** (Suppl.): 60.
4. Reisner, D. 1961. *Amer. Rev. Resp. Dis.* **96**: 361.
5. James, D. G. 1961. *Amer. Rev. Resp. Dis.* (Suppl.) **84**: 66.

An Attempt to Quantify the Factors Affecting the
Prognosis of Sarcoidosis

M. Odaka[1], Y. Hosoda[1], Y. Fukuda[1], Y. Maeda[1] M. Yamamoto[2],
M. Matsuda[3], T. Tachibana[4],I. Shigematsu[5]
T. Kosuda[6] AND N. Shigematsu[7]

There have been a number of reports concerning the factors affecting the prognosis of sarcoidosis. The object of this study is to investigate those of greatest importance for the prognosis, using Hayashi's quantification theory.

The subjects for study were the 242 histologically confirmed sarcoidosis cases which had revealed BHL at the time of discovery and which had been observed for 2 years or more (Fig. 1). As shown in the authors' previous study, in which the chest X-ray findings had cleared more frequently during the first 2 years of the disease than during the period after that, the tendency for recovery seems to have a critical point within the 2-year period. From these results, the cases showing cleared chest X-ray findings during the first 2 years were regarded as favourable cases and the cases where the chest X-ray findings had persisted beyond this period, as unfavourable cases. One hundred and seventy cases were placed in the former category, and 72 other cases in the latter. One hundred and fifty-four BHL cases accompanied by lung parenchymal lesions were analysed separately from those not having them in order to investigate the progress of the lung involvements. According to Hayashi's quantification analysis, a correlation ratio (η^2) is sought and a metric value can be introduced into the quantitative patterns. Let α_i be the numerical value given to the i-th case and quantify the categories so as to maximise the correlation ratio. If the correlation is large, the pattern can be treated quantitatively by using X_{jk}.

$$\alpha_i = \sum_{i=1}^{R} \sum_{k=1}^{Kj} X_{jk} \, \delta i(jk)$$

R: number of factors

K: the k-th category in the j-th factor

$\delta_i(jK)=1$ if the i-th case responds to the k-th

$=0$ otherwise

We have $\sigma^2 = \dfrac{1}{n} \sum_{i=1}^{n} (\alpha_i - \alpha)^2$ as the total variance with respect to elements, where $\bar{\alpha} = \dfrac{1}{n} \sum_{i=1}^{n} \alpha_1$. Now we want to quantify the subcatogories so as to maximise the correlation ratio $\eta^2 = \dfrac{\sigma_b{}^2}{\sigma^2}$ where $\sigma_b{}^2$ is the variance between strata. This is generally

1) JNR Central Health Institute, Tokyo, Japan.
2) Nagoya City University School of Medicine, Nagoya, Japan.
3) Center for Adult Diseases, Osaka, Japan.
4) Osaka Prefectural Hospital, Osaka, Japan.
5) National Institute of Public Health, Tokyo, Japan.
6) Kanto Chuo Hospital, Tokyo, Japan.
7) Research Institute of Chest Disease, Kyushu University, Fukuoka, Japan.

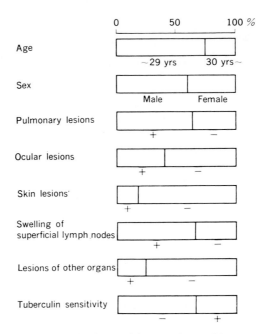

FIG. 1.   Background factors of the subject.

factor	1			2			......	R		
Category	C_{11}	C_{12} ...... C_{1K}		C_{21}	C_{22} ...... C_{2K2}			C_{R1}	C_{R2} ...... C_{RKR}	
Case$_1$	V				V				V		
Case$_2$		V		V						V	
Case$_3$		V			V				V		
⋮											
Case$_n$			V	V							V

Outside variable

V Means the response category each element checks only 1 category in each factor.

FIG. 2.   Pattern of cases responding to the category in each factor.

a reasonable method of quantification, because η^2 is considered to be a fairly good measure of discriminative power by items, that is, a measure of the efficiency of the classification in the case in question. If η^2 is large in the quantification, we can quantitatively treat the pattern using X_{jk}. Thus we can introduce a metric value into the quantitative patterns. In this case, it is possible to obtain the largest correlation ratio by partially differentiating η^2 with respect to X_{jk} ($j=1,......R$, $k=1......Kj$) and making it zero.

As shown in Fig. 1, the following factors were analysed: age, sex, the presence or absence of lung parenchymal lesions, eye lesions, skin lesions, swollen lymph nodes and other involvements such as occur in the parotid glands, nerves etc. and also tuberculin sensitivity. The item of corticosteroid treatment was too difficult to analyse because it has been administered to most of the patients in greatly varying doses. Figure 3 shows the accumulated η value viewed from the progress of BHL. The presence of eye lesions, age

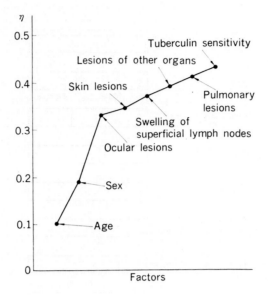

FIG. 3. Square-root correlation ratio (η) concerning with the course of BHL. (242 cases).

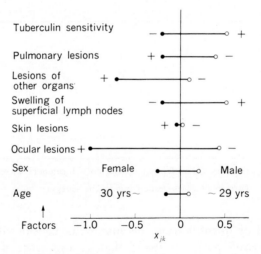

FIG. 4. The numerical value (x_{jk}) given to each category in factors affecting to the course of BHL. (242 cases).

and sex were indicated as major factors. Figure 4 shows X_{jk} calculated from the above η value according to the categories (over 30 years old, male, absence of eye lesions) in each factor (age, sex, presence of eye lesions). If X_{jk} is given as positive, the prognosis tends favourable, and if negative, the prognosis tends to be unfavourable. By way of example, in respect of the age factor, the 29-or-less age group showed a favourable prognosis and the 30-or-more age group, an unfavourable one. Figure 5 shows the distribution of total gain α_i in each X_{jk} is separated at the P point centering at -0.275 in α_i, showing the

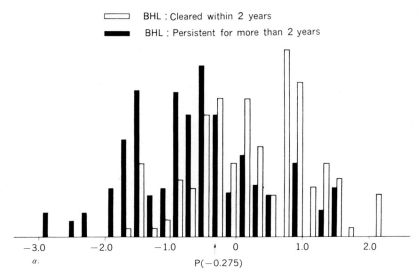

FIG. 5. Distribution of subjects by the numerical value (αi).

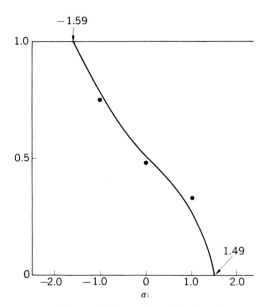

FIG. 6. The curve suggesting possibility of anticipating the course of BHL by the numerical value at the onset of sarcoidosis. (242 cases).

favourable and unfavourable prognoses. The probability of BHL disappearing within 2 years is high in cases whose α_i exceeded -0.275, whereas in cases whose α_1 was smaller than -0.275, the probability is low. Figure 6 shows a predictable rate of prognosis using the α_i value. There is a 100% accuracy rate in predicting bad prognosis in cases with an α_i of less than -1.59, and also good prognosis in cases with α_i larger than 1.49. The cases whose α_i values were between 1.49 and -1.59 showed an average predictability of about 70%.

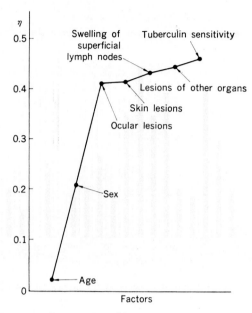

FIG. 7. Square-root correlation ratio (η) concerning with the course of pulmorary lesions. (154 cases).

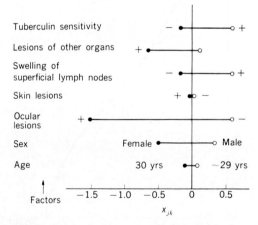

FIG. 8. The numerical value (x_{jk}) given to each category in factors affecting to the course of pulmonary lesions.

The above observations proved that the predictability of the prognosis, or the progress of BHL, can be derived from a_i, the sum of the numericals X_{jk}, according to factors such as age, sex, clinical findings etc. Of these factors, the presence of eye lesions, age and sex were shown to be quite important. Regarding the progress of lung parenchymal lesions, similar results were obtained, as shown in Figs. 7, 8, 9 and 10.

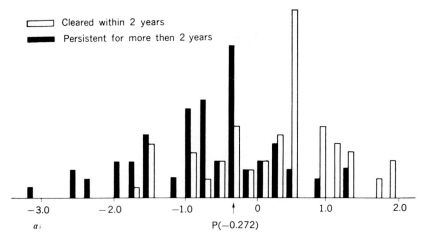

Fig. 9. Distribution of subjects by numerical value (αi) pulmonary lesions.

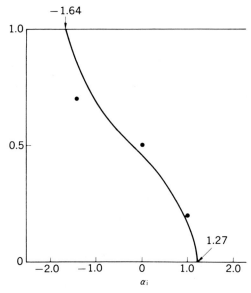

Fig. 10. The curve suggesting pL possibility of anticipating the course of pulmonary lesions by the numerical value at the onset of sarcoidosis. (154 cases).

ACKNOWLEDGEMENT

The authors of this paper are greatly indebted to Dr Hayashi for his help in calculating the data according his original quantitative analysis method.

REFERENCES

1. C. Hayashi 1961. Sample Survey and Theory of Quantification. *Bull. Int. Statist. Instit. XXXVIII* Part **iV**: 506.
2. Y. Hosoda, H. Osada, Y. Hiraga, M. Odaka, and T. Hashimoto. 1971. Factors Affecting the Prognosis of Sarcoidosis. *Lung and Heart* **18**: 1, 46.

DISCUSSION

Chairmen: C. JOHNS AND T. G. VILLAR

DR WURM: Erythema nodosum is a very characteristic symptom of Löfgren's syndrome, but not exclusively so. I have observed erythema nodosum about 5 times in cases of chronic sarcoidosis, not in the beginning but during the course of the disease.

DR TEIRSTEIN: Yes, we have 1 such patient—Dr Israel tells me he has another patient—and it is true that occasionally erythema nodosum will occur late in the course of sarcoidosis. In our instance, the patient had neurological sarcoidosis which cleared and then 8 years later, she experienced another "attack" of sarcoidosis, when she suddenly blossomed with erythema nodosum and hilar nodes. Of course, it is always possible that the late erythema nodosum may be evidence of some other illness, for example a drug sensitivity, and not sarcoidosis.

DR ISRAEL: I cannot agree with Dr Teirstein that most investigators find that erythema nodosum does not influence the prognosis of sarcoidosis. Most studies summarized in Scadding's monograph indicate that patients with erythema nodosum have a much greater chance of recovery within 2 years.

DR TEIRSTEIN: I was referring specifically to Professor Stavenow's papers at the Copenhangen meeting, where he presented a group of patients in whom he could accurately date the onset of sarcoidosis radiographically. He then compared that group of new bilateral hilar lymph node enlargement with a group of patients who had erythema nodosum and bilateral hilar lymph node enlargement. And in these 2 groups the course was rather similar, and therefore we could then take erythema nodosum as a marker of the onset of sarcoidosis, since he had already shown the correlation between new BHL cases and erythema nodosum.

DR JOHNS: I certainly wanted to express appreciation for Professor Turiaf's report where he tells of experiences similar to ours. I will describe some of those in my paper tomorrow where there are significant numbers of patients who require very prolonged treatment, and will relapse every time that steroids are discontinued. I also agree with his comments about how important it is to follow the patients carefully, including pulmonary function evaluation.

DR TACHIIRI: I would like to express my opinion about chest roentgen examination in sarcoidosis.

As all clinical and laboratory examinations have become more precise and detailed, the roentgenological examination of sarcoidisis should be more developed and precise, too.

We have many problems about the correlation between X-rays and other data. Among these, the most important is, whether the X-ray findings after any treatment are "normal" or change of sarcoidosis are "completely disappeared".

According to my opinion, it is very difficult to interpret chest X-ray as normal. If the chest could be examined more precisely, for example, by means of "magnification radiography", you might sometimes or frequently find some abnormal signs of fibrotic changes, especially in case of parenchymal dissemination.

Our criteria for the existence of pulmonary fibrotic changes of not so high grade are:
1. Irregular contour of vascular shadows,
2. Irregular running course and irregularly arranged diameters of vascular shadows, as well as peripheral bronchial shadows, especially by means of magnification radiography and bronchography,

3. Abnormal, localized, faintly increased translucencies, etc.

It is necessary to examine, not only the reduction or disappearance of BHL, small nodulation and reticular shadow, but also more precise changes of vascular shadows, I think.

* The following points were not mentioned previously, due to lack of time, and since nothing is negligible in disccussing X-ray findings, I would like to add some remarks here.

If the chest X-ray holds an important position in diagnosis of sarcoidosis and in evaluation of the effect of treatment, we should define the method of radiography internationally, just as in the case of pneumoconiosis.

For example:

1. Routine examination
   a. Frontal-plane radiography,
   b. kV, Focus-film-distance,
   c. Exposure time,
   d. With or without grid, etc.
2. Precise (Accurate) examination
   a. High-voltage radiography,
   b. Bilateral radiography,
   c. Tomography,
   d. Magnification radiography,
   e. Bronchography and
   f. Pneumoangiography
3. Gross and detailed criteria for interpretation of sarcoidosis and fibrotic changes of the lung—considering the method of examination.

DR VILLAR: A lot has been said about the prognosis of sarcoidosis but, when one comes down to the individual patient, it is difficult to tell exactly what he can expect as far as the prognosis of his sarcoidosis is concerned. From all we have heard in this session I believe the plan presented in Professor Turiaf's paper is the most positive contribution in this direction. After a 3-month dynamic radiologic study and a complete functional assesment, he divides his patient's, as to prognosis, into 3 groups: those that he does not treat, those that he treats for 2 years and those that he treats all their life. This work was supported by Professor

Viskum's paper in which he showed us how important a complete lung function study can be in determining the prognosis of sarcoidosis. I think these were the positive facts that came out in this session. I believe the use of erythema nodosum to mark the beginning of sarcoidosis, as Dr Teirstein showed us, has very marked geographical variations. Professor Wurm told us he sees comparatively few cases of erythema nodosum. In Lisbon, when we see a case of erythema nodosum we think of tuberculosis, streptococcal infections etc. Only 7% of our few cases of sarcoidosis present with erythema nodosum. Thus, although erythema nodosum is a good marker for the beginning of sarcoidosis in New York it may not be as useful in other parts of the world.

This is why, for the type of sarcoidosis patient I see, Professor Turiaf's paper fits in best.

DR TEIRSTEIN: I obviously have confused some of you here today. The purpose of my paper was not to talk about erythema nodosum. The purpose of the paper was to show that if one looks at the beginning of sarcoidosis, and erythema nodosum was the best available means for dating the onset of the disease, one finds that there is a great deal of sarcoidosis that goes undiagnosed. The reason why all the prognostic statistics, as Dr Israel points out, are so good for erythema nodosum is because the prognosis, in general, is good for sarcoidosis. Reaffirming that patients who present with erythema nodosum reflect the true course of sarcoidosis. Probably at least 90% of the patients who have sarcoidosis never know they have the disease. They do not see a doctor; they do not have a chest X-ray; they have no symptoms, and they recover spontaneously from their disease. The patients with erythema nodosum behave like this 90%. We are then left with 10% of the patients who really comprise the patient population this meeting is all about. It has been shown, in everybody's studies, something approaching two-thirds of these pateints will improve, no matter what we do or don't do. So we are now talking about two-thirds of 10%, and we are getting down to a very small number of patients, some of whom die, some of whom improve spontaneously, and some of whom need therapy. As yet, I do not believe any of us can predict, in that small group of patients, which will need therapy and which will not need therapy.

X CHILDHOOD SARCOIDOSIS

Sarcoidosis in Childhood

Teruo Tachibana and Kazuhiko Aratake

Osaka Prefectural Hospital, Osaka, Japan

Shizuo Okada

Japan Antituberculosis Association (Osaka Branch), Osaka, Japan

Yoshitake Yamamoto

National Ehime Sanatorium, Osaka, Japan

AND

Shiro Kato and Matao Naito

Research Institute for Microbial Diseases, Osaka University, Osaka, Japan

As reports concerning sarcoidosis in childhood are rather few in medical literature,[1-6] we should like to report on this topic.

Epidemiological

From 1960 to June 1972, 20 children with sarcoidosis were detected by us. Most of them were asymptomatic and detected by the annual mass radiographic survey, mainly in the Osaka area, covering both tuberculin-positive and -negative children. Mean incidence rate per 100,000 was 0.3 in primary school, 0.5 in middle school, and 1.8 in high school.

Clinical picture at detection

Sex, age, mode of detection and chest X-ray changes are shown in Table 1. In parenthesis are data found during a nationwide survey in 1964. Extrathoracic lesions are shown in Table 2. The central column represents biopsy results. Hepatic lesions were demonstrated by peritoneoscopy and liver biopsy and were characterised in half of these

TABLE 1. Twenty cases of sarcoidosis in children.

1.	Sex	
	male	12 (50)
	female	8 (36)
2.	Age	
	less than 10	1 (9)
	10~15	19 (77)
3.	Mode of detection	
	subjective complaint	2 (15)
	mass X-ray examination	18 (71)
4.	Intrathoracic lesion on chest film	
	BHL	14 (56)
	BHL with Parenchymal lesion	6 (28)

TABLE 2. Extrathoracic lesions

Eye		(14)
uveitis	2	
uveitis with retinal lesion	1	
Skin	0	(6)
Superficial lymph node	3 in 3	
R. scalene node	9 in 11	
Tonsil	1 in 3	
Liver	6 in 7	
Pituitary, suspected	1	
CNS, suspected	1	

TABLE 3. Tuberculin reaction at detection.

negative	11 (32)
doubtful positive	7 (17)
positive	2 (20)
Total cases	20 (69)

positive cases by normal hepatic functions. As already reported in the last conference, 1 case had a lowered growth hormone level and abnormal Metopirone test which suggested anterior pituitary lesions. Furthermore, epileptic attacks began to occur, since detection of BHL on chest film, in another case. Both cases also had other marked extrathoracic lesions, namely eye, liver and extrathoracic lymph node lesions were revealed by lymphography. Tuberculin reaction at detection is shown in Table 3. Before detection it was positive in all cases which were confirmed by the yearly mass survey.

CLINICAL COURSE

1) Radiographic course. Most of the cases had shown a good radiological course. Thirteen of 20 cases had moderate or marked improvement after 3 months, and 12 of 18 cases after 6 months. But thereafter, 3 cases relapsed: 2 had eye and marked hepatic lesions and 1 relapsed after a short period of steroid treatment.

2) Persistence of sarcoid nodules in the liver. In 2 cases with marked hepatic lesions but without abnormal hepatic function, a second or third peritoneoscopy and liver biopsy were done after marked improvement in chest X-ray. In 1 case sarcoid nodules were found on the liver surface and fibrosed sarcoid nodules in a liver biopsy specimen. In the other case, where the same examination prosedures were carried out, after radiographic improvement was observed after a relapse, similar findings were revealed.

3) Changes in tuberculin reaction (after improvement of chest X-ray findings). Three negative and 2 doubtful positive out of 8 cases did not convert to positive after improvement of chest X-ray changes.

Antibody titers to EB virus
As already reported in a paper titled "Clinical course of patients with sarcoidosis

Table 4. Antibody titer to EBV in sera taken once or 4 times
from chidren with sarcoidosis.

Patient No.	Age	Sex	Chest radiograph	Anti-EBV titers			Sampling interval (months)
				At detection	Under treatment	After chest radiographic improvement	
1	9	F	BHL	640	2560	640, 40	6, 5, 8
2	14	M	BHL	160	160, 160, 2560		11, 7, 13
3	13	M	BHL	160			
4	13	F	BHL+ Parenchymal lesions	160			
5	12	M	BHL+ Parenchymal lesions	640		160, 160, 40	14, 13, 7
6	11	F	BHL+ Parenchymal lesions	640		640, 640, 160	25, 27, 3

Extrathoracic lesions : No. 2 Eyes, tonsils, liver
No. 3 Liver
No. 4 Liver
No. 5 Eyes, liver
No. 6 Liver

with hepatic lesions," in this conference, antibody titers to EB virus were higher in sarcoidosis patients than in normal controls and patients with other diseases. These titers became lower after chest radiographic improvement. A similar tendency was also observed in 6 other children with sarcoidosis (Table 4).

DISCUSSION

It must be emphasized that if the above procedures are performed in the case of children, the systemic lesions of sarcoidosis will be found in these children. For instance, we could detect a high percentage of hepatic lesions by peritoneoscopy and liver biopsy. Extrathoracic lymph node lesions detected by lymphography will be discussed in this conference by Dr Ishida.

As for the radiographic course of these children, most improved, but 2 symptomatic cases with marked extrathoracic lesions became worse.

SUMMARY

1) Since 1960, 20 children with sarcoidosis were detected by us. Mean incidence rate per 100,000 was 0.3 in primary school and 0.5 in middle school in the Osaka area.

2) Most of them are asymptomatic and their clinical course was good. But some of them showed marked extrathoracic lesions and relapsed.

REFERENCES

1. Kendig, E. L. 1962. *J. Ped.* **61**: 269.
2. Mandi, L. 1964. *Acta Tuberc. Scand.* **45**: 256.
3. Niitsu, Y. 1967. La Sarcoidose. Paris: Masson et cie. p. 392.

4. Jasper, P. L., and Denny, F. W. 1968.   *J. Ped.* **73**: 499.
5. Siltzbach, L. E., and Greenberg, G. M. 1968. New Engl.   *J. Med.* **279**: 1239.
6. Niitsu, Y., et al. 1969.   *Fifth Int. Conf. on Sarcoidosis.* 1969. p. 506.
7. Tachibana, T. et al. 1969.   *Fifth Int. Conf. on Sarcoidosis.* 1969. p. 554.

Intrathoracic Sarcoidosis in Children

Yasutaka Niitu, Masahiro Horikawa, Tomiko Suetake, Sumio Hasegawa, Hideo Kubota and Shigeo Komatsu

Department of Pediatrics, The Research Institute for Tuberculosis, Leprosy and Cancer, Tohoku University, Sendai, Japan

In foreign countries, cases of intrathoracic sarcoidosis in children have been reported: 13 cases by Kendig,[1] 8 cases by Beier,[2] 22 cases by Jasper,[3] 18 cases by Siltzbach,[4] 22 cases by Vojetek,[5] 48 cases in Milan district, Italy, by Giobbi,[6] and 41 cases in Hungary by Mandi.[7] The cases reported by Giobbi and Mandi were found by chest X-ray surveys; most cases reported by other authors were found in the clinic. The reason why intrathoracic sarcoidosis was not frequently observed in children as compared with adults may have been that X-ray surveys are not widely made among children in foreign countries.

In Japan, mass chest X-ray surveys have been widely carried out in primary and middle schools, and the recognition of intrathoracic sarcoidosis by doctors has stimulated them into finding more cases. One hundred and seventy-nine cases of intrathoracic sarcoidosis in children were reported before the end of 1969 according to the surveys by the Japan Sarcoidosis Committee.[8] 50 cases were reported by Niitu,[9] 9 cases by Matsushima,[10] and 15 cases by Tachibana.[11]

Here we will report clinical, laboratory, and epidemiological findings observed in intrathoracic sarcoidosis in children.

We have observed 55 cases of intrathoracic sarcoidosis in children with ages ranging from 8 to 15 years. Thirty-five were male and 20 were female. All cases were found in mass chest X-ray surveys in primary and middle schools and had no complaints. Thirty-eight cases were found by routine annual X-ray surveys in Sendai and 3 cases by extra surveys in Sendai. The other 14 cases were found by surveys in other districts and subsequently visited our clinic.

X-ray findings showed bilateral hilar lymphadenopathy in all of the 55 cases and additional lung involvement in 6 cases. Superficial lymph nodes were palpable in 44% of the cases and iridocyclitis was noted in 1 case. No involvements of other organs were noted.

Diagnosis of sarcoidosis was made in 25 cases (45%) from clinical findings, i.e., X-ray findings, confirmation of the development of the X-ray findings within 1 year, and negative or weak tuberculin reaction. Diagnosis was made in 30 cases (55%) from histopathological findings and/or positive Kveim test in addition to the clinical findings.

Positive results were obtained in 86% of 22 samples of biopsied scalene lymph nodes and 3 of 5 samples of biopsied peripheral lymph nodes. Biopsy of follicles of conjunctiva was performed in 18 cases and gave positive results in 56% of them. This follicle biopsy is rather simple and is recommended for wide use, if follicles are observed.

Because of the wide administration of BCG vaccination, over 90% of the schoolchildren in Sendai have shown positive tuberculin reaction. With sarcoidosis cases, the tuberculin reaction was negative in 84% of the 55 cases, as tested within 3 months after detection. In 17 cases it was positive at the first test but soon became negative. Twenty three cases negative to 1 : 2,000 OT or 0.005 γ of PPD were tested with a higher concentration of tuberculin, 1 : 100 OT or 0.05 γ of PPD, and positive reaction was obtained in 61% of them, showing that the depression of tuberculin reactivity was not very strong in sarcoidosis. In 16 cases positive to the tuberculin test, the reaction was weak and showed only redness and no induration.

Leukocyte and lymphocyte counts of peripheral blood were less in mean values for sarcoidosis as compared with the normal mean values reported in corresponding ages in Japan,[12] showing that lymphocyte counts decreased in sarcoidosis (Table 1). The levels of serum protein and gammaglobulin showed higher mean values in sarcoidosis as compared with normal values reported in corresponding ages in Japan,[13,14] demonstrating that they were increased in sarcoidosis (Table 2). Blood sedimentation rate was not accelerated over 25 mm an hour in the 55 cases tested. Eosinophilia was observed in 25% of 40 cases studied. Increase in serum uric acid over 6 mg/dl was observed in 38% of 42 cases studied. Uric acid in 24-hour urine over 1 g was observed in only 1 of 16 cases studied. Increases in calcium content in serum and in 24-hour urine were observed in only 1 case. Thus, hypercalcemia or hypercalciuria was very rare in the present cases.

With lung function tests of vital capacity, lung volume, residual volume to total lung capacity, and diffusion capacity, though values outside normal ranges were observed in 5 to 21% of cases, higher grades of impairment were not observed in any case.

Regarding the prognosis, 1 year after the detection of the disease, the X-ray findings had been restored to normal in 92% of 48 cases studied. Forty-nine cases were followed up for more than 1 year. Abnormal X-ray findings remained in 2 cases, 1 and 5 years after detection, and had been restored to normal in 47 other cases within 2 years after detection. One patient became blind. The results reveal that the prognosis of intrathoracic sarcoidosis in children, as found in mass chest X-ray surveys is fairly good, as

TABLE 1.   Leukocyte and lymphocyte counts in sarcoidosis at detection, as compared with normal values by age reported in Japan.

Age	No. of cases	Leukocyte count (mean)		Lymphocyte count (mean)	
		Sarcoidosis	Normal value* by age	Sarcoidosis	Normal value* by age
8–10 years	9	7,777	7,435–7,950	2,627	3,082–3,806
11–15 years	32	5,887	6,680–7,310	2,118	2.774–3,353

* Oya[12] (1967).

TABLE 2.   Total protein and gammaglobulin of sera in sarcoidosis at detection, as compared with normal values reported in Japan.

	Age in years	No. of cases	Total protein of serum (g/dl)	Gammaglobulin of serum protein (%)
Sarcoidosis	8–15	33	7.5*(6.6~8.3)	15.3 (7.9~23.8)
Normal values {Momma[13] (1967)	5–10	27	7.1 (5.9~8.3)	10.3 (5.9~14.7)
	11–14	18	6.9 (5.9~7.9)	11.1 (6.3~15.9)
Hara[14] (1970)	5–10	73	6.9±0.6	12.0±3.9
	11–14	28	6.8±0.6	13.1±4.0

* ≧8.0 g/dl in 8 cases (24%).

previously reported by Niitu and associates,[9,15,16] in contrast to the results reported by Siltzbach,[4] who observed mainly cases of children with complaints.

Epidemiological observations were made on the 38 Sendai cases found in the routine annual X-ray surveys made on all school children with ages ranging from 6 to 15 years. Table 3 shows the annual incidence of intrathoracic sarcoidosis found in the surveys from 1953 to 1972. The rate was lower in primary schools and higher in middle schools. The recent incidence among middle schools was 1.0 per 10,000. The rate has been

TABLE 3. Incidence of intrathoracic sarcoidosis found in routine mass chest X-ray surveys among school children in Sendai.

Year	Primary school (6~11 years of age)		Middle school (12~14 years of age)	
	No. of X-rays surveyed	New cases No. per 10,000	No. of X-rays surveyed	New cases No. per 10,000
1953	39,926	1 0.3	17,753	
1954	42,929		19,436	
1955	44,850		20,515	
1956	64,860		21,814	
1957	49,134		21,267	
1958	51,653	1 0.2	19,471	
1959	53,143		18,093	
1960	49,673		21,206	1 0.5 ⎫
1961	47,110		25,240	4 1.5 ⎪
1962	44,421		27,981	1 0.4 ⎪
1963	42,620		27,059	5 1.8 ⎬ 1.1
1964	41,426		25,605	3 1.2 ⎪
1965	41,469	3 0.7	24,036	2 0.8 ⎭
1966	41,700		22,249	
1967	42,500		21,173	4 1.9 ⎫
1968	43,462	1 0.2	20,767	3 1.4 ⎪
1969	43,931		20,609	3 1.5 ⎪ 1.0
1970	44,351	2 0.5	20,741	1 0.5 ⎬
1971	45,499	1 0.2	21,098	1 0.5 ⎪
1972	47,102	1 0.2	21,184	⎭

Total 38 cases.

TABLE 4. Age and sex of 38 children with intrathoracic sarcoidosis found in the routine chest X-ray surveys in primary and middle schools in Sendai (1960-72).

Sex	Age in years								Total
	8	9	10	11	12	13	14	15	
Male	1 ⎫		⎬	2 ⎫	6	5	8	1 ⎬	23 (61%)
		1				22			
Female	4 ⎫	1	1 ⎬	1 ⎫	3	3	2 ⎬		15 (39%)
		6				9			
Total	5 ⎫	1	1 ⎬	3 ⎫	9	8	10	1 ⎬	38
		7 (18%)				31 (82%)			

Clinic of Sarcoidosis in Children

Branislav Djurić and Vojin Bašičević

*Institute of Tuberculosis and Chest Diseases and Institute for Maternity
and Child Care, Novi Sad, Yugoslavia*

It is known that sarcoidosis in children has been rarely described so far. In the last 2 decades McGovern and Merritt, Kendig, Mándi and Niitu have described sarcoid changes in a number of children.

TABLE 1. Our patients. Sex and age of the patients at the time diagnosis was established.

	Age groups				Total
	0–3	4–7	8–10	11–14	
Male	—	6	—	1	7
Female	—	3	2	1	6
Total	—	9	2	2	13

At the time when diagnosis was established, the age of our patients ranged from 5 to 14. Age distribution was as follows: 2 boys aged 5 (they were our youngest patients), 1 boy aged 6, 3 boys and 3 girls aged 7, 1 girl aged 9, 1 girl aged 10, 1 boy aged 11 and 1 girl aged 14. Clinical signs and symptoms are usually of a mild nature: cough, dyspnoea, asthenia, loss of appetite, pains in the abdomen, thorax and joints. Most often the children are afebrile, less frequently subfebrile.

In 1 patient with diagnosis established at the age of 5, predominant symptomatology developed in the third year of his life and later on the symptoms progressed and new ones occurred.

At the time diagnosis was established, tuberculin allergy was found negative in all 13 children. Only 1 patient showed a positive tuberculin reaction (10×10 mm) to increased PPD concentration subsequently, and BK was negative. In the other child, negative even to high PPD concentrations, positive tuberculin allergy developed 2 years later. BK was not found even after repeated studies.

Records on earlier TB patients in the family were found in 3 children. At the time this diagnosis was established no known sources of infection in the presented patients were found.

Erythema nodosum was not recorded in any of our patients.

Erythrocyte sedimentation rate was normal in most cases; in 4 children it was slightly accelerated. In most cases the leucocyte count of the blood picture was normal; in 2 children it was lightly increased and in 3 slightly reduced. Serum calcium level was investigated in 8 patients and it was within normal limits. Gammaglobulins were increased in half of the examined cases.

Predominant pathologic changes indicating sarcoidosis were enlarged lymph nodes in the hilus, first degree BHL and, in 1 patient, second degree BHL.

In addition to the clinical picture, diagnosis of sarcoidosis was made in 12 children on the basis of a positive Kveim test, in 1 child by prescalene lymph node biopsy (Kveim test was not performed in this case).

In 1 patient (a 5-year-old boy with sarcoid edema of the locomotor apparatus) slightly more complete histopathologic diagnostics comprising skin biopsy, subcutaneous tissue, synovia, striated muscles (m. quadriceps), peripheral lymph nodes, liver and Kveim test were performed. All the results obtained agreed reasonably well.

In 12 patients, localization of sarcoidosis was found in hilar lymph nodes. In addition, changes in peripheral lymph nodes were found in 4 patients. In 1 child, as mentioned above, pathologic changes in liver, spleen, skin, subcutaneous tissue and in the locomotor apparatus were found.

Treatment was carried out in 6 patients with corticoids; therapy was conducted long-

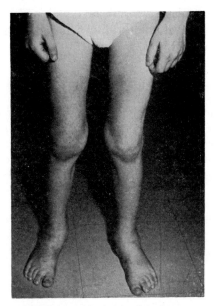

Fig. 1.   A 5-year-old boy with sarcoid edema of the locomotor apparatus-histologically proved.

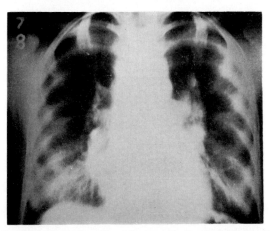

Fig. 2.   This shows intrathoracic sarcoidosis of a 14-year-old girl.

er than 2 months in 4 children and was done regularly. Prednisolone dose was 1 mg/1 kg pro die. In 1 child, 6-month corticoid therapy was preceeded by Resochine for 2 months. The best succes was obtained in this child with the above therapy (changes in the locomotor apparatus with T, edema of joints, enlarged spleen and liver).

The illness got worse in the girl (aged 14) with enlargement of the hilar nodes. The patient refused therapy with Prednisolone.

SUMMARY

Thirteen children with sarcoidosis were presented. The youngest was 5-year-old. All children were found to be tuberculin negative. Kveim tests were performed in 12 children and found positive. Calcium in serum was normal in all children while gammaglobulins were increased in half of the examined cases. In 12 children enlarged hilar lymph nodes, and in 4 cases enlarged peripheral lymph nodes, were observed. The case of a 5-year-old child is of especial interest, in whom sarcoid granulomas were found in the joint synovia, liver, skin and skeletal muscles.

REFERENCES

1. Levine 1956. Sarcoidosis in Childhood. *Advances Pediatrics* **8**: 97.
2. Kendig, E. 1960. Sarcoidosis in Children *Amer. Rev. Resp. Dis.* **5**: 49–51.
3. Mandi, L. 1964. Sarcoidosis in Childhood. *Acta Med. Scand.* Supp. **325**: 216–217.
4. Niitu, Y. 1966. Intrathoracic Sarcoidosis found among School Children in Sendai in Mass X-ray Surveys of the Chest. *La Sarcoidose*, Paris. p. 392–399.

Sarcoidosis Among Children in the United States

Edwin L. Kendig, Jr.

5801 Bremo Road, Richmond, Virginia 23226, U.S.A.

Since February, 1953, there have been only 4 series of cases of sarcoidosis in children under 15 years of age reported in the United States. One of these was a group of 8 cases of rather atypical sarcoidosis reported from Utah and Idaho, an area in which sarcoidosis in adults appears to be extremely rare. The others included 18 cases reported by Siltzbach and Greenberg in New York, 25 cases reported by Jasper and Denny (hereinafter referred to as the North Carolina group) and the 7 cases previously reported at the Medical College of Virginia. To date there have been 19 cases so diagnosed at the Medical College of Virginia. This presentation will include a comparison of 3 of the reported United States' series in an attempt to provide a picture of the "typical" case of sarcoidosis among children in the United States.

The most commonly involved organ is the lung—with the typical lesion, bilateral hilar lymphadenopathy, with or without parenchymal involvement. You will note that 60 of the 62 cases (97%) had such involvement.

Next in frequency is peripheral lymph node involvement which occurred in 43 of 62 cases (69%).

Eye lesions were relatively frequent, 25 of 62 (37%) and often serious with blindness occurring in 5 cases (22% of those with eye lesions).

Skin lesions occurred in 31% (19 of 62) of the cases and there was bone involvement in only 10% (6 of 62).

The liver was palpable in 40% (25 of 62) of the cases and the spleen was enlarged in 32% (20 of 62).

The most common laboratory finding was hyperglobulinemia, which occurred in 75% (46 of 61) of the cases. This is really the only significant laboratory finding.

Next in frequency among the laboratory findings is eosinophilia (above 4%), which occurred in exactly one-half of the 44 cases in which the statistics are available.

Leukopenia (white blood cell count below 5,000) was present in 37% (7 of 19) of the Medical College of Virginia cases.

The incidence of both hypercalcemia and elevated alkaline phosphatase varied greatly. Hypercalcemia was present in one-third of the cases tested (19 of 57) and the incidence of elevated alkaline phosphatase was the same (6 of 18 cases).

The typical pediatric patient diagnosed as sarcoidosis in the United States is a preadolescent or adolescent (9 to 15 years of age in 61 of 62 cases), black (44 of 62 cases), who has bilateral hilar lymphadenopathy (97%), frequent eye lesions (23 of 62) which are often serious (5 with blindness), and hyperglobulinemia (46 of 61 cases).

DISCUSSION

Chairmen: E. L. Jr. Kendig and R. Mikami

Dr Matusima: Since 1962, 15 cases of sarcoidosis under 15 years of age were observed at Maebashi. There were 9 boys and 6 girls. Four cases were 7–9 years and 11 cases were 10–15 years.

Diagnosis was made by biopsy and/or Kveim test in 9 cases, clinically in 6 cases. Tuberculin reaction was negative in 11 cases. In all these 11 cases it was positive prior to the onset of sarcoidosis. Thirteen cases were asymptomatic and found in routine chest X-ray surveys. The other 2 cases complained of ocular symptoms, and visited ophthalmologists first.

Enlargement of bilateral hilar lymph nodes were found in all cases, and faint mottling of the lungs in 6 cases. Uveitis was found in 6 cases. In 2 cases it was severe or moderate with blurring of vision, in the others minimal and asymptomatic. Superficial lymph nodes were markedly enlarged in 3 cases. It seems noteworthy that 2 of these 3 cases showed broad mediastinal shadows suggesting thymic largement, which I reported in the session 'Extrathoracic sarcoidosis'. Swelling of parotid gland was found in 1 case. Skin lesions and bone lesions were found in no cases. Serum calcium level was normal. Gammaglobulin was elevated only in 1 case.

Although the prognosis of childhood sarcoidosis is very good, as Niitu pointed out, I tried short-term administration of corticosteroid, in order to shorten its course. Prednisolone was administered for a short period of 6 to 8 weeks in 14 cases. In 6 cases hilar lymph node enlargement regressed rapidly and subsided in a short time without relapse. In the other 8 cases the administration of steroid seemed to have scarcely any influence on the natural course of the disease.

Prognosis was good. Chest X-ray findings cleared in all cases within 2 years. But in 1 case uveitis of 1 eye resulted in loss of vision due to cataract formation after one and half years.

Dr Kendig: A few years ago, Dr Siltzbach remarked to me that he thought the low incidence of sarcoidosis in children was reflected by the fact that there was no routine mass radiography in this age group. It certainly seems that he is correct in that. However, I did note that Dr Djuric showed a much lower age limit and perhaps somebody might like to comment on that.

Dr Israel: It seems to me that the extremely thorough X-ray surveys performed in Japan have disclosed a low frequency of sarcoidosis below the age of 10, and have established that in fact sarcoidosis is extremely rare before adolescence. Dr Putkonen has informed me that experience in Finland is that the Kveim reaction is usually negative in children with sarcoidosis. This has been true in the only 3 cases of childhood sarcoidosis that I have tested. I wonder whether the speakers can present any data on Kveim tests in children with sarcoidosis.

Dr Niitu: We performed Kveim tests in 13 childhood sarcoidosis and obtained positive results in 5 of them.

Dr Stork: I wonder if some of these cases with rather prominent hilar lymphadenitis in the young—around 6–7 years old—which we see in our chest clinic, and with a negative tuberculin test, are sarcoidosis? Most of these show leukopenia, and never come to biopsy because they are not sick, and in approximately 3 to 4 months the adenitis has practically all faded and nothing more is done about it. I wonder if we are overlooking a mild case of sarcoidosis in these children? I would like your comments, Dr Kendig. How long does the hilar lymphadenitis in children with sarcoidosis last?

DR KENDIG: We don't have many cases, but I would say I have seen 10 in the past year. I think that is probably a significant number. In our own area, a glandular enlargement which persists longer than a month is followed up or the node is excised for examination.

DR JOHNS: We have had a very similar experience at Johns Hopkins to yours Dr Kendig and I have seen about 15 such children. I wonder if anyone else has had a comparable experience in that 2 of them had thrombocytopenic purpura of clear and marked magnitude. This obviously could be the coincidental idiopathic type, but one wonders whether it might be related to sarcoid. All of these children had very clear pictures of rather typical sarcoidosis.

DR KENDIG: That is very interesting. We had no such experience. Has anybody else?

DR HOSODA: I have a question to put to Professor Niitu. You showed an area in which a large number of sarcoidosis cases were concentrated. Is there any difference in incidence rate between that area and other areas?

DR KENDIG: It is interesting that there is a certain area in the country in which there is more sarcoidosis than in others: there is 1 county (district) in Virginia in which there is an incidence of presumptive sarcoidosis of 500 per 100,000 population.

DR NIITU: This slide shows the incidence rate of pulmonary sarcoidosis in each of 23 middle schools in Sendai for last 11 years. In this particular school, 6 cases of pulmonary sarcoidosis were found and the incidence rate was 5.9 per 10,000, showing the highest value. In some schools, nearly 20,000 children were surveyed but no cases were found. The incidence rate varied greatly among schools. This clearly shows the local accumulation of sarcoidosis.

We have observed that about 30% of childhood cases with Mycoplasma pneumoniae infections show hilar lymphadenopathy with or without lung lesions and that some of them show only bilateral lymphadenopathy. The lymphadenopathy associated with Mycoplasma pneumoniae infections disappears within 1 to 2 months. I think that lymphadenopathy in these cases must not be mistaken for sarcoidosis.

DR VILLAR: In Portugal, where sarcoidosis is rare, we did find a case of sarcoidosis out of 11 children with bilateral hilar lymphadenitis. The most curious feature of this case was the very evident multisystemic localizations of the disease. There were granulomas in random biopsies of the bronchi, in the liver and there were eye lesions. It was clearly a very serious form of sarcoidosis that cleared up very nicely on steroids. She also had a negative Kveim test.

DR KENDIG: I think the finding of so many cases, particularly in those areas where mass radiography of children is utilized, now provides a much better opportunity for the study of the disease in children. This has been particularly exemplified by the work of Dr Niitu, Dr Tachibana and Dr Djuric.

XI THERAPY

Results of Treatment with Lampren and Prolixan (Azapropazone) in Sarcoidosis

K. WURM

University of Freiburg, Freiburg, Federal Republic of Germany

Generally, corticoid therapy is considered today as the method of choice in the treatment of sarcoidosis, but on account of various other effects, particularly in long-term therapy, it is not without problems and risks. We are, therefore, still searching for medicaments suitable for the treatment of sarcoidosis.

Leprosy and sarcoidosis are very similar to each other from the histomorphological point of view. Recently, Lampren as a monotherapeutic as well as in combination with corticosteroids, has shown excellent results in the treatment of leprosy.

Lampren, the riminophenazine derivate of clofazimine (B 663), is a compound of a chemical group which so far has not been therapeutically used and has significant anti-inflammatory (antiproliverative) properties. It is well-tolerated and nontoxic. The only side effect is a red-brown discoloration of the skin.

Therefore, it has been of interest to include Lampren in the treatment of sarcoidosis. In the last 2 years we treated 45 cases of sarcoidosis of stages I, II, and III with Lampren alone or in combination with corticosteroids. The daily dose in all cases was 1 capsule (=100 mg).

We could observe neither a roentgenological improvement of the lung manifestations nor a therapeutic effect of Lampren in sarcoidosis, as shown in Table 1.

James[1] reported positive results with *Tanderil* (oxyphenbutazone) in the treatment of pulmonary sarcoidosis. For that reason we started trials with the presently well-appraised *azapropazone* (Prolixan (R) 300), a compound developed from an alkaline flavine. As the table shows, Prolixan 300 has been used so far in 35 sarcoidosis patients, of whom 11 used Prolixan exclusively and 24 in combination with triamcinolone. The daily dose was in each case 900 mg Prolixan orally. The period of treatment was several weeks minimum, and in 50% of the cases more than 3 months.

Eight patients out of 11 treated exclusively with Prolixan showed roentgenological improvement. This is a rate which excludes coincidental spontaneous remission. The therapeutic effect with Prolixan was demonstrated most obviously in the group using combined therapy, namely 24 cases treated with Prolixan plus corticosteroids and 19 with Lampren plus corticosteroids. The smaller Lampren group showed 4 failures and 1 deteriorating in the therapeutically favourable stage II, whereas in the larger Prolixan group only 1 failure (in the hard-to-influence stage III) and no deterioration in any case could be observed.

Based on these preliminary results *we are concluding that Prolixan 300 represents an effective and a very well-tolerated sarcoidosis therapeutic*, although somewhat less effective than corticosteroids. When used in combination, a corticosteroid-sparing effect is possible. As a monotherapeutic it is a particularly indicated in the secondary phase of treatment in the sense of a recidive prophylactic agent after remission following earlier therapy.

TABLE 1. Clinical trials in sarcoidosis of the lung.

a) Lamprene alone (Clofazimin, B 663)

Stage	Duration (Months)	Number	Improvement					Worsening	Side effects
			0	?	+	++	+++		
I	<3	4	2		1			1	
	3–6	8	6		1			1	twice
	>6	7	5	1					
II	<3	2	1	1					once
	3–6	2	1	1					
	>6	1	1						
III	3–6	1				1			
	>6	1	1						

b) Lamprene and Steroids

Stage	Duration (Months)	Number	Improvement					Worsening	Side effects
			0	?	+	++	+++		
I	<3	5	2		1	2			
	>6	2				2			
II	<3	7	2				4	1?	twice
	3–6	3				3			
	>6	1				1			
III	>6	1				1			

c) Azapropazone alone (Prolixan® 300)

Stage	Duration (Months)	Number	Improvement					Worsening	Side effects
			0	?	+	++	+++		
I	<3	7	2		2	2	1		
	3–6	2		?	1				
II	<3	1	1						
	3–6	1				1			

d) Azapropazone combined with steroids

Stage	Duration (Months)	Number	Improvement					Worsening	Side effects
			0	?	+	++	+++		
I	<3	1			1				
	3–6	5		1	2	2			
II	<3	6			3	2	1		once
	3–6	6			2	4			once
	>6	3				2	1		
III	<3	3	1		1	1			

In particular, it can be recommended in all forms of sarcoidosis, acute as well as chronic, if there are pains in the joints, in the back, in the muscles or in the ligaments. These clinical observations are the basis for some general thoughts. It is apparent from the negative results with Lampren and the positive effect with Prolixan that, based on the histomorphology, no conclusion can be drawn as to the possible effect of a drug. It is a general principle that the effect of a compound is based on an enzymatic interaction. We know that every inflammation is caused by disorders of the various lysosomal enzymes and that the enzymatic situation is specific to a disease.

In the trials made thus far,[2] we could observe a significant increase of collagen peptidase as a feature of sarcoidosis. According to further findings, steroids show a strong inhibitory effect on the activity of collagen peptidase. Prolixan also inhibits this enzyme, although in a lesser degree.

There is a significant correlation between the therapeutic effect and the decrease in the activity of collagen peptidase: the quicker and lower the decrease in the enzyme activity, the better the therapeutic effect. The lower therapeutic effect of Prolixan correlates with its lesser reduction of the enzyme activity and this can be evaluated as a real pharmacodynamic effect.

Further experiments will show whether the determination of collagen peptidase is a general informational test for the clinical investigation of new drugs in the treatment of sarcoidosis. However, the *final* evaluation of investigational drugs should be based on clinical data. An international agreement would be highly appreciated, and I would like to propose the following criteria for further discussion.

1) Selection

a) Only diagnostically clear cases, confirmed by biopsy or Kveim reaction or sarcoid-specific roentgenological stages[3] without any evidential complications not belonging to sarcoidosis should be considered.

b) Acute courses (Loefgren's syndrome) are not suitable for testing medication because of coincidence with spontaneous remission, as well as present gravidity.

2) Stages

The therapeutic effectiveness for sarcoidosis is dependent on the stage. It is therefore necessary to differentiate the test cases by their stages.

3) Course tendency

According to the course of sarcoidosis before administering a medication, the effect of the therapeutic agent will be different. Therefore, the test cases should be divided into stationary, progressive and regressive cases and separately evaluated in accordance to their course during the earlier period without treatment.

4) Duration test

In cases of sarcoidosis with lesions of the skin, peripheral lymphomas, tumors of parotid and uveitis anterior, the effect of corticoid medication will show within 2–3 weeks. In cases of pulmonary sarcoidosis, a radiological improvement occurs in 3 to 4 weeks. This duration should also be the basis for the evaluation of test preparations.

An effective therapy with drugs will be assumed if during a treatment of only several weeks an improvement can be seen, but only in cases where the disease showed previously during months or years a stationary or even progressive course.

5) Recidivity test

An efficacious effect can be assumed in cases where, after initial improvement, the medication is discontinued and afterwards a relapse occurs within 1 to 3 months. In case of spontaneous remission, relapses are not to be expected or perhaps extremely rarely and after a much longer space of time. The ensuing relapse excludes a spontaneous remission and consequently proves the therapeutic effect.

6) Iridocyclitis test

A highly sensitive and quick test is indicated in cases of iritis nodosa. In this case the ophthalmologist can, by means of his instruments, almost under microscopic conditions, and administering peroral corticoid medication, note a decrease in the cell flow in the aqueous humour and a decrease of the nodules in the iris within a few days. Because of its sensitivity, this test is very suitable for the determination of the minimum effective dose (dosis efficax minima).

Only the criteria 5 and 6 justify the evaluation of the single case referring to the therapeutic effectiveness of the medication. In general, the effectiveness of a medication for sarcoidosis should only be taken for granted when similar results have been observed in a larger number of analogous cases: i.e., course, stages and tendency. In this way, possible coincidental spontaneous remissions and erroneous post hoc conclusions will be avoided.

REFERENCES

1. James, D. G. 1969. *Internist* **19**: 316.
2. Stojan, B., Müller, W., Wurm, K., and Tariverdian, M. T. 1972. *Schweiz. Rundschau Med.* (Praxis) **61**: 591.
3. Wurm, K. 1971. *Fifth Int. Conf. on Sarcoidosis*. Prague: Univ. Karlova. p. 483.
4. Wurm, K. 1967. *Mschr. Tuberk. Bekpf.* **10**: 57.

A Follow-up Study of Treated and Untreated Early Pulmonary Sarcoidosis

Olof Selroos, Markus Niemistö and Nils Riska

Fourth Department of Medicine,Helsinki University Central Hospital,
Helsinki, and Mjölbolsta Hospital, Finland

This report is concerned with the results obtained in a follow-up examination of patients with early pulmonary sarcoidosis. During the years 1960–1966, we diagnosed 132 patients with a duration of disease known to be less than 1 year before diagnosis. A total of 115 patients took part in the follow-up study made in 1971. Three patients had died, 1 from myocardial infarction, 1 from malignant hypertension with cerebral palsy, and 1 from gastric carcinoma. Fourteen patients did not participate. The age and sex distributions of the final series are indicated in Table I. In all 115 cases, the clinical picture was consistent with sarcoidosis. The diagnosis was also supported in every case by a positive Kveim test (79 patients) or positive biopsy specimen (83 patients). The initial chest radiographic findings were found to be stage I in 67 cases (26 in combination with erythema nodosum), and stage II in 48 cases (6 in combination with erythema nodosum).

Because of a change in attitude towards indications for corticosteroid therapy in sarcoidosis, it has been possible to divide the total material into 2 parts: primarily treated patients, diagnosed in 1960–1963, and primarily untreated patients diagnosed in 1963–1966. Corticosteroid treatment was given with an initial prednisone dose of 30–50 mg per day for 2–4 weeks, gradually decreased to a maintenance dose of 7.5–10 mg for 3–12 months (mean duration of treatment, 6 months).

At the follow-up examination in 1971, 89 of the 115 patients were subjectively in good health. Nineteen patients had symptoms or signs of diseases other than sarcoidosis, and 7 had a sarcoid disease that was still active.

Figure 1 illustrates the development of the chest radiographic findings of those patients with changes that were initially stage I. Forty-three of the 46 primarily untreated patients recovered. In 3 cases, steroid treatment was begun because of the ap-

TABLE 1. Age at diagnosis and sex distribution of 115 patients with early pulmonary sarcoidosis.

Age group (in years)	No. of patients		Total
	Women	Men	
15–19	1	—	1
20–29	11	13	24
30–39	23	12	35
40–49	28	6	34
50–59	18	1	19
60–	2	—	2
Total	83	32	115

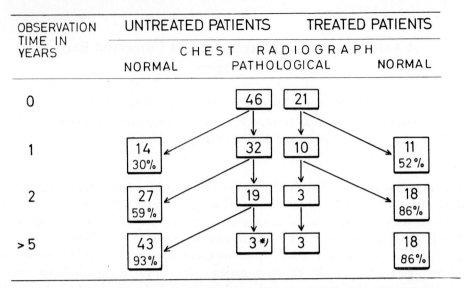

FIG. 1. Development of chest radiographic findings in primarily untreated and treated sarcoidosis patients with initially stage I changes. x) Treatment with corticosteroids started because of progressive pulmonary infiltrations.

pearance of progressive pulmonary infiltrations during the time of observation. Although these cases are now inactive, residual changes are observable in the chest radiographs. The primarily treated patients exhibited more rapid normalization of their radiographs. After observation for 1 and 2 years, the percentage of cured patients was higher in this group than in that of untreated patients. Nevertheless, the final result was no better. After observation for at least 5 years, 86% had recovered, as compared with 93% in the group of untreated patients. Of the 3 patients with a pathological radiograph, 2 have an inactive disease but with residual changes, and 1 patient has a still-active sarcoidosis, with general multisystem involvement. Of the 18 patients with a normal chest radiograph in 1971, 5 had had stage II parenchymal infiltrations during the course of the disease after the initial treatment had been discontinued. In 4 cases, the radiograph cleared up after a second course of treatment, and did so without treatment in the fifth case.

Figure 2 indicates the course of the patients with changes that were initially stage II. Of the 23 primarily untreated patients, only 10 had recovered after 2 years of observation, but 20 (87%) had done so after at least 5 years. In 3 cases, rapidly deteriorating ventilatory function led to the beginning of therapy. At the moment, 1 of these patients has an inactive disease, but with residual pulmonary infiltrations; 2 patients have an active disease with multisystem involvement. Of the 25 patients initially treated with steroids, 20 fully recovered after a period of at least 5 years. In 6 cases, the relapses occurred after the treatment had been discontinued, but after a second course of treatment—and in 1 case after a third course—the radiograph was normalized. In 5 cases, the radiograph is still pathological. Four of these patients have developed multisystem sarcoidosis that is still active.

The above figures are valid for the total series. When analysing different parameters it was noticed that the prognosis was better in patients initially suffering from erythema nodosum as compared with patients without erythema nodosum. The same was ap-

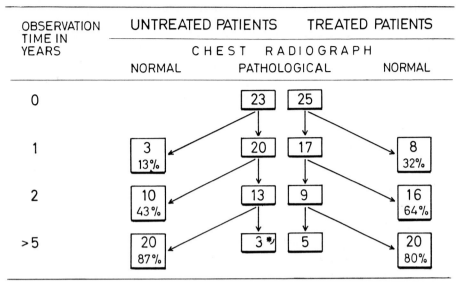

FIG. 2. Development of chest radiographic findings in primarily untreated and treated sarcoidosis patients with initially stage II changes. x) Treatment started because of progressive pulmonary infiltrations.

parent for patients with a high tuberculin sensitivity (positivity to 0.1–1 TU) as compared with patients with initially more depressed tuberculin sensitivity (positivity to 10–100 TU or tuberculin negativity to 100 TU), for patients below the age of 40 as compared with older patients and finally for the female sex as compared to the male sex.

The series in question is not particularly large, and treatment was not started by the application of any alternative-case regimen. However, it is noteworthy that of the 7 patients who did not recover during the time of observation, 5 belonged to the group of patients initially treated with steroids. Moreover, recurrences are more common in the treated group. Accordingly, the results obtained support earlier observations that treatment with corticosteroids is of minor prognostic value in sarcoidosis with pulmonary changes of stage I and II, but without extrapulmonary manifestations.[1–5]

Mention should also be made of some findings in laboratory studies made during the investigations. Determinations of the total serum protein concentration and the electrophoretic fractions during the active and cured stages of the disease were as follows. In the active phase, diminished albumin and elevated α_2-, β- and γ-globulin fractions were observable. They were all normalized in the cured state.

Persistently elevated serum calcium values were noted in 12 patients during the active phase (stage I, 6 patients, stage II, 6 patients); 7 of them had received prednisone treatment. All the patients were normocalcemic in the cured state.

Table 2 contains a summary of some immunological investigations. A positive Latex fixation test was detected in 8 females of the 38 tested during the active phase, but in no male patient of 20 tested. Six of the patients with an initially positive test were also positive after recovery. Twelve other female patients, negative during the active phase, were found to be positive at the follow-up examination. Of the 18 Latex-positive patients, 2 were suffering from clinically active rheumatoid arthritis. The remaining 16 patients were Waaler-Rose-negative, and did not display any signs of rheumatoid disease.

TABLE 2. Immunological investigations in patients with early pulmonary sarcoidosis.
(No. of pathological tests / No. of tests performed.)

Investigation	Active stage	Inactive stage
Latex fixation	8/38 females	18/78 females
	0/20 males	0/29 males
Antistreptolysine titer	16/86	2/103
Antistaphylolysine titer	1/32	1/103
Immunofluorescent nuclear antibodies		
Polyvalent antiserum		8/43 females
		0/15 males
IgG antiserum		5/43 females
IgM antiserum		5/43 females
Direct Coombs' test		1/58

Sixteen patients of 86 tested had an elevated antistreptolysin titer in the active phase; this was also observable after the precipitation of lipids. Nuclear antibodies were demonstrated by the application of immunofluorescent technique in 8 female patients of 43 tested; 3 patients had an elevated IgG titer, 3 an elevated IgM titer, and 2 had elevated titers of both IgG and IgM. These immunological reactions were observable in both treated and untreated patients, and their clinical significance is still obscure.

CONCLUSION

The prognosis of early pulmonary sarcoidosis of stages I and II is favourable in Finland. The initial occurrence of erythema nodosum, high tuberculin sensitivity, age below 40 years and female sex favour an especially good prognosis. The utility of corticosteroids is no more than suppressive during the initial phase of the disease, and leads to a false conception of its favourable effect. Moreover, it seems probable that the risk of recurrence and of chronicity of the disease increases if steroids are administered, particularly if they are given for only 4–6 months.

REFERENCES

1. Hapke, E. J., and Meek, J. C. 1971. Steroid treatment in pulmonary sarcoidosis. *Fifth Int. Conf. on Sarcoidosis*. Prague: Univ. Karlova. p. 621.
2. Israel, H. L., and Beggs, R. A. 1971. Prednisone treatment of sarcoidosis. A controlled study. *Fifth Int. Conf. on Sarcoidosis*. Prague: Univ. Karlova. p. 617.
3. Scadding, J. G. 1967. Sarcoidosis. London: Eyre and Spottiswoode.
4. Sharma, O. P., Colp, C., and Williams, M. H. 1966. Course of pulmonary sarcoidosis with and without corticosteroid therapy as determined by pulmonary function studies. *Amer. J. Med.* **41**: 541.
5. Young, R. L., Harkleroad, L. E., Lordon, R. E., and Weg, J. G. 1970. Pulmonary sarcoidosis: a prospective evaluation of glucocorticoid therapy. *Ann. Internal Med.* **73**: 207.

A Controlled Trail of Prednisone Treatment of Sarcoidosis

HAROLD L. ISRAEL, D. W. FOUTS AND ROBERT A. BEGGS

Departments of Medicine and Preventative Medicine, Jefferson Medical college,
Thomas Jefferson University, Philadelphia, U.S.A.

The action of corticosteroids on the lesions of sarcoidosis has seemed prompt and consistent in pathologic, physiologic, radiologic, and clinical studies.[1-5] However, a recent controlled study[6] showed no significant effects and whether these drugs alter the eventual outcome of the disease has never been established. Authorities differ as to whether adrenal steroid therapy should be confined to relief of symptoms or extended more widely in the hope of averting pulmonary fibrosis and other major complications.[7,8]

A controlled clinical trial of corticosteroids in sarcoidosis was instituted in 1961, and a preliminary report[9] of the results was presented in 1969; the present evaluation (Table 1) is based on study of patients observed at a mean interval of 5 years after the trial.

TABLE 1. Clinical, radiologic and spirographic evaluation of 83 patients in controlled trial of prednisone therapy of sarcoidosis.

		Improved	Unchanged	Worse
Evaluation at end of 3-month trial		32	44	7
Stage I	Placebo	6	10	1
	Prednisone	11	4	5
Stage II–III	Placebo*	4	21	0
	Prednisone*	11	9	1
Evaluation 5.3 years after trial		44	25	14
Stage I*	Placebo	9	6	2
	Prednisone	14	6	0
Stage II–III*	Placebo	11	10	4
	Prednisone	10	3	8

* Significant difference : $p < 0.05$.

Three-month evaluation

Stage I   On completion of treatment 59% of patients in the steroid group and 35% of controls were improved; the difference is not significant.

Stages II and III   Fifty-three % of treated patients were improved and 41% were unchanged. In contrast, 17% of controls improved while 83% were unchanged. The difference between treated and control groups is significant ($P = <0.025$).

Long-term evaluation

Stage I   After a mean observation interval of 5.2 years, 70% of treated patients and 53% of controls were classified as improved.

Stages II and III   Definite improvement was noted in 48% of treated patients and 44% of the controls at the end of a mean observation interval of 5.3 years. The difference in outcome between patients originally receiving prednisone and those receiving placebo was not significant (P=>0.1).

The outcome in those with pulmonary involvement at the onset of the trial was significantly worse than in those with mediastinal adenopathy alone (P=<.05).

DISCUSSION

The patients who completed the present trial represent a sample typical of sarcoidosis in the United States. Evaluation of the 83 patients, treated and untreated, at the end of a mean observation period of over 5 years, shows complete clearing in 37%, improvement with residuals in 16%, and worsening in 17%, while 30% were classified as unchanged. These figures are similar to those observed in a previously reported study[10] of patients in Philadelphia, and in a large clinic population in New York.[11]

Six-month trials of medication have been used by other investigators.[6,12-14] These studies in smaller groups and shorter periods of observation have given varying results. Only James, Trowell and Carstairs[12] have reported significant improvement as the result of treatment, not only in patients receiving prednisone but also in those given oxyphenbutazone. McLean and Carter's study of 16 patients with advanced disease gave equivocal results.[13] Hopke and Meek[14] followed 11 matched pairs for 4 years; radiologic and physiologic studies revealed no differences between those originally treated for 6 months and the controls. Young and his associates[6] studied the effect of 60 mg of prednisone for 1 month and 20 mg for 5 months in 25 military personnel with impaired respiratory function. Treated and control groups showed no difference in response during treatment or after 1 to 2 years follow-up.

Our observations support the view that corticosteroids have significant and important palliative effects while medication is given but are unsuccessful in averting pulmonary fibrosis or serious extrathoracic manifestations of sarcoidosis. The controlled studies reported, despite their limitations, offer no encouragement for routine administration of corticosteroids to patients with sarcoidosis in the absence of distressing symptoms, hypercalcemia or ocular involvement.

Deenstra and Van Ditmars[8] reported a high recovery rate from prolonged use of high doses of corticosteroids in a large series of patients in the Netherlands. There is no way of establishing that this approach gave better results than those obtained by administration of corticosteroids on a symptomatic basis.

The patients included in the present study are a representative sample, including many patients detected in radiographic surveys (31 cases), as well as patients seeking medical attention because of skeletal,[2] ocular,[5] cutaneous,[9] and respiratory (34) symptoms. Only a single patient had erythema nodosum. The greater frequency of erythema nodosum in Europeans and the better prospects associated with this manifestation, are familiar but unexplained facts. The outcome was significantly more favorable among patients who did not have pulmonary involvement on admission to the study, but disappearance of hilar and mediastinal adenopathy was not as frequent or rapid as European reports[7] indicate. It has been suggested that the apparent greater frequency of progressive disease in the United States is the result of ethnic influences. However, a recent analysis[15] of Veterans Administration data which included large numbers of black and white men revealed no ethnic difference in mortality.

An unexpected observation in the present investigation was the frequency of chronic forms of sarcoidosis. In earlier studies of the course of the disease, a relatively small percentage was classified as " unchanged " and it was assumed that since patients in this category had been followed for relatively short periods, recovery or progression would occur within a few years. In the present material, after a mean interval of observation of more than 5 years, almost a third of the patients were neither definitely better nor worse. One-third of patients admitted to the study with stage I disease have had persistent lymphadenopathy, and have shown no significant changes in symptoms or in ventilatory function. A sixth of patients who had pulmonary infiltration at the time of admission to the study remained essentially unchanged in clinical, radiologic and ventilatory status 5 years later. It is evident that a sizeable number of patients have extremely chronic or torpid sarcoidosis.

Eight patients received chlorambucil therapy. Since this agent was administered only to patients who appeared to have severe progressive disease not responding to prednisone it is noteworthy that 3 patients recovered fully and 1 was markedly improved. Two patients are classified as unchanged and 2 progressed. In view of these favorable late results, further trials of immunosuppressive therapy in sarcoidosis are indicated.

SUMMARY

Ninety patients with sarcoidosis were enrolled in a randomized trial of the effect of 3 months of prednisone therapy. Eighty-three patients completed treatment and were followed for at least a year. In 37 patients with hilar lymphadenopathy alone on admission to the study, no significant difference between treated and control groups was noted either at the end of the treatment period or after a mean interval of 5.2 years. In 46 patients with pulmonary infiltration on admission to the study, significant improvement was evident at the end of the treatment period but no differences between treated patients and controls were demonstrable after a mean interval of 5.4 years. The prognosis was significantly better in patients entering the study with hilar adenopathy alone. These observations support the views, widely but not universally held, that prednisone exerts little influence on the eventual outcome of sarcoidosis but is ameliorative in patients with pulmonary involvement.

REFERENCES

1. Sones, M., Israel, H. L., Dratman, M., and Frank, J. H. 1951. Effect of cortisone in sarcoidosis. *New Engl. J. Med.* **244**: 20.
2. Siltzbach, L. E. 1952. Effects of cortisone in sarcoidosis. *Amer. J. Med.* **12**: 139.
3. Scadding, J. G. 1961. Prognosis of intrathoracic sarcoidosis in England. *Brit. Med. J.* **2**: 1165.
4. Sharma, O. P., Colp, C., and Williams, M. H. 1966. Course of pulmonary sarcoidosis with and without corticosteroid therapy as determined by pulmonary function studies. *Amer. J. Med.* **41**: 541.
5. Hoyle, C., Smyllie H., and Leak, D. 1967. Prolonged treatment of pulmonary sarcoidosis with corticoseroids. *Thorax.* **22**: 519.
6. Young, R. L., Harkleorad, L. E., Lordon, R. E., and Weg, J. G. 1970. Pulmonary sarcoidosis. A propsective evaluation of glucocorticoid therapy. *Ann. Internal Med.* **73**: 207.
7. Scadding, J. G. 1967. Sarcoidosis. London: Spottiswoode and Eyre.

8. Deenstra, H., and Van Ditmars, M. J. 1968. Sarcoidosis. *Dis. Chest* **53**: 57.

9. Israel, H. L., and Beggs, R. A. 1971. Prednisone treatment of sarcoidosis. A controlled study. *Proc. Fifth Int. Conf. on Sarcoidosis*. Prague: Univ. Karlova. p. 617.

10. Sones, M., and Israel, H. L. 1960. Course and prognosis of sarcoidosis. *Amer. J. Med.* **29**: 84.

11. Siltzbach, L. E. 1967. Sarcoidosis: clinical features and management. *Med. Clin. No. Amer.* **51**: 483.

12. James, D. G., Trowell, J. M., and Carstairs, L. S. 1967. Treatment of Sarcoidosis. Controlled therapeutic trial. *Lancet* **2**: 526.

13. McLean, R. L., and Carter, F. M. 1967. A controlled trial of corticosteroids in pulmonary sarcoidosis. *La Sarcoidose*. Paris: Masson et cie.

14. Hapke, E. J., and Meek, J. C. 1971. Steroid treatment in pulmonary sarcoidosis. *Proc. Fifth Int. Conf. on Sarcoidosis*. Prague: Univ. Karlova.

15. Keller, A. Z. 1971. Hospital, age, racial occupation, geographical, clinical and surviorship characteristics in the epidemiology of sarcoidosis. *Amer. J. Epid.* **94**: 222.

A Double-Blind Controlled Trail on the Effect of Corticosteroid Therapy in Sarcoidosis

R. Mikami[1], Y. Hiraga[2], K. Iwai[3], T. Kosuda[4], H. Mochizuki[5],
H. Homma[5], H. Osada[6], Y. Chiba[6], R. Soejima[7], M. Odaka,[8],
Y. Hosoda[8], T. Hashimoto[8], H. Yanagawa[9],
I. Shigematsu[9] and K. Nakao[10]

Japan Sarcoidosis Committee

The effectiveness of corticosteroids for sarcoidosis is generally accepted, but opinions are divided on the indication, dosage and the period of medication. This study was made to reach some conclusion about the value of corticosteroid therapy in the treatment of sarcoidosis with bilateral hilar adenopathy. Cases, drawn from all over the country, were assigned at random to steroid and placebo groups and observed by the double-blind method. Pregnant cases or severe cases were withdrawn.

MATERIALS AND METHODS

The method of medication and items of examination are shown in Table 1. Drugs were given for 6 months. The doses of predonisolone were 30 mg a day for the first 4 weeks, followed by 20 mg for 4 weeks, 10 mg for 4 weeks and 5 mg for the remaining 12 weeks. The same number of placebo tablets was given to the control cases. X-rays were taken before, during and after medication; namely, before treatment, at 2, 4, 8, 12, 16, 20, 24 and 30 weeks, and then at 12 months. The period of observation is so far limited to 1 year. The registered cases in this trial totalled 141. During the study, however, 40 cases were excluded for various reasons. Thus this study was performed on the remaining 101 cases; 50 cases in the steroid group and 51 cases in the placebo group. Both groups were matched in age distribution, showing the highest frequency in the 20-year age group (Fig. 1). As for the sex, the placebo group contained more female cases than the steroid group.

Figure 2 illustrates the locations of lesions involved in sarcoidosis expressed as number of cases. Beside BHL and pulmonary involvements, ocular involvement was seen most frequently, in about 40% of cases. There were also a few cases with cutaneous and osseous involvement. There was no marked difference between the steroid and placebo

1) *Tokyo University School of Medicine, Tokyo, Japan.*
2) *JNR Sapporo Hospial, Sapporo, Japan.*
3) *Japan Antituberculosis Association Research Institute, Tokyo, Japan.*
4) *Kanto-Chuo Hospital, Tokyo, Japan.*
5) *Toranomon Hospital, Tokyo, Japan.*
6) *JNR Central Hospital, Tokyo, Japan.*
7) *Kumamoto University Medical School, Kumamoto, Japan.*
8) *JNR Central Health Institute, Tokyo, Japan.*
9) *National Institute of Public Health, Tokyo, Japan.*
10) *Jiji Medical School, Tochigi, Japan.*

TABLE 1. Method of study.

Subject : 101 adult cases of sarcoidosis with BHL confirmed with biopsy
Medication : Randomly administered " Steroid " or " Placebo "
　" Steroid " : (50 cases) 5 mg tab. of Prednisolone (" Donisolone " Sankyo)
　" Placebo " : (51 cases) Tablets with the same taste and appearance as " Donisolone "
Doses of drugs and items of examinations :

Period	0 w	2 w	4 w	8 w	12 w	16 w	20 w	24 w	30 w	1 yr
Doses (tab.)		6	4	2		1				
Chest X-ray	O	O	O		O	O	O	O	O	O
Blood exam.	O	O	O		O			O		
Immunoglobulin	O							O		
Urinalysis	O				O			O		
Tuberculin	O				O			O		
Kveim test	O									
Ophthalmology	O				O			O		
Dermatology	O				O			O		

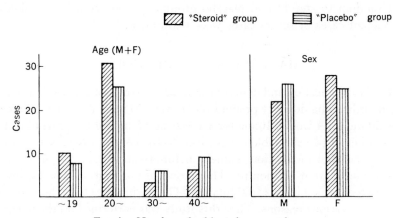

FIG. 1. Number of subjects by age and sex.

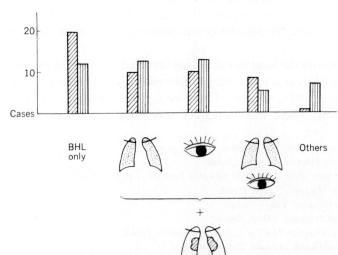

FIG. 2. Involvement of sarcoidosis.

TABLE 2. Method of evaluation of X-ray findings.

1	Comparison between "before treatment" and 2, 4, 12, 24 weeks after treatment
2	Criteria of evaluation
	Slightly improved: 10–50% improved of total findings
	Markedly improved: 50–90%
	Cleared: More than 90%
	Unchanged: Less than 10% changed
	Worsened: New shadows or enlargement
3	Improvement rate: All improved and cleared cases/total cases
	Marked improvement rate: Markedly improved and cleared/total
	Clearing rate: Cleared cases/total

groups. The effect of medication was evaluated as follows (Table 2). The X-ray film before treatment was compared with the film 2, 4, 12, 24 weeks after treatment. The criteria of the course of X-ray findings were; slightly improved, markedly improved, cleared, unchanged and worsened. The rate of improvement or clearing was calculated as shown in Table 2.

RESULTS

The improvement rate and clearing rate of BHL was investigated. In Fig. 3, the upper curve of the shaded area of each group shows the improvement rate when all the "medication-suspended" cases were excluded from the analysis. The lower curve of the shaded area means that all these withdrawn cases were taken and included in the group showing no improvement. Thus the improvement rate should be somewhere within the shaded area. The larger shaded area in the placebo group means that more cases dropped out from the latter group than from the steroid group. The improvement rate was better in the steroid group than in the placebo group at 2, 4 and 8 weeks. These differences are statistically significant. There was no such difference after 12 weeks. Concerning the clearing rate, the steroid group exceeded the placebo group. At 8 weeks the difference is once more statistically significant. Again after 12 weeks or so, there was no difference between the 2 groups.

The improvement rate and clearing rate of lesions in lung parenchyma are shown in Fig. 4. The steroid group had a higher improvement rate than the placebo group for the first 12–24 weeks. The differences are statistically significant at 4, 8 and 12 weeks. However, the difference disappeared after 24 weeks. As for the clearing rate, the steroid group was higher for the first 24 weeks than the placebo group. The difference is statistically significant at 12 weeks. After 24 weeks, the difference was no longer discernible.

Figure 5 represents the clearing rate of all the involvements in sarcoidosis, such as the clearing rate of BHL, lung lesion, ocular involvement and so on. At 3 months, the steroid group looks better than the placebo, but the difference has no statistical significance. In 6 months or later, the clearing rates of both groups were very close to each other. The clearing rate in 1 year ranged from 50% to 70% in both groups. The worsening of the initial involvement or new appearance of lesions is summarized in Table 3. In the placebo group, worsening of the initial lesion was noted in 16 cases and new lesions appeared in 4 cases, as shown in parentheses. On the other hand, in the steroid group, worsening was

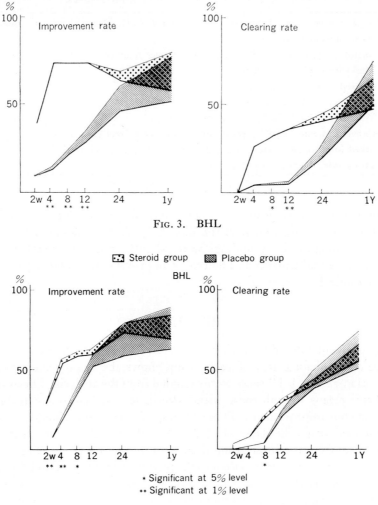

FIG. 3.   BHL

FIG. 4.   Pulmonary lesions.

noted only in 8 cases and new lesions appeared in 2 cases. In particular, in the period up to 8 weeks, worsening or new lesions were observed in none of the steroid group. Thus steroid therapy was effective against worsening of the initial lesion and suppressed the appearance of new lesions, at least for the first 1 to 2 months of treatment. Thereafter, no difference was noted in the 2 groups. Table 4 shows the number of cases withdrawn in each group for the above reasons. In the placebo group, most of them were dropped as a result of worsening or no improvement, while none were withdrawn for reasons relevant to the steroid group during treatment.

Undesirable side effects are given in Table 5. In 36% of the cases in the steroid group there were complaints such as moon face, obesity, acne, hypertrichosis, and vomiting; 15.7% of the cases in the placebo group had such complaints as moon face, obesity and acne. Herpes zoster occurred in 1 case in both groups. In 1 case in the steroid group, steroid was discontinued because of melena, and 2 cases were dropped from the placebo group due to vomitting and epigastralgia.

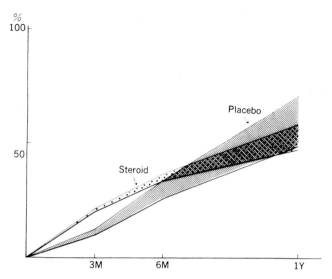

FIG. 5.   Clearing rate of all involvements.

TABLE 3.   Worsening of initial involvement or new appearence.

Lesion / Period	"Steroid" group		50 cases	"Placebo" group		51 Cases
2W				1	4(1)	1
~4W					1(1)	
~8W					2	1
~12W		1(1)			1	1(1)
~24W		2			1(1)	1
~1Y	1	3(1)	1		2	

(   ): New Appearance
(Secondary Mention)

TABLE 4.   Medication-suspended cases.

Period	Reasons	Steroid group	Placebo group
During treatment	Worsening	0	6
	No improvement	0	3
	Side effect	1	2
	Others	2	2
After treatment	Worsening	3	1
	No improvement	2	2
	Total	8	16

TABLE 5. Undesirable side effects.

	" Steroid " group	" Placebo " group
Cases with side effects	18 (36.0%)	8 (15.7%)
Moon face	6	2
Obesity	7	1
Acne, Hypertrich.	4	3
Herpes zoster	1	1
Vomiting	1	1*
Epigastralgia	2	1*
Melena	1*	

* Dropped cases.

CONCLUSION

Double-blind study revealed the following results. Treatment with prednisolone for 6 months accelerated the improvement of bilateral hilar lymphadenopathy (BHL) and pulmonary lesions, especially during the first month of the treatment; or it prevented further worsneing. However, after 1 year the overall improvement rate in the steroid group was no different from that of the placebo group being around 50%–70%. Therefore, steroid therapy should be indicated for those patients whose pulmonary involvement was progessive, for the purpose of averting fibrosis.

REFERENCES

1. Scadding, J. G. 1967. Sarcoidosis. London: Eyre and Spottiswoode. p. 520.
2. Israel, H. L., and Beggs, R. A. 1971. Prednisolone treatment of sarcoidosis. A controlled study. *Fifth Int. Conf. on Sarcoidosis.* Prague: Univ. Karlova. p. 529–531.
3. Bolecek, O. 1971. Development of sarcoidosis in seventy-two patients treated with corticotherapy in the first stage of the disease. *Fifth Int. Conf. on Sarcoidosis.* Prague: Univ. Karlova. p. 539–540.
4. Hapke, E. J., and Meek, J. C. 1971. Steroid treatment in pulmonary sarcoidosis. *Fifth Int. Conf. on Sarcoidosis.* Prague: Univ. Karlova. p. 621–625.

Long-Term Study of Corticosteroids in Pulmonary Parenchymal Sarcoidosis

Carol Johnson Johns, James B. Zachary, Mary C. Riley,
Sami Brahim and Wilmot C. Ball, Jr

*Department of Medicine, The Johns Hopkins University School of Medicine
and Hospital, Baltimore Md., U.S.A.*

This study reports our experiences with a consecutive series of 152 patients with symptomatic pulmonary parenchymal sarcoidosis treated with corticosteroids. The patients have been followed both clinically and with serial measurements of pulmonary function. It represents an extension of our earlier series of 60 patients reported in 1966.[1]

MATERIALS AND METHODS

The study includes all patients with incapacitating or progressive pulmonary parenchymal sarcoidosis followed at the Johns Hopkins Hospital and treated with corticosteroids during the past 10 years. During this time, approximately 500 patients with sarcoidosis have been evaluated. The present group consists of 152 patients of whom 139 (92%) are black, 11 (7%) are white and 2 are American Indians. Females predominated with 112 (74%) and 40 (26%) were males.

All patients had a compatible clinical picture as well as histologic support of the diagnosis by biopsy of lymph node, liver, skin, lung or Kveim test. There was no supportive evidence for other recognized causes of granulomatous disease.

Almost all patients received 300 mg of isoniazid daily as prophylaxis in this area with a high incidence of tuberculosis.

Significant pulmonary symptoms were the major indication for treatment in all but a few patients and all had objective evidence of pulmonary parenchymal disease. The treatment schedules were individualized according to the clinical situation, but the most frequently used program with prednisone is outlined in Table 1.

Table 2 indicates the age of the patients at the time treatment began. Seventy-seven

TABLE 1. Prednisone treatment schedule.

40 mg, 30 mg (divided doses)	2 wks each	
25 mg single 8 a.m. daily dose	2 wks	6½ months
20–15 mg single 8 a.m. daily dose	5 months	
12.5, 10.0, 7.5, 5.0, 2.5 mg.	2 wks each......2½ months	
Careful observation during tapering		
Retreat if relapse occurs.		

Alternate day equivalents for maintenance and tapering, if desired.

Supported in part by grants from the Maryland Tuberculosis Association and the Eudowood Women's Board.

TABLE 2. Age when steroids begun.

Years	No. of patients	% patients
15 or less	4	3%
16–20	14	9%
21–30	77	51%
31–40	34	22%
41–50	15	10%
Over 50	8	5%
	152	

(51%) were in the third decade, with 73% included in the third and fourth decades combined.

Serial pulmonary function studies were carried out on all patients. Ventilatory studies consisted of a forced vital capacity using a Stead Wells 10-liter spirometer. The predicted normal values were those of Goldman and Becklake.[2] Steady-state resting carbon monoxide diffusion studies have been performed serially on all patients seen since 1962, using the method of Bates, with end-tidal sampling.[3]

All pulmonary function data (approximately 1000 studies) since 1963 were available for computer storage, analysis and retrieval, and were correlated and coordinated with prednisone dosage.

RESULTS

Pulmonary Function Studies

The computer analysis of these studies are summarized in Table 3–10. The statistical analysis was possible for varying numbers of patients, depending on the specific parameter defined. Table 3 identifies groupings of the patients with respect to severity of reduction of vital capacity at 3 points in time: the earliest, the study at the time of maximal vital capacity (" best ") and the most recent study (" latest "). After treatment the decreased frequency of severe reduction in vital capacity is indicated, with change from 54% to only 17% at the time of maximal response. However, with the passage of time, this again increases to 33% but this still represents improvement. Similarly, the mildly affected groups increased significantly, but again the improvement is not fully sustained. Similar observations are documented in Table 4 with regard to the magnitude of loss of diffusing capacity.

The base line was defined as that study just prior to the initiation of corticosteroid treatment.

TABLE 3. Patient distribution (145 patients).

Vital capacity % pred.		Earliest		Best		Latest	
Less than 55%	(Severe)	31	54%	5	17%	15	33%
55–64%	"	23		12		18	
65–74%	(Moderate)	26	26%	28	28%	26	26%
75–84%	(Mild)	15	20%	32	55%	24	41%
85% or more	"	5		23		17	
		100%		100%		100%	

TABLE 4. Difference between predicted and measured diffusing capacity
(ml CO/min/mm Hg).

Diffusing capacity	Earliest		Time of max VC		Latest	
Loss of >10 (Severe)	22⎫	60%	6⎫	35%	9⎫	43%
Loss of 6–10 „	38⎭		29⎭		34⎭	
Loss of 4–6 (Moderate)	17	17%	24	24%	19	19%
Loss of 2–4 (Mild)	11⎫	23%	18⎫	41%	18⎫	38%
Loss of <2 „	12⎭		23⎭		20⎭	
	100%		100%		100%	

TABLE 5. Time from base-line pretreatment to highest vital capacity
(99 patients).

	% patients
Less than 6 months	31%
6–12 months	28
1–2 years	21
2–3 years	13
More than 3 years	7

TABLE 6. Increase in vital capacity (88 patients).

Liters	Base line to best (%)			Base line to latest		
less than 0.25	21			36		
0.25–0.49	27			23		
0.50–0.99	42⎫	52	79	32⎫	41	64
1.0 or more	10⎭			9⎭		

TABLE 7. Maximal pulmonary function improvement (81 patients).
(Base line to best)

Change in vital capacity	Change in diffusing capacity			
	<2.0	2.0–3.9	4.0 or more	
<0.25 l	15 pts.	2	2	23%
0.25–0.49 l	15	5	2	27%
0.50–0.99 l	10	9	13	40%
1.0 or more	1	2	5	10%
	51%	22%	27%	

Analysis of the time interval from this base line to that of maximal observed percent of predicted vital capacity (Table 5) reveals that 31% reached this value within the first 6 months and 59% within the first year. However, significant numbers achieved their highest vital capacity after 2 years. For most, improvement is prompt but others demonstrate more gradual change.

Table 6 reveals the amount of increase in vital capacity for 88 patients for whom good " base-line " data could be identified. An increase of 500 ml or more is demonstrated in

52% and 79% show increases of 250 ml or more. The falloff with time is again noted.

Table 7 compares the improvement in vital capacity and diffusing capacity between the earliest study and that at the time of the " *best* " vital capacity. Here 50–77% showed significant increases of at least 0.5 l or 0.25 l respectively. Simultaneously, the diffusing capacity showed definite increases in only 27%, though was suggestive in 49%. In 51%, there was no significant increase in the diffusing capacity.

Table 8 compares the base-line diffusing capacity and the most recent study (" latest ") in 94 patients. Approximately half show no significant change, with 36% at least suggestively improved: 15% show a decrease.

Table 9 compares the changes in pulmonary function between the base line and most recent studies in the 82 patients on whom adequate data was available for computer analysis. Significant gains in vital capacity are almost twice as frequent as significant improvement in diffusing capacity.

Table 10 presents an overview for the entire group, indicating the final outcome for both vital capacity and diffusing capacity at the time of the latest study. These are categorized and indicated as % of the total group and compared with the earliest study groupings indicated in parentheses. Definite trends toward improvement are indicated in both vital capacity and diffusing capacity.

TABLE 8.　Change diffusing capacity base line to latest (94 patients).

Decrease of more than 2	15%	(Worse)
±2	49%	(No change)
Increase 2–4	17% } 36%	(Better)
Increase more than 4	19%	

TABLE 9.　Pulmonary function change : base line to latest.

Vital capacity	Diffusing capacity				Total
	Loss	±	Gain 2.1–4.0	Gain >4.0	
<0.25 l	9	17	1	2	29 (35%)
0.25–0.49 l	2	15	2	1	20 (24%)
0.50–0.99 l	2	7	6	10	25 (30%)
1.0 or more l	0	2	3	3	8 (10%)
Total	13 (16%)	41 (50%)	12 (15%)	16 (19%)	82 patients

TABLE 10.　Patient distribution (earliest) latest study.

Vital capacity	Diffusing capacity				% Earliest	% Latest
	<8.0	8.0–11.9	12.0–15.9	>16		
<55%	13 pts	7	1	0	(31)	15
55–64	10	11	3	2	(23)	18
65–74	6	9	15	7	(26)	26
75–84	4	11	11	8	(15)	24
85%+	0	7	9	9	(5)	17
(Earliest) %	(23)	(38)	(26)	(12)		
Latest	21	33	28	18		

REVIEW OF CLINICAL COURSE

Table 11 indicates the total time period from earliest treatment to most recent treatment in the study period. More than half the patients have been treated and observed for more than 2 years (51%). Twenty-five % have required treatment for 5 or more years. Multiple courses of treatment have frequently been required, as shown in Table 12, with 13% requiring 3 or more courses, and 39% 2 or more courses. The prolonged duration and multiple courses are necessitated by symptomatic and objective relapses when treatment is withdrawn. A " course " is defined as a period of treatment followed by an interval without treatment. Many other relapses occurred as the dose was reduced and increased dosage was required.

At the time of review of the most recent patient data (Table 13) 95 of the 152 (62.5%) were apparently still on prednisone treatment. The clinical status was uncertain in 17 of these who had been lost to follow-up. Fifty-seven (37.5%) were off treatment. Of these 29, or approximately one-fifth had remained well after a good response to treatment.

TABLE 11.   Period of treatment.

	No. patients	(% patients)
Less than 1 year	30	(20%)
1–2 years	44	(29%)
2–5 years	40	(26%)
5–10 years	31	(20%)
More than 10 years	7	(5%)
Total	152	

TABLE 12.   Number of courses of treatment.

	No. patients	%
1	93	61
2	39	26
3	12	8
4	4	3
5	2	1
6 or more	2	1
Total 245 course	152 patients	

TABLE 13.   Recent status.

	No. patients
Treatment continued	
Clinically improved	78 ⎱ 95
Uncertain	17 ⎰
Off treatment	
Improved-no relapse	29 ⎫
Uncertain	12 ⎪ 57
No Effect	2 ⎬
Dead	14 ⎭
Total	152 patients

TABLE 14. Deaths–152 patients–10 years.

Pulmonary insufficiency	7
Aspergillosis	2
Hemoptysis massive	1
Intercurrent pneumonia	1
Sudden death ? cause	1
Hypertensive CVD	2
Total deaths	14

TABLF 15. Recent status.

	No. patients	% patients
Clinically improved	107	71
Uncertain	29	19
No effect	2	1
Dead (earlier benefit)	14	9
Some benefit	150	99
No effect	2	1

There were 14 deaths in this group of 152 patients over this 10-year period of study (Table 14). The most frequent cause of death was pulmonary insufficiency in 7 and related pulmonary problems in 4 additional patients. Two of these had terminal disseminated aspergillus infection.

In summary, (Table 15), review of the recent status indicates that 71% of the patients were clinically improved with less than 10% dead. Review of the entire series over the period of 10 years shows that all but 2 patients demonstrated clinical benefit at least earlier in the study.

DISCUSSION

This study has provided both the opportunity for day-to-day participation in the care of these patients and retrospective analysis of their course and serial pulmonary function data. Direct clinical observations provide a strong impression of the favorable influence of prednisone treatment upon their course. Repeated well-documented relapses occurring even after 10 years of treatment strongly suggest that the treatment was having significant impact upon the course of the disease.

The severity of the disease in these patients, because this is a hospital population, distinguishes this group from other series comprising mild, relatively asymptomatic cases. In such a series, it is clearly difficult to demonstrate significant benefits from treatment. The vast predominance of blacks may influence the course and prognosis in this series. Progressive relapsing disease seems more frequent in Negro patients than in Caucasians.

Corticosteroids are usually by no means the perfect cure for sarcoidosis. At best, they significantly suppress the inflammatory reaction, thereby often abolishing symptoms and returning the patient towards normal. A few patients respond to treatment and remain well with no further evidence of activity of their disease. If such a remission continues for a few weeks or months after treatment is discontinued, it is unlikely that subsequent relapse will occur.

If continued corticosteroid therapy is required to suppress disease activity, an obvious relapse becomes apparent shortly after treatment is discontinued or as the dose is tapered. Reinstitution of low-dose prednisone usually again rapidly reverses the process. It appears that when a patient has demonstrated 1 relapse, the likelihood of repeated relapses is increased and extended low-dose maintenance therapy may be indicated. However, periodic gradual attempts to withdraw treatment are certainly justified and indicated.

The serial use of simple noninvasive measurements of pulmonary function is of great assistance in following the course of disease and response to treatment. Although the pulmonary function improves, and the patient may be without symptoms, residual evidence of impairment is often noted. Changes in vital capacity usually reflect quite accurately the course of the disease. The vital capacity increases more frequently and significantly in response to treatment than the diffusing capacity. The latter more frequently remains reduced. Changes in breathing pattern and ventilation introduce significant variation in the determination of the steady-state carbon monoxide diffusing capacity, making it more difficult accurately to determine and assess. In some patients, and perhaps more frequently in Caucasians, there may be significant radiographic changes with little or no abnormality of pulmonary function measurements.

With computer analysis of the measurements of pulmonary function of the approximately 1,000 studies, the gradual decline with time, compared to the point of maximal improvement becomes evident. This doubtless represents a number of different factors. These include possible progressive disease, in spite of treatment, inadequate periods or delinquencies in treatment, or simply the ravages of time.

Complications were infrequent and usually not serious. A cushinoid state with excessive weight gain was most frequently observed, especially in females. A few developed diabetes, especially in association with significant liver disease. Multiple fungus balls were observed in 7 patients. Five of these are still living and without evidence of invasive disease, though 3 are of known duration of 4–8 years. Problems related to these fungus balls have been limited to occasional small hemoptyses, similar to those in patients with bronchiectasis, even though it has proved necessary to continue corticosteroid treatment to control the sarcoid. Other complications included reversible exacerbation of underlying psychiatric disorders. There was 1 patient who demonstrated tuberculosis several months after isoniazid had been discontinued. The most frequent problems were those of repeated bronchopulmonary infections and pulmonary insufficiency in those patients with severe fibrocystic changes.

SUMMARY

Previous studies are extended with a consecutive series of 152 patients with incapacitating pulmonary parenchymal sarcoidosis treated with corticosteroids. Ninety-two % of the patients were black and 74% females. Clinical response was almost uniformly favorable but often not complete or sustained. Prolonged treatment periods of 2–10 or more years were often required because of recrudescence of the disease process. Low-dose prednisone treatment (10–15 mg) appeared to prevent relapse. Twenty % remained well after the initial course of treatment, but 62.5% required continued treatment: 9% died.

Serial pulmonary function measurements to assess response to treatment revealed increases in vital capacity in two-thirds of the patients with only 33% with persistent significant reduction at the most recent study. The diffusing capacity was increased in one-third, with persistent significant reduction in 43%. Maximal responses usually occurred within 6–12 months. Prolonged follow-up revealed a trend towards reduction with the progress of time as determined in the most recent study.

Complications were infrequent and mild with the relatively low doses of prednisone required. Long-term corticosteroid therapy is strongly recommended for treatment of symptomatic pulmonary sarcoid in Negro patients to eliminate symptoms, improve pulmonary function, and suppress activity of the disease process, thereby reducing progressive damage. Although attempts to terminate treatment are indicated, the frequency of relapse necessitates careful observation during and after tapering. Reinstitution of treatment is often necessary.

REFERENCES

1. Johns, C. J., and Ball, W. C., Jr. 1967. Steroids in pulmonary parenchymal sarcoidosis with serial measurements of pulmonary function. *La Sarcoidose. Rapp. IV Conf. Int.* Paris: Masson et cie.

2. Goldman, H. I., and Becklake, M. R. 1957. Respiratory function tests: normal values at median altitudes and the prediction of normal results. *Amer. Rev. Tuberc.* **79**: 457.

3. Bastes, D. V., et al. 1962. Chronic bronchitis. A report on the first two stages of the coordinated study of chronic bronchitis in the Department of Veterans Affairs. Canad. *Med. Ser. J.* **18**: 211.

Long-Term Corticosteroid Treatment of Pulmonary Sarcoidosis

Olav Refvem

Medical Department A, Aker Hospital, Oslo, Norway

Any treatment program with a fair chance of succeeding, has to pay due attention to the crucial point in the natural course of sarcoid granuloma, namely its tendency to a more-or-less complete fibrotic transformation from about 2 years. Age differences between sarcoid nodules make development of lung fibrosis a steadily progressing process during active disease. Corticosteroids act on nonfibrotic and probably on early fibrotic infiltration. *The principle of treatment*, therefore, obviously must be to suppress reversible tissue changes and prevent relapses until the disease activity has ceased. Ideally, treatment should start before any fibrosis has developed.

Figure 1 gives a schematic presentation of the expected course of a single case with disease activity lasting 8 years—(A) when treated continuously from the nonfibrotic stage; end result: clear lungs;—(B) when treated continuously after some fibrosis has developed; end result: slight fibrosis;—and (C) when not treated; end result: extensive fibrosis.—It seems logical to assume that pauses, as practiced in intermittent treatment, will increase the danger of developing fibrosis, since during relapses parts of the granulomas will reach their fibrosing age.

Main indication for treatment is nonfibrotic infiltration of some extent and duration showing a stationary or progressive trend. To avoid the inclusion of many cases undergoing early spontaneous regression, treatment is not started until 14 to 18 months of

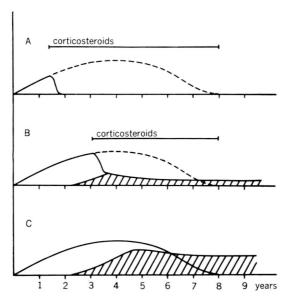

Fig. 1.   Effects of corticosteroid treatment.

547

infiltration. Massive densities call for earlier treatment. Infiltration of unknown duration is treated as soon as a nonregressive trend is clear. The same applies to partially fibrotic infiltration. Entirely fibrotic infiltration may be treated for symptomatic effect. Dyspnoea often is an indication for treatment, regardless of the extent or duration of the process.

Practical implementation

Prednisolone was used in practically all patients. Initial dose as a rule was 15 mg/day, if necessary 20 to 30 mg. For maintenance the lowest effective dose was used with 2.5–5 mg added for subradiological infiltration. Allowance had to be made for individual tolerance. In every patient a high-level physical activity was aimed at, to prevent osteoporosis and muscle wasting. The continuous medication was interrupted only about every second year by a short pause to explore disease activity. This was done by reducing stepwise prednisolone to zero through 4–5 weeks and controlling chest X-ray every month. Relapse indicated restarting prednisolone immediately. In this way, each patient served as his own control. Such pauses were tolerated unexpectedly well.

The material consisted of 76 patients, 38 females and 38 males. Duration of treatment is shown in Table 1. The effects on lung infiltration emerge from Table 2. In no case did infiltration increase during treatment. Special interest attaches to the outcome in 33 who had completed their treatment (Table 3).

Figure 2 is a contribution to the clarification of the important question: How long can the start of treatment be postponed without endangering results? Excellent results can be

TABLE 1. Duration of treatment.

Treatment	Cases	Treatment duration years		
		Total	Mean	Range
Completed	33	117	$3\frac{6}{12}$	$\frac{7}{12}-10\frac{8}{12}$
Continuing	43	161	$3\frac{9}{12}$	$\frac{4}{12}-12\frac{6}{12}$
Total	76	278	$3\frac{8}{12}$	$\frac{4}{12}-12\frac{6}{12}$

TABLE 2. Treatment effects on infiltration.

Pretreatment age of infiltration		Worse	Unchanged	Fair	Good	Excellent
$\leqq 2$ ys	25 cases				4	21
>2 ys	40 cases		9	9	13	9
Unknown	11 cases			2	3	6
Total	76 cases	0	9	11	20	36

TABLE 3. Treatment effects on infiltration.

Treatment completed	Worse	Unchanged	Fair	Good	Excellent
Total 33 cases	0	3	6	7	17

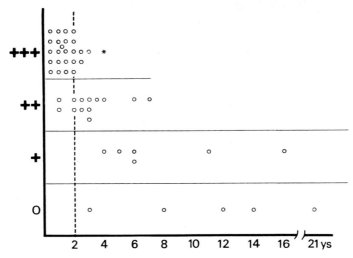

FIG. 2. Results related to age of infiltration before treatment in 49 cases.

TABLE 4. Effects of treatment on ventilation.

	Unchanged normal	Worse	Unchanged reduced	Improved
69 cases	38	4	8	19

achieved in some patients even when prednisolone is instituted as late as 3 years after the start of infiltration. On the other hand, an exceptional case may already prove refractory to treatment after 3 year's delay. Marked by an asterisk is a woman who achieved clear lungs in spite of not starting on prednisolone till 4 years of infiltration; obviously contributing to this result was the fact that she had had 2 full pregnancies during those 4 years. Chances of achieving full therapeutic effects decrease rapidly on starting later than 2 or 2½ years. Preferably, treatment should start some time before the critical limit in order to have sufficient " prefibrotic " time left for subsequent pauses necessary for assessing disease activity.

Ventilation was examined in 69 patients before and during treatment, using vital capacity, FEV_1'' and MVV or PEF (see Table 4). In 4 patients ventilation got worse, all of them having moderate or extensive fibrosis; in 1, low-dose medication was exclusively symptomatic. One of those 4 stopped treatment for 14 months. During that pause an irreparable, mainly obstructive deterioration of his ventilation occurred, and this fits in well with simultaneous increase of shrinkage on the chest X-ray.

Subjective complaints (dyspnoea, cough, stridor, mucus production) occurred in 46 patients prior to treatment, and of these 40 were improved. Side effects were few and mild. No patient developed tuberculosis or diabetes.

May I conclude by showing 2 X-rays of the patient with the longest treatment time, 12½ years up to now. When first discovered, in 1959 (Fig. 3), the duration of his extensive infiltration was unknown, but it reacted favourably to prednisolone, relapsing at every attempt to stop. This X-ray (Fig. 4) was taken this summer; it shows very slight fibrosis and is identical with that showing the early maximal response.

To summarize, continuous prednisolone treatment as described has a very good sup-

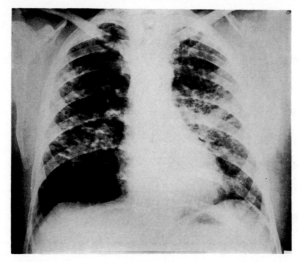

FIG. 3.

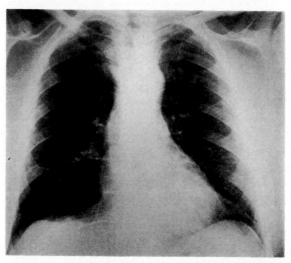

FIG. 4.

pressive effect on nonfibrotic and perhaps early fibrotic lung infiltration. Most interesting is the observation that, during treatment, infiltration from the minimum did not increase later (except just temporarily during probing pauses), not even in cases who had to continue on prednisolone for many years. If this means that a good primary result can be maintained indefinitely, or until the disease has reached its inactive stage, treatment will certainly improve the final prognosis. This investigation does not show whether primarily treatment-resistant cases exist.

Experience with the Treatment of Aspergillosis Complicating Sarcoidosis

Harold L. Israel

Department of Medicine, Jefferson Medical College, Thomas Jefferson University, Philadelphia, U.S.A.

In recent years the most common infection complicating sarcoidosis has proven to be aspergillosis. In most instances the infection occurs in cysts resulting from destruction of the lung by sarcoidosis, and assumes the form of an aspergilloma; in 19 such cases in our series the clinical problem has been that of pulmonary hemorrhage. In 3 instances the infection took the form of a fluid collection within the cysts and was clinically manifested by fever. Invasive pulmonary aspergillosis has been infrequent but was observed in 1 patient who required high doses of prednisone following lobectomy for an aspergilloma. One patient had diffuse bronchitis and 1 patient developed meningitis due to aspergillosis.

The problem of bleeding due to the intracavitary fungus balls has been a serious one, 6 of our patients having died of hemorrhage. Bleeding from aspergillomas may be extremely severe and there can be little question concerning the wisdom of surgical resection when the source of the hemorrhage is unilateral and readily identified. However, in sarcoidosis the pulmonary damage is usually symmetrical, the cyst formation is usually bilateral, and it is often extremely difficult to determine which side is the source of bleeding. Moreover extensive pulmonary damage make many patients incapable of withstanding resectional surgery.

Since surgical therapy has not been feasible in many of our cases with sarcoidosis, we have had to resort to symptomatic therapy or chemotherapy. It should be emphasized that aspergillosis healed in 3 patients without specific treatment. This experience demonstrates that not all patients with aspergillosis have progressive and life-threatening disease, and it appears wise to adopt a fairly conservative approach to surgical resection. Two hemorrhages should lead to a recommendation for surgical resection if the patient is a good or fair surgical risk. The use of 5-fluorocytosine pre- and postoperatively offers some promise of reduction in postoperative infectious complications but 1 patient developed an empyema despite use of this drug. Medical therapy alone with 5-fluorocytosine or amphotericin has not been consistently helpful in the reducing of bleeding due to aspergillomas, presumably because diffusion into the cyst of these agents is limited. One patient who had both infection and hemorrhage showed remarkable improvement while taking 5-fluorocytosine, but in 4 other patients no benefit was evident. In patients with febrile aspergillosis and aspergillus bronchitis and pneumonitis, 5-fluorocytosine has been consistently effective and has replaced amphotericin as the initial treatment of invasive aspergillosis. In patients who fail to respond, combined amphotericin and 5-fluorocytosine therapy has been employed. Our experience with clotrimazole (Bayer 5097) is limited to 1 terminal case, and I am unable to evaluate this drug which appears to be more toxic than the agents we have used.

TABLE 1. Treatment of 22 patients with sarcoidosis and aspergillosis.

	Symptomatic			Chemotherapy		Surgery	
	No.	Success	Failure	Success	Failure	Success	Failure
Aspergilloma	19	3	8	1	3	2	2
Infected cyst	3	1	0	1	1	0	1
Pneumonia	1	—	—	1	0	—	—
Meningitis	1	—	—	1	0	—	—
Diffuse bronchitis	1	—	—	1	0	—	—

The most impressive evidence of the effectiveness of 5-fluorocytosine has been in the patient with aspergillus meningitis. Three positive cultures were obtained prior to the start of therapy. Within 6 weeks spinal fluid changes had disappeared. The patient completed a 3-month period of treatment and has gone 18 months since without recurrence, despite the need for continued corticosteroids because of ocular disease.

The seriousness of the aspergillosis problem in patients with severe sarcoidosis is shown in Table 1. There have been 9 deaths, 6 from pulmonary hemorrhage in patients with extensive pulmonary fibrosis. Two patients who recovered spontaneously and 1 who had lobectomy subsequently died of cardiorespiratory failure; in these 3 instances necropsy revealed no evidence of aspergillosis. It might be concluded that our therapy for aspergillosis is more effective than our therapy for sarcoidosis which has been the major factor in the terrible death toll in this group of patients.

Necrosis of the Femoral Head and Side Effects of the Steroid Treatment of Sarcoidosis

K. Wurm

University of Freiburg, Freiburg, Federal Republic of Germany

The growing frequency of idiopathic ischemic necrosis of the femoral head (IINFH) was the reason for detailed studies of its pathogenesis. It had been noticed that disturbances of the capillary blood circulation were the cause of necrosis of the bony tissues of the femoral head, which are especially subject to great pressure and stress. In analogy to the pathogenesis of the myocardial infarction, the expression " coronary disease of the hip " had also been used. As causing and/or favouring factors the following had been discussed: previous illnesses in combination with disturbances of the metabolism of fat and sugar (especially hyperlipemia); illnesses with tendency to osteoporosis; general and localized stress and finally, antiphlogistic medicaments, which inhibit, retarding the fibroblastic activity, the osteogenesis. In this view, oral *corticoid medication* is considered as frequent noxa. The amount of the daily dosage is more important than total amount of the dosage. Necrosis of the femoral head is a complication of which rheumatologists especially are afraid. But it deserves our special interest because we have to use corticoids in sarcoidosis therapy.

After an IINFH due to steroids, this question arose in connection with myself, when 1 of my patients treated with steroids sustained a bilateral IINFH following which he sued me for damages. Extensive catamnestic examinations of our sarcoidosis patients, who in previous years have received corticoids over a considerable period, make us able to contribute to this problem which has so much importance for all of us. The results of examinations of sarcoidosis patients treated with steroids are shown in Table 1. As far as

TABLE 1. Corticosteroid therapy and bone modifications in 2577 sarcoidosis patients.

| Age | Number | Duration of corticosteroid medication (years) | | | | | Modifications resp. complaints in the bone system | | | | | |
| | | | | | | | Osteoporosis | | | Frac-ture | Femur necro-sis | Rheu-matism |
		1/2	1	2	4	4	?	Questi-onable	Evi-dent			
<25	733	374	136	93	63	67	7	1	0	0	0	5
♀	64	30	15	9	3	7	0	0	0	0	0	1
♂	140	83	31	7	5	14	0	0	0	0	0	1
26–40	1249	545	225	151	156	172	17	6	0	0	0	18
♀	149	77	20	22	13	17	1	1	0	0	0	5
♂	205	110	39	31	12	13	4	1	0	0	0	2
>40	595	198	100	95	73	129	21	4	1	4	1*	19
♀	144	58	33	22	17	14	4	0	0	2	1*	5
♂	46	14	11	9	5	7	0	1	1	0	0	0

* Patients with congenital dislocation of the hip-joint, not due to corticosteroids!

the corticoid dosage is concerned, we start the therapy in almost all cases with an agressive initial daily dosage of at least 40 mg of Prednison or with an equivalent dosage of other corticoids and after several weeks we gradually reduce to a maintenance dosage, on which we remain, above the Cushing threshold dose. Only in very few cases, or after a long period of time we do decrease this dosage. The incorporated total amount of corticoids may be estimated by the duration of treatment.

There are 2,577 cases of sarcoidosis who have been treated by us with steroids some years ago and who have been controlled as regards the further course of disease. Femoral head necrosis is known in only *one* 55-year-old female patient, but long before her sarcoidosis, a coxarthrosis existed in consequence of congenital hip luxation. In this case a causal connection with the corticoid therapy can be refuted. Lesions of bone structures are taken into consideration by a total of 61 cases, of which 45 are only suspected. 30 cases i.e., 50% are in patients more than 40 years old whilst their group amounts to only 23% of the total number. A geriophysiological factor of osteoporosis, independent of sarcoidosis and steroids is therefore evident. The cases registrated as " rheumatism " are uncharacteristic complaints, which cannot be related to bone lesions.

Further, about 3,000 subsequent cases of sarcoidosis, treated with corticoids could not be analysed up to now. Beyond these we meet 3 male patients of 31 to 38 years of age with femoral head necrosis. It is emphasized that all 3 patients informed us at once. The clinical picture of femoral head necrosis is subjectively so impressive and objectively so characteristic, that it does not pass latently, and will always be diagnosed. Therefore it is not probable that you will find in the group which is still not evaluated a larger number of unknown cases of femoral head necrosis. Thus we may assume the frequency of femoral head necrosis as a maximum of 1: 1000 in a total of 5000 cases of sarcoidosis treated with steroids.

DISCUSSION

When discussing the cause of an IINFH in a case of sarcoidosis, treated with corticoids, it must be considered that it does not concern previously healthy individuals; in other illnesses treated with antiphlogistic medicaments with subsequent IINFH, the question remains unanswered as to whether the necrosis of bone is caused by the basic illness or by antiphlogistic drugs, or by an accumulation effect of both.

It is known on the one side that sarcoidosis may lead to bone changes, less regarding minor cysts than the diffuse rarefications of the trabecular structure. These are easier to identify at the phalanges of hands and feet than at the larger bones, deeply situated. Often in sarcoidosis the metabolism of calcium and uric acid is disturbed. On the other hand it is known that corticoids may cause an increased disposition to thrombosis, as well as petechial skin hemorrhages, i.e., a vascular alteration. Both factors must be taken into causal consideration. In connection with this it can be stated that frequent occurence of hypercholesterinemia in our steroid-treated patients was not found, and for this reason we cannot comment on this problem.

Though these theoretical considerations lead us to expect the occurence of bone necrosis in sarcoidosis patients treated with corticoids, the results of our catamnestic statistics show that an IINFH in connection with sarcoidosis cannot be caused only by corticoid therapy.

Further more direct observations, in view of today's knowledge of the pathogenesis of

IINFH may lead to more precise elucidation of this subject than is presently possible with our catamnestic method.

Besides this, the modern *Strontium scintigraphic* method makes it possible to examine the influence of corticoids on the bone structures in an early stage before the occurence of subjective complaints and before the radiological manifestation of bone lesions—so that the therapeutical consequences can be detected in time. Results of such examinations are not yet available.

DISCUSSION

Chairmen: E. WILLIAMS AND M. YAMAMOTO

DR WILLIAMS: Using ability to work as a parameter of morbidity, some wage earners with Stage 1 do not feel well enough to work. Dr Refvem said "I never treat Stage 1" and I would ask Dr Selroos, Dr Israel and Dr Mikami if they would be inclined to persuade Dr Refvem to treat some of these patients.

DR ISRAEL: I believe that all of the views that were expressed this morning, and all the evidence that was presented this morning lead us to the conclusion that the proper indication for treatment is symptoms. In the absence of symptoms, I would not treat any patient, stage I or stage II.

DR SELROOS: I fully agree with Dr Israel. The fact that we in the early 1960's were treating patients with pulmonary lesions of stage I depended on the opinion that all patients should be treated with steroids. Subsequent studies with and without steroid medication have clearly indicated that treatment is unnecessary in uncomplicated stage I disease and even in patients with pulmonary lesions of stage II if they are symptom-free and the ventilatory function is within normal limits. However, an unchanged or deteriorated radiographic finding after 4 months' observation represents an indication for starting with steroids in order to prevent the development of persisting fibrosis.

DR JAMES: Thus far we have concentrated on corticosteroid therapy for pulmonary sarcoidosis. I wish to widen the discussion to include phenylbutazone as an anti-inflammatory agent for acute sarcoidosis, chloroquine and potassium paraminobenzoate for chronic fibrotic disease, azathioprine as an immunosuppressive agent, effervescent phosphate and possibly calcitonin for the abnormal calcium metabolism, and also perhaps most significant of all, transfer factor for the reconstitution of cellular immunity. We should not overlook these other therapeutic approaches.

DR VILLAR: I was particularly interested in Dr Israel's paper on aspergilloma in sarcoidosis. In Lisbon we see a lot of aspergillomas and, out of approximately 700, 2 occurred in our few cases of sarcoidosis· To begin with, I would like to ask Dr Israel if his cases that developed aspergillomas were on corticosteroid therapy and, especially on long-term corticosteroid therapy, and if any developed invasive aspergillosis as we have seen in some cases of leukemia.

As for the fluid levels Dr Israel showed on his X-rays, they are a characteristic radiological finding and correspond to the liquefaction of the fungus ball, generally because of associated infection. Quite often, if the cavity's drainage bronchus is open, they will clear up spontaneously by eliminating the remains of the fungus ball.

In 400 operative specimens examined, and against all our expectations, our pathologist found that the great majority of the cavities inhabited by the fungus were bronchial cavities, i.e., dilated bronchi. Of course, most of our cases developed in residual upper lobe tuberculous lesions. In a patient I had treated 20 years before for a tuberculous upper lobe cavity, an aspergilloma developed radiologically in exactly the same place. I thought the fungus had invaded the reopened cavity, but examination of the resected specimen showed the scar of the old tuberculous cavity and the fungus ball in an enormously dilated bronchus quite near it. This has therapeutic implications, especially when one tries chemotherapy. We have tried catheterizing the invaded cavity through the upper airways and maintaining a continuous drip of amphotericin B or pimaricin in the cavity for several days. In the few cases we have tried, we had good results as there was no systemic involvement and no complications unless one gets the catheter too nicely into the cavity when one may get hemoptysis because of granulation tissue and the mobilization of the fungus ball. Killing the fungus alone does not help, since as it dies it often calcifies and the ball becomes more traumatic.

We are trying 5-fluor-cytosine in a case of allergic aspergillosis. This drug has given splendid results in 2 cases of *Candida albicans* infection and in a case of pulmonary crypto-coccosis. The most important features of this new antifungal drug are its good absortion in the digestive tract, its perfect tolerance and low complication rate. We think there is a great future for this drug.

DR ISRAEL: Many of these patients had had steroids in the past, because of dyspnea due to pulmonary sarcoidosis, but in none was aspergilloma formation directly related to steroid therapy. Invasive aspergillosis was precipitated by use of prednisone in only 1 case, a young man who had a lobectomy for hemorrhage. He also had myocardial sarcoi-dosis, and required very high doses of pred-nisone postoperatively and he did develop fungal pneumonia, responding to ampho-tericin-B. Very large doses may encourage in-vasion, but in the vast majority of our cases using small doses, prednisone had not been a precipitating factor. In fact, many patients require continued steroid therapy and have received it for long intervals without recur-rence of aspergillosis.

DR VILLAR: I would like to state most emphatically that the great majority of our patients with aspergillomas had never taken corticosteroids in their life.

DR TURIAF: C'est à propos de la com-munication de notre collègue Harold Israel que je voudrais souligner les inconvénients des statistiques concernant les résultats du traitement de la sarcoïdose réunissant en un seul groupe les stades II et III ainsi qu'a procédé Harold Israel. En effet l'action des corticostéroïdes au stade II et au stade III n'est pas la même. Au stade II de granulomatose on obtient des résultats sub-stantiels, tandis qu'au stade III de fibrose les

résultats sont très modestes de sorte que si l'on confond dans un même groupe stade II et stade III les résultats finaux sont inexacts on ne peut pas conclure clairement.

J'estime qu'au stade I quand il n'y a pas d'association de lésions oculaires, cutanées, spléniques, hépatiques ou du système ner-veux, on ne doit pas traiter avant la première année d'évolution parce que dans environ 70% des cas la régression se fait spontanément. Ce n'est qu'après une année, si les adéno-pathies persistent, que le traitement se trouve indiqué.

DR LUNDAR: The way she has been treating sarcoidosis in the John Hopkins Hosptal is precisely the same as I am doing it in Oslo. And I think the results were also precisely the same.

DR YAMAMOTO: Could I ask Dr Refvem to speak on this question? There seems to be some difference of opinion on the question of whether stage I should be treated or not.

DR REFVEM: I do not treat stage I. I do not treat stage II before 14 or 18 months have elapsed, because there is a very strong tendency towards spontaneous complete re-solution during stage I and early stage II. But, if there is not a spontaneous regression before that time, I treat continuously for 2 years before pausing to see if infiltration will relapse or not. If it does not relapse, as judged by monthly X-ray control for half a year, treatment is stopped definitively. On the other hand, relapse indicates restarting treat-ment immediately. I think there will be tremendous differences in results according to the selection of patients for treatment.

I do not quite agree with Dr Israel, who is not treating before symptoms are evident, for instance, dyspnea, because dyspnea often comes on late, perhaps not till the patient has developed a widespread fibrosis which will not react to treatment at all.

DR JOHNS: I think we are all agreed that we do not want to treat asymptomatic stage I disease. I think most of us would agree that we want to treat stage II disease when it is symptomatic and incapacitating so that the patients are not able to work or not able to lead their normal life, If the stage II patients have persistent diffuse infiltrations after a period of a year even though they may still be asymptomatic, I would agree with Dr Refvem that we then have to consider seriously the need for treatment. Here, I believe, there is a marked difference between Negro patients and other races. Negroes demonstrate dyspnea very early, very consistently, and symptoms usually correlate very well with the radiographic appearance. In Caucasians, this does not seem to be the case, where you can see very marked infiltration, and no symptoms. There, I think, we have to pay some attention, if it shows no signs of spontaneous remission, after a period of a year, even though the patient may still be asymptomatic.

XII FUTURE ASPECTS

Epidemiology

Itsuzo Shigematsu

Department of Epidemiology, Institute of Public Health, Tokyo, Japan

The assignment given to me is to talk about future aspects of epidemiology in sarcoidosis, based upon present knowledge in this field.

In this conference 11 papers were presented on epidemiological problems, but 3 speakers could not read their papers because of their absence. To begin with, it would be worthwhile to mention that the first epidemiological information on sarcoidosis appeared from Asian countries such as Korea, Taiwan and Thailand.

In Korea the estimated prevalence rate of this disease among railroad employees seemed to be as high as that among corresponding workers in Japan, but in the other 2 countries it was assumed that the frequency of this disease might be very low, although available data were still limited.

From other countries such as Finland, Italy, Yugoslavia and Japan, more detailed epidemiological data were presented in terms of incidence and prevalence, contributing to the study of the epidemiology of this disease.

Considering the number of papers presented, 11 in this conference was the fewest; compared with 21 in Prague 1969; 18 in Paris 1966 and 39 in Stockholm 1963. Of course, quantity is not necessarily more important than quality, yet it can not be denied that there seems to be some slowdown in the progress of epidemiological studies on this disease.

Frankly speaking, as an epidemiologist, I am not satisfied with the epidemiological studies on sarcoidosis which have been conducted by many researchers including ourselves. As already pointed out by the chairmen of the epidemiology sessions, almost all the data presented here were mainly concerned with the frequency of sarcoidosis, though divided into incidence and prevalence, and very few with the causal factors which epidemiology primarily should deal with.

Frequency itself is not only fundamental for comparative epidemiological studies but is also indispensable for assessing the size of the problem in a population group. However, it is my feeling that the epidemiology of sarcoidosis has come to the point where the causal problems related to the occurrence of this disease should be studied more deeply.

In this connection, I should like to mention 3 points as examples of epidemiological studies which should be further promoted. These are case control studies, migrant studies and theoretical studies.

CASE CONTROL STUDIES

Today it is not difficult to obtain a sufficient number of new sarcoidosis cases in a limited period, so that we shall be able to conduct case control studies regarding the various factors supposedly related to the occurrence of sarcoidosis if clinicians cooperate with epidemiologists concerning this matter. In Japan this type of study has already been carried out by the Japanese National Railways (JNR) group, although still on a small scale. In this case, 36 patients with sarcoidosis were subject to study simultaneously with 72 healthy control persons who were matched with the patients in such respects as sex, age, job, place of work, height and weight. Many host and environmental factors were comparably investigated.

If forms of questionnaire and items of examination could be standardized, international cooperative studies would be possible.

MIGRANT STUDIES

The importance of this type of study has already been pointed out in the previous conferences and also in this one. Studies based on migrants are useful in measuring the effect on health of the environment, either of the place of origin or of the host country, and of changes in habits that follow migration.

In this sense, migrant studies, both intra- and intercountry, are one of the most attractive methods for epidemiologists. However, it should be kept in mind that migrants are usually not random samples of the mother country and may be biased in terms of physical, mental and social conditions.

This type of study also requires international cooperation, for which, we hope our international committee would take the initiative.

THEORETICAL STUDIES

This type of study should be one of the proper duties of epidemiologists. More reliable data concerning the frequency of sarcoidosis by time, place and person are now being accumulated sufficiently to be analyzed theoretically. Theoretical analysis of familial and geographical aggregation of sarcoidosis should be carried out and also time-space relationships of sarcoidosis can be studied. Mathematical models including simulation of the frequency and distribution of this disease may be attempted in the near future.

I am sure that these theoretical studies will be useful for elucidating the mechanisms of the epidemiological behavior of this disease.

In conclusion, I should like to stress that in order to accomplish these studies, active participation of epidemiologists is desired in close cooperation with other specialists in various fields.

Granulomatous Diseases

Harold L. Israel, Bernard Bowman, Ward Bullock, H. S. Lawrence,
George B. Mackaness, J. G. Scadding and Byron Waksman

*Report of the Panel on Granulomatous Lung Disorders, Task Force on Research
in Respiratory Diseases, National Heart and Lung Institute,
Washington, D.C., U.S.A.*

INTRODUCTION

The National Heart and Lung Institute organized in 1971 a task force to plan clinical and laboratory investigation in the field of respiratory diseases. Among the 11 panels instituted was one on the noninfectious granulomatous diseases. This panel, which included clinical investigators, immunologists, pathologists and microbiologists with special interest in sarcoidosis and other granulomatous lung disorders surveyed current research approaches and made recommendations for future studies. The full reports will be published in the future, but it appeared that a presentation to the Sixth International Conference on Sarcoidosis of the recommendations of the panel regarding research priorities might stimulate and expedite exploration of these projects.

PRIORITIES FOR FUTURE RESEARCH

Immunology

The development of a reliable and specific in vitro test for sarcoidosis will represent a major clinical advance of importance not only to the many patients who have sarcoidosis, but to physicians and surgeons in virtually every speciality for whom sarcoidosis is a frequent diagnostic consideration. It is likely also to represent an immunologic breakthrough which will advance the understanding of many other illnesses as well as of normal defense mechanisms. A prime need is for a Kveim test antigen which does not react in patients with inflammatory gut disease, disseminated lupus and adenopathies of diverse etiology and which can be generally distributed for investigative and diagnostic purposes with monitoring to ensure that potency and specificity of test materials are maintained. Commercial production would undoubtedly soon be undertaken because of the wide demand for Kveim test materials.

Kveim test preparations used in the past have been prepared from lymph nodes and spleens. Since tissue antigens may be responsible for the granulomatous response, an important step would be the preparation and testing of extracts of other tissues, such as sarcoid lung or liver, as well as spleens and lymph nodes diffusely involved by granulomas of other etiology.

Immunochemical procedures should be used to the fullest extent possible in an effort to establish the source and nature of the Kveim test antigens. If environmental constituents were demonstrated, this should prove an important clue to the etiology of this disorder. Failure to demonstrate exogenous factors would strengthen the concept that sarcoidosis is an immunologic over-reaction to trivial or miscellaneous environmental insults. Increased reactants to histocompatibility antigens have been recognized in patients with lymphomatous, leukemic and collagen diseases, and investigation is indicated to determine whether HLA antigens may be involved in the Kveim reaction.

Further identification of the nature of the antigen should be pursued by immunofluorescence studies which may provide evidence as to whether these factors are endogenous, that is of tissue origin, or exogenous, that is of environmental origin.

Ethical objection to transfer of cells from 1 patient to another should be minimized if both patients have the same disease. It would be most informative to ascertain whether administration of transfer factor from Kveim-positive patients to Kveim-negative patients with sarcoidosis will induce reactivity. Conversely, if transfer factor from Kveim-negative cases abolished the reaction of Kveim-positive cases, therapeutic benefits might be obtained.

The list of immunologic investigations applicable in sarcoidosis is long: extension of blast transformation studies, T and B cells counts and measurement of their life span in granulomatous lungs; study of the various lymphokines; examination of sarcoid sera for immunosuppressive factors; analysis of the HL-A histocompatibility system. Proficiency in all of these approaches cannot be anticipated in a single institution. It would appear more profitable for a center focused on clinical and immunologic study of sarcoidosis to serve as a bank or clearing house, providing cells, sera and tissues to investigators developing the techniques enumerated above. In every field of immunologic research, the availability of specimens from carefully studied and classified patients with sarcoidosis should be of great value.

Since improved in vitro techniques for measurements of lymphocyte responses are essential to make rapid and precise diagnosis of sarcoidosis possible when standardized antigens are available, investigation in this field should be intensified.

Experimental pathology

Macrophage nodulization at sites of antigen deposition to form granulomas is immunologically directed by sensitized lymphocytes. Bronchopulmonary lavage should be employed in an effort to obtain specifically reactive lymphocytes which may be more numerous in diseased tissues than in the blood stream, and more numerous in the lung since reactive cells may be trapped in the pulmonary capillaries.

It would appear useful to expose primates to a variety of inhalation exposures in an effort to produce granulomas with an anatomic distribution and behavior consistent with sarcoidosis. This would provide an opportunity also for ascertaining whether the immunologic alterations characteristic of sarcoidosis are essential to the formation or dissemination of the granulomas.

Cell culture of sarcoid tissues has been attempted with occasional success. Further attention should be given this approach in the hope of securing antigens or evidence of an infectious agent in cell lines derived from granulomas in various tissues. Enzyme biochemistry at the electron microscopic level may identify the function and activity of these cells.

Microbiology

It appears safe to conclude that microbiologic study in the past has been adequate and has excluded infectious agents with the exception of slow viruses and host-dependent bacteria. Further study of a possible etiologic role of these types of infection is indicated.

Epidemiology

Study is indicated in an effort to determine possible late consequences of the immunologic abnormalities present in sarcoidosis; the frequency in sarcoidosis patients and controls should be determined of allergic disorders, viral infections, bacterial infections, fungal infections, neoplasia and autoimmune diseases.

It would also be of interest to determine the immunologic status of subjects prior to the onset of manifest sarcoidosis. Such studies should include measurements of antibody responses to immunization, delayed hypersensitivity tests, storage of frozen sera, etc. Several population groups should be considered for such studies: (a) Offspring and younger siblings of patients with sarcoidosis. (b) Student nurses and medical students, since these groups have a higher likelihood of recognition of sarcoidosis. (c) Comparable ethnic groups in the rural South and urban North to determine possible effects of air pollution and other geographic differences. There should be further study of genetic mechanisms in the familial occurrence of sarcoidosis, and an attempt made to determine whether the concentration of sarcoidosis in the third and fourth decades is a reflection of constitutional factors or of exposure to infectious agents.

Physiology

The most promising physiologic approaches at present would appear to be those involving study of the metabolic and defense functions of the lung.

Clinical features

Prevention and more satisfactory methods of treatment must await discovery of the etiology and pathogenesis of the disease. Although a great mass of observations have been accumulated regarding the clinical features of the granulomatous diseases, there is need for interpreting these data in immunologic, pathologic and physiologic terms.

RECOMMENDATION

The highest priority in terms of likelihood of success based on presently available knowledge and tools should be given to development of an in vitro test for the diagnosis of sarcoidosis. This will require a center with access to large numbers of patients with sarcoidosis, where a multidisciplinary effort can be organized, employing immunochemical, immunologic and clinical approaches to define and refine the antigens present in splenic extracts; prepare and test in vivo and in vitro antigens derived from various granulomatous tissues; carry out transfer factor studies in patients with sarcoidosis to ascertain whether reactivity can be transferred from Kveim-positive to Kveim-negative cases and vice versa in the same fashion as tuberculin hypersensitivity; develop reproducible in vitro methods of measuring lymphocyte sensitization to antigens; provide to other investigators tissues, sera and cells from carefully studied and classified examples of the pulmonary granulomatoses.

Thanks are due Drs Louis E. Siltzbach and Charles Carrington who served as consultants to the Panel.

Immunology

T. H. HURLEY

Royal Melbourne Hospital, University of Melbourne, Victoria, Australia

A purpose of these final sessions is to look into the future in an attempt to define those areas which may, over the next few years, be ones in which further studies may lead to advances in our understanding of this intriguing disorder we call sarcoidosis. In doing this, I intend to be deliberately provocative.

Any attempt to forecast future advances in the immunology of sarcoidosis immediately raises very basic questions—Is sarcoidosis due to an infection? and are the immunological changes associated with it a reflection of this? Our answer to these questions very largely determines the way in which we view possible future developments. Let us look briefly then at the evidence that sarcoidosis represents the deployment of the immunologic mechanism of the patient to repel invasion by an infective agent. Undoubtedly the strongest evidence for this has been that of Dr Mitchell, who has produced sarcoid lesions in immunologically deficient animals with inoculations of sarcoid tissues—an observation which has now been confirmed. This is challenging indeed but it is well to remember that using the same model, apparent transmission has occurred of such disorders as multiple myeloma and even leukaemia, and many of us might be reluctant to accept these conditions as manifestations of infections or at any rate infections transmitted in the usual 'horizontal' fashion.

What other evidence have we that the disorder we call sarcoidosis is due to an infectious agent? The answer, I believe, is very little. It could truly be said that, especially in recent years, our understanding and thinking about sarcoidosis has grown up in the shadow of tuberculosis and it is very easy to see why this should be so. This has inclined us to start with the premise that sarcoidosis is due to a single infective agent whereas in fact, as I hope to indicate, there is little evidence to support this supposition.

If sarcoidosis is due to an infectious agent, like tuberculosis, superficially there are a number of points of resemblance. Let us look briefly at just 3 of these. Firstly, there is evidence from pathology that the pattern of inflammation in sarcoidosis closely resembles that seen in certain diseases which are clearly due to an infective agent, such as tuberculosis or histoplasmosis, and the more closely the structure of the cells concerned is examined the closer the resemblance becomes. On the other hand however we have the very disconcerting fact, mentioned frequently during our meetings this week, that an identical histologic appearance may be found at certain times in diseases such as carcinoma, lymphoma, rheumatoid arthritis and systemic lupus erythematosus, which we are reluctant to accept as infections in the traditional sense of the word. To the believer of what J. K. Galbraith would refer to as the 'conventional wisdom' this difficulty presents no problems—one simply has to learn to recognise the 'sarcoid reaction' and to distinguish this from the disease sarcoidosis. However, until such time as a specific etiological process is identified to characterise sarcoidosis from the other disorders, this distinction remains a theory. Such cases, as were mentioned this week of the patient who presented initially with tuberculous adenitis, then developed apparent sarcoidosis and finally died with lymphoma, provide us with a challenge to be fitted into the system somewhere.

The second point of resemblance between sarcoidosis and tuberculosis, of course, is that both conditions affect the lungs and related tissues very commonly. It is known that this is early in the course of tuberculosis and it is presumed that it is also the case with the disorder we call sarcoidosis. In both, the pulmonary lesions frequently resolve without residual disability and in both, the alternative course is a progressive one which may be associated with considerable fibrosis. These observations easily incline us to the view that sarcoidosis, like tuberculosis, may well be due to an infective agent acquired, as in the case with tuberculosis, by inhalation. This may be the case but if it is so there are a number of observations which we might expect to make and yet do not. If sarcoidosis is due to an infectious agent why is there so little evidence of person-to-person infection? Why do we not see ' microepidemics ' in closed groups and communities as we do with tuberculosis? If it is argued that this is due to the fact that a very widespread infectious agent is involved, that many acquire it in a form which is not manifest clinically (like poliomyelitis), this still fails to explain the baffling lack of evidence of epidemic spread within communities. The other fact difficult to fit into this theory is the curious age incidence of the disorder, occurring as it does predominantly in young adult life with, as Sven Lofgren has reminded us, an onset often associated with alterations in endocrinologic patterns, e.g. the menarche and after childbirth. This type of pattern suggests that sarcoidosis may represent the expression of a process or pattern of much longer standing than a recently acquired infection. What I am saying now of course, is not new and a theory of etiology along these lines was proposed by Burnet as long ago as 1959. He suggested that many of the immunologic features of sarcoidosis could be explained on the basis of the persisting presence intracellularly of either an L. form of a mycobacterium or a low-grade virus and that this entry into the cell may long precede the manifest condition of sarcoidosis. In recent years we have become accustomed to the concept that the occurrence of disease may reflect an altered balance between the host and a virus and the occurrence of manifest disease may reflect a failure of immunologic surveillance which had previously provided a check to its florid expression. We are coming to believe that such processes are probably involved in the genesis not only of the so called slow virus infections but also of neoplasia and especially neoplasms of lymphoreticular tissues. Animal models of leukaemia and lymphoma show that disease which may not be manifest for some considerable time after birth may have its origin in viral nucleoprotein accepted into the genome and transmitted from parent to offspring in the so-called ' vertical ' method of transmission. The time of expression of diseases of this type may be influenced by environmental factors which influence surveillance mechanisms, such as irradiation, hormonal factors, drugs or infections. Although such a method of transmission has not as yet been determined in human leukaemia it has been demonstrated in animals; this type of mechanism may explain those cases of human leukaemia which follow exposure to irradiation or those lymphomas which are encountered in patients given immunosuppressive therapy or antilymphocyte serum.

I do not wish to be misunderstood and I am not proposing a similar etiology for sarcoidosis and lymphoma. What I am saying is that the mechanism involved in the genesis of disease becomes more, rather than less, complex with the acquisition of new knowledge. In the case of a disease such as sarcoidosis, where we really have no clear picture of the etiology, it is important to retain an open mind receptive to the possible occurrence of even the most unlikely or improbable mechanisms. However, in this regard it is important to remember that a number of similarities exist between the clinical and immunologic features of sarcoidosis and some lymphomas. Two of the papers presented this week have a possible bearing on these aspects. They were the report from Professor Wurm's group of the aggregation of HLA antigen groups in patients with sarcoidosis, an observation already made in relation to Hodgkin's disease—I think this is a most exciting observation and one which should be confirmed. The other papers which were extremely interesting in this regard were the reports of familial occurrence of sarcoidosis from Sweden and from Japan. The striking occurrence of sarcoidosis in 3 generations, as was shown in 1 family, raises again the possible importance of inherited factors in the development of, or predisposition to, sarcoidosis.

I started off by saying that our thoughts about sarcoidosis had grown up in the shadow of tuberculosis and I have mentioned 2 aspects where I believe this has influenced our thoughts about sarcoidosis. The third and perhaps most important aspect deals with the tuberculin test and the Kveim test. The tuberculin reaction clearly is the very pattern of specific delayed-type hypersensitivity and it is very tempting to regard the Kveim test as being in some way similarly related to sarcoidosis. Although Dr Izumi was not able to get a direct answer to his question " Is the Kveim Test an Immunologic one? " many, if not most of us, probably 'believe' that it is. It is with this belief that the various new in vitro techniques have evolved in recent years and one of the highlights of thisConference has been the reports of the various in vitro techniques using sarcoid tissue as an 'antigen' to demonstrate various patterns of lymphocyte reactivity. These have been intriguing and have contributed to the thought that there may infact be a specific factor or antigen, like tuberculin, involved and that once this is discovered and purified at last we will have within our grasp the elusive etiologic agent of sarcoidosis. This may well be so and clearly this is a theory capable of being tested. One such way would be to transfer Kveim sensitivity from positive to negative Kveim reactors in a manner similar to that which has been achieved with tuberculin sensitivity. If previous observations in this regard can be confirmed and strengthened, more substantial evidence for the presence of an antigen in sarcoid tissue will have been established. Two aspects of the Kveim test as one due to the effect of a specific antigen are at the moment somewhat disturbing. The first is that to date no one has been able to isolate an active soluble fraction either in the in vivo reaction or in vitro. This is curious. The second basic problem is that although in vitro Kveim tests do show reactivity in sarcoidosis there are now quite a number of reports of similar activity occurring in in vitro tests (using sarcoid tissue from quite a number of sources) in reactions with lymphocytes from patients with diseases such as Crohn's disease, coeliac disease and dermatitis herpetiformis, which are very distinct from sarcoidosis. These are, it seems to me, very important observations and progress in the immunology of sarcoidosis in the next 3 years may well be advanced by the perfection of more specific in vitro techniques and the recognition of the factor or factors responsible for these reactions. Whether or not we will then find in our hands the antigen associated with a specific infective agent still remains to be seen.

General Aspects and Possible Causes

D. GERAINT JAMES

Royal Northern Hospital, London, Great Britain

Harold Israel and I are the only two participants who have been to all the conferences and that allow us as very old friends, to be the knock-about, comedian, nitty-gritty men throughout this week. I was asked to comment on possible causes. As we understand more of the immunology, we shall learn more of the etiology, for they are interwoven. It seems likely, in our present state of knowledge, that the agent, whatever it is, causes an eclipse of the thymus-mediated T cells, when at the same time there is evidence of a lymphoproliferative disorder with overactivity of the B cells. We must try to understand the interaction between T and B cells.

T AND B CELL HYPOTHESIS

An antigenic insult, whether by an infective agent or chemical or even vegetable matter is met by a reticulo-endothelial response in which both thymus-mediated (T) cells and bursa-dependent plasma (B) cells participate. The T cells are transformed, possibly by undergoing antigenic alteration on their cell surface, and become depleted. Depletion may be due not only to T cell transformation but also from T cell interaction against transformed T cells. Depletion results in depression of delayed-type hypersensitivity, which is recognised by cutaneous anergy and by in vitro lymphocyte transformation tests. At the same time there is vigorous lymphoproliferation, and the B cell response is recognizable by an increase in circulating immunoglobulins. This phase of expansive lymphoproliferation with T cell eclipse is represented histologically by granuloma formation in all organ systems. During this same phase, transformed T cell immune complexes are responsible for such clinical phenomena as erythema nodosum and uveitis. The antigenic insult is probable airborne, for bilateral hilar lymphadenopathy is such a frequent mode of onset. The more acute the onset and the more active the reticulo-endothelial response, the more likely will there be spontaneous remission with full restoration of T cell function. If this does not occur spontaneously, then it may be induced by corticosteroids, which may overcome T cell eclipse and restore nomal T cell function.

The antigen responsible for lymphoproliferation, T cell transformation and granuloma formation almost certainly resides in Kveim-Siltzbach antigen, possibly linked to and altered by transformed T cells into an immune complex responsible for the granuloma formation which characterizes this distinctive skin test.

ICEBERG SYNDROME

I regard sarcoidosis as an iceberg which we must continue to investigate more deeply for hidden aspects. In order to do so, it is essential to organise a weekly sarcoidosis clinic.

It is too difficult to do it any other way, and I would advise those of you who are interested to set up a weekly, not a monthly, sarcoidosis clinic, so that you can review the material, and other granulomatous disorders which present at this clinic. As you dig deeper you will start finding various immunological upsets, and during this decade we shall reach an exciting level of molecular biology.

The International Committee on Sarcoidosis met this week and decided that the next conference will be held in New York City under the organisation and chairmanship of Louis Siltzbach between now and then, you have got to dig. The motto is " Search for Sarcoid ". Go back home to Sendai, Oslo and all the other places and write across your heart, " Search for Sarcoid! " When you wake up in the morning and shave, have, on the mirror, " Search for Sarcoid to-day! " And that will be the road that will take you to New York City and to Dr Siltzbach.

KVEIM-SILTZBACH TEST

Call it the Kveim-Siltzbach Test. Dr Kveim would be the first man, if he were alive, to pay homage to Dr Siltzbach who has done a tremendous amount of work right round the world in trying to understand his fascinating immunological reaction. He has really put it on an admirable footing as a safe, specific, outpatient test. By calling it the Kveim-Siltzbach test I draw attention to the rigid and strict criteria laid down by Dr Louis Siltzbach in this Conference.

VISIT OTHER CENTERS

One of the features of this week's Conference is that the pioneers are still strongly in the field. Harold Israel, Professor Turiaf and Professor Wurm are obviously still working hard, having laboured for a long time in this field. And it's exciting to see a splendid lot of new, young Japanese workers emerging with new ideas, which will obviously be fruitful. I hope that all workers will visit each other's Sarcoidosis Clinics. I want you all to come to see me at the Royal Northern Hospital, London, and then to see Dr Jones Williams in Cardiff and so on. I think that this is a most important way of breaking down international barriers in medicine, as we have done over the years.

Once again, may I, on behalf of all the overseas participants, congratulate and thank you very much Mr President, Mr Secretary, the Japanese Organising Committee and all your co-workers. By that, I mean you young ladies on the projection and recording apparatus, and the persons who mounted such beautiful exhibits upstairs. Indeed, I include everybody on stage and backstage who has worked unsparingly to ensure the undoubted tremendous success of this particular Congress.

SUMMARY

Chairmen: H. HOMMA AND W. JONES WILLIAMS

DR JONES WILLIAMS: Mr. Chairman, when it was suggested that I might say something about future developments in pathology, I found it very difficult, in that this is a very large subject. Every paper has future advances in pathology, and this is the message, I think, that we have heard, that there are so many new and exciting laboratory tools that we can use. We have also had the message put very strongly, that it is not just in a laboratory that we may find an answer. We need better and more thorough epidemiological studies, better, more thorough and new immunological techniques. Even old-fashioned microscopy can still tell us quite a lot, and I am delighted to say how nice it is to see all these aspects being done by so many excellent workers in Japan. I think this is really wonderful, and this is why we need to meet each other and to compare our results, and to have people in each country working in all these various fields.

I would like to suggest that this slide of the emblem of the royal family of Japan—the chrysanthemum, with its lines radiating towards the centre—is a good model of sarcoidosis. This illustrates the many different factors to consider in the search for the causative agent(s) and the many disciplines and types of investigations required to solve the problems. As a pathologist I obviously like to think that we can contribute to a further understanding of the underlying mechanisms which, once understood, will link up sarcoidosis with many other granulomatous, lymphoproliferative and even neoplastic diseases.

So, in conclusion, I would like to thank our hosts very warmly for a most wonderful, excellent conference. We are all going back tired, but very happy.

CLOSING CEREMONY

J. TURIAF

Hospital Bichat, Université Paris VII, Paris, France

Monsieur le Président,
Messieurs les Membres du Comité National Japonais de la Sarcoïdose,
Mesdames, Messieurs,

C'est pour moi un très agréable devoir au terme de cette VIe Conférence de vous remercier au nom du Comité International sur la Sarcoïdose et en particulier de son Secrétaire Général, le Professeur Louis Siltzbach retenu à New-York par une récente indisposition de santé.

Laissez-moi d'abord vous exprimer notre gratitude pour l'accueil chaleureux, charmant, j'ajouterai amical que vous nous avez réservé. Pas un instant nous n'avons éprouvé un sentiment de dépaysement. Vous avez su nous entourer de telle sorte que notre séjour soit le plus agréable possible. De cela nous vous sommes très reconnaissants. Nous avons enregistré avec admiration la merveilleuse organisation de Mr le Dr Hosoda et de son Comité d'Organisation. Vous aviez composé un excellent programme de travail; son accomplissement fut remarquable à la fois sur le plan de l'ordonnance et de la hiérarchisation. Je mesure quant à moi la somme d'efforts accumulés pour obtenir un tel résultat. La plupart des grands problèmes que posent la sarcoïdose notamment ceux qui sont imparfaitement ou non encore résolus, y furent placés aux premières places et discutés dans des rapports ou communications de qualité. Je retiendrai au passage les granulomatoses expérimentales et leurs relations avec la sarcoïdose, les travaux sur l'immunologie, le traitement et le pronostic et surtout l'irritante question du test de Kveim toujours d'actualité quant à sa spècificité. Si des conclusions définitives n'ont pas été énoncées au terme de nos débats, des progrès ont été accomplis dans la connaissance de divers aspects encore mal définis de cette maladie, dont le mystère de l'étiologie et les inconnues de la physio-pathologie demeurent les thèmes principaux de ces recherches et de nos réunions périodiques. Nous avons fait ici à Tokyo de l'excellent travail, dans le domaine de la recherche médicale, mais aussi et cela n'est pas moins important nous avons cohabité pendant 4 jours, cela sur le plan humain est capital. Désormais nous nous connaissons mieux. Nous n'oublierons pas votre belle cité, sa merveilleuse activité et ses réalisations qui en font l'égale de nos plus grandes métropoles occidentales.

Nous garderons dans nos mémoires les fastueuses et fort agréables réceptions que nous ont réservées Monsieur le Gouverneur de la Cité de Tokyo et Monsieur le Président de la VIe Conférence Internationale sur la Sarcoïdose. Nous y avons gouté le charme et la délicatesse des épouses de nos collèques Japonais qui de même que de nombreuses jeunes-filles ont aidé à la réalisation et au succès de cette Conférence. Elles lui ont apporté une note de fraicheur, de gaité et de distinction qui nous a ravis.

La Conférence de Tokyo fera date dans l'histoire des Conférences sur la Sarcoïdose.

Puissions-nous revenir à Tokyo pour travailler, pour revoir nos amis Japonais, leur exprimer à nouveau nos remerciements et leur dire que nous serons heureux de les recevoir chez nous.

Y. Chiba

Vice-Chairman of the Sixth International Conference on Sarcoidosis

Japanese National Railways Central Hospital, Tokyo, Japan

Ladies and Gentlemen, we are deeply grateful that the Sixth International Conference on Sarcoidosis has ended so successfully, thanks to the fruitful efforts of the International Committee on Sarcoidosis, and all the particiapnts who have given eminent presentations and discussions.

In spite of the severe time limitation, due to the number of papers, the conference was able to proceed as scheduled. This too was made possible by presenting your many years of research in a relevant and well-organised fashion. Our deep thanks to you again, for at tending this Conference. I believe this Conference has made deep probes into substantial areas of the causes of sarcoidosis; and I am certain that future discoveries are not far off. We wait with great expectancy for the fruits of our next conference. Until then, let us continue our mutual efforts for further development. Finally, let us meet again at the next World Conference for the further progress of our studies.

RELATED EVENTS

1. Slide Conference on the Kveim Reactions
2. Exhibition
3. The Post-Conference Kyoto Meeting
4. Other Meetings

Slide Conference on the Reading of Kveim Reactions
14th September, Thursday, 1972

Chairmen: R. Fukushiro and W. Jones Williams

This meeting was held in a small conference room of Tokyo Bunka Kaikan under the chairmanship of Drs W. Jones-Williams and Ryoichi Fukushiro at lunch time (12: 45–14: 00) in order to discuss differences of opinion sometimes encountered in the reading of Kveim reactions and to discuss how to resolve such differences.

Before the meeting, 9 members (Table 1) inspected carefully 10 selected Hemotoxylin-Eosin sections of Kveim reactions and recorded their readings with comments (Table 2).

TABLE 1. Readers.

Fukushiro, R.	Japan	Jones-Williams, W.	Great Britain
Hirako, M.	Japan	Mitchell, D.N.	Great Britain
Hongo, O.	Japan	Shigematsu, N.	Japan
Hurley, T.H.	Australia	Turiaf, J.	France
Iwai, K.	Japan		

TABLE 2. Summary of readings.

Sec-tion No.	Presenter of sections	Diagnosis of cases	Antigen	Fukushiro	Hirako	Hongo	Hurley	Iwai	Jones Williams	Mitchell	Shigematsu	Turiaf	+	±	−	?
1	Wurm	Sarcoidosis	Own	±	+	±	+	±	?	±	+	±	3	5	0	1
2	Fukushiro	Sarcoidosis (BHL, skin)	JPN-NIH No. 21	−	−	−	+	−	−	±	±	±	1	3	5	0
3	Turiaf	Tuberculosis	Own (lymph node)	+	±	±	+	+	−	±	+	+	5	3	1	0
4	Jones-Williams	Tuberculosis	Own (lymph node)	?	+	±	±	−	−	−	+	−	2	2	4	1
5	Hongo	Sarcoidosis (BHL)	JPN-NIH No. 20	−	−	−	−	−	−	±	+	±	1	2	6	0
6	Mitchell	Sarcoidosis (stage I)	K 12 Lot 5	±	−	−	−	±	−	±	?	−	0	3	5	1
7	Wurm	Crohn's disease	Own	−	−	−	+	−	−	+	±	+	3	1	5	0
8	Jones-Williams	Sarcoidosis (stage I)	—	?	?	+	+	?	+	±	?	+	4	1	0	4
9	Fukushiro	Leprosy ?	JPN-NIH No. 6	±	+	±	−	+	−	±	?	+	3	3	2	1
10	Turiaf	Sarcoidosis (stage II)	Own	±	±	−	−	±	−	−	+	±	1	4	4	0

* +, positive; ±, equivocal; −, negative; ?, undiagnosed.

At the meeting, with about 20 participants, features in each of the sections were projected on a screen with a microprojector. These features, the above readings and the grounds for the readings were discussed. Some of the features are illustrated in the following microphotographs (Figs. 1 to 9).

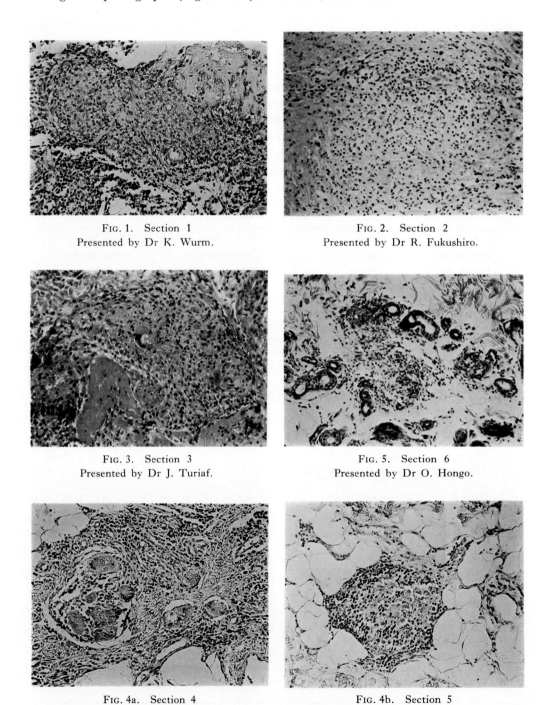

FIG. 1. Section 1
Presented by Dr K. Wurm.

FIG. 2. Section 2
Presented by Dr R. Fukushiro.

FIG. 3. Section 3
Presented by Dr J. Turiaf.

FIG. 5. Section 6
Presented by Dr O. Hongo.

FIG. 4a. Section 4
Presented by Dr W. Jones-Williams.

FIG. 4b. Section 5
Presented by Dr W. Jones-Williams.

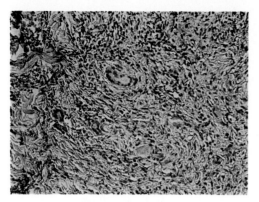

FIG. 6.   Section 7
Presented by Dr K. Wurm.

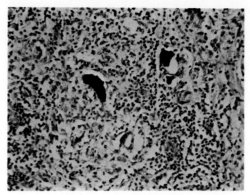

FIG. 7.   Section 8
Presented by Dr W. Jones-Williams.

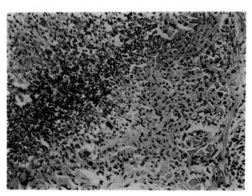

FIG. 8.   Section 9
Presented by Dr R. Fukushiro.

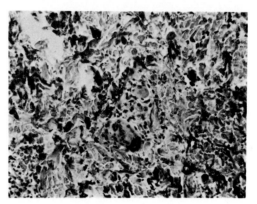

FIG. 9.   Section 10
Presented by Dr J. Turiaf.

EXHIBITION

Incidence of Sarcoidosis in Denmark, 1962–1971

O. HOROWITZ

TABLE 1. Incidence of saroidosis in Denmark 1962–71.

Age in years	Hilar adenopathy*		Lung lesion only		All cases**	
	No.	Annual No. per 100,000	No.	Annual No. per 100,000	No.	Annual No. per 100,000
0–4	—	—	—	—	—	—
5–14	30	0.4	1	0.0	31	0.4
15–19	120	3.2	13	0.3	134	3.5
20–24	465	10.9	57	1.3	523	12.3
25–29	363	11.2	67	2.1	434	13.3
30–34	223	7.8	44	1.5	267	9.3
35–44	272	4.7	86	1.5	363	6.3
45–54	245	4.1	128	2.1	373	6.3
55–64	206	3.8	101	1.9	310	5.7
65–75	57	1.5	51	1.4	111	3.0
75 or more	9	0.5	8	0.4	17	0.9
Total	1,990	4.1	556	1.1	2,563	5.3

* The group includes patients who had a lung lesion in addition to hilar adenopathy.
** Including 17 patients with unknown X-ray status.

TABLE 2.   Incidence of "primary" and "post-primary" sarcoidosis in Denmark 1962–71.

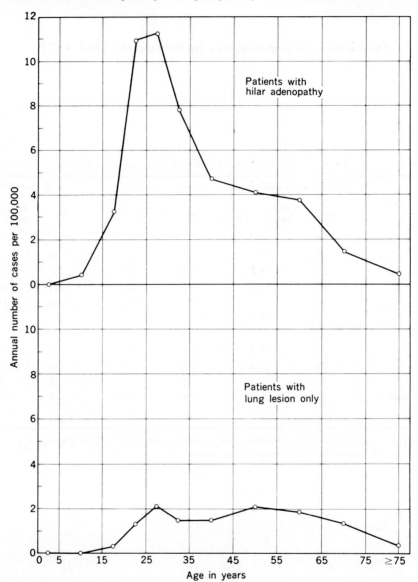

TABLE 3.   Incidence of sarcoidosis in Denmark 1962–71.

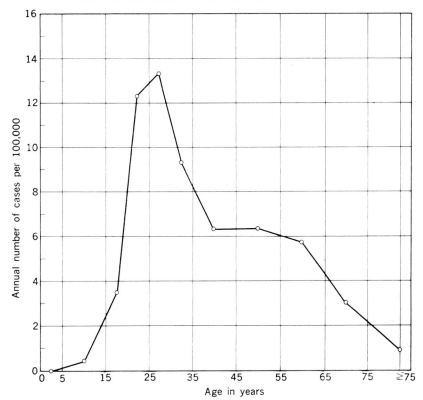

Scar Infiltration in Sarcoidosis

Ryoichi Fukushiro, Hiroshi Ishizaki and Yoshichika Eryu

Department of Dermatology, Kanazawa University School of Medicine, Kanazawa, Japan

Observations of 69 patients with sarcoidosis, all of whom underwent systematic dermatological examinations, revealed cutaneous sarcoid in 11 patients and scar infiltration in 10 others. Some clinical and histological findings of scar infiltration in 4 select patients (Table 1) are presented in the form of photographs (Figs. 1 to 15).

TABLE 1.   Summary of patients presented.

Patient No.	Age (Yr)	Sex	BHL	Scalene node involvement	Ocular change	Tuberculin test	Kveim test	Location of infiltrated scar
1	52	F	+	+	+	−	+	Left eyelid, arm and knees
2	40	M	+	−	+	−	−	Knees
3	28	M	+	−	−	−	+	Left 2. finger
4	22	M	+	+	−	−	−	Forehead (subcutaneous)

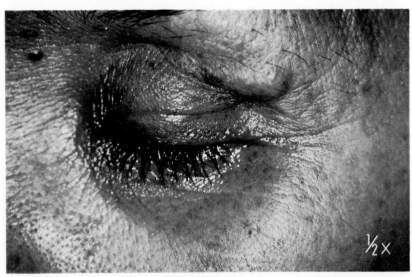

FIG. 1.   Nodular swelling of a linear scar on the left upper eyelid (case 1).

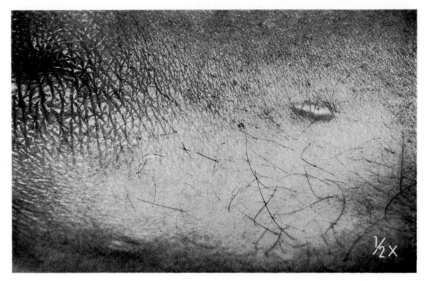

FIG. 2. Minute linear scar with partial swelling on the left forearm (case 1).

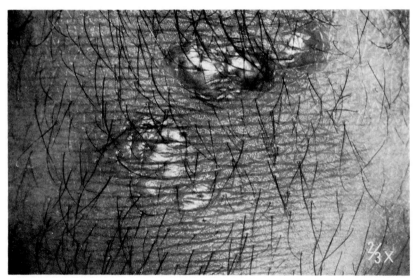

FIG. 3. Three nodular lesions on the left knee (case 1).

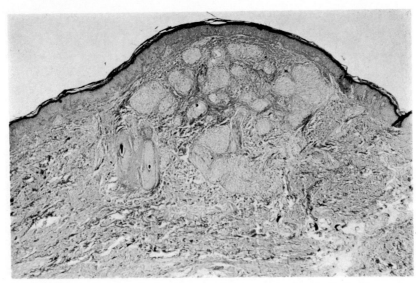

Fig. 4.   Biopsy of scar on the forearm, showing aggregate of epithelioid cell granulomas in upper dermis.   Azan, Mag. ×20 (case 1).

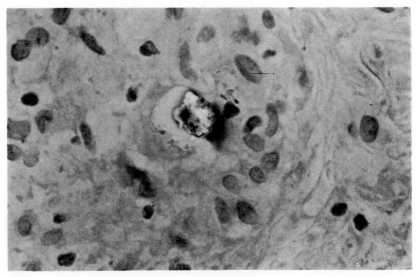

Fig. 5.   Same biopsy as in Fig. 4.   Glass-like foreign body within the epithelioid cell granuloma.   Hematoxylin-eosin, Mag. ×504.

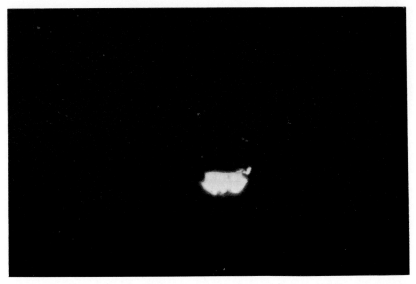

FIG. 6. Same section as in Fig. 5. Foreign body more clearly seen by polarized light. Mag. ×400.

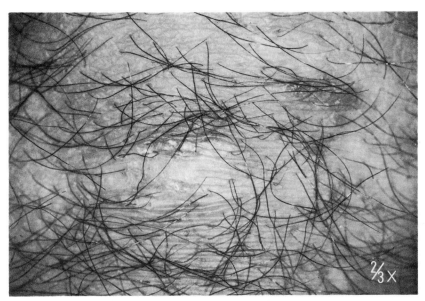

FIG. 7. Slight infiltration of a scar on the right knee (case 2).

R. FUKUSHIRO ET AL.

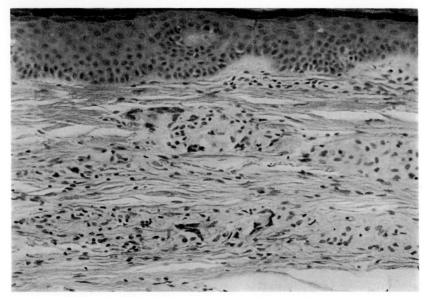

FIG. 8.   Biopsy of scar showing fibrosis intermingled with epithelioid cell granulomas in the upper dermis.   Hematoxylin-eosin, Mag.   ×125 (case 2).

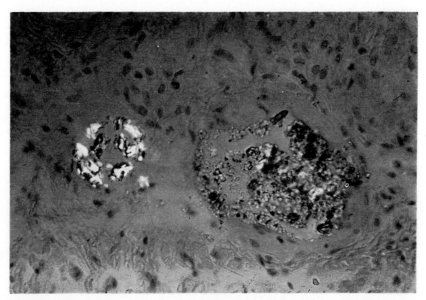

FIG. 9.   Same section as in Fig. 8.   Aggregates of crystallized foreign bodies revealed by filtered polarized light.   Mag. ×200.

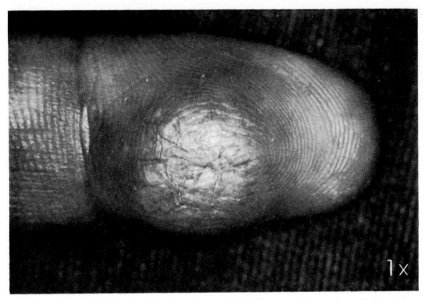

FIG. 10. Nodule with cicatrized surface on the left second finger (case 3, dentist).

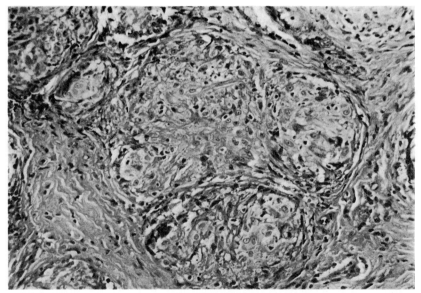

FIG. 11. Biopsy of the nodule showing epithelioid cell granulomas surrounded by fibrosis in the subcutaneous tissue. Azan, Mag. ×125 (case 3).

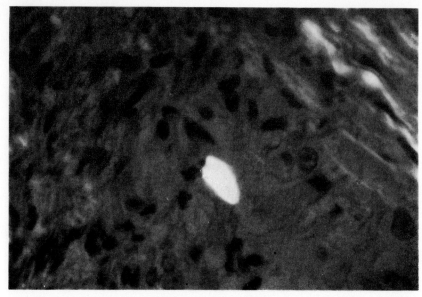

FIG. 12. Same section as in Fig. 11. Minute foreign body visualized by polarized light. Mag. ×600.

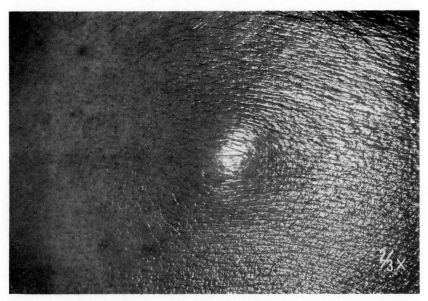

FIG. 13. Subcutaneous nodule on the forehead (case 4).

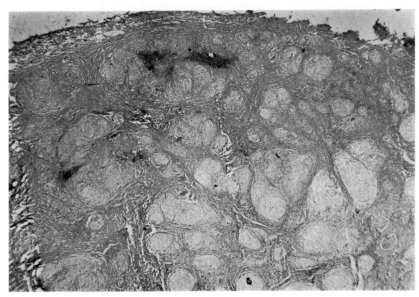

FIG. 14. Biopsied nodule consisting of numerous epithelioid cell granulomas and fibrosis. Azan, Mag. ×20. (case 4).

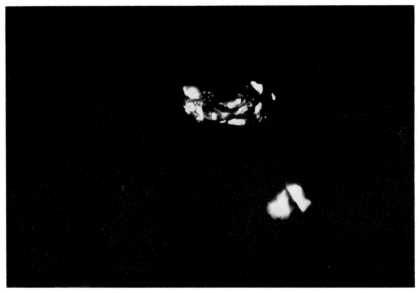

FIG. 15. Same section as in Fig. 14. Aggregates of foreign bodies revealed by polarized light. Mag. ×200.

Sarcoidosis Involving the Nervous System

topsy and 3 clinical cases (including 1 surgical case)—

Y. Matsui and N. Yoshimizu

Japan Red Cross Medical Center, Tokyo, Japan

N. Tanaka

Chiba Cancer Center, Research Institute, Japan

S. Naoe

St. Malianna School of Medicine, Kawasaki, Kanagawa, Japan

H. Imai

Shionogi Research Laboratory

AND

I. Dohi

Japanese National Railways Central Hospital, Tokyo, Japan

Systemic sarcoidosis rarely involves the nervous system and its incidence, as given in the literature, varies between 2 and 9%. In Japan such cases are as high as approximately 3%. Japanese cases of neurosarcoidosis show a high incidence of complication by uveitis. Sarcoidosis of the nervous system is clinically divided into 2 varieties as follows;

1. Central nervous system
2. Peripheral nervous system
   a. Cranial nerves
   b. Spinal nerves

However, many combined cases are found. Cases 1 and 2 are each type 2 (a+b), case 3 is of types 1+2, and case 4 is type 1 (meningoencephalitic type). The present report comprises 2 clinical cases, 1 autopsy and 1 surgical case.

CASE PRESENTATION

Case 1 (Fig. 1) and Case 2 (Fig. 2) were 35-year-old and 48-year-old females, respectively. Case 1 showed Heerfordt's syndrome with polycranio- and peripheral neuropathies.

Case 2 also showed polycranio- and peripheral neuropathies. Spinal tap always showed elevation of protein content and pleocytosis in moderate degree, and lymphocytes were dominant in both cases.

Case 3 (Fig. 3) was a 31-year-old male, hospitalized in Dec. 1971 because of dizziness, tinnitus, headache, nausea and vomiting. Ten months prior to admission, he suddenly complained of dizziness, facial palsy, trigeminal neuralgia on the left side, and deafness. He was treated at a hospital under the diagnosis of Meniere's syndrome.

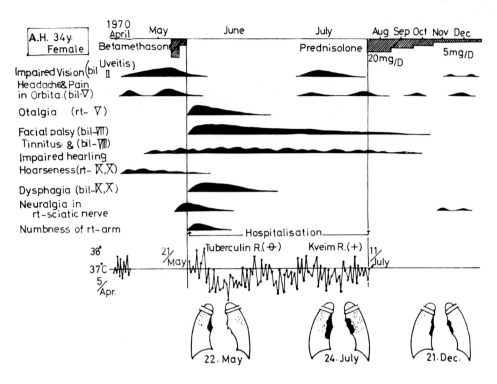

FIG. 1.   Clinical course of case 1.

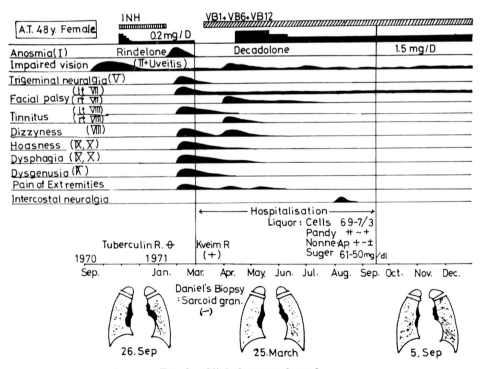

FIG. 2.   Clinical course of case 2.

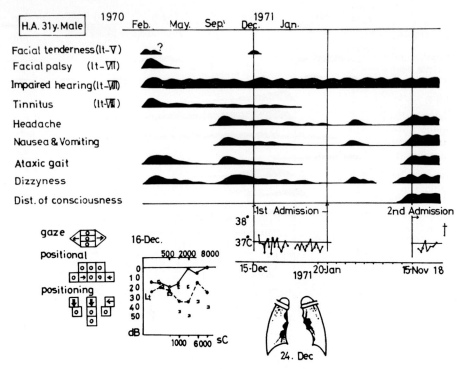

FIG. 3.   Clinical course of case 3.

One month prior to sudden death, headache and dizziness had become severe, and cerebral signs appeared. The chest X-ray film showed slight BHL and pulmonary mottling.

Upon autopsy, the cause of death was found to be a myocardial sarcoidosis. Advanced meningoencephalitic-type sarcoidosis was observed in association with marked internal hydrocephalus, especially significant in the fourth ventricle besides widespread systemic sarcoidosis. A significant finding was that the thoracic duct was severely involved by sarcoidosis (Figs. 4, 5, 6, 7, 8, 9).

Case 4 (Fig. 10) was a 28-year-old male, who had been suffering from headach and vomiting for a year. Frontal lobectomy was performed on the left side in our hospital for release of cerebrospinal hypertention of unknown etiology. The pachymeninges were found to be thick and turbid. Histological examination revealed perivascular epitheloid cell granulomas with lymphocytic infiltration in the leptomeninges and cerebral parenchyma (Figs. 11, 12).

The present case was difficult to diagnosis exactly prior to operation because of negative Daniel's biopsy, absence of BHL and positive Mantoux test. After operation, his complaints completely disappeared. Thereafter sarcoid granulomas were detected by liver needle biopsy. The Kveim test was positive. Corticosteroid therapy is being given continuously.

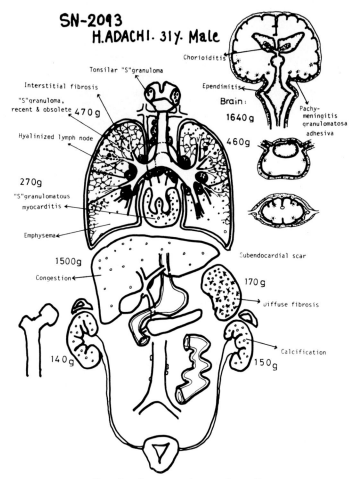

FIG. 4. Autopsy schema of case 3.

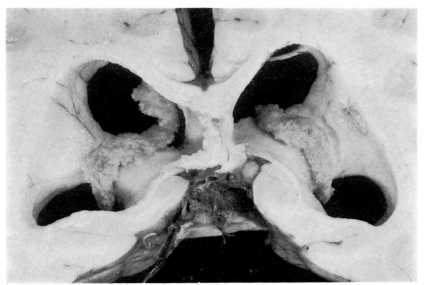

FIG. 5. Dilatation of lateral ventricle, edemtous granular ependym, sclerotic thickning of plex. chorioideus.

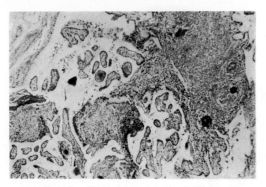

FIG. 6.   Granulomatous chorioiditis.

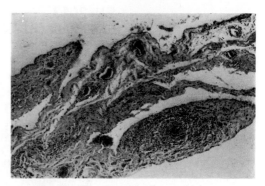

FIG. 9.   The thoracic duct, which was severely involved by sarcoidosis.

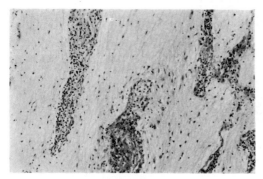

FIG. 7.   Perivascular granuloma with lymphocytic cuffing (N. opticus).

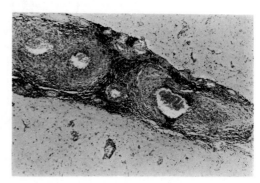

FIG. 11.   Perivacular epitheloid cell granuloma with lymphocytic infiltraticn in the leptmeninges.

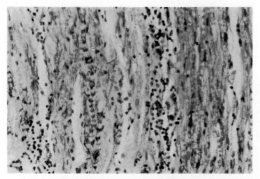

FIG. 8.   Degeneration of myelin sheath with lymphocytic infiltration (lt. N. facialis).

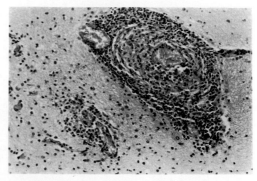

FIG. 12.   Perivascular epitheloid cell granuloma with lymphocytic cuffing in cerebral parenchyma.

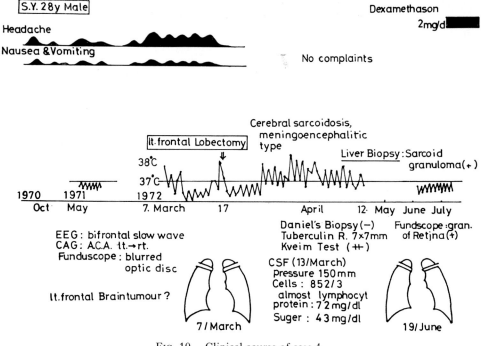

FIG. 10.   Clinical course of case 4.

COMMENT

In neurosarcoidosis, the peripheral nerve disorders usually improve spontaneously, in the majority of instances. Hence, neuropathological evidence of peripheral nerve lesions of sarcoidosis is difficult to find in autopsy cases. Thus, interpretation of the etiology of various peripheral nerve disorders in sarcoidosis is still speculative. A considerable degeneration of the myelin sheath detected only in the left facial nerve of the third case appears to be a significant finding. It shows an irregular, tigroid-striated pattern. This finding has never previously been described in the literature (Fig. 9). On the other hand, multiple patchy perivascular sarcoid granulomas were found in various cranial nerves; optic, oculomotorius etc., although they fail to show any clinical neural manifestations. They do not involve and damage the nerve fibers and are not always associated with relevant clinical manifestations.

The course of CNS sarcoidosis is generally chronic and slowly progressive extending over many years. Clinical dignosis of sarcoidosis of CNS is particularly difficult when the signs of systemic sarcoidosis are obscure. It is of interest to note that neurological symptoms are frequently among the first to appear. Sometimes cranial surgery is the best procedure for the diagnosis of CNS. In this respect, case 4 is a valuable example.

Zeman (1958) has classified sarcoidosis of the CNS from the pathological aspect, as follows;

1.   Meningoencephalitis
   a.   Localized form, tumor-like
   b.   Diffuse-disseminated form
2.   Diffuse metastatic focal encephalitis

3. Angitic and arteritic form

Case 3 is compatible with Zeman's classification 1b, and case 4 is nearly compatible with class 1b+3.

Addendum

The case No. 4 has developed spastic paresis of the leg, bilateral, with incotinence of urinary discharge from May 1973, which is gradually progressing in Aug. 1973.

Gastric Sarcoidosis

Teruo Tachibana and Yoshio Murata
Osaka Prefectural Hospital, Osaka, Japan

Kaoru Kitano
Otemae Hospital, Osaka, Japan
AND
Hiroshi Taketani
Osaka Kosei Nenkin Hospital, Osaka, Japan

In 1971 Liehr reviewed the literature concerning 38 cases of gastric sarcoidosis reported previously.[1]

The present report is about 2 cases of gastric sarcoidosis; 49 years old (case 1) and 29 years old (case 2), both females. They were clinically diagnosed as gastric cancer from endoscopic and roentgenographic findings, and received gastrectomy; they showed no abnormalities on their chest films.

The surgical specimen from the resected stomach tissue histologically showed epithelioid cell granulomas in both the stomach and the regional lymph nodes, but no evidence of carcinoma. In 1 case (case 1) granulomatous lesions were also found in the liver and the Kveim reaction was positive. Findings in the 2 cases are illustrated in Figs. 1–8.

Twelve cases of surgically resected gastric sarcoidosis have been reported in Japan.

1. Age
    0–10 yrs.: 0
    21–30 yrs.: 4
    31–40 yrs.: 3
    over 41 yrs.: 5
2. Sex
    Male: 3
    Female: 9
3. Preoperative Diagnosis
    Gastric Ulcer 5
    Gastric Cancer 7
4. Intrathoracic Lesion (BHL) 0
5. Extrathoracic Lesion
    Regional Lymph Node 6
    Liver 1
6. Negative Tuberculin Reaction 7/9
7. Positive Kveim Reaction 2

REFERENCES

1. Liehr, H. 1971. *Med. Klinik* **66**: 418.

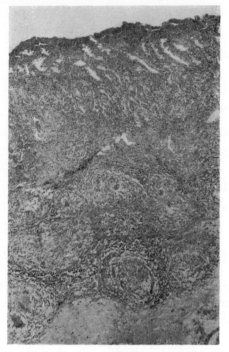

FIG. 1. Case 1. Sarcoid nodules in the gastric mucosa and submucosa, HE stain.

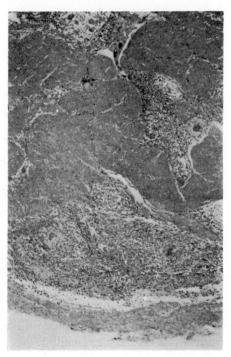

FIG. 2. Case 1. Sarcoid nodules in the gastric muscle layer and subserosa, HE stain.

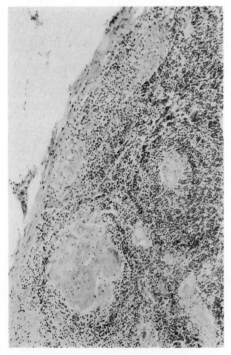

FIG. 3. Case 1. Sarcoid nodules in the perigastric lymph node, HE stain.

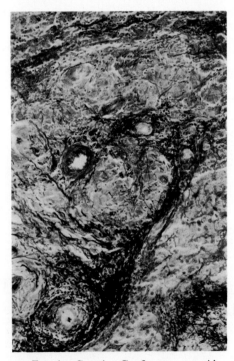

FIG. 4. Case 1. Confluent sarcoid nodule in the portal triad, Azan Mallory stain.

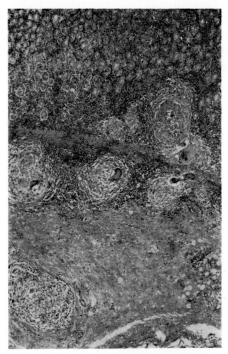

FIG. 5. Case 2. Sarcoid nodules in the gastric mucosa and submucosa, HE stain.

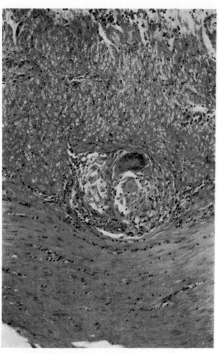

FIG. 6. Case 2. Sarcoid nodule in the gastric muscle layer, HE stain.

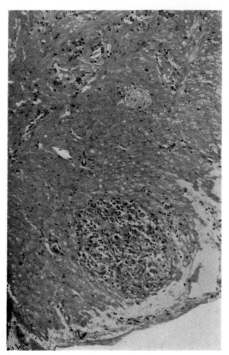

FIG. 7. Case 2. Sarcoid nodule in the gastric subserosa, HE stain.

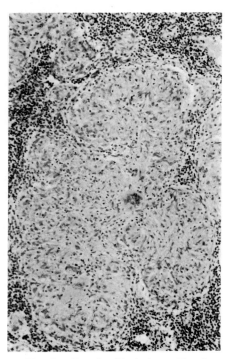

FIG. 8. Case 2. Typical sarcoid nodule in the perigastric lymph node, HE stain.

Pulmonary Sarcoidosis with Multiple Noncircumscribed Lesions Simulating Metastatic Neoplasm

Kenkichi Shikanai, Ryosuke Saheki and Sachiko Narita

Seirei Hospital, Hamamatsu City, Shizuoka, Japan

A 24-year-old man was refered to Seirei Hospital in July 1971 for evaluation of abnormal shadows in his chest X-ray.

The patient had always been healthy. In May 1970, his miniature X-ray film was interpreted as normal (Fig. 1). However, at admission, the chest film revealed multiple non-circumscribed infiltrations in both lung fields. These shadows suggested metastatic neoplasm in the lung areas (Figs. 2, 3, 4).

Physical examination and laboratory findings showed no abnormality data. (Table 1) His bronchogram was normal (Fig. 5).

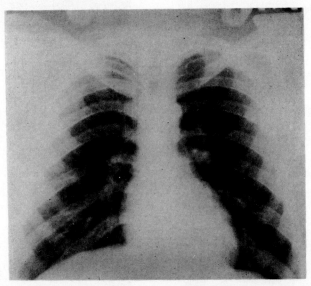

Fig. 1. May, 1970.

Table 1. Laboratory findings.

Tuberculin reaction: $\dfrac{0}{6 \times 6}$ Kveim Test: negative,

B.S.R. 27 mm/h, Leucocyte count 7600, Urine and Feces: normal

Liver function tests: Icterus Index 4.0, Z.T.T. 7.7, Cholesterol 124, GOT 12, GPT 11, Al-ph 6.0 (K-A.), γ-glob. 14.9%,

Electrolytes: Na. 136, K. 3.8, Cl. 103, Ca. 4.6,

Sputum: Tubercle Bacilli (——), Fungi (——), Malignant Cells (——),

E.C.G: normal

Pulmonary function tests: V.C. 4290, %V.C. 104.4%, %FEV$_{1.0}$ 87.4%, DLco 34.3 ml/min./mmHg, %DLco 98.0%,.

Po$_2$ 76 mmHg, Pco$_2$ 36mmHg, PH 7.44

In september 1971, open lung biopsy was performed, and numerous gross, yellow-grayish flecks on the lung surface and marked enlargement of mediastinal and hilar-lymphnodes were seen.

Microscopically, these specimens revealed noncaseating granulomas and typical sarcoid findings. (Fig. 6: Lung tissue; Fig. 7 Lymph nodes.)

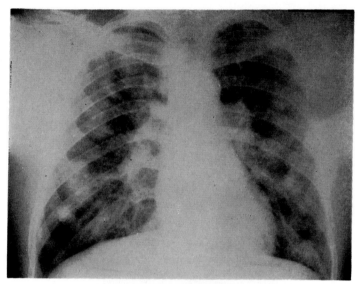

FIG. 2.   July, 1971.

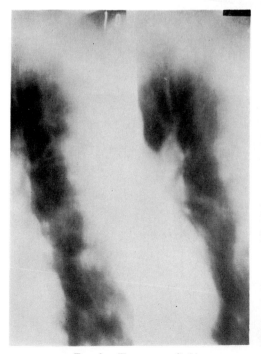

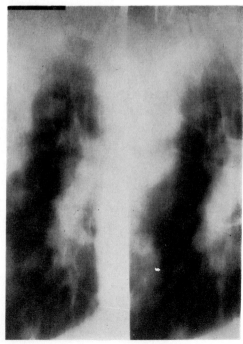

FIG. 3.   Tomogram (left).   FIG. 4.   Tomogram (right).

The patient did not receive corticosteroid or other special therapy for his pulmonary sarcoidosis during hospitalization, but nonetheless, his abnormal chest X-ray shadows improved remarkably (Fig. 8: 1 month after open-lung biopsy) and 3 months later, disseminated infiltrations in both lung fields had disappeared completely (Fig. 9).

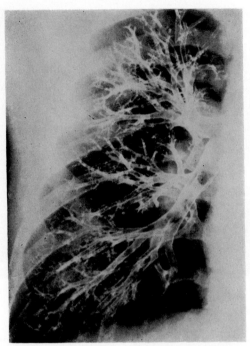

FIG. 5.   Bronchogram.

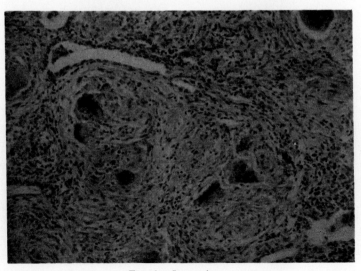

FIG. 6.   Lung tissue.

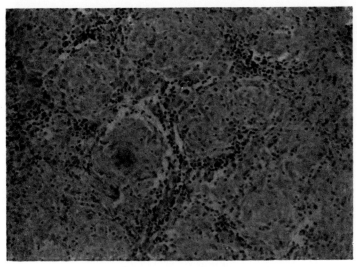

FIG. 7.   Lymph nodes.

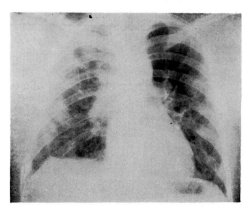

FIG. 8.   One month after open-lung biopsy.

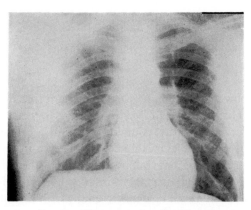

FIG. 9.   Three months after Fig. 8.

Sarcoidosis or Tuberculosis?

Tzihiro Takahasi

Heatlth Control Institute, Ajinomoto Co. Inc., Kawasaki, Japan

AND

Teruhisa Kurokawa

Kitasato Institute Hospital, Tokyo, Japan

Case

S.M., 44-year-old male, a company director (Fig. 1).

Mr. S.M. 44-year-old male, a company director. Tuberculin test was positive when aged 13. No BCG vaccination was made.

1955: Abnormal shadow in the right lung.

1957: Visual disturbance with central scotoma.

Fig. 1.

Family history

His father died of a disease of the liver and his mother of a cerebral homorrhage. His brother, wife and son are in good health.

Past history

Tuberculin test was positive when aged 13. No BCG vaccination was made. The patient happened to be X-rayed in July 1955 and in July 1960 (Fig. 2) an abnormal shadow of the right lung was detected. In 1957 and 1959, he complained of visual disturbance with central scotoma.

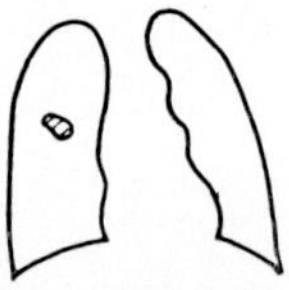

Fig. 2.   1960: Jul. 13.

Status

From February to November 1960, he worked so hard that his body weight fell from 85 kg down to 74.5 kg. His height was 175 cm. A chest X-ray taken on 14 November 1960 revealed unilateral hilar adenopathy containing 2 small calcified lesions in the left adenopathy and an oval shadow (A) of about 24 by 14 mm in the right lower lobe (segment 6b) (Fig. 3). On admission on 18 November 1960, the following laboratory examinations were in normal limits; urinanalysis, blood hemoglobin concentration, erythrocyte count, total and differential leucocyte count with 2% of eosinophil leucocytes, erythrocyte sedimentation rate, sulfabromphthalein retention, and Thorn's test. Gamma-

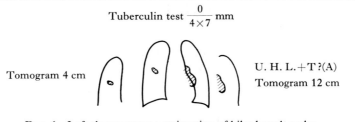

Tuberculin test $\dfrac{0}{4\times7}$ mm

Tomogram 4 cm

U. H. L.+T ?(A)
Tomogram 12 cm

Dec. 6   Left thoracotomy ; extirpation of hilar lymph nodes.

FIG. 3.   Admission, Nov. 14.

1961 :   Feb. 19 Discharge.

FIG. 4.   Sarcoid granulomas were demonstrated by photomicrographs in colour.

(After discharge no special treatment was given.)

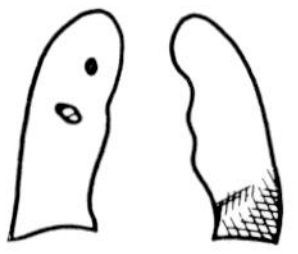

FIG. 5.   Apr. 7.

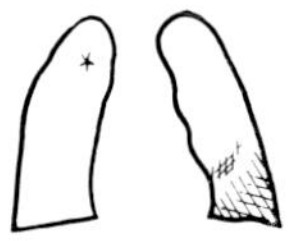

FIG. 6.   1962 : Apr. 18.

globulin in the serum was 22.3%, a little higher than normal. Wasserman serum reaction was negative. Laryngeal swab culture was negative for tubercle bacilli. Bronchoscopy gave no stenotic findings. Exfoliative examinations of sputum as well as bronchial washings by bronchoscopic procedures were negative for cancer. Bronchography showed a normal pattern. A tuberculin test using 1: 2,000 dilution of old tuberculin showed a redness of 4 by 7 mm at the 48-hour reading on 9 November 1960. On suspicion of tumor of the lung, left thoracotomy was performed on 6 December. Fifteen of the enlarged hilar lymph nodes were extirpated but no lung lesions were palpable. The size of the extirpated hilar lymph nodes ranged from about 5 by 5 mm to about 20 by 20 mm. The adhesion of lymph nodes to the surrounding tissues was not very strong. These lymph nodes showed a negative culture for tubercle bacilli. They contained many epitheloid cell granulomas compatible with sarcoidosis (Fig. 4). After the operation, a total of 74 mg of Dexamethasone was given for 10 weeks, though radiographically unchanged. Ophthalmological examination on 25 January 1961 gave no sarcoid findings except for coloboma chorioideae congenita. He was discharged on 19 February 1961 (Fig. 5). After 1 year and a half, the abnormal shadow disappeared (Figs. 6 and 7). During this period no special treatment was given. Since discharge he has been in good health. On 17th August 1972, his body weight was 86 kg and blood pressure showed 170/80 mmHg. A chest X-ray revealed no abnormal shadow in either lung (Fig. 8). A tuberculin test showed a redness

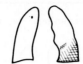

FIG. 7. 1963 : Aug. 5.

Tuberculin test $\dfrac{+}{16 \times 14}$ mm

FIG. 8. 1963 : Dec, 1972 : Aug.

of 16×14 mm with induration, i.e., positive reaction. The following laboratory examinations were within normal limits; urinanalysis, blood hemoglobin concentration, erythrocyte count, total and differential leucocyte count with 4% of eosinophil leucocytes; calcium (5.0 mEq/l), total protein, albumin and globulin in serum. The serum gamma-globulin was 20.7%, a little higher than normal.

It may be presumed that the cause of the lesion was sarcoidosis, and not tuberculosis, i.e., natural healing of sarcoidosis.

Sarcoidosis in Japan

The Japan Sarcoidosis Committee

EPIDEMIOLOGY

Cooperative studies on sarcoidosis in Japan began in 1960, when Dr Nobechi reported 94 collected cases under the title " The Epidemiology of Sarcoidosis in Japan " at the second International Conference on Sarcoidosis in Washington.

Over the last decade, the Japan Sarcoidosis Committee has conducted 4 nationwide surveys of this disease, in 1960, 1961, 1964, and 1969, and in 1967 made a follow-up study on 416 histologically confirmed cases.

Nationwide surveys

Table 1 shows the number of questionnaires, and responses to questionnaires, and the number of cases reported to the Committee.

The data on these patients was recorded on personal registration cards, patients being carefully checked to avoid duplicated registration.

TABLE 1. Nationwide surveys.

Survey	Questionnaires sent	Answers		Cases registered
		received	%	
1 st. (1960)	783	343	43.8	94
2 nd. (1961)	3016	716	23.7	188
3 rd. (1964)	2579	1163	45.0	418
4 th. (1969)	2742	1146	42.0	1052
Total	9140	3368	37.0	1752

Annual number of new cases with sarcoidosis

The annual number of newly detected sarcoidosis patients over the last decade, as shown in Fig. 1, has been increasing at a remarkable rale, both in histologically confirmed and clinically diagnosed cases.

Reason for discovery of sarcoidosis

Of the total cases, 50% were detected by mass survey, and 38% of cases as a result of visiting hospitals with complaints.

Incidence rate of sarcoidosis in a defined working group

The number of sarcoidosis patients, has been showing a marked increase year by year (Fig. 1), but the annual incidence rate of the disease among over 400 employees of the Japan National Railways seems to have remained almost unchanged except for 1968–1969 (Fig. 3). It may be said that the remarkable increase in the number of newly

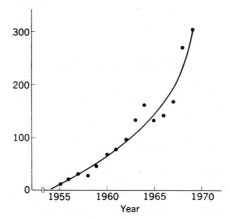

FIG. 1.   Aunual number of new cases with sarcoidosis (1955–1969) (J.S.C.).

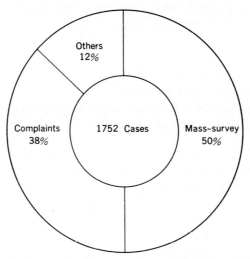

FIG. 2.   Reason for discovery of sarcoidosis (J.S.C., 1969).

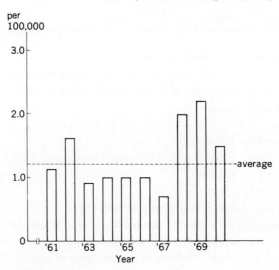

FIG. 3.   Aunual incidence of sarcoidosis (1961–1970) (Y. Hosoda et al.).

detected sarcoidosis cases has mainly been due to a growing interest among doctors in this disease.

Geographical distribution

The geographical distribution of the cases shows that the northern districts had a higher incidence rate than the southern in Japan.

The rate in Hokkaido was 3 times higher than that in the Chugoku-Shikoku-Kyushu districts.

Site of lesions at the onset (1752 Cases) (J.S.C.)

Figure 5 shows a particular feature of sarcoidosis in Japan. In the chest involvement, BHL with or without lung lesions is distinctly predominant. Lung lesions without BHL

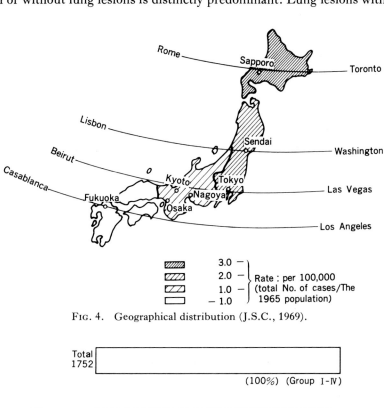

FIG. 4.   Geographical distribution (J.S.C., 1969).

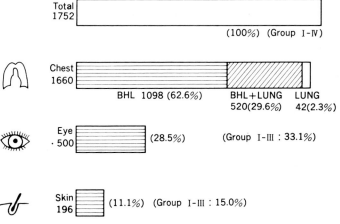

FIG. 5.   Site of lesions at the onset (1752 Cases), (J.S.C.).

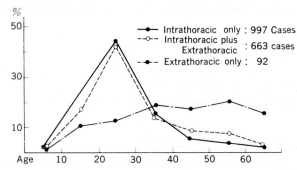

FIG. 6. Age distribution by types of the disease (1752 Cases), (J.S.C.).

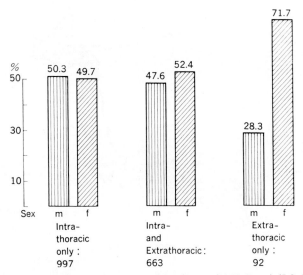

FIG. 7. Sex difference by types of the disease (1752 Cases) (J.S.C.).

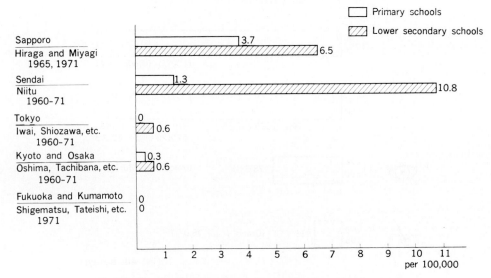

FIG. 8. Frequency of childhood sarcoidosis, based on annual mass survey.

accounted for only 2.3% of the cases. These facts suggest the majority of sarcoidosis cases in Japan belong to the early stage.

The frequency of ocular lesions was relatively high.

The frequency of skin sarcoidosis (11.1%), in Japan is almost similar to, or slightly lower than that reported in Europe.

Age distribution by types of the disease

Figure 6 represents the age distribution of sarcoidosis patients. In the " Intrathoracic only " cases, the 20–29 age group shows a high peak accounting for 44%. However, in the " extrathoracic only " cases, the 50–59 age group, represents the peak, although it is lower than that of the " intrathoracic only " cases.

Sex difference by types of disease

With regard to sex difference " intrathoracic only " cases showed an equal sex distribution. " Extrathoracic only " cases, on the other hand, revealed a distinct female predominance accounting for 71%.

These characteristic features concerning sex and age were distinct particularly in patients suffering from skin sarcoidosis without any chest lesions.

CHILDHOOD SARCOIDOSIS IN JAPAN

The frequency of childhood sarcoidosis based on annual mass X-ray surveys has been reported (Fig. 8).

Almost all Japanese schoolchildren and university students have been mass X-rayed at least once a year. This accounts for the large number of childhood sarcoidosis cases discovered in this country. The rate of newly discovered cases showed a decrease from the north to the south, with the exception of Sendai lower secondary schools, where it reached 10.8 per 100,000

FAMILIAL SARCOIDOSIS IN JAPAN

There have been 16 instances of familial sarcoidosis so far reported in Japan. The disease has occurred in siblings in 14 families, in mothers and their offspring in 2 families, and in a married couple in both partners. The observed incidence rate of familial sarcoidosis seems to be significantly higher than the expected rate.

TUBERCULIN SENSITIVITY

All cases had been tuberculin-tested with more than 1 measured record. The prior strong reactors never showed negative reversion during the course of the disease, though some of them became medium reacters. The prior medium reacters were negative in 46% of cases at the onset, remaining negative in 7.7% after recovery. The prior weak reactors changed to negative in 50% of cases at the onset, remaining negative in 30% after recovery. It seems that depression of tuberculin sensitivity in sarcoidosis depends on prior tuberculin sensitivity.

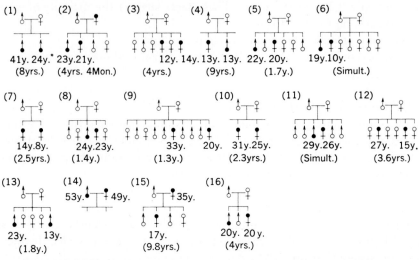

* :   the age of patient.
( ):   the interval of onset between the first, second and third patients.
Reporters: (1) Yamada, N.   (2) Kinoshita, Y.   (3) Sugiyama, S.   (4) Sugiyama, S.
   (5)   Hirasawa, I.   (6) Arai, T   (7) Arai, T.   (8) Gomi, T.   (9) Yamamoto, M.
   (10) Tachibana, T.   (11) Ito, Y.   (12) Niitsu, Y.   (13) Tuchiya, Y.   (14) Ito, Y.
   (15) Kawabe, H.   (16) Hiraga, Y.

FIG. 9.   Familial sarcoidosis in Japan (1972).

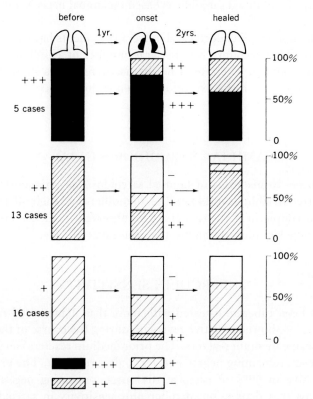

FIG. 10.   Tuberculin sensitivity before the disease, at the onset and after healing
(1969 Y. Hosoda).

INTRATHORACIC SARCOIDOSIS

Radiological classification of pulmonary sarcoidosis (J.S.C.)
The morphological classification of the X-ray findings of pulmonary sarcoidosis proposed by the Japan Sarcoidosis Committee is as follows.

TABLE 2. Morphological classification.

I. Lymph Node

H : Hilar

M : Mediastinal
   Size 0 : No enlargement
        1 : Less than 1.4 cm
        2 : Less than 2.4 cm
        3 : More than 2.5 cm

H 1-3   M 1-3

II. Lung Field

Character
    n : Nodular
   nc : Nodular confluent
    l : Linear
    f : Linear contracted or fibrotic

n   nc   l   f

Extent
    0 : No dissemination
    1 : Under half of the whole lung field
    2 : Over half of the whole lung field
    3 : Whole lung field

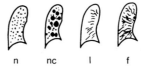

1   2   3

Dissemination
    a : Sparse
    b : Profuse

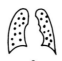 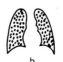

a   b

The radiological course of intrathoracic sarcoidosis

In order to clarify the radiological course of intrathoracic sarcoidosis, a follow-up study was made by the Japan Sarcoidosis Committee.

One hundred and fifty-five histologically confirmed cases of sarcoidosis were followed for a period of more than 2 years. These 155 cases were divided into 3 groups according to the initial chest X-ray findings, namely, a group of 59 BHL cases of, a group of 88 BHL cases with lung parenchymal lesions and a group of 8 cases with lung parenchymal lesions only.

BHL disappeared within 3 years of the observation period in about 50% of cases in the BHL-only group and in 50% of cases in the BHL group with lung parenchymal lesions.

BHL remained unchanged during the observation period in about 20% of cases in the BHL-only group and in the some percentage of cases in the BHL group with lung parenchymal lesions.

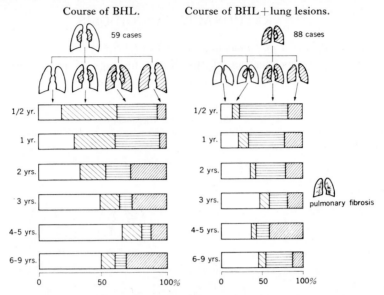

FIG. 11.   Radiological course of intrathoracic sarcoidosis (J.S.C. 1971).,

Pulmonary fibrosis was not found in the BHL-only group, but was detected in 5% of cases in the BHL group in the lung parenchymal lesions in the third year or later.

EXTRATHORACIC SARCOIDOSIS

Ocular lesions

This represents the distribution of 252 sites in 159 to sarcoidosis cases with ocular lesions, observed over a period of about 5 years on average.

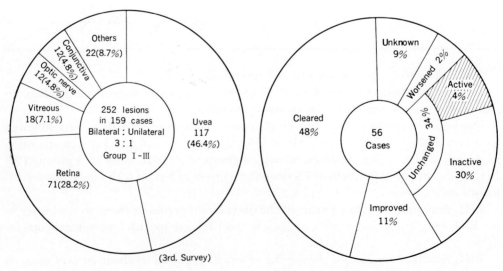

FIG. 12.   Types of ocular lesions (J.S.C., 1964).

FIG. 13.   Prognosis of ocular sarcoidosis after 2.6 years on average.

Prognosis of ocular sarcoidosis

Among 38 patients with initially active ocular changes, 27 (48%) showed clear improvement, 6(11%) improved with no impairment of vision but were unstable. Two remained active and 1 had inactive lesions with moderate impairment of vision. Two cases were lost during the follow-up study. Eighteen cases with initially inactive lesions remained inactive.

Lesions in the liver and spleen

Hepatic lesions were found by peritoneoscopies and/or liver biopsies in 37 of 50 asymptomatic cases with normal hepatic functions (T. Tachibana).

Skin lesions

Skin manifestations of sarcoidosis were classified in Japan by Fukushiro and Niki (1960) into 4 types: (1) nodular type, (2) plaque type, (3) diffuse infiltration, and (4) subcutaneous type. The incidence of erythema nodosum in sarcoidosis in Japan is very rare, only about 1%. Figure 14 represents the incidence rate of each type of skin manifestation of sarcoidosis in Japan.

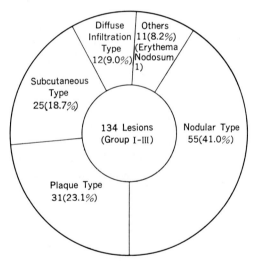

FIG. 14. Types of skin lesions (J.S.C., 1964).

TABLE 3. Course of skin lesions in 43 cases of sarcoidosis
during 5.7 years on average (J.S.C.).

		No. of Cases	Course			
			Cleared	Improved	Unchanged	Worsened
Total No. of cases		43 (100%)	26 (60%)	10 (23%)	5 (12%)	2 (5%)
Types of skin lesion	Nodular type	20	14	2	2	2
	Plaque type	5	1	4	0	0
	Diffuse infiltration	10	4	3	3	0
	Subcutaneous type	5	4	1	0	0
	Erythema nodosum	2	2	0	0	0
	Erythroderma	1	1	0	0	0

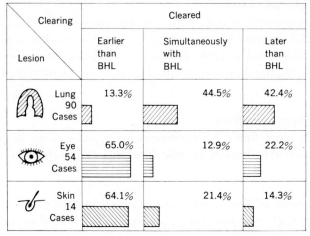

Clearing \ Lesion	Cleared		
	Earlier than BHL	Simultaneously with BHL	Later than BHL
Lung 90 Cases	13.3%	44.5%	42.4%
Eye 54 Cases	65.0%	12.9%	22.2%
Skin 14 Cases	64.1%	21.4%	14.3%

(1st-3rd. Surveys)

FIG. 15. Clearing time of involvements in relation to BHL.

Course of skin lesions

Table 3 shows the course of skin lesions in the 43 cases of sarcoidosis during 5.7 years on average. Kosuda et al. (1969) reported that the frequency of skin manifestations of sarcoidosis was higher in females than in males, especially among patients aged above 40.

Clearing time of involvements in relation to BHL

The clearing of the lung involvements seems to be later than that of BHL.

About 65% of ocular and skin lesions cleared earlier than the disappearance of BHL. On the other hand, 42% of lung lesions remained after the disappearance of BHL.

PROGNOSIS

Prognosis of intra- and extrathoracic sarcoidosis

Table 4 presents the prognosis of sarcoidosis during an average observation period of 5.5 years. In the group of " intrathoracic only " cases, 61% of 225 cases became clear, while only 35% of 131 " Intra- and extrathoracic " cases and 33% of 12 " extrathoracic

TABLE 4. Prognosis of intra- and extrathoracic sarcoidosis.

(Follow-up study in 1967)

	No. of Cases	Cleared (%)	Remained (%)	Dead (%)
Intrathoracic only	225	61	39	—
Intra- and extrathoracic	131	35	58	7
Extrathoracic only	12	33	67	—
Total	368	54	44	2

Average observation period : 5.4 years.

only " cases cleared. Therefore, the " intrathoracic only " group showed a greater number of recoveres than eithertle the " intra- and extrathoracic " or the " extra-thoracic only " groups.

Deaths were included only in the " intra- and extrathoracic " group. The prognosis of sarcoidosis was shown to be worse than had previously been respected.

Autopsy and cause of death

From the observation of 32 autopsy cases, sarcoid granulomas of the lung were shown in all cases except 1, in which only a small portion of the lung had been examined. The myocardium, the spleen and the liver were the next most highly affected organs (88%,

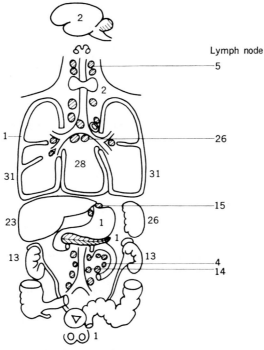

Deep-lying lymph nodes were systematically examined in 26 of 32 autopsy cases.

FIG. 16.   Distribution of sarcoid granulomas (32 autopsy cases), (J.S.C., 1972).

TABLE 5.   Cause of death (32 Autopsy cases).

Sarcoidosis	25(6)*
Myocardial	20(2)
Pulmonary	4(4)
Cerebral	1(0)
Other than sarcoidosis	7(2)**
Total	32(8)

* The cases diagnosed as sarcoidosis prior to death are placed in parentheses.

** Cases of rupture of the aneurysm, agranulocytosis, encephalitis, postoperative death, uremia, hemoptysis etc.

81%, and 72%, respectively). The kidney revealed sarcoid lesions in 39% of the cases. The deep-lying lymph nodes showed different behaviour from the lymph stream system. The hilar and mediastinal lymph nodes were affected in all of the 26 exammined cases; while the pancreaticolienal lymph nodes, the para-aortic lymph nodes, the mesenteric lymph nodes, and the neck lymph nodes showed involvements in 15, 14, 4 and 5 cases, respectively. The frequency of involvement of each lymph node system seemed to be influenced by the degree of involvement in the regional organs (Fig. 16).

The most frequent cause of death in sarcoidosis patients was myocardial involvement which had been diagnosed as sarcoidosis in only 2 out of 20 cases during life. On the other hand, all of the 4 cases in which death had occurred from cor pulmonale, had been diagnosed as sarcoidosis before death (Table 5).

CONCLUSION

During the period 1960–1969, the Japan Sarcoidosis Committee (J.S.C.) conducted nationwide surveys 4 times, and collected a total of 1752 registered cases.

This report, based on a study of these registered cases, reveals several features of sarcoidosis as it has occurred in Japan.

1) Extrathoracic lesions (ocular, skin, bone, etc.) were significantly more prevalent and persistent in females than in males, while intrathoracic lesions were equally distributed in both sexes.

2) Childhood sarcoidosis was not infrequent.

3) The incidence of ocular changes was quite high while that of erythema nodosum was very low.

4) Ocular lesions were found not only in the uvea and the conjunctiva but also, rather more frequently, in the retina.

5) It usually required at least 3 years after the time of the onset for the initial lung infiltrations to develop fibrosis.

6) Myocardial lesions were a frequent cause of death in the fatal cases autopsied.

7) The classification of the radiographic appearance of pulmonary changes proposed by the J.S.C. was useful in recording the course, or evaluating the effect, of treatment.

Familial Occurrence of Sarcoidosis

LARS-GÖSTA WIMAN

Department of Lung Diseases, University Hospital, Umeå, Sweden

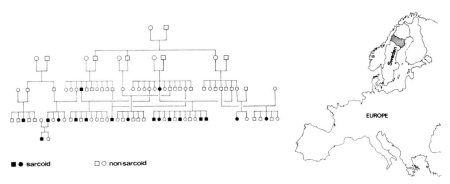

■ ● sarcoid   □ ○ non sarcoid

EUROPE

Sweden

Area : 411,405 square km

Population : 8,013,696 inhabitants

Capital : Stockholm

Sarcoidosis rates (Prevalence) : 64 Cases per 100,000 mass chest radiographies (in Northern Sweden 100–150/100,000)

Tuberculosis rate (Prevalence) : 310 Cases per 100,000 inhabitants (in Northern Sweden 487/100,000)

THE POST-CONFERENCE KYOTO MEETING

organized by
Chest Diseases Research Institute
Kyoto University

16th September, Saturdy, 1972
Kyoto Hotel

PROGRAMME

Opening Remarks by S. Tsuji

SYMPOSIUM I
On the Etiology of Sarcoidosis

Chairmen: W. Jones Williams (Great Britain)
K. Yasuhira (Japan)

Opening Remarks by Dr K. Yasuhira

Designated Speakers: H. Takamatsu (Japan)
M. Yamamoto (Japan)
D. N. Mitchell (Great Britain)
A. Hanngren (Sweden)
J. Turiaf (France)

General Discussion

SYMPOSIUM II
On the Treatment of Sarcoidosis

Chairmen: H. L. Israel (U.S.A.)
H. Homma (Japan)

Designated Speakers: D. G. James (Great Britain)
K. Wurm (German Federal Republic)
C. J. Johns (U.S.A.)
R. Mikami (Japan)
T. Tachibana (Japan)

General Discussion

Opening Remarks

S. Tsuji

Chairman of the Kyoto Conference
Chest Disease Research Institute, Kyoto University, Kyoto, Japan

Ladies and gentlemen: It is a privilege for me to give an opening address at the International Symposium on Sarcoidosis in Kyoto. First of all, I must extend a sincere welcome to all of you distinguished researchers on sarcoidosis who have already attended the symposium in Tokyo, and have now also come to Kyoto to attend this symposium. This symposium is sponsored by the Chest Disease Research Institute, Kyoto University and also by the Japan Sarcoidosis Committee. I wish to thank Professor Kitamura and other members of the Committee most warmly for their kind support in preparing this symposium. You have had many papers and discussions in Tokyo, but I think you may have had little opportunity for concentrated discussions on one specific subject in sarcoidosis. This is the reason why we and the Japan Sarcoidosis Committee have decided to hold a symposium-type meeting in Kyoto to consider 2 important subjects, the etiology and treatment of sarcoidosis. Unfortunately, time is limited and I am afraid that this will not allow us to discuss fully these important problems. Nevertheless, I believe that your enthusiasm may bring fruitful results even from such a small meeting. I again welcome all of you most heartily, and I trust that you will find time to enjoy the traditional atmosphere of Kyoto, the old capital of Japan when the meeting is over.

Thank you.

Sarcoidosis and Mycobacterial Infection

Masahiko Yamamoto

Nagoya City University Medical School, Nagoya, Japan

Since the time of Besnier, there has been much debate concerning the etiological implication of mycobacterial infection for sarcodosis. However, the problem remains unsolved.

In this symposium, the results of 2 analyses supporting a close relationship between mycobacterial infection and the etiology of sarcoidosis will be reported: 1 on the analysis of family and previous history of tuberculosis and the other on the analysis of the results of atypical mycobacterial tuberculin tests.

1) From analysis of 100 cases of sarcoidosis, it was revealed that 24% had a family history of tuberculosis and 13% had a previous history, and that in 36%, calcified foci and in 21% pleural thickness was found in the chest roentgenogram. These percentages were rather higher than in 286 cases of moderately advanced tuberculosis.

The prognosis of the cases with these positive factors in mycobacterial infection was poorer than the others.

2) Skin reaction tests with atypical mycobacterial tuberculin were performed on 57 cases of sarcoidosis. Atypical mycobacterial tuberculin employed here was purified tuberculin, made from each of 3 speices of atypical mycobacteria, namely M. kansasii, M. scrofulaceum and M. intracellulare. Each patient was given 3 intradermal injections of the above 3 types of atypical mycobacterial tuberculin. A control injection was given with an equivalent dose of human-type tuberculin simultaneously. The results were read 48 hours later and erythematous reactions greater than 10 by 10 mm were judged to be positive. They were considered to be significant when the reaction to the atypical mycobacterial tuberculin was more than 1.25 times that of human tuberculin.

The percentage of cases which showed significant reaction to M. kansasii tuberculin was 9.7% in sarcoidosis, 1.5% in healthy persons and 1.6% in pulmonary tuberculosis; to M. scrofulaceum tuberculin 15.6%, 1.0% and 0.1% and to M. intracellulare tuberculin, 21.6%, 5.7% and 3.3%, respectively. As for the reaction to M. scrofulaceum and M. intracellulare tuberculin, statistically significant differences were observed in the sarcoidosis cases as opposed to healthy persons or pulmonary tuberculosis cases.

3) In conclusion, many cases of sarcoidosis were found infected with mycobacteria, i.e., tubercle bacilli or atypical mycobacteria, and it may be supposed that immunodeficiency in sarcoidosis may be related to mycobacterial infection.

DISCUSSION

Dr James: You read your skin test at 48 hours. Did you also read them at 1 month? Because, if you are using lipopolysaccharide, I will predict at 1 month small nodules, and granuloma reproducing the Kveim test. If you have not done so, it is worth looking over these patients.

DR YAMAMOTO: Thank you for your suggestion. I did not do that.

On the Etiology

D. N. Mitchell

MRC Tuberculosis and Chest Diseases Unit, Brompton
Hospital, London, Great Britain

AND

R. J. W. Rees

National Institute for Medical Research, London, Great Britain

In 1969 we presented evidence of a transmissible agent for normal and immunologically deficient (T/900r) mice from human sarcoid tissue (1969. Lancet 2: 81). In subsequent experimental animal studies we have used normal in preference to immunologically deficient mice, since these had shown no significant advantages in our earlier studies.

The results of these further controlled experiments were presented at an earlier session of this Conference, and confirmed our earlier findings. Thus, normal mice inoculated with fresh homogenates from human sarcoid tissue into foot pads, intraperitoneally or intravenously, have yielded local and disseminated sarcoid granulomas associated with positive Kveim tests in the ear. Conversely, identically prepared fresh nonsarcoid and autoclaved or irradiated (2.5 mega. r) sarcoid homogenates inoculated by these same routes, yielded none of these changes after similar intervals of time following inoculation.

Moreover, in other controlled experiments, mice receiving a first or a second passage of ' sarcoid ' mouse foot pad homogenate into foot pads or intravenously, again yielded evidence of local sarcoid and disseminated granulomas associated with positive Kveim tests in the ear. Conversely, mice receiving a first or a second passage of mouse foot pad homogenate prepared from foot pads after an identical interval but following the injection of human nonsarcoid homogenates, and mice receiving a homogenate prepared from normal mouse foot pads by these same routes, showed no evidence of granulomas and all had negative Kveim tests in the ear after corresponding and prolonged intervals following inoculation.

Thus, we were able to show that the transmissible agent for mice derived from human sarcoid tissue is viable, since it can be passaged successfully and is inactivated when the human sarcoid or mouse foot pad ' sarcoid ' homogenates are autoclaved or irradiated.

More recently, we have again turned our attention to the use of the immunologically deficient animal, using mice prepared by adolescent thymectomy followed by whole-body irradiation, (600r) but without subsequent partial syngeneic mouse bone-marrow cell replacement. Six (T/600r) mice were each inoculated with cells (8×10^6) derived from a freshly removed sarcoid lymph node. Thus far, 4 of these mice have been examined after an interval of only 68 days following inoculation; 3 showed granulomas in the lung with associated granulomatous changes in the hilar lymph nodes and spleen. Kveim tests made in the ears of these 4 mice 33 days after initial intravenous inoculation of sarcoid lymph node cells, showed no histological evidence of Kveim reactivity when the mice were killed 4 weeks later. However, in our earlier work using normal and immunologically deficient (T/900r) mice, Kveim reactivity appeared late and followed the prolonged interval required for the development of characteristic sarcoid granulomas 9–24 months after initial foot pad, intravenous, or intraperitoneal inoculation of sarcoid homogenates.

Although much remains to be elucidated, it seems probable that our further exploration of the potential of this animal model (T/600r) in these and other similar controlled experiments, may allow the establishment of sarcoid lesions after a much shorter interval of time following inoculation. If so, we should then be afforded the greater part of the life span of the mouse during which to study the natural history of sarcoidosis and the development of Kveim reactivity.

DISCUSSION

DR JONES WILLIAMS: Thank you very much, Dr. Mitchell. It is most interesting and most fascinating and very provocative. I am sure we must have more time for discussion to go into this. I think I might proceed and go on to the next paper.

Sarcoidosis
—An immunological reaction with disturbed T/B cell ratio—

Å. Hanngren, E. Hedfors, B. S. Nilsson and E. Ripe

Karolinska Hospital, Stockholm, Sweden

The immune system consists of 2 cell types:

1)   Bone marrow- or Bursa equivalent-derived lymphocytes, so-called B cells, which are responsible for humoral antibody production.

2)   Thymus-derived lymphocytes, so-called T cells, which are responsible for the delayed-type immune reactions.

To summarize our paper presented at the Tokyo meeting, we think that the essential pathogenetic event in sarcoidosis is a disturbance in the balance of these 2 components of the immune system, the T and B lymphocytes. The imbalance between the 2 components is characterized by a depression of T cells and a stimulation of B cells.

We have chosen a virus infection to explain *T cell depression*. The reasons are:

1)   A more-or-less transient depression of the PPD skin reactivity occurs in infectious mononucleosis,[1] an EB virus infection, as well as in some other viral diseases. Earlier in vitro studies have shown that lymphocytes from these patients could not be stimulated by PHA, a T cell stimulator.[2] On the other hand the B cell function seems to be undisturbed as judged from increased immunoglobulin levels and production of heterophile antibodies.

2)   Sarcoidosis patients show signs of infection with EB virus and/or other viruses belonging to the herpes group.[3, 4]

As the *B cell stimulator* we have proposed tuberculoproteins from a BCG vaccination, a common event in Sweden, or a tuberculous infection. This latter proposal needs perhaps some explanation. We are used to consider tuberculin as a T cell stimulator, since the expression of delayed hypersensitivity seems to be intimately linked to the thymus function. However, it has recently been shown that tuberculin is a strong B cell stimulator.[5, 6] In nonimmunized mice of 2 different strains, spleen cells responded strongly to PPD stimulation. The same stimulatory effect was also found in both newborn and adult guinea pigs, and in mice having only B cells. Furthermore, these cells show signs of immunoglobulin production.[6] PPD-stimulated cells can be stained for intracellular immunoglobulin by the immunofluorescence technique.

In tuberculin-negative humans we find a lymphocyte response profile to PPD which looks very much the same as the response in mouse B cells.[7] This type of response is in sharp contrast to that found in tuberculin-positive humans.[7] Consequently we may speculate that the PPD response found in tuberculin-negative humans is in fact a B cell response. In lymphocytes from sarcoidosis patients we find the same dose-response profile as in negative healthy persons.[8] Also using other specific B cell markers, which time does not permit me to go into detail about, we have found suggestive evidence for B cell predominance in sarcoidosis.[9]

The idea that products from tubercle bacilli act as a general stimulator of antibody production is, for a chest physician, nothing new and you all know about the adjuvanticity of mycobacteria both in tuberculous patients and in experimental situations, where a generalized antibody formation can be found. This fits very well with the B cell-stimulating effect of tuberculin, whether this substance is really purified or contains lipopolysacharides.

Integrating the evidence for T cell depression in sarcoidosis and the B cell stimulating properties of products from tubercle bacilli a hypothesis on the etiology can be formulated as follows: A virus infection, for example an EB infection, depresses the T cell function but leaves the B cell function undisturbed, resulting in depressed tuberculin reactivity but with normal response in antibody production. A BCG vaccination or a tuberculous infection may induce an atypical immune response due to the defective T cell function. Instead of a normal T cell response the B cell-stimulating property of the tuberculoproteins will dominate. The stimulated B cells (whole population of B cells) may give rise to immunoglobulins found in stage I sarcoidosis, (clinically also expressed in an increase of ESR). The hyperergic reaction erythema nodosum, which for the clinician has been in contrast to the hypoergic condition of negative tuberculin reaction may be explained by an antigen-antibody-complement reaction. This reaction fits well with an overall B cell stimulation. Fever and arthralgia sometimes seen in stage I may also be attributed to the B cell stimulation. The generalization of the disease may be explained if we accept that tuberculoproteins (not bacilli) are spread throughout the whole body after a BCG vaccination[10] or a tuberculous infection and the epitheloid cell granuloma without necrosis can be explained by stimulated macrophage activity but without any transformation of T cells to killer cells that otherwise causes necrosis. The T cells are depressed by viral infection. Finally the defective T cell function explains the depressed PPD reactivity.

If we accept this reasoning some other findings are reasonable:

1) No findings of tubercle bacilli in most cases. 2) No effect of antituberculous drugs. 3) Certain effect of corticosteroids. 4) Difficulties in transferring the disease to animals. 5) The difference in epidemiology between tuberculosis and sarcoidosis and in sarcoidosis epidemiology between different countries, ages and social groups.

We have chosen the virus-BCG interaction to explain the pathogenesis but we certainly realize that other combinations of one agent causing depression and another causing stimulation of the 2 components of the immune system are possible.

REFERENCES

1. Lantorp, K., Wahren, B., and Hanngren, Å. 1972 Depression of the tuberculin reaction in infectious mononucleosis. Brit. Med. J. 4: 668.
2. Rubin, A. D. 1966. Lymphocyte RNA synthesis in infectious mononucleosis. The response to phytohaemagglutinin in vitro. *Blood* 28: 602–605.
3. Hirshaut, Y., Glade, P., Viera, L. O. Ainbender, E., Dvorak, D., and Siltzbach, L. E. 1970. Sarcoidosis, another disease associated with serologic evidence for herpes-like virus infection. *New Engl. J. Med.* 283: 502–506.
4. Wahren, B., Carlens, E., Espmark, Å. Lundbeck, H., Löfgren, S., Madar, E., Henle, G., and Henle, W. 1971. Antibodies to various herpesviruses in sera from patients with sarcoidosis. *J. Nat. Cancer Inst.* 47: 747–756.
5. Sultzer, B. M., and Nilsson, B. S. 1972 PPD-tuberculin, a B cell mitogen. *Nature,* 240: 198–200.

6. Nilsson, B. S., Sultzer, B. M., and Bullock, W. W. 1973 PPD tuberculin induces immunoglobulin production in normal mouse spleen cells. *J. Exp. Med.* **137**: 127–139.

7. Nilsson, B. S. 1972. The response of lymphocytes from tuberculin positive or negative humans to various doses of PPD tuberculin in vitro. *Cell. Immunol.* **3**: 493–500.

8. Hedfors, E., and Nilsson, B. S. The response of lymphocytes in sarcoidosis to various doses of PPD tuberculin in vitro. Manuscript in preparation.

9. Hedfors, E., and Nilsson, B. S. The lymphocyte response to various doses of lipopolysacharides in sarcoidosis. Manuscript in preparation.

10. Gormsen, H. 1956. On the occurence of epitheloid cell granulomas in the organs of BCG-vaccinated human beings. *Acta Path. Microbiol. Scand.* Suppl. **111**: 117.

DISCUSSION

Dr James: I agree completely with every point in Dr Hanngren's idea. He uses the interaction of virus and chosen mycobacterium. But I would like to expand it to include not just mycobacterium but lipopolysaccharide. One example is pine pollen, which is not a mycobacterium, but is full of lipopolysaccharide. When we had the Congress in Washington, the whole story in those days was that lipopolysaccharide in pine pollen behaves like mycobacterium. I am sure this is the right way to look at these problems.

Dr Hanngren: If you do laboratory experiments for B cell stimulation, you can buy commercial lipopolysaccharide. This is, I think, manufactured from Coli bacterium. Comparing commercially available lipopolysaccharide with the effect of tuberculin, tuberculin is much more efficient and the most efficient B cell-stimulating agent found at present.

Dr Selroos: I would like to ask Professor Hanngren what strength of PPD you used in tuberculin skin tests. Because in my material, for example, 24 patients were negative for 100 TU, and many of them had in vitro response.

Dr Hanngren: Skin reactivity was measured with 2 and 20 TU. Each time you measure the reactivity, you must increase the strength by 10 times. I don't think this provides any evidence for B cell activity, if you don't know what the skin reactivity is due to.

About the Etiology of Sarcoidosis

J. Turiaf

Bichat Hospital, University of Paris, Paris, France

Of all attempts to reproduce sarcoidosis experimentally, those using FCA are the least disappointing. Following several authors[1] we have shown that intravenous injection of FCA frequently provokes in laboratory animals, especially the rat[2] a diffuse granulomatosis sometimes severely involving the lungs. This granulomatosis has the histological character of sarcoid lesions, i.e., a cell population composed principally of epithelioid cells and a few giant cells without caseous necrosis. Pearson and Waksman[3] established also that intradermal injection of FCA can provoke an inflammatory and transient polyarthritis in the rat after some latency; sometimes uveitis or other inflammatory eye lesions occur as well as cutaneous papules and nodules. These facts, as interpreted by authors who described them, suggest an intervention of allergic and immunological phenomena induced by FCA. But it is essential that the adjuvant should be complete, because the mycobacterial fraction alone is ineffective.

Chase,[4] injecting experimental guinea pigs intramuscularly with killed KB suspended in mineral oil, obtained various genital and cutaneous lesions with the same pathological pattern as in sarcoidosis. But these lesions only occur in animals unable to develop tuberculin allergy, which leads us to believe, with Chase, in a particular kind of allergic reaction to mycobacterial antigens. It should be emphasized that this reaction, as regards pathological aspects, is not specific to allergic reactions or immunological disorders brought about by antigens of mycobacterial origin or by substances derived from them. The same is observed in berylliosis, which in its chronic and generalized form affects numerous organs: lungs, liver, lymph nodes, spleen, etc . . . The part played by allergy is sufficiently shown in this disease by the positiveness and specificity of the beryllium cutaneous test.

Zirconium dermalitis, although very localized, is also a sarcoid-type lesion related to an allergic reaction.

In both examples, skin tests with zirconium and beryllium are strictly specific.

Such is the Kveim test for sarcoïdosis. We shall not recall the arguments about the Kveim-test specificity. This reaction happens exceptionally to be positive in diseases distinct from sarcoidosis. The reactogen should be prepared from a tissue (lymphadenopathy or splenomegaly) rich in sarcoid granulomas.

Sarcoidosis can be considered as a state betraying a reaction of the organism to one or several still unknown agents. Specificity of their biophysical or biochemical nature is likely, as suggested by the Kveim test data.

Race may intervene as a predisposing factor, particularly in cross-breeding.

Immunological disorders, i.e., decrease of cellular immunity, disturbances of immunoglobulins, are symptoms of sarcoidosis, as well as radiological and clinical signs. Most of them disappear on recovery.

REFERENCES

1. Laufer, A., Tal, C., and Behar, A. J. 1959. Effects of adjuvant (Freund's type) and tis components on the organs of various animal species: a comparative study. *Brit. J. Exp. Path.* **40**: 1.
2. Basset, F., Soler, D., Fiez-Vandal, D. Y., Basset, G., and Turiaf, J. 1972. Granulomatose diffuse des poumons induite experimentalement chez le rat. *Ann. Med. Intern.* **123**: 1, 71.
3. Pearson, C. M., Waksman, B. H., and Sharp, J. T. 1961. Studies of arthritis and other lesions induced in rats by injections of mycobacterial adjuvant. Changes affecting the skin and mucous Membranes'. *J. Exp. Med.* **113**: 485.
4. Chase, M. W. 1959. Disseminated granulomata in Guineapig, Mechanism of hypersensitivity. Boston: Shaffer-Lagrippe and Chase. p. 673.

DISCUSSION

DR JAMES: This is a very important slide (asking to see the last slide in the presentation by Dr Turiaf) for epidemiologists. As with Caribbean people in Paris, the same thing is observable in many different communities such as Puerto Ricans in New York and Irish people coming to London. The epidemiologist should be thinking along racial lines as a predisposing factor for the disease.

DR MITCHELL: I would like to bring out 2 points.   Firstly about immunology, restricted primarily to the Kveim test. Specific skin reaction in the zirconium story is commonly recognized, but in the case of the Kveim test, it is reported that there is 1.5 to 5% positivity among a wide variety of diseases other than sarcoidosis. The second point is with regard to the etiology of sarcoidosis. It is generally recognized among patients presenting with Löfgren's syndrome or radiologically stage I disease, about 25% will be tuberculin-positive to 10 TU, and probably about 50 or even 54% patients of erythema nodosum with Löfgren's syndrome. We know very well among progressive sarcoidosis with granulomata all over, not less than 7 or 8% will be quite strongly tuberculin-sensitive to a 10 TU test or even weaker tuberculin dilution. This also occurs in patients with hypogammagloburinemia, in whom multisystem sarcoidosis has been demonstrated.

GENERAL DISCUSSION

Chairmen: W. Jones Williams and K. Yasuhira

Dr. Jones Williams: There are large number of points which come out from these fascinating speeches. I will just mention very briefly 1 or 2 points about these speeches. First is histology, with very beautiful slides by Professor Takamatsu of his data on exudative, proliferative and productive types of granuloma. I would like to ask him what he found regarding changes of the lymphocytes around granuloma as the lesions change from exudative to productive and to proliferative. Going on to the second paper, Dr. Yamamoto gave a very interesting discussion and introduction to the difficult topic of the meaning of abnormal skin reaction to atypical tuberculin. Lots of similar work, as you know, has been done by Dr Chapmann in Texas and others. They are also looking at the same sort of problem in pneumoconiosis in coal workers who have massive lesions in the lung and as to whether atypical mycobacterium are involved. How much of this is really applicable to sarcoidosis? Perhaps it is just measuring again T—or may be B—cell function. Going on to the third paper read by Dr. Mitchell, he reminded us about the variety of views that have been expressed in the past and what the epithelioid cell does. I tend to think now, it is a biosynthetic cell producing something. I was very impressed by Dr Mitchell's report trying out amyloid in skin reaction. Then going on to the next paper of Professor Hanngren, this raises a number of questions as to how we distinguish T cells or B cells, and the relationship of T cells to B cells. Perhaps one cell contains the other. Finally, Professor Turiaf's paper. Dealing with Freund's complete adjuvant, he produced very beautiful sarcoid-like lesions and again raises the question of how does this sort of experiment help us to understand what is happening in sarcoidosis. I would like briefly to show 2 or 3 slides. In discussions on the etiology of sarcoidosis, many people show similar slides. We think of this large variety of agents in trying to induce sarcoid granuloma, and we should seek such agents in patients with clinically and radiologically confirmed sarcoidosis. The clinicians have nice clear pictures usually of what constitutes sarcoidosis. But really to be sure, I think, one ought to try in every case to find these various agents. Then, what worries me is Professor Hanngren's work. It is extremely exciting and very interesting. In the divergent findings one gets with these various tests, tests of T cells, we get very mixed results. Sometimes, they are positive and sometimes they are negative. The next slide is again on differences of opinion. This is macrophage inhibition factor. Three or 4 authors here and others in the Tokyo Conference find that we can stimulate B cells. If the cells are T cells, then we are proving stimulation and not depression.

Fractionation of Kveim test material may not give us the cause of sarcoidosis: it may give us agents that provoke the sort of reaction in many different diseases. Mucopolysaccharide in the mature epithelioid cell, I think, might be produced by epithelioid cells and might be the Kveim agent, though this is not necessarily what starts sarcoidosis, because the same sort of reaction occurs in such a variety of conditions. At the moment, we think that the lymphocytes transform to activated lymphocytes and epithelioid cells. We know that the monocyte becomes the macrophage. But what we have to remember is the cross-linking between the cells. The T and B cell concept is not at all absolute. The cells can easily change their function, change their morphology. Now I would like open general discussion. Dr Israel Would you like to ask any questions on this fascinating topic of what has mycobacterial got to do with sarcoidosis?

DR ISRAEL: I should like to ask Professor Hanngren whether his concept does not suppose that an immunologic defect preceeds sarcoidosis. The same point was illustrated in Dr Turiaf's diagram. What evidence is there for an immunologic defect prior to the onset of sarcoidosis? As you know we proposed a few years ago that inability to develop and maintain tuberculin sensitivity antedated sarcoidosis. I must admit we have never been able to find any support for that thesis. Most evidence, I believe, is the other way around.

DR HANNGREN: When we are looking at the lymphocytes of sarcoid patients, we found predominantly B cell lymphocytes. So there must be either enormous stimulation of B cell lymphocyte or depression of T cells. Most likely, it is both B cell stimulation and T cell depression.

DR MITCHELL: I would like to respond to Professor Israel's question. In the Medical Research Council's Clinical Trial of Tuberculosis Vaccines, 52,239 young adults were followed from age 14 for a decade or more. They were divided into 5 groups according to their initial skin test and vaccination studies. Over the decade 52 of these young people developed early intrathoracic sarcoidosis: these were shared fairly equally between the 5 groups and clearly the onset of sarcoidosis was quite irrespective of prior tuberculin sensitivity or vaccination studies. What is more, the evidence for depression of delayed-type sensitivity, eg to tuberculin among those tested shortly after onset of the disease was much less than one might expect.

DR SELROOS: As Dr Jones Williams showed in his slide the blood lymphocytes of sarcoidosis patients have a spontaneous transformation capacity. This must be noticed when we culture the lymphocytes in the presence of PPD. Furthermore, culture studies with lymphocytes from patients with normal renal function and various degrees of impaired function and with PPD as mitogen have shown, that a negative skin reaction to 10 TU does not necessarily indi-

cate tuberculin negativity. Incubated with PPD the lymphocytes of these "negative" patients may exhibit DNA synthesis and undergo blastic transformation. This means that when we are talking about tuberculin negativity the skin reaction must be negative to at least 100 TU of PPD. This is of importance also when we are dividing our series into tuberculin positive and negative groups.

DR HANNGREN: There were different studies from that Dr Jones-Williams referred to, in which different B cells in the lymphocyte stimulation were considered to be Kveim stimulators. There are different results reported concerning this point. You are observing the response in exactly the same types of patients in the same stages who either do not respond at all or who do respond well to Kveim. Were all these patients in the same stage?

DR JONES WILLIAMS: We related our results to the duration of the disease. I am sorry, I cannot give you exact figures of stage I, II or III. Patients in our study were stage I or II and there were no stage III in our cases. But, B cells with this sarcoid test were thought to be T cells, and yet in vitro they respond with this technique.

DR HANNGREN: You already answered this problem, because you spoke of interaction between T and B cells. I agree. This is mainly why I misunderstood the question a moment ago. In healthy normal persons with negative skin reaction, all lymphocytes responding to PPD stimulation may not be B lymphocytes, but may include some T lymphocytes. They are always a mixed lymphocyte culture. But the evidence that B lymphocytes are responsible for most of the response is supported during LPS stimulation. LPS only stimulates B cells. If you use PPD, you will find that they are very slightly stimulated.

DR JONES WILLIAMS: You are using lymphocytes from the spleen in some of your animal experiments. They are a mixture of T and B cells.

DR HANNGREN: For distinguishing T and B lymphocytes, you can see in spleen culture, almost 60% are B cells. In thymus and thoracic lymph nodes, they are mostly T cells.

DR TSUJI: I have some comments regarding tuberculosis. Among mycobacterium, tuberculosis bacilli may have some significance in induction of sarcoidosis. But I think it is not only mycobacterium. As we reported in Tokyo, we have found 4 or 5 strains of Nocardia from sarcoid tissue. This may have some role, too, in the production of sarcoid tissue reaction.

DR UESAKA: I don't know whether Nocardia, which we isolated, have any relation to sarcoidosis or not. About 4 years ago, we first isolated an organism from sarcoid tissue. We repeated the isolation and found 8 strains of Nocardia from 65 specimens, as I reported in Tokyo.

DR IZUMI: I would like to have some comments. In experimental sarcoidosis, I think, we must have several check points: the first is histological change with epithelioid tubercles, the second, immunological changes, i.e., the depression of T lymphocyte reaction and normal or elevated B lymphocyte reaction. The third is that the experimental lesion has the possibility of showing spontaneous regression.

DR YASUHIRA: In my experience with lipopolysaccharide from mycobacteria, we can cause sarcoid-like lesions in animals. But these lesions regress within several weeks without any treatment. If the organism is alive and the component of the bacilli is produced continuously, the lesion may remain as long as the action has continued. However, in the case of human beings, lesions which have continued for several years, may finally regress as you all know. So chemical factors of bacterial agent may play some role in the sarcoid.

DR JONES WILLIAMS: One also knows that in a variety of lesions such as in the intestinal tract and liver, one can find sarcoid granuloma. When one does histochemistry on this, phospholipid and also mucopolysaccharide and a variety of other similar related complex, mucolipoproteins are demonstrated. No doubt, these types of material contribute to granuloma.

I would like just to quote the title of an excellent paper by Professor David in Boston, who has done so much work on lymphocyte function. The title of the paper, in J. Allergy 1971, is "The elusive humors of the lymphocyte mediators of delayed hypersensitivity". The lymphocyte is not a simple little black dark cell. Now we find not only that it can pass information to monocytes, perhaps to macrophages, but also that it can itself introduce a substance which can effect macrophages.

I would like, at the end of session, to thank all of you on the panel and the floor.

SYMPOSIUM II

ON THE TREATMENT OF SARCOIDOSIS

Drugs for the Treatment of Sarcoidosis

D. Geraint James

Royal Northern Hospital, London, Great Britain

INDICATIONS FOR CORTICOSTEROID THERAPY

Ocular Involvement

Topical corticosteroids should always be administered for iridocyclitis in the form of eye drops applied frequently during the day, reinforced with a corticosteroid eye ointment at night. If there is no substantial and continuing improvement during 10 days, then the concentration of corticosteroid in the anterior segment of the eye may be increased by a local subconjunctival depot of cortisone. Oral corticosteroids are indicated if local treatment does not lead to a rapid response or if ophthalmoscopy reveals posterior uveitis. In addition, the inflamed iris should be rested by local atropine eye drops to maintain a dilated pupil.

Abnormal chest radiograph

An abnormal chest radiograph which does not show any spontaneous improvement in the course of 6 months should be treated. Bilateral hilar lymphadenopathy is likely to subside without treatment and this is particularly so if it is associated with erythema nodosum. On the contrary, pulmonary infiltration which remains static or worsens during the course of 6 months is an indication for oral steroids in an effort to prevent the development of irreversible pulmonary fibrosis. Substantial improvement in the chest radiograph is related to the length of time before treatment is given. Results are considerably better in those treated within 1 year of the onset of the disease.[1]

Breathlessness

If this symptom is present, then the patient has already reached a stage of irreversible pulmonary fibrosis or disturbed gas transfer. Oral steroids provide symptomatic relief but do not influence the natural history of the disease or its grave prognosis at the irreversible stage of breathlessness.

Persistent hypercalciuria

Steroids will prevent excessive gastrointestinal absorption and excessive urinary excretion of calcium. Instead, calcium is diverted to a harmless fecal excretion within days of the exhibition of oral steroids.

Disfiguring skin lesions

When lupus pernio or other unsightly lesions distress patients, oral and local corticosteroids may correct the deformity. Unfortunately small doses of steroids must be continued indefinitely if the cosmetic improvement is to be maintained. In order to minimise the side effects of oral corticosteroids, local intralesional triamcinolone acetonide (Lederle) or chloroquine or both are helpful alternatives. Potaba (Glenwood Laboratories) makes fibrotic skin more supple and is yet another alternative worth trying for chronic skin lesions.

Neurological involvement

The more acute the disease, the more likely is it that it will respond to systemic corticosteroids, which should be administered as soon as the diagnosis has been established. Resolution of neurosarcoidosis is more likely to occur in younger patients whose sarcoidosis has an explosive sudden onset. The response to treatment is better in those with accompanying erythema nodosum rather than chronic skin lesions, or with acute rather than chronic uveitis; and with hilar adenopathy rather than old diffuse pulmonary infiltration.[2]

Glandular involvement

Glandular involvement should be treated, particularly if there is disordered function, e.g. dry eyes due to lacrimal gland involvement, dry mouth due to salivary gland enlargement, and hypersplenism due to sarcoidosis of the spleen. The indication for treatment is disordered function rather than anatomical enlargement of the gland in question.

Myocardial involvement

It is easy to include involvement of the heart in a theoretical list of indications for corticosteroid therapy, but much more difficult, in practice, to recognise myocardial sarcoidosis. It is, of course, suspected and treated when a patient with multisystem sarcoidosis develops cardiac arrhythmia or bundle branch block.

WHAT ALTERNATIVE DRUGS ARE AVAILABLE IF CORTICOSTEROIDS ARE CONTRAINDICATED?

Treatment may be necessary when there are contraindications to corticosteroid therapy, or it has proved fruitless. Under these circumstances it is worth considering treatment with oxyphenbutazone (Tanderil), chloroquine or Potaba (Glenwood Laboratories).

Oxyphenbutazone

In a blind controlled trial comparing oxyphenbutazone, prednisolone and a placebo in the management of pulmonary sarcoidosis, both active drugs were significantly better than the placebo. Prednisolone and oxyphenbutazone were equally effective. Whereas 1 in 6 patients showed spontaneous regression of pulmonary sarcoidosis in 6 months, this trial showed that the number is increased by oxyphenbutazone or prednisolone to 1 in 2 patients.[1]

Chloroquine and hydroxychloroquine

The way in which the chloroquines act is unknown, but they control some instances of chronic fibrotic sarcoidosis involving lungs (3, 4) and skin. Such treatment is particularly helpful in the management of lupus pernio and pulmonary fibrosis, commencing with a dose of 250 mg daily for 3 months and thereafter 250 mg twice daily for 6 months. It may lead to irreversible retinopathy with blindness, or to reversible keratitis particularly if used in large doses for over 1 year, so its ocular toxicity should always be kept in mind.

Potaba

Potassium para-aminobenzoate (Glenwood Laboratories) is known to have an anti-fibrotic effect in Peyronie's disease, scleroderma and rheumatoid arthritis. It is worth considering in pulmonary fibrosis and lupus pernio due to sarcoidosis. Three-gram envules should be taken by mouth 4 times daily for several months. This form of treatment is an alternative to corticosteroids and chloroquine, and giving all 3 in rotation helps to overcome the undesirable long-term complications of any 1 drug.

Azathioprine (Imuran)

We have observed clinical improvement in 4, chest clearing in 2, and improved respiratory function in 1, out of a group of 10 patients given azathioprine. These 10 patients had already failed to respond to corticosteroids, oxyphenbutazone and chloroquine, so they can be regarded as hard-core chronic fibrotic sarcoidosis which has resisted all other therapy. Harold Israel (Philadelphia) has come to the same conclusion following the use of chlorambucil and methotrexate. To date, there have been no trials of the effect of antilymphocytic serum in sarcoidosis.

ABNORMAL CALCIUM METABOLISM

This is brought swiftly under control by oral corticosteroids. If there are contraindications to steroids, then sodium phytate or an oral phosphate preparation is a good alternative. For the phosphate, Sandoz effervescent tablet forms a palatable solution, providing 500 mg elemental phosphorus. Oral administration of inorganic phosphate in this way prevents overabsorption of calcium, eliminates hypercalciuria and leads to normal serum calcium levels.

REFERENCES

1. James, D. G., Carstairs, L. S., Trowell, J., and Sharma, O. P. 1967. Treatment of Sarcoidosis. *Lancet* **2**: 526.
2. James, D. G., and Sharma, O. P. 1967. Neurosarcoidosis. *Proc. Roy. Soc. Med.* **60**: 1169.
3. Siltzbach, L. E., and Teirstein, A. S. 1964. Chloroquine therapy in 43 patients with intrathoracic and cutaneous sarcoidosis. *Acta Med. Scand. Suppl.* **425**: 302.
4. British Tuberculosis Association. 1967. Chloroquine in the treatment of sarcoidosis. *Tubercle, Lond.* **47**: 257.

The Problems and Limitations of Corticoid Therapy in the Treatment of Sarcoidosis
(preliminary abstract)

K. WURM

University of Freiburg, Freiburg, Federal Republic of Germany

Fourteen years ago a new era began in the treatment of sarcoidosis by introduction of corticoid therapy. With this era came new problems in the treating of the disease. It is well known that corticoids have been used with great success, but there are also problems associated with their use.

This report is designed to point out these problems.

The optimum result in corticoid therapy is achieved not only by mastering the treatment technique, but also by application only when precise indications are present.

The knowledge of sarcoidosis stages offers valuable factors for the therapeutical indications.

When the indications exist, then corticoid therapy over a long period is indispensable, and it can extend over many months, or over a number of years.

The specific point at which a long-term treatment should be ended depends entirely on the individual case and this requires great experience on the part of the doctor.

Side effects of corticoids

The side effects often result in a falling short of a possible therapeutical improvement, because the treatment often has to be stopped. The side effects are many and well-known, but they vary in gravity from case to case. Because of ignorance or fear of these side effects, corticoids are sometimes not given for long enough, or in too small doses, so that the therapeutic result is poor or the disease does not come to a standstill.

The characteristic steroid effects.

The topographical position of the lymphoma influences the effect of steroids. A lymphoma on the periphery reacts more quickly than a lesion within the thorax; on the other hand a lesion in the upper part of the mediastinum reacts more favourably than one found in the central hilar region.

Corticoids have little or no effect on tumors of the spleen.

Changes in the lung parenchyma are better influenced by corticoids than the mediastinal lesions; and for that reason, the steroid effect is greater in stage II than in stage I. In stage I massive lesions of both hilar lymphnodes often become completely intractable but with the further development into stage II, the results become more favourable.

Resistance to corticoids

Sometimes, although the indications point definitely to corticoid therapy, effective therapeutic results are not achieved. We have to differentiate between the following:

An apparent corticoid resistance to which has anatomical causes may be present, for instance atelectase, a thickening of the pleura, calcification, hyalinose or sclerosis.

A real resistance to Corticoids may exist. The cause is unknown, but may be hormonal antagonism.

Treatment of Sarcoidosis (summary statement)

CAROL JOHNSON JOHNS

Johns Hopkins University and Hospital, Baltimore Md., U.S.A.

Sarcoidosis is a disease which may be associated with no symptoms or incapacity. An incidental finding of hilar adenopathy on chest radiograph requires no treatment beyond reassurance and serial observations. Spontaneous remissions are frequently observed in such patients.

Other patients may have a relatively mild clinical disease, with some incapacity which may be controlled with salicylates while awaiting a spontaneous remission (i.e., with fever and arthralgias often associated with erythema nodosum). If the patient worsens, or symptoms cannot be controlled, treatment may be indicated to hasten the patient's return to normal activity.

Patients with significant incapacity and threatening organ involvement usually require treatment. Occasionally, it is advisable to withhold treatment for a period of observation of 6 weeks to 6 months. This will identify the likelihood of a spontaneous remission or occasionally enable the completion of other diagnostic studies, such as the Kveim reaction, which might otherwise be inhibited by corticosteroid therapy. There is no evidence that irreversible fibrosis will occur in a period of a few weeks or months.

The degree of incapacity and site and extent of organ involvement may dictate a need for prompt initiation of treatment. This is most commonly the case with incapacitating pulmonary parenchymal disease, severe ocular disease not responding to local steroid treatment, significant hypercalcemia, central nervous system involvement with serious functional impairment (especially with evidence of meningeal involvement), thrombocytopenic purpura, or progressive and incapacitating hepatic disease.

Corticosteroid therapy is usually dramatically and promptly clinically effective in reversing evidence of the inflammatory process. Initial daily divided doses of 40 mg tapered over a period of 6–8 weeks to single daily 8 a.m. maintenance doses of 15–20 mg prednisone are recommended. Treatment should be continued for at least 6 months, and then gradually tapered over 2–3 months, with close serial observations. Approximately two-thirds of the patients may demonstrate objective relapse and require treatment for 2–5 or more years. Some patients, with repeated relapses, seem to require lifetime maintenance with 10–15 mg prednisone.

No forms of treatment more effective than corticosteroids have been identified. Complications are infrequent, though a mild Cushinoid state frequently results. Diabetes develops more frequently in association with liver disease. Aseptic bone necrosis is occasionally encountered. Some response has been observed with chloroquine (especially in cutaneous sarcoid) and hydroxyphenbutasone. Immunosuppressive agents warrant further study, especially where corticosteroids are contraindicated. Combinations of corticosteroids and immunosuppressive agents should be studied in the few patients with relentless progressive disease.

Antituberculous therapy alone is ineffective, but may be indicated if the diagnosis of tuberculosis remains in question. At least 2 antituberculous drugs must be used if clinically active tuberculosis is suspected. Isoniazid prophylaxis to accompany corticosteroid treatment is usually indicated for Negro patients with significant pulmonary disease and especially in areas with high risks of exposure to tuberculosis. Such prophylaxis is always indicated when the tuberculin reaction is positive.

Prednisolone Treatment of Sarcoidosis

R. Mikami

Tokyo University School of Medicine, Tokyo, Japan

Before entering the main subject, I would just like to mention quickly the follow-up study done in 1967 by the Japan Sarcoidosis Committee. A total of 209 cases were studied (Fig. 1), and all of them were confirmed to have sarcoidosis histologically. The average observation period was 5.2 years: 87% were treated, mostly with steroids. The outcome or prognosis is shown on the lower right of Fig. 1 pulmonary fibrosis was revealed in 6%, of the cases worsening of ocular lesions in 15%, including 6 cases of severe visual disturbance. Chest complications obscured included pulmonary abscess, aspergillosis and pulmonary tuberculosis. Pulmonary abscess and aspergillosis occurred during steroid therapy of more than 1 year.

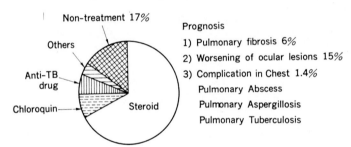

209 histologically confirmed cases.
The average observation period : 5.2 years

Non-treatment 17%
Others
Anti-TB drug
Chloroquin
Steroid

Prognosis
1) Pulmonary fibrosis 6%
2) Worsening of ocular lesions 15%
3) Complication in Chest 1.4%
   Pulmonary Abscess
   Pulmonary Aspergillosis
   Pulmonary Tuberculosis

FIG. 1.   Follow-up study of sarcoidosis (Japan Sarcoidosis Committee, 1967).

TABLE 1.

Initial \ Last	healed	H M / H M	n1,nl1,l1 l2,l3a (inactive)	n2,nl2, n3, nc (active)	l3b,f pulmonary fibrosis	n1,nl1,l1, l2,l3a (inactive)	n2,nl2 n3, nc (active)	l3b,f pulmonar fibrosis
59	35 (59.5%)	9	2	4	0	4	5	0
88	46 (52.5%)	6	9	4	1	14	5	3
8	0	0	0	0	0	2	1	5
	81 (52.5%)	15 (9.7%)	11 (7.1%)	8 (5.2%)	1 (0.6%)	20 (12.9%)	11 (7.1%)	8 (5.2%)

CAUSES OF PULMONARY FIBROSIS

Table 1 illustrates the relationship between the initial lesions shown on the left and the final lesions shown in the top column. The results were already reported at the Fifth International Conference on Sarcoidosis. In short, 9 cases had pulmonary fibrosis on the final chest X-ray film. Now the fact that I would like to point out is, that all of these 9 observed cases had pulmonary involvement as the initial lesion, that is, none of the cases having only BHL, deteriorated into pulmonary fibrosis. I have to add also, that pulmonary fibrosis was found mostly in those patients who were never on steroid therapy. From the results shown here, the patients who have only BHL as a manifestation of sarcoidosis are not likely to end up with pulmonary fibrosis.

COURSE OF OCULAR LESIONS

Figure 2 shows the course of ocular lesions in a total of 99 cases. In 15% of these, worsening of the lesion was observed. Delay in diagnosis, and incomplete or interrupted steroid therapy could be the reason for this worsening. Now, from the results shown here, steroid therapy should be restricted only to the prevention of pulmonary fibrosis or to the treatment of ocular lesions. Also, extra-thoracic lesions other than ocular lesions, should be treated with steroids. Now I will go on to the main subject. Double-blind study on prednisolone therapy by the Japan Sarcoidosis Committee gave the following results.

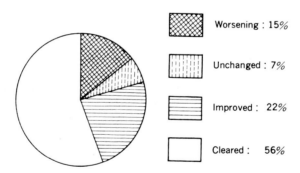

Worsening : 15%

Unchanged : 7%

Improved : 22%

Cleared : 56%

FIG. 2. Course of ocular lesions : 99 cases.

DOUBLE-BLIND STUDY OF CORTICOSTEROID THERAPY

Treatment with prednisolone for 6 months accelerated the improvement of bilateral hilar lymphadenopathy (BHL) and pulmonary lesions especially during the first month of the treatment, or it prevented further worsening. However, after 1 year the overall improvement rate in the steroid group was no different from that in the placebo group, being around 50–70% of cases. Therefore, steroid therapy should be indicated for those patients whose pulmonary involvement is progressive, for the purpose of averting fibrosis. And, for the patient with only BHL, I favour the general opinion that steroids should not be administered.

Figure 3 demonstrates the improvement rate and clearing rate of the pulmonary

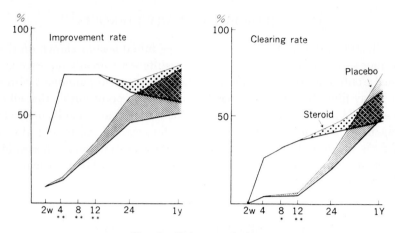

FIG. 3. Pulmonary lesions.

lesions. Here the dotted area shows the result in the steroid group and the dark area, the placebo group. As you can see in the figures, the rates were better in the steroid group than the placebo group, up to 12 months. However, at 1 year, no difference was observed between the 2 groups. This might be due to insufficient dosage and duration of steroid therapy or other unknown factors. In about 30–50% of the patients, the pulmonary lesions disappeared quickly in response to steroid therapy. However, there were some patients whose pulmonary lesions resisted at steroid therapy and progressed during the steroid treatment.

A CASE WHICH RESISTED PREDNISOLONE TREATMENT

Here, I will present an interesting case (Fig. 4). He was a patient of Dr Osada's at the Japanese National Railways Central Hospital. In this 22-year-old male, BHL and pulmonary lesions on the bilateral middle lung fields were discovered for the first time in July, 1969, at the time of a mass survey. He also had uveitis. From Sept., 1969, he was placed on steroid therapy by the double-blind test. In 6 months, the ocular lesions improved. However, his chest X-ray film was not changed at all. Tuberculin reaction which had been++ initially was negative at this time and the absolute peripheral lymphocyte count dropped markedly to around 600 from the initial value of 1,680. After 6 months' treatment with prednisolone, dexamethasone was further administered for another 10 months, but the pulmonary lesions did not improve and a recent chest X-ray film showed the fibrotic process. Tuberculin reaction was false-positive and lymphocyte count remained low. Here, the interesting point is that the rate of lymphoblastic transformation stimulated by PHA was 17% at the end of 6 months of prednisolone therapy and was 14.4% and 26%, thereafter. All of these values were very low. One of the reasons for the deterioration observed in this patient might be the fact that steroids further decrease the cellular immune reaction in sarcoidosis. Upon treating patients with sarcoidosis, I think that the adverse effect of steroids should be taken into account.

Figure 5 shows the change in tuberculin reaction before and after treatment. In the placebo group, more cases gave positive reaction after treatment. On the other hand, in

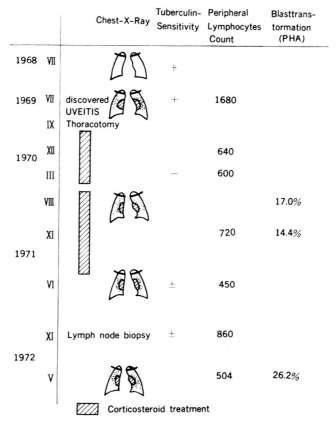

FIG. 4.   A 22-year-old male (at discovery).

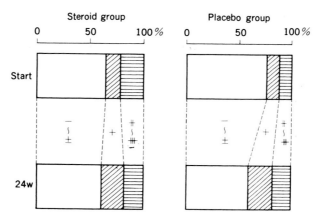

FIG. 5.   Course of tuberculin sensitivity.

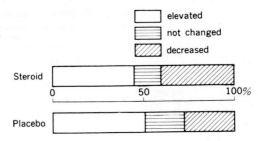

Fig. 6.   Change in lymphocyte count.

the steroid group, cases with negative reaction remained negative after treatment. Thus, steroids might suppress a positive reaction.

Figure 6 shows the changes in lymphocyte count in peripheral blood before and after each treatment. Lymphocyte count decreased more frequently in the steroid group than in the placebo group.

A CASE IMPROVED BY PREDNISOLONE TREATMENT

Such a case is shown in Fig. 7. The patient was a 19-year-old male. He visited a physician because of chest pain, inguinal lymph node enlargement, general malaise, weight loss and a nonproductive cough of a few months' duration. His chest X-ray film revealed BHL and fine nodular dissemination in both pulmonary fields. Generalized lymph node enlargement was apparent as well as splenomegaly. The diagnosis of sarcoidosis was confirmed by lymph node biopsy. Tuberculin reaction was negative. White blood cell count was 5,400 and the lymphocytes were markedly decreased to 540. Hypergammaglobulinemia was also present. Prednisolone was administered in an ini-

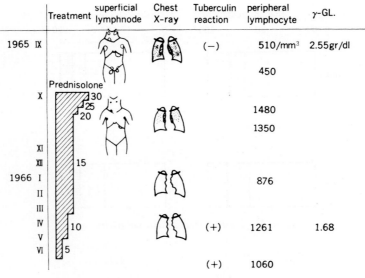

Fig. 7.   A-19-year-old male (M. K.).

tial amount of 30 mg. Four weeks after the treatment, his subjective complaints and objective findings were remarkably improved. At the same time, lymphocytes in his peripheral blood increased to 1,480 and 1,350. Thereafter he improved uneventfully. Lymph node swelling, BHL and pulmonary lesions disappeared in 12 weeks, and lymphocyte count increased to more than 1,000. Hypergammaglobulinemia returned to normal and tuberculin reaction was positive 24 weeks after the initiation of prednisolone. Steroid therapy was stopped at 7 months, and no recurrence of the lesions has been observed since then.

Hoffbrand stated that steroid therapy should be indicated for those patients whose lymphocytes were low in peripheral blood. Indeed, in this patient, steroid therapy seemed to increase the lymphocyte count, and the improvement of the symptoms and X-ray findings coincided with the increase in lymphocyte count.

CONCLUSION

Thus the effect of steroid therapy in sarcoidosis differs from case to case. It sometimes favours improvement, at least in the early days of treatment or it sometimes suppresses the immune mechanism and thus accelerates the worsening of the lesions.

The underlying immune abnormality in sarcoidosis might differ from case to case or from stage to stage even in 1 patient. Therefore steroid therapy should be performed with these facts in mind. For sarcoidosis where pulmonary fibrosis progresses despite steroid therapy, some other effective methods of treatment are seriously needed.

REFERENCES

1. Hoffbrand, B. I. 1968.: Occurence and significance of lymphopenia in sarcoidosis. *Amer. Rev. Resp. Dis.* **98** : 107.
2. Israel, H. L. 1971.: Effects on chlorambucil and methotrexate in sarcoidosis, *Proc. Fifth Inte. Conf. on Sarcoidosis*, Prague ; Univ. Karlova. p. 632–634.
3. Sharma, O., Hughes, D.T.D., James, D. G., and Naish, P. 1971,: Immunosuppressive therapy with azathioprine in sarcoidosis, *Proc. Fifth Inte. Conf. on Sarcoidosis*, Prague : Univ. Karlova, p. 635–637.

Treatment of Sarcoidosis

Teruo Tachibana
Osaka Prefectural Hospital, Osaka, Japan

INDICATION FOR STEROIDS

It is desirable to treat those patients with marked extrathoracic lesions even if their chest film showed BHL alone or with only a slight parenchymal lesion. These extrathoracic lesions may be inapparent, but they may be disclosed by appropriate procedures. For example, a marked hepatic lesion may exist even in BHL cases and it can be proved by peritoneoscopy and liver biopsy. The clinical course in some of these cases was worse, compared with those without or with a slight hepatic lesion.

DURATION OF TREATMENT

In those cases with inapparent hepatic lesions disclosed by peritoneoscopy and liver biopsy, hepatic lesions were still found after the improvement or clearing of chest film findings. Furthermore, relapse often occurs when the duration of treatment is short. If the patients have marked extrathoracic lesions, relapse may occur even after a long period of treatment. I think it is desirable to continue the treatment rather longer in these cases, even if the chest film finding shows improvement.

CHLOROQUINE TREATMENT

More than 50 patients were treated with chloroquine by us. Without any severe side effects, chloroquine showed a definite therapeutic effect.

GENERAL DISCUSSION

Chairmen: H. L. Israel and H. Homma

Dr Homma: As Co-chairman, I would like to ask for concentrated discussion on a few problems in the treatment because of the limited time. I would like to raise 3 questions. The first one is: Is it true that steroid can prevent the development of fibrosis? If so, to what extent? Concerning this question, do you acknowledge the preventive use of steroid? The second one is: Which do you favor: long-term, permanent, life-long therapy or short-period therapy, and how long should the initial dose of 40 mg of predonisolone be given, 4 weeks or 12 weeks? Finally, is there any procedure to find cases resistant to steroids very early in order to prevent the patients from losing time and money?

Dr James: There is a plenty of evidence that steroids can prevent fibrosis. In the days before steroids, I used to look out for the patients with chronic fibrotic uveitis, and now one can prevent this chronic fibrotic uveitis. Steroids have changed the natural history of sarcoid uveitis. In the old days, the patients used to go blind. With adequate, early steroid, the patient does not go blind. About the long-term or short-term steroid treatment, I think long-term treatment is better than lots of short-term treatment. Certainly, there are steroid-resistant case, but I just think these cases are in the late stage and they are fibrotic patients who do not respond well. If any of you worry about long-term steroid treatment, do routine slit lamp examination of the eyes of all your patients. One of the very common complications from long-term steroid treatment is posterior cortical cataract. If you use long-term steroid eye drops you will get high incidence of raised intraocular pressure and secondary glaucoma.

Dr Johns: As regards whether cortico-

steroids can prevent fibrosis, in the patient whom I showed, who had recurrent infiltrations, when steroids were stopped even over a ten year period I think that had she not had the steroid, she would have gone on to very advanced fibrosis. As regards long-term or short-term, I think we all prefer short-term treatment, and I think it is important to try to take the patients off the steroid after a reasonable period of time. I usually like to treat them for at least 6 months with therapeutic doses on the schedule I indicated. Then, I think, we are obliged to try to reduce the dose and take them off, because about one-fifth of the patients who had significant systematic disease will remain well. Then if they relapse, I seek no steroid treatment alternative, but to continue more I am convinced, there are some patients who require very long-term treatment, perhaps for life. As regards how long one should use 40 mg, I only give 40 mg for 2 weeks, then I reduce it to 30 mg for 2 weeks, 25 mg for 2 weeks and then maintain them on 15 or 20 mg. In none of the patients have I seen any relapse at any dose of 15 mg or above with a schedule such as that. I don't think you have to continue very high doses for very long.

Dr Mikami: At the fibrotic stage, it is very difficult to anticipate any effect of steroid, but at the granulomatous stage, steroid therapy is indicated. Offen it is very difficult to differentiate granulomatous lesions from fibrotic lesions.

Dr Turiaf: Cortisone can clear up the X-ray image of so-called fibrotic sarcoid, but it is not necessarily a fibrotic lesion. I think one cannot make radiological diagnosis of pulmonary fibrosis because I saw so many pulmonary fibrosis cases clearing up either spontaneously or on treatment. It is impossible to maked diagnosis without pulmonary biopsy. So this is an explanation for different results on cortisone treatment of so-called fibrotic sarcoidosis. Response to the treatment in so-called fibrotic sarcoidosis is not due to fibrotic lesion, but due to other lesions of sarcoidosis. If you add a pulmonary function test, you can have a general idea of whether gas exchange in the tissue is involved in the process, and if so, you have a better chance to make this diagnosis. This, I find, is very important when you start to evaluate the patient, and in treatment of so-called fibrotic sarcoidosis in particular.

DR TACHIBANA: I would like to ask professor Turiaf or Dr Johns about pulmonary function. How many fibrotic patients do you have in whom the diffusion capacity became normal or near normal after steroid treatment?

DR JAMES: If there is fibrosis and depression of diffusion capacity, it does not go back to normal. I note that you call it diffusion capacity, because we, in England, are beginning to call it transfer factor.

DR TACHIBANA: I have some patients who showed BHL or BHL with slight lung mottling and lowered diffusion capacity. After steroid treatment, their diffusion capacity returned to normal.

DR DJURIĆ: I had a patient who had small, diffuse miliary-like lesions in the lung without any evident hilar change. After each stop in the steroid treatment, 2 or 3 weeks later, miliary lesions in the lung relapsed and peripheral lymph nodes enlarged. I repeated the reduction of steroid 4 or 5 times in the last 4 years, but always observed the same responses when the dose of the steroid went under 10 or 5 mg. How can we treat such patients? How long should we give steroid?

DR JAMES: In the treatment of sarcoid, we need one more drug. When we have relapse, we may give steroid again, or may give chloroquine or potassium para-amino-benzoate. But we still need one more active agent. You are now getting lingering effects with the steroid-relapse-chloroquine-relapse-para-aminobenzoate sequence.

DR JOHNS: I want to respond to the question about patients who relapsed every time the dose got below 10 mg. I agree with Dr James' opinion, that we need something that is better than corticosteroid. But lacking that, I think that 10 mg maintenance dose of prednisolone is not a bad treatment. We get into very little difficulty with this low dose and I think it prevents relapse in such patients. I, at this point, would simply continue 10 mg of predonisolone or predonisolone. After about 3 relapses I begin to lose enthusiasm for stopping the treatment.

DR SBAR: I would like to ask a question perhaps more related to prognosis than therapy. I wonder how many of you have seen patients who had spontaneous clearing from stages 1 or 11 and subsequently relapsed.

DR ISRAEL: Could any of you comment on Dr Sbar's question? I have seen 3 such cases. Two of the 3 were in association with pregnancy. That's very rare.

DR TURIAF: I have seen only 1 patient who was in stage 1 for 5 years and recovered. It is very rare.

DR VISKUM: How do you treat patients who show shortness of breath and definitely have established fibrosis? Steroids, or just symptomatic treatment?

DR SULAVIK: I would like to mention 1 interesting case, of a female physician, who developed BHL with parenchymal lesions in 1963, stage 11, diagnosed histologically. She recovered and showed a perfectly normal chest X-ray by 1966. I saw her in 1969 because she was developing increasing fatigue. On this occasion, the X-ray showed bilateral mottling without BHL. The most interesting point in this patient was an increased PBI. She was obviously hyperthyroid at that time. She was treated for her hyperthyroids, and not sarcoidosis. Within about 6 weeks she became euthyroid and her chest X-ray showed total clearance.

DR YAMAMOTO: I have a question for Dr Johns. I agree with your recommendation for long-term treatment with steroid. Could you suggest some index for stopping long-term steroid treatment other than pulmonary function test?

Dr Johns: I am very much influenced by the patients symptoms. If the patient has no symptoms and seems to be very stable, and the X-ray seems stable, then I think it is reasonable to try to stop the steroid. I think the pulmonary function test does not have to be a very complicated one. I believe that just the vital capacity is a very reasonable and easily performed parameter which is helpful in documenting relapse.

Dr Kosuda: I think BHL itself is not an indication for sterioid treatment. However, it is also true that other harmful organ lesions will develop following BHL. If we try steroid therapy early, even in stage I, is it really possible to prevent the development of these harmful involvements and subsequently to avoid the miserable end results of sarcoidosis.

Dr Johns: My feeling is one might well wait until there is at least a significant symptom, because of the frequent occurrence of spontaneous remission in which treatment is not required. I would rather wait, and that would be my choice rather than treat lots of patients unnecessarily. I think it should be noted that when you examine the lung of a BHL patient, you do indeed find microscopic granuloma. So we should not worry too much whether stage 1 is totally without pulmonary disease, as this is probably unusual.

Dr Tachibana: I had 1 patient who had marked hepatic lesion with elevation of GOT and GPT. His X-ray finding was BHL and slight lung mottling. With long-term steroid treatment, GOT and GPT got back to normal.

Dr James: At the stage of BHL, sarcoid granuloma are already right through the lung, right through the liver and the muscle. The only sign is BHL and we can't see the other findings on X-ray. But granuloma are there though they are not dense enough to show up on X-ray in this stage. If sarcodosis is associated with erythema nodosum, you can be quite certain that things will clear up without treatment. Erythema nodosum is a passport to clearing. Your problem is in the group without erythema nodosum. I also just wait hopefully as Dr Johns suggested. If they have uveitis, of course, you must treat uveitis.

Dr Israel: I think it is very interesting that Dr James, Dr Siltzbach, Dr Johns and our own clinic in Philadelphia, have almost identical figures for the percentage of patients treated with steroid, one-third. In Japan, 60% of patients received prednisolone. I would like to hear from Dr Selroos and Dr Viskum what percentage of patients in Scandinavia are now treated with steroid?

Dr Selroos: In Finland we do not treat patients with pulmonary stage I disease. These patients constitute more than 50% of all our sarcoidosis patients. In stage II we determine the ventilatory function (vital capacity and/or diffusion capacity) and if this is normal or almost normal we follow the patient without therapy. In about one-third of the patients with stage II disease we never need to start with steroids, and the radiographic changes disappear. However, if the ventilatory function is reduced or deteriorates we start the treatment and give steroids for at least 6 months, sometimes for a much longer period. As I mentioned in Tokyo the best is when we can wait for spontaneous recovery. Then the recurrencies are really rare. If treatment is started the duration must be sufficiently long. After steroid therapy for 3 months only, the risk of recurrency is much higher than if the treatment has been continued for 6–12 months. Finally, to answer the question of Dr Israel: we treat much less than one-third of all our sarcoidosis patients.

Dr Viskum: The percentage is between 10 and 15. But our material is a little different from that observed in New York and London. . . .

Dr Selroos: I would like to comment on the indication of steroid therapy from another point of view. We know that chronic sarcoidosis sometimes is complicated by renal involvement, also in cases without disturbances in the calcium metabolism. In such normalcemic and normocalciuric patients with pulmonary disease of stage I or II we have performed percutaneous renal biopsies. In acute cases with erythema nodosum we have seen the picture of an acute interstitial nephritis, sometimes combined with proteinuria. In about 5% of the cases we have found sarcoid granulomas in the renal parenchyma, also in cases without signs of renal disease. We think that this is an indication for long-term medication with steroids. If these patients are left untreated they may represent the group taking a chronic course with therapy-resistance and multisystem involvement. This is only one example but it shows that there are patients with BHL as the only obvious sign of sarcoidosis, but in fact with a widespread disease which requires steroid therapy. We have to learn more how to detect these patients in the early phase of the disease.

DR JONES WILLIAMS: Regarding the role of steroids, there was nice work done in 1950 by an Australian, Professor Magariee, who is now in Sidney. According to his work, the effect of steroid on silicotic fibrotic nodules, makes them swell, become gelatinous, and change with depolymerisation of collagen fibers. Then when it was halted, it sclerosed again. This is very interesting in relation to the radiological changes with steroid. How does the steroid act? This reminds me of the work of Professor Perkonenn. Steroid action, at least, one of its many actions, is supposed to be on cell membranes. In the presence of steroid, there is a defect of fusion of the membrane in the cell with the cell outer membrane. It stops material getting out and accumulates it in the cell. Then perhaps, it depresses the sarcoid picture. The best Kveim reaction may come with sarcoid tissue of patients on steroid. So it may be that the steroid is just a concentrating agent in the cell.

OTHER MEETINGS

SOCIAL PROGRAMME

MONDAY 11th, 1972

9:50   Opening Ceremony at the conference site.

19:00   Cocktail Party at Daiichi Hotel (Invitees only).
Magic tricks and traditional Japanese dance will be performed by a participant, Dr. M. Shimoda.

WEDNESDAY 13th

13:30–15:50   Tokyo sight-seeing by coach. To be included in ladies programme. Pick-up service in front of Ueno Seiyoken Restaurant.

16:00   Kimono Fashion Show at Isetan. Overseas participants will be guests. (See Ladies Programme.)

THURSDAY 14th

19:00   Tokyo Governor Reception at Palace Hotel in front of the Imperial Palace.

FRIDAY 15th

13:40   Closing Ceremony at the conference site.

OTHERS

MONDAY 11th

12:45–14:00   International Committee on Sarcoidosis Executive Committee meeting at Ueno Seiyoken Restaurant.

WEDNESDAY 13th

14:00–15:00   Tokyo Igakukai (The Tokyo Society of Medical Sciences) Sarcoidosis meeting at the Faculty of Medicine, University of Tokyo.
Moderators: Dr. Kawamura, T. and Dr. Fujita, S.
Speakers: Dr. Turiaf, J. and Dr. Wurm, K.

LADIES PROGRAMME

Japanese doctors' wives will greet overseas ladies at the conference lobby during registration hour.

MONDAY 11th, 1972

9:00– 9:50   Registration.

9:50–10:50   Opening Ceremony.

11:00–12:45   "Let's join tea ceremony" hour on 4th floor of the conference site.

12:45–14:00   Lunch (free of charge).

14:00–15:00   "Let's join flower arrangement" hour (same site as above).

19:00   Cocktail Party at Daiichi Hotel (See Social Programme).

TUESDAY 12th

10:20   Tokyo Day Tour. Pick-up service at Imperial Hotel. Barbecue lunch will be served.
Tour will end ot 17:30.

WEDNESDAY 13th

13 : 00–16 : 00   Tokyo sight-seeing. (See Social Programme)

16 : 00   There will be a Kimono fashion show at Primula Restaurant at Isetan, one of Tokyo top level department store. Shopping hour will follow.

18 : 00   Return bus service from the side entrance of Isetan.

THURSDAY 14th

19 : 00   Reception by Tokyo Governor at Palace Hotel (Invitees only).

FRIDAY 15th

13 : 40   Closing Ceremony at the conference site.

LIST OF LADIES PROGRAMME PARTICIPANTS

Mrs. Berqvist, Sven, Sweden
Mrs. Carlens, Erik, Sweden
Mrs. Chusid, E. Leslie, U.S.A.
Mrs. Dalen, Anders, Sweden
Mrs. Figueroa-Lebron, Ramon E., U.S.A.
Mrs. Kendig, Edwain L., U.S.A.
Mrs. Miller, Albert, U.S.A.
Mrs. Nieschultz, Otto, F.R.G.
Mrs. Patterson, John R., U.S.A.
Mrs. Sbar, Sidney, U.S.A.
Mrs. Stavenow, Sven, Sweden
Mrs. Teirstein, A. S., U.S.A.
Mrs. Villar, T. G., Portugal
Mrs. Widström, Olle, Sweden
Mrs. Wurm, Karl, F.R.G.
Mr. Wurm, H.
Mrs. Young, Roscoe, C., U.S.A.
Mr. Young, Roscoe C. III, U.S.A.
Mr. Young, Peter J., U.S.A.

Mrs. Fujita, Shinnosuke, Japan
Mrs. Furuta, Mamoru, Japan
Mrs. Hiraga, Yomei, Japan
Mrs. Homma, Hiomi, Jopan
Mrs. Hosoda, Yutaka, Japan
Mrs. Hongo, Osamu, Japan
Mrs. Kitamura, Kanehiko, Japan
Mrs. Kataoka, Tetsuro, Japan
Mrs. Kosuda, Tatsuo, Japan
Mrs. Mikami, Riichiro, Japan
Mrs. Ohira, Ichiro, Japan
Mrs. Shigematsu, Itsuzo, Japan
Mrs. Takahara, Tadashi, Japan
Mrs. Takahashi, Hakko, Japan

AUTHORS INDEX